1-23-58

The Critical Reader

THE Critical Reader

Poems ⁂ *Stories* ⁂ *Essays*

Compiled and Edited by

WALLACE DOUGLAS
NORTHWESTERN UNIVERSITY

ROY LAMSON
WILLIAMS COLLEGE

HALLETT SMITH
CALIFORNIA INSTITUTE OF TECHNOLOGY

W · W · NORTON & COMPANY · INC · *New York*

PRINTED IN THE UNITED STATES OF AMERICA
FOR THE PUBLISHERS BY THE VAIL-BALLOU PRESS, INC.

Acknowledgments

For suggestions and advice in the preparation of this book the editors wish to thank the staff of English 1–2 at Williams College, and especially Professor Robert J. Allen. The Williams College Library has cheerfully fulfilled many requests. For help in preparing the manuscript we are grateful to Miss Mary O'Brien, Miss Edith Warren, Miss Catherine Winn, and Mrs. Francis Goodale. Throughout, Addison Burnham has given freely of his advice and experience.

Contents

The selections that are analyzed or provided with exercises are marked with an asterisk.

The Stories

The Essays

> ". . . nothing can permanently please, which does not contain in itself the reason why it is so, and not otherwise."
>
> Coleridge, *Biographia Literaria*, XIV

Introduction

THE CRITICAL READER is a book of poems, short stories, and essays designed for the course that emphasizes the critical analysis of the aims, methods, and results of works of literature. Sample analyses of a few poems and short stories, together with some questions, are included in order to illustrate how analysis may lead up to judgment and appreciation. The analyses of the essays and the questions are included partly to suggest a method of getting at the qualities of a prose style, but also to indicate that, even in the perhaps less strictly organized literary form of the essay, an author's habit of mind has its influence on the formal relations among the words he uses, and that a full reading of an essay necessarily involves an understanding of the "tone and spirit of unity, that blends, and (as it were) fuses" the different parts of a work into a unified whole.

The editors are aware of the many motives for reading and of the many ways of reading, any one of which may be momentarily satisfactory. But they assume that a full reading should bring into activity at least as much of the mind as Coleridge supposed was at work in the act of composing poetry. If Coleridge was right when he maintained that nothing will permanently please which does not contain within itself the reason why it is so, and not otherwise, the student of literature must sooner or later study the reasons within any given work why it is so; if, that is, he intends to understand the work and not merely to read it. The editors do not, however, mean that this understanding can be reached through only one system. They have not committed themselves either to the classifying impulse of a new Aristotelianism or to the anxious search for paradox and irony. The editors believe that the meaning of a work of literature can be reached by reading it carefully and completely, according to the demands which the work itself sets up, and by giving due attention to the mode in which it was composed and to such historical information as is necessary to understand the language and general context of the work.

The editors know, of course, that students like nothing better than a stock response, unless it is a historical fact or gossipy reference that they can substitute for a simple and accurate knowledge of the work they are supposed to be reading. An effort has been made, therefore, to avoid encumbering the book with material that would entice the student's wandering eye from the text; and in the analyses the editors have tried to direct the student's attention to the elements of writing which, when understood and evaluated, provide bases for proper critical judgment: those elements of language, imagery, and form, of style, scope, approach to material, attitude, proportion, and emphasis which reveal what we sometimes call, by a convenient fiction, the "intention" of the work. The proper end of such study is a reader who has learned to recognize and discount his own prejudices, whether as to form or as to content, and has learned to test his impulses and responses against an honest and thorough examination of what the writer before him is trying to do and how he tries to do it.

Criticism will of course never be standardized, nor should it be. But it is desirable that critics who differ should be able to account for their differences, and it is desirable also that a reader know when he is responding to something within a work of literary art and when he is responding to something outside it—in his own experience and memory, in his environment, or perhaps even in a misunderstanding of the work before him.

The ability to read critically is developed by doing it, not by having it done for one. Therefore the editors consider that the most valuable exercise in critical reading is the writing of a paper on a poem, story, or essay without any significant help except what comes from the form, style, and scope of the piece itself. In a story as simple as Galsworthy's *Spindleberries*, for example, there is the question of the attitude the reader is intended to take toward the painter in the story; a satisfactory description of this attitude must draw on the form of the story, on Galsworthy's style, and on the disposition of the episodes as well as on the obvious direct characterization. Robinson's *Miniver Cheevy* is not a difficult poem, but no account of the character of Miniver or the poet's attitude toward him can neglect the repetition in

> Miniver thought, and thought, and thought,
> And thought about it.

A reader who is willing to commit himself in judgment on a work and to back up his commitments with a relevant and searching examination of method and manner is enlarging his own experience. He is the kind of reader the best writers want.

Finally, we should take some notice of the oft-repeated prejudice that critical analysis ruins appreciation of the content of a work of art. Applied more directly to the critical reading of poems, short stories, and essays, such a prejudice involves opposition to careful attention to technique—a much-abused word. But Mark Schorer has pointed out in a recent essay "that it is only when we speak of the *achieved* content, the form, the work of art as a work of art, that we speak as critics. The difference between content, or experience, and achieved content, or art, is technique." ("Technique as Discovery," in *The Hudson Review*, Spring, 1948.) To study technique, then, as the editors have used the word in this volume, is not merely to examine the means used to organize the basic content of literary accomplishments.

but to explore and evaluate the whole subject and meaning of the work. To read in this way is to be a critical reader whose ideal objective is the fullest possible understanding and appreciation of the work before him.

The Poems

THE READER who is trying to develop his critical understanding usually finds his greatest opportunity in reading poems, which by their nature are the most conspicuously planned and integrated forms of communication in literature. Very often this experimenting reader has attitudes or prejudices which come between him and the enjoyment or the understanding of poems. Perhaps he begins with an indifference or hostility toward poems; he may feel that an interest in poems is a specialized interest, for those of a poetic temperament but not for him. Such a reader might begin reading the poems in *The Critical Reader* by comparing the first and last: Housman's "Terence . . ." and Marianne Moore's "Poetry." In the first he will find a humorous and wistful attack on mooning, mournful, sad poetry and a defense of drinking as a superior way to meet life's troubles. In the other he will find a poet admitting that there is much reason to condemn poetry; but asserting that if you are interested in the literal, in raw experience in all its rawness, if you are interested in the genuine, then you are in fact, whether you realize it or not, interested in poetry.

A more stubborn reader is one who says he likes poetry, but who really means that he likes one kind of poem, or one or another quality of poems. He may like melodious words and insist that it is a poet's business not to think but to sing. Such a reader might begin by examining his reactions to Keats' ode "To Autumn" and to Marvell's "The Garden," which are, of course, made up of melodiously arranged and beautiful words, but words which, at the same time, carry within themselves meanings which cannot be accounted for only in terms of verbal pyrotechnics, and meanings, moreover, of which no reader can be wholly unaware. For however much he may wish to exclude it from his "reactions," a reader must be aware of the meaning which arises when words are arranged in sentences, and when sentences are arranged in an order.

Another type of reader may be constantly looking for doctrine in the poetry he reads. There is value, he says, in Tennyson's "Light Brigade" or in Shelley's "Ozymandias," because they tell him things that he can repeat. But what good is there in Shakespeare's "Spring" and "Winter," which tell him nothing, or at least not at once? There is also the reader who thinks poems must be full of the atmosphere of nature, and will not admit Pope's "Of the Characters of Women": and there is the reader who insists upon conventional meters and rhyme schemes; he snorts at Jeffers' "The Eye" or Spender's "I Think Continually." These readers too may find, from the sixty poems that we have laid before them, that there is more to a poem than they had supposed.

In fact, all the clinical disorders of our reading habits should appear somewhere in the responses to these poems. Sometimes they may appear negatively, as in an admiration of Elizabeth Barrett Browning's "When Our Two Souls" or of Rupert Brooke's "The Great Lover" which is based not on the poems themselves but upon what these poems are supposed to be about. At other times they may reveal themselves positively in failure to respond to one or more of the poem's main constituents—the metrical effect, the imagery, the *unstated* attitudes or *tone* implicit in the poem.

What a poem says, what it means, what final effect it produces—these are by no means easy questions. Language is both direct and oblique. And the language of poems works with a full realization of this fact. Coleridge described this quality of poetry in the twenty-second chapter of *Biographia Literaria:*

In poetry, in which every line, every phrase, may pass the ordeal of deliberation and deliberate choice, it is possible, to attain that *ulti-*

matum which I have ventured to propose as the infallible test of a blameless style,—its *untranslatableness* in words of the same language without injury to the meaning. Be it observed, however, that I include in the *meaning* of a word not only its correspondent object, but likewise all the associations which it recalls. For language is framed to convey not the object alone, but likewise the character, mood, and intentions of the person who is representing it.

There could hardly be a better introduction to the reading of poetry than this paragraph. But it must not be misunderstood. The fact that a successful poem is ultimately untranslatable does not mean that it is impossible to say anything about it. An understanding of the greatness of a poem consists in an understanding of just *why* it is untranslatable, and that realization is something to which every reader must come himself. No expert is in a position to tell him; he can only suggest questions which start the reader on the right path, a path which, incidentally, will vary from poem to poem.

Probably the best way to understand just how much of a poem one is responding to is to write out one's observations and perceptions; in other words, to try to analyze the reactions and responses involved in reading, beginning where one does begin, with the pleasure, which Coleridge said was the immediate end of a poem. If done systematically, this exercise will eventually convince even the most skeptical that it is possible not only to describe but also to analyze the pleasure (and its sources) provided by a poem.

Any sensitive reader who takes to heart Coleridge's wisdom on the subject of meaning and words will soon find that as he reads poems, he is uncertain where to draw the line at the inclusion of associations. "All the associations which it recalls," says Coleridge. But surely some associations in the mind of every one of us are accidental and irrelevant, not really a part of the language of the poem at all. "How can I be sure I'm not reading *into* the poem something that isn't there—or that *you're* not reading into it?" It is a valid question. And the answer is difficult. One can only say that to test his own reading, his own series of suggestions and association called up by the poem, the safest way is to study what is sometimes called the poem's "strategy"—its form, organization, size, and scope; its approach to the reader through its diction and verse form; its symmetry and proportion. These elements of the poem, properly studied, supply a control over the amount of association admitted. Finally, the critical reader needs a native tact in these matters, and it is to remind him of this that we have included in our essay section Theodore Spencer's amusing parody, "How to Criticize a Poem."

It should not be necessary to refute the hoary and disreputable claim that critical analysis of a poem destroys the reader's pleasure in it; quite the contrary is true. We are all lazy, even about enjoyment, and in our laziest moments we sometimes maintain that a thinner pleasure with less effort is what we want. But the rewards of the most complete enjoyment of poetry are so great that it takes only one or two experiences of them to make us look down on the easy and superficial response to a single and simple reading of a poem as somehow cheap and unsatisfying.

However thorough the analysis, one should finally come back to the poem itself. For a poem exists, not primarily to offer us exercise for our critical faculties, any more than it exists to give us biographical information about the poet or historical information about his times. It exists to arouse and discipline the imagination, to sharpen the senses and to organize our world of thought, feeling, and observation for us. A poem may serve for a time as an opportunity for criticism, but we should finally return to it as an experience itself, unified, complete, and unique.

Terence, This Is Stupid Stuff

A. E. HOUSMAN (1859–1936)

"Terence, this is stupid stuff:
You eat your victuals fast enough;
There can't be much amiss, 'tis clear,
To see the rate you drink your beer.
But oh, good Lord, the verse you make,
It gives a chap the belly-ache.
The cow, the old cow, she is dead;
It sleeps well, the hornèd head:
We poor lads, 'tis our turn now
To hear such tunes as killed the cow.
Pretty friendship 'tis to rhyme
Your friends to death before their time
Moping melancholy mad:
Come, pipe a tune to dance to, lad."

Why, if 'tis dancing you would be,
There's brisker pipes than poetry.
Say, for what were hop-yards meant,
Or why was Burton built on Trent?
Oh, many a peer of England brews
Livelier liquor than the Muse,
And malt does more than Milton can
To justify God's ways to man.
Ale, man, ale's the stuff to drink
For fellows whom it hurts to think:
Look into the pewter pot
To see the world as the world's not.

And faith, 'tis pleasant till 'tis past:
The mischief is that 'twill not last.
Oh, I have been to Ludlow fair
And left my necktie God knows where,
And carried half-way home, or near,
Pints and quarts of Ludlow beer:
Then the world seemed none so bad,
And I myself a sterling lad;
And down in lovely muck I've lain,
Happy till I woke again.
Then I saw the morning sky:
Heigho, the tale was all a lie;
The world, it was the old world yet,
I was I, my things were wet,
And nothing now remained to do
But begin the game anew.

Therefore, since the world has still
Much good, but much less good than ill,
And while the sun and moon endure
Luck's a chance, but trouble's sure,
I'd face it as a wise man would,
And train for ill and not for good.
'Tis true, the stuff I bring for sale
Is not so brisk a brew as ale:
Out of a stem that scored the hand
I wrung it in a weary land.
But take it: if the smack is sour,
The better for the embittered hour;
It should do good to heart and head
When your soul is in my soul's stead;
And I will friend you, if I may,
In the dark and cloudy day.

There was a king reigned in the East:
There, when kings will sit to feast,

They get their fill before they think
With poisoned meat and poisoned drink.
He gathered all that springs to birth
From the many-venomed earth;
First a little, thence to more,
He sampled all her killing store;
And easy, smiling, seasoned sound,
Sate the king when healths went round,
They put arsenic in his meat
And stared aghast to watch him eat;
They poured strychnine in his cup
And shook to see him drink it up:
They shook, they stared as white's their shirt:
Them it was their poison hurt.
—I tell the tale that I heard told.
Mithridates, he died old.

Two Tramps in Mud Time

ROBERT FROST (1875-)

Out of the mud two strangers came
And caught me splitting wood in the yard.
And one of them put me off my aim
By hailing cheerily "Hit them hard!"
I knew pretty well why he dropped behind
And let the other go on a way.
I knew pretty well what he had in mind:
He wanted to take my job for pay.

Good blocks of beech it was I split,
As large around as the chopping block;
And every piece I squarely hit
Fell splinterless as a cloven rock.
The blows that a life of self-control
Spares to strike for the common good
That day, giving a loose to my soul,
I spent on the unimportant wood.

The sun was warm but the wind was chill.
You know how it is with an April day
When the sun is out and the wind is still,
You're one month on in the middle of May.
But if you so much as dare to speak,
A cloud comes over the sunlit arch,
A wind comes off a frozen peak,
And you're two months back in the middle of March.

A bluebird comes tenderly up to alight
And fronts the wind to unruffle a plume,
His song so pitched as not to excite
A single flower as yet to bloom.
It is snowing a flake: and he half knew
Winter was only playing possum.
Except in color he isn't blue,
But he wouldn't advise a thing to blossom.

The water for which we may have to look
In summertime with a witching-wand,
In every wheelrut's now a brook,
In every print of a hoof a pond.
Be glad of water, but don't forget
The lurking frost in the earth beneath
That will steal forth after the sun is set
And show on the water its crystal teeth.

The time when most I loved my task
These two must make me love it more
By coming with what they came to ask.
You'd think I never had felt before
The weight of an ax-head poised aloft,
The grip on earth of outspread feet,
The life of muscles rocking soft
And smooth and moist in vernal heat.

Out of the woods two hulking tramps
(From sleeping God knows where last night,
But not long since in the lumber camps).
They thought all chopping was theirs of right.
Men of the woods and lumberjacks,
They judged me by their appropriate tool.
Except as a fellow handled an ax,
They had no way of knowing a fool.

Nothing on either side was said.
They knew they had but to stay their stay
And all their logic would fill my head:
As that I had no right to play
With what was another man's work for gain.
My right might be love but theirs was need.
And where the two exist in twain
Theirs was the better right—agreed.

But yield who will to their separation,
My object in living is to unite
My avocation and my vocation
As my two eyes make one in sight.
Only where love and need are one,
And the work is play for mortal stakes,
Is the deed ever really done
For Heaven and the future's sakes.

Miniver Cheevy

EDWIN ARLINGTON ROBINSON (1869–1935)

Miniver Cheevy, child of scorn,
Grew lean while he assailed the seasons;
He wept that he was ever born,
And he had reasons.

Miniver loved the days of old
When swords were bright and steeds were prancing;
The vision of a warrior bold
Would set him dancing.

Miniver sighed for what was not,
And dreamed, and rested from his labors;
He dreamed of Thebes and Camelot,
And Priam's neighbors.

Miniver mourned the ripe renown
That made so many a name so fragrant;
He mourned Romance, now on the town,
And Art, a vagrant.

Miniver loved the Medici,
Albeit he had never seen one;
He would have sinned incessantly
Could he have been one.

Miniver cursed the commonplace
And eyed a khaki suit with loathing;

He missed the mediæval grace
    Of iron clothing.

Miniver scorned the gold he sought,
    But sore annoyed was he without it;
Miniver thought, and thought, and thought,
    And thought about it.

Miniver Cheevy, born too late,
    Scratched his head and kept on thinking;
Miniver coughed, and called it fate,
    And kept on drinking.

Boy-Man

KARL SHAPIRO (1913–)

England's lads are miniature men
To start with, grammar in their shiny hats,
And serious: in America who knows when
Manhood begins? Presidents dance and hug
And while the kind King waves and gravely chats
America wets on England's old green rug.

The boy-man roars. Worry alone will give
This one the verisimilitude of age.
Those white teeth are his own, for he must live
Longer, grow taller than the Texas race.
Fresh are his eyes, his darkening skin the gauge
Of bloods that freely mix beneath his face.

He knows the application of the book
But not who wrote it; shuts it like a shot.
Rather than read he thinks that he will look,
Rather than look he thinks that he will talk,
Rather than talk he thinks that he will not
Bother at all; would rather ride than walk.

His means of conversation is the joke,
Humor his language underneath which lies
The undecoded dialect of the folk.
Abroad he scorns the foreigner: what's old
Is worn, what's different bad, what's odd unwise.
He gives off heat and is enraged by cold.

Charming, becoming to the suits he wears,
The boy-man, younger than his eldest son,
Inherits the state; upon his silver hairs
Time like a panama hat sits at a tilt
And smiles. To him the world has just begun
And every city waiting to be built.

Mister, remove your shoulder from the wheel
And say this prayer, "Increase my vitamins,
Make my decisions of the finest steel,
Pour motor oil upon my troubled spawn,
Forgive the Europeans for their sins,
Establish them, that values may go on."

Moral Essays: Epistle II, To a Lady
Of the Characters of Women

ALEXANDER POPE (1688–1744)

Nothing so true as what you once let fall,
"Most women have no characters at all."
Matter too soft a lasting mark to bear,
And best distinguish'd by black, brown, or fair.
How many pictures of one nymph we view,
All how unlike each other, all how true!
Arcadia's countess here, in ermin'd pride,
Is there Pastora by a fountain side;
Here Fannia, leering on her own good man,
And there a naked Leda with a swan.
Let then the fair one beautifully cry,
In Magdalen's loose hair and lifted eye,
Or, dress'd in smiles of sweet Cecilia shine,
With simp'ring angels, palms, and harps divine;
Whether the charmer sinner it, or saint it,
If folly grow romantic I must paint it.
  Come then, the colours and the ground prepare!
Dip in the rainbow, trick her off in air;
Choose a firm cloud, before it fall, and in it
Catch, ere she change, the Cynthia of this minute.
  Rufa, whose eye quick-glancing o'er the park,
Attracts each light gay meteor of a spark,
Agrees as ill with Rufa studying Locke
As Sappho's di'monds with her dirty smock;
Or Sappho at her toilet's greasy task,
With Sappho fragrant at an ev'ning mask:
So morning insects that in muck begun
Shine, buzz, and fly-blow in the setting sun.

How soft is Silia! fearful to offend,
The frail one's advocate, the weak one's friend:
To her Calista prov'd her conduct nice,
And good Simplicius asks of her advice.
Sudden, she storms! she raves! You tip the wink,
But spare your censure; Silia does not drink:
All eyes may see from what the change arose,
All eyes may see—a pimple on her nose.
Papillia, wedded to her am'rous spark,
Sighs for the shades—"How charming is a park!"
A park is purchas'd, but the fair he sees
All bath'd in tears—"Oh, odious, odious trees!"
Ladies, like variegated tulips, show;
'Tis to their changes half their charms we owe;
Fine by defect, and delicately weak,
Their happy spots the nice admirer take;
'Twas thus Calypso once each heart alarm'd,
Aw'd without virtue, without beauty charm'd;
Her tongue bewitch'd as oddly as her eyes,
Less wit than mimic, more a wit than wise;
Strange graces still, and stranger flights she had,
Was just not ugly, and was just not mad;
Yet ne'er so sure our passion to create,
As when she touch'd the brink of all we hate.
Narcissa's nature, tolerably mild,
To make a wash, would hardly stew a child;
Has ev'n been prov'd to grant a lover's pray'r,
And paid a tradesman once to make him stare;
Gave alms at Easter, in a Christian trim,
And made a widow happy, for a whim.
Why then declare good-nature is her scorn,
When 'tis by that alone she can be borne?
Why pique all mortals, yet affect a name?
A fool to pleasure, yet a slave to fame:
Now deep in Taylor and the Book of Martyrs,

Now drinking citron with his Grace and Chartres:
Now conscience chills her, and now passion burns;
And atheism and religion take their turns;
A very heathen in the carnal part,
Yet still a sad, good Christian at her heart.
  See Sin in state, majestically drunk;
Proud as a peeress, prouder as a punk;
Chaste to her husband, frank to all beside,
A teeming mistress, but a barren bride.
What then? let blood and body bear the fault,
Her head's untouch'd, that noble seat of thought:
Such this day's doctrine—in another fit
She sins with poets through pure love of wit.
What has not fir'd her bosom or her brain?
Cæsar and Tall-boy, Charles and Charlemagne.
As Helluo, late dictator of the feast,
The nose of *haut-gout*, and the tip of taste,
Critiqu'd your wine, and analyz'd your meat,
Yet on plain pudding deign'd at home to eat;
So Philomedé, lect'ring all mankind
On the soft passion, and the taste refin'd,
Th' address, the delicacy—stoops at once,
And makes her hearty meal upon a dunce.
  Flavia's a wit, has too much sense to pray;
To toast our wants and wishes, is her way;
Nor asks of God, but of her stars, to give
The mighty blessing, "while we live, to live."
Then all for death, that opiate of the soul!
Lucretia's dagger, Rosamonda's bowl.
Say, what can cause such impotence of mind?
A spark too fickle, or a spouse too kind.
Wise wretch! with pleasures too refin'd to please;
With too much spirit to be e'er at ease;
With too much quickness ever to be taught;
With too much thinking to have common thought:

You purchase pain with all that joy can give,
And die of nothing but a rage to live.
  Turn then from wits; and look on Simo's mate,
No ass so meek, no ass so obstinate.
Or her, that owns her faults, but never mends,
Because she's honest, and the best of friends.
Or her, whose life the church and scandal share,
Forever in a passion, or a pray'r.
Or her, who laughs at hell, but (like her Grace)
Cries, "Ah! how charming, if there's no such place!"
Or who in sweet vicissitude appears
Of mirth and opium, ratafia and tears,
The daily anodyne, and nightly draught,
To kill those foes to fair ones, time and thought.
Woman and fool are two hard things to hit;
For true no-meaning puzzles more than wit.
  But what are these to great Atossa's mind?
Scarce once herself, by turns all womankind!
Who, with herself, or others, from her birth
Finds all her life one warfare upon earth:
Shines in exposing knaves, and painting fools,
Yet is whate'er she hates and ridicules.
No thought advances, but her eddy brain
Whisks it about, and down it goes again.
Full sixty years the world has been her trade,
The wisest fool much time has ever made.
From loveless youth to unrespected age,
No passion gratified except her rage.
So much the fury still outran the wit,
The pleasure miss'd her, and the scandal hit.
Who breaks with her, provokes revenge from hell,
But he's a bolder man who dares be well.
Her ev'ry turn with violence pursu'd,
No more a storm her hate than gratitude:
To that each passion turns, or soon or late;

Love, if it makes her yield, must make her hate:
Superiors? death! and equals? what a curse!
But an inferior not dependent? worse.
Offend her, and she knows not to forgive;
Oblige her, and she'll hate you while you live:
But die, and she'll adore you—Then the bust
And temple rise—then fall again to dust.
Last night, her lord was all that's good and great;
A knave this morning, and his will a cheat.
Strange! by the means defeated of the ends,
By spirit robb'd of pow'r, by warmth of friends,
By wealth of follow'rs! without one distress,
Sick of herself through very selfishness!
Atossa, curs'd with ev'ry granted pray'r,
Childless with all her children, wants an heir.
To heirs unknown descends th' unguarded store,
Or wanders, Heav'n-directed, to the poor.
  Pictures like these, dear Madam, to design,
Asks no firm hand, and no unerring line;
Some wand'ring touches, some reflected light,
Some flying stroke alone can hit 'em right:
For how should equal colours do the knack?
Chameleons who can paint in white and black?
  "Yet Chloe sure was form'd without a spot"—
Nature in her then err'd not, but forgot.
"With ev'ry pleasing, ev'ry prudent part,
Say, what can Chloe want?"—She wants a heart.
She speaks, behaves, and acts just as she ought;
But never, never, reach'd one gen'rous thought.
Virtue she finds too painful an endeavour,
Content to dwell in decencies forever.
So very reasonable, so unmov'd,
As never yet to love, or to be lov'd.
She, while her lover pants upon her breast,
Can mark the figures on an Indian chest;

And when she sees her friend in deep despair,
Observes how much a chintz exceeds mohair.
Forbid it Heav'n, a favour or a debt
She e'er should cancel—but she may forget.
Safe is your secret still in Chloe's ear;
But none of Chloe's shall you ever hear.
Of all her dears she never slander'd one,
But cares not if a thousand are undone.
Would Chloe know if you're alive or dead?
She bids her footman put it in her head.
Chloe is prudent—Would you too be wise?
Then never break your heart when Chloe dies.
One certain portrait may (I grant) be seen,
Which Heav'n has varnish'd out, and made a queen;
The same forever! and describ'd by all
With truth and goodness, as with crown and ball.
Poets heap virtues, painters gems at will,
And show their zeal, and hide their want of skill.
'Tis well—but, artists! who can paint or write,
To draw the naked is your true delight.
That robe of quality so struts and swells,
None see what parts of nature it conceals:
Th' exactest traits of body or of mind,
We owe to models of an humble kind.
If Queensberry to strip there's no compelling,
'Tis from a handmaid we must take a Helen.
From peer or bishop 'tis no easy thing
To draw the man who loves his God, or king:
Alas! I copy (or my draught would fail)
From honest Mah'met, or plain Parson Hale.
But grant, in public men sometimes are shown,
A woman's seen in private life alone:
Our bolder talents in full light display'd;
Your virtues open fairest in the shade.
Bred to disguise, in public 'tis you hide;

There, none distinguish 'twixt your shame or pride,
Weakness or delicacy; all so nice,
That each may seem a virtue, or a vice.
  In men, we various ruling passions find;
In women, two almost divide the kind;
Those, only fix'd, they first or last obey,
The love of pleasure, and the love of sway.
  That, Nature gives; and where the lesson taught
Is but to please, can pleasure seem a fault?
Experience, this; by man's oppression curst,
They seek the second not to lose the first.
  Men, some to bus'ness, some to pleasure take;
But ev'ry woman is at heart a rake:
Men, some to quiet, some to public strife;
But ev'ry lady would be queen for life.
  Yet mark the fate of a whole sex of queens!
Pow'r all their end, but beauty all the means:
In youth they conquer, with so wild a rage,
As leaves them scarce a subject in their age:
For foreign glory, foreign joy, they roam;
No thought of peace or happiness at home.
But wisdom's triumph is well-tim'd retreat,
As hard a science to the fair as great!
Beauties, like tyrants, old and friendless grown,
Yet hate repose, and dread to be alone,
Worn out in public, weary ev'ry eye,
Nor leave one sigh behind them when they die.
  Pleasures the sex, as children birds, pursue,
Still out of reach, yet never out of view;
Sure, if they catch, to spoil the toy at most,
To covet flying, and regret when lost:
At last, to follies youth could scarce defend,
It grows their age's prudence to pretend;
Asham'd to own they gave delight before,
Reduc'd to feign it, when they give no more:

As hags hold sabbaths, less for joy than spite,
So these their merry, miserable night;
Still round and round the ghosts of beauty glide,
And haunt the places where their honour died.
See how the world its veterans rewards!
A youth of frolics, an old age of cards;
Fair to no purpose, artful to no end,
Young without lovers, old without a friend;
A fop their passion, but their prize a sot;
Alive, ridiculous, and dead, forgot!
Ah! Friend! to dazzle let the vain design;
To raise the thought and touch the heart, be thine!
That charm shall grow, while what fatigues the Ring,
Flaunts and goes down, an unregarded thing:
So when the sun's broad beam has tir'd the sight,
All mild ascends the moon's more sober light,
Serene in virgin modesty she shines,
And unobserv'd the glaring orb declines.
Oh! blest with temper, whose unclouded ray
Can make to-morrow cheerful as to-day;
She, who can love a sister's charms, or hear
Sighs for a daughter with unwounded ear;
She, who ne'er answers till a husband cools,
Or, if she rules him, never shows she rules;
Charms by accepting, by submitting sways,
Yet has her humour most, when she obeys;
Let fops or fortune fly which way they will;
Disdains all loss of tickets, or codille;
Spleen, vapours, or smallpox, above them all,
And mistress of herself, though china fall.
And yet, believe me, good as well as ill,
Woman's at best a contradiction still.
Heav'n, when it strives to polish all it can
Its last best work, but forms a softer man;
Picks from each sex, to make the fav'rite blest,

Your love of pleasure, our desire of rest:
Blends, in exception to all gen'ral rules,
Your taste of follies, with our scorn of fools:
Reserve with frankness, art with truth allied,
Courage with softness, modesty with pride;
Fix'd principles, with fancy ever new;
Shakes all together, and produces—You.
Be this a woman's fame: with this unblest,
Toasts live a scorn, and queens may die a jest.
This Phœbus promis'd (I forget the year)
When those blue eyes first open'd on the sphere;
Ascendant Phœbus watch'd that hour with care,
Averted half your parents' simple pray'r;
And gave you beauty, but denied the pelf
That buys your sex a tyrant o'er itself.
The gen'rous god, who wit and gold refines,
And ripens spirits as he ripens mines,
Kept dross for duchesses, the world shall know it,
To you gave sense, good-humour, and a poet.

Critical Analysis

THE SUBTITLE "Of the Characters of Women" describes generally Pope's poem, but the first five-sixths of the epistle is a satirical portrait gallery in verse, and the last part is an enthusiastic favorable portrait—a compliment to the Lady of the title, Martha Blount. Pope contrasts her character, manner, and disposition to an array of eighteenth-century court women. No one in the group is named except the Duchess of Queensberry (line 193), but they are given distinguishing classical names, some of which suggest particular features or qualities.

The poem develops as a series of illustrations of the truth of Martha Blount's remark, "Most women have no characters at all." What this means is that women, unlike men, are not controlled by a ruling passion or principle; they are changeable, self-contradictory, inconsistent. Any definite description you apply to a woman is immediately contradicted by something else in her behavior or temperament. This complaint, by no means original with Pope or Martha Blount, of course, is made fresh and vivid by the metaphor of painting portraits. Most society ladies, says Pope, have to be portrayed in a series of roles—as a countess in court costume and as a shepherdess; as a good and loving wife and as the naked pagan Leda with her swan-lover; as the immoral Magdalen and the pure St. Cecilia. How then is the poet to capture them in a single verse portrait apiece? This is the all but impossible task Pope sets himself, and the answer he gives to the question of how to do it develops the painting metaphor and incidentally characterizes his own style and manner:

> Come then, the colours and the ground prepare!
> Dip in the rainbow, trick her off in air;
> Choose a firm cloud, before it fall, and in it
> Catch, ere she change, the Cynthia of this minute. (17–20)

The idea that the material itself is evanescent is of course a phrasing of the main theme, but the suggestion that the treatment is to be all delicate and airy is in part a deliberate deception of the reader: he is all the more shocked when he finds that very frequently the ladies are sketched not with cloud-stuff and rainbow tints, but with acid, sharply and firmly etched. But Pope's model in this poem and others like it is Horace, and the epistles of Horace are satires which are never heavy-footed and violent, but witty, urbane, and smooth. The conventional "epistle" or letter gives an air of informality, and the poet is not setting himself up as the formal indignant castigator of the vices and follies of mankind. The instrument of this kind of satirist is the rapier and not the whip.

But neither "rapier" nor "paintbrush" adequately conveys an idea of Pope's technique. It is first of all a kind of thinking, and the intellectual power of the poem should not be underestimated. Take Calypso, for example, she who

> once each heart alarm'd,
> Awed without virtue, without beauty charm'd; (45–46)

what is the mysterious source of her attractiveness? If she is neither good nor beautiful, what is it that she has? Pope pretends that it is a mystery, but he shows by his manner of describing it that he knows that we are sometimes drawn or attracted by those things that are just this side of the repulsive:

> Strange graces still, and stranger flights she had,
> Was just not ugly, and was just not mad;
> Yet ne'er so sure our passion to create,
> As when she touch'd the brink of all we hate. (49–52)

For all the emphasis on female vanity, on social foibles, on fashionable affectations, this epistle is fundamentally a Moral Essay; it probes deeply into the relationship between motives and deeds. Narcissa is not a "bad" woman; she wouldn't stew a child, in the fashion of witches making their broth, just to prepare a cosmetic "wash" for her face; she is even generous, if you recite some of her deeds—but what about the motives? She

> Has ev'n been prov'd to grant a lover's pray'r,
> And paid a tradesman once to make him stare;
> Gave alms at Easter, in a Christian trim,
> And made a widow happy, for a whim. (55–58)

As a matter of fact, she is another example of that combination of irreconcilable opposites which constitutes the female character:

> Now conscience chills her, and now passion burns;
> And atheism and religion take their turns;
> A very heathen in the carnal part,
> Yet still a sad, good Christian at her heart. (65–67)

Pope's moral insight is exhibited even more impressively in the rhetoric and logical syntax of passages which appear on the surface to be mere wit:

> See Sin in state, majestically drunk;
> Proud as a peeress, prouder as a punk; (69–70)

Here the paradox in the phrase "majestically drunk" not only expresses contempt for the degradation of majestic qualities in drunkenness; it also prepares the reader's mind for some such phrase as "drunk as a lord." And the phrase follows, satisfyingly: "Proud as a peeress," but by a verbal trick Pope converts what seems like a superlative into a mere positive, and the comparative "prouder as a punk" explodes in a marvelous anticlimax. The rhetorical progression in the description of Flavia, the epicurean, reveals the same degree of profundity:

> Wise wretch! with pleasures too refin'd to please;
> With too much spirit to be e'er at ease;
> With too much quickness ever to be taught;
> With too much thinking to have common thought:
> You purchase pain with all that joy can give,
> And die of nothing but a rage to live. (95–100)

The thrice-repeated "with too much . . ." and the metaphor of purchasing develop a sense of opulence and wealth to give a terrible significance to the word "nothing" in the last line.

To temper this moral seriousness and to keep the poem on the level of the well-bred, cultivated letter from one friend to another, to suggest a tone of gallant frankness rather than zealous misogyny, Pope returns, after one hundred and fifty lines, to a comment on his technique:

> Pictures like these, dear Madam, to design,
> Asks no firm hand, and no unerring line;
> Some wand'ring touches, some reflected light,
> Some flying stroke alone can hit 'em right: (151–154)

Any analysis of Pope's style might take this passage as its point of departure. Is there really no firm hand or unerring line in these portraits? Are they really just flying strokes?

The versification of this poem is of course connected with its wit. But the iambic pentameter couplet which Pope so polished and developed, which he made so capable of variety and so fluent in a poem of almost three hundred lines, is not to be considered the source of the wit. It is the sharpening of something which already cuts. So many illustrations offer themselves to show Pope's skill in the technique of versification that it is hard to make a choice. Is he most remarkable for his variation of the normal iambic movement to make a sudden special effect, as in the second line of

> A very heathen in the carnal part,
> Yet still a sad, good Christian at her heart. (67–68)

or is he to be praised for the compactness of his summarizing couplets, when he conveys the matter of an epic in an epigram?

> From loveless youth to unrespected age,
> No passion gratified except her rage. (125–126)

One might point out the extraordinary precision in the choice of the specific detail to contrast with a general emotion:

> She, while her lover pants upon her breast,
> Can mark the figures on an Indian chest;
> And when she sees her friend in deep despair,
> Observes how much a chintz exceeds mohair. (167–170)

This is in reality a perfect realization of balance, intellectually and imaginatively, and the same poise is evident in Pope's prosody. The quotability of his general statements is often due to this balance:

> In men, we various ruling passions find;
> In women, two almost divide the kind;

Those, only fix'd, they first or last obey,
The love of pleasure, and the love of sway. (207–210)

Here the unbalance of the third line, in the placing of caesuras, prepares the ear for the satisfaction of the perfect balance of the fourth, and even the parallel structure of the first and second lines, with the early caesura, has its effect on the last line.

The end of the poem, progressing from the character of "Queensberry" through some general reflections on the female sex, leads up to the good advice and gallant compliment paid to Martha Blount. Yet in paying this compliment Pope does not retract his general contention about the contradictions in feminine character; he only makes it clear that one combination of disparate traits, the best from each sex, has resulted in the creation of an ideal woman and friend. As the poet makes his exit, he separates Martha Blount from the women of the world he has been describing. She has beauty but not wealth; hence she is unspoiled. And in the final lines, as he shows the compensations for lack of wealth, he produces the same retarding effect in the last line that we are accustomed to at the end of a piece of music:

The gen'rous god, who wit and gold refines,
And ripens spirits as he ripens mines,
Kept dross for duchesses, the world shall know it,
To you gave sense, good-humour, and a poet. (289–292)

Anyone who walks through an art gallery and looks at the portraits of eighteenth-century ladies by Lely, Kneller and Reynolds is not quite satisfied until he goes up to the pictures of the ladies, in their roles as the goddess Diana, the Tragic Muse, or St. Cecilia, to read on the little brass plates the names of the actual subjects of the pictures. So, in Pope's poem, it may be of some interest to know that Philomede is supposed to represent Henrietta, Duchess of Marlborough, in succession to her father, the first Duke; Atossa is traditionally supposed to be Sarah, Duchess of Marlborough, widow of the first Duke; Chloe is thought to be the Countess of Suffolk (Mrs. Howard), a neighbor of

Pope's at Twickenham and formerly mistress to King George II. There is some point to "dross for *duchesses*" in the next-to-last line.

Sir Patrick Spence

ANONYMOUS

The king sits in Dumferling toune,
  Drinking the blude-reid wine:
"O whar will I get guid sailor,
  To sail this schip of mine?"

Up and spak an eldern knicht,
  Sat at the kings richt kne:
"Sir Patrick Spence is the best sailor
  That sails upon the se."

The king has written a braid letter,
  And signd it wi his hand,
And sent it to Sir Patrick Spence,
  Was walking on the sand.

The first line that Sir Patrick red,
  A loud lauch lauchèd he;
The next line that Sir Patrick red,
  The teir blinded his ee.

"O wha is this has don this deid,
  This ill deid don to me,
To send me out this time o' the yeir,
  To sail upon the se!

"Mak hast, mak haste, my mirry men all,
  Our guid schip sails the morne":
"O say na sae, my master deir,
  For I feir a deadlie storme.

"Late late yestreen I saw the new moone,
  Wi the auld moone in hir arme,
And I feir, I feir, my deir master,
  That we will cum to harme."

O our Scots nobles wer richt laith
  To weet their cork-heild schoone;
Bot lang owre a' the play wer playd,
  Thair hats they swam aboone.

O lang, lang may their ladies sit,
  Wi thair fans into their hand,
Or eir they se Sir Patrick Spence
  Cum sailing to the land.

O lang, lang may the ladies stand,
  Wi thair gold kems in their hair,
Waiting for thair ain deir lords,
  For they'll se thame na mair.

Haf owre, haf owre to Aberdour,
  It's fiftie fadom deip,
And thair lies guid Sir Patrick Spence,
  Wi the Scots lords at his feit.

Edward

ANONYMOUS

"Why dois your brand sae drap wi bluid,
Edward, Edward,
Why dois your brand sae drap wi bluid,
And why sae sad gang yee O?"
"O I hae killed my hauke sae guid,
Mither, mither,
O I hae killed my hauke sae guid,
And I had nae mair bot hee O."

"Your haukis bluid was nevir sae reid,
Edward, Edward,
Your haukis bluid was nevir sae reid,
My deir son I tell thee O."
"O I hae killed my reid-roan steid,
Mither, mither,
O I hae killed my reid-roan steid,
That erst was sae fair and frie O."

"Your steid was auld, and ye hae got mair,
Edward, Edward,
Your steid was auld, and ye hae got mair,
Sum other dule ye drie O."
"O I hae killed my fadir deir,
Mither, mither,
O I hae killed my fadir deir,
Alas, and wae is mee O!"

"And whatten penance wul ye drie for that,
Edward, Edward,

And whatten penance will ye drie for that?
My deir son, now tell me O."
"Ile set my feit in yonder boat,
Mither, mither,
Ile set my feit in yonder boat,
And Ile fare ovir the sea O."

"And what wul ye doe wi your towirs and your ha,
Edward, Edward?
And what wul ye doe wi your towirs and your ha,
That were sae fair to see O?"
"Ile let thame stand tul they doun fa,
Mither, mither,
Ile let thame stand tul they doun fa,
For here nevir mair maun I bee O."

"And what wul ye leive to your bairns and your wife,
Edward, Edward?
And what wul ye leive to your bairns and your wife,
Whan ye gang ovir the sea O?"
"The warldis room, late them beg thrae life,
Mither, mither,
The warldis room, late them beg thrae life,
For thame nevir mair wul I see O."

"And what wul ye leive to your ain mither deir,
Edward, Edward?
And what wul ye leive to your ain mither deir?
My deir son, now tell me O."
"The curse of hell frae me sall ye beir,
Mither, mither,
The curse of hell frae me sall ye beir,
Sic counseils ye gave to me O."

Lord Randal

ANONYMOUS

"O where hae ye been, Lord Randal, my son?
O where hae ye been, my handsome young man?"
"I hae been to the wild wood; mother, make my bed soon,
For I'm weary wi hunting, and fain wald lie down."

"Where gat ye your dinner, Lord Randal, my son?
Where gat ye your dinner, my handsome young man?"
"I din'd wi my true-love; mother, make my bed soon,
For I'm weary wi hunting, and fain wald lie down."

"What gat ye to your dinner, Lord Randal, my son?
What gat ye to your dinner, my handsome young man?"
"I gat eels boiled in broo; mother, make my bed soon,
For I'm weary wi hunting, and fain wald lie down."

"What became of your bloodhounds, Lord Randal, my son?
What became of your bloodhounds, my handsome young man?"
"O they swelld and they died; mother, make my bed soon,
For I'm weary wi hunting, and fain wald lie down."

"O I fear ye are poisond, Lord Randal, my son!
O I fear ye are poisond, my handsome young man!"
"O yes! I am poisond; mother, make my bed soon,
For I'm sick at the heart and I fain wald lie down."

The Charge of the Light Brigade

ALFRED, LORD TENNYSON (1809–1892)

Half a league, half a league,
Half a league onward,
All in the valley of Death
  Rode the six hundred.
  "Forward, the Light Brigade!
Charge for the guns!" he said.
Into the valley of Death
  Rode the six hundred.

"Forward, the Light Brigade!"
Was there a man dismayed?
Not though the soldier knew
  Some one had blundered.
Theirs not to make reply,
Theirs not to reason why,
Theirs but to do and die.
Into the valley of Death
  Rode the six hundred.

Cannon to right of them,
Cannon to left of them,
Cannon in front of them
  Volleyed and thundered;
Stormed at with shot and shell,
Boldly they rode and well,
Into the jaws of Death,
Into the mouth of Hell
  Rode the six hundred.

Flashed all their sabres bare,
Flashed as they turned in air
Sabring the gunners there,
Charging an army, while
All the world wondered:
Plunged in the battery-smoke
Right through the line they broke;
Cossack and Russian
Reeled from the sabre-stroke
Shattered and sundered.
Then they rode back, but not,
Not the six hundred.

Cannon to right of them,
Cannon to left of them,
Cannon behind them
Volleyed and thundered;
Stormed at with shot and shell,
While horse and hero fell,
They that had fought so well
Came through the jaws of Death,
Back from the mouth of Hell,
All that was left of them,
Left of six hundred.

When can their glory fade?
O the wild charge they made!
All the world wondered.
Honor the charge they made!
Honor the Light Brigade,
Noble six hundred!

The Chariot

EMILY DICKINSON (1830–1886)

Because I could not stop for Death,
He kindly stopped for me;
The carriage held but just ourselves
And Immortality.

We slowly drove, he knew no haste,
And I had put away
My labour, and my leisure too,
For his civility.

We passed the school where children played,
Their lessons scarcely done;
We passed the fields of gazing grain,
We passed the setting sun.

We paused before a house that seemed
A swelling on the ground;
The roof was scarcely visible,
The cornice but a mound.

Since then 'tis centuries; but each
Feels shorter than the day
I first surmised the horses' heads
Were toward eternity.

THE CHARIOT by Emily Dickinson is reprinted from *The Poems of Emily Dickinson*, edited by Martha Dickinson Bianchi and Alfred Leete Hampson, by permission of Little Brown & Company.

The Scholar-Gypsy

MATTHEW ARNOLD (1822–1888)

Go, for they call you, shepherd, from the hill;
  Go, shepherd, and untie the wattled cotes!
    No longer leave thy wistful flock unfed,
  Nor let thy bawling fellows rack their throats,
    Nor the cropped herbage shoot another head.
      But when the fields are still,
  And the tired men and dogs all gone to rest,
    And only the white sheep are sometimes seen
    Cross and recross the strips of moon-blanched green,
  Come, shepherd, and again begin the quest!

Here, where the reaper was at work of late—
  In this high field's dark corner, where he leaves
    His coat, his basket, and his earthen cruse,
  And in the sun all morning binds the sheaves,
    Then here, at noon, comes back his stores to use—
      Here will I sit and wait,
  While to my ear from uplands far away
    The bleating of the folded flocks is borne,
    With distant cries of reapers in the corn—
  All the live murmur of a summer's day.

Screened is this nook o'er the high, half-reaped field,
  And here till sun-down, shepherd! will I be.
    Through the thick corn the scarlet poppies peep,
  And round green roots and yellowing stalks I see
    Pale pink convolvulus in tendrils creep;
      And air-swept lindens yield
  Their scent, and rustle down their perfumed showers

Of bloom on the bent grass where I am laid,
And bower me from the August sun with shade;
And the eye travels down to Oxford's towers.

And near me on the grass lies Glanvil's book—
Come, let me read the oft-read tale again!
The story of the Oxford scholar poor,
Of pregnant parts and quick inventive brain,
Who, tired of knocking at preferment's door,
One summer-morn forsook
His friends, and went to learn the gypsy-lore,
And roamed the world with that wild brotherhood,
And came, as most men deemed, to little good,
But came to Oxford and his friends no more.

But once, years after, in the country-lanes,
Two scholars, whom at college erst he knew,
Met him, and of his way of life inquired;
Whereat he answered that the gypsy-crew,
His mates, had arts to rule as they desired
The workings of men's brains,
And they can bind them to what thoughts they will.
"And I," he said, "the secret of their art,
When fully learned, will to the world impart;
But it needs heaven-sent moments for this skill."

This said, he left them, and returned no more.—
But rumors hung about the country-side,
That the lost Scholar long was seen to stray,
Seen by rare glimpses, pensive and tongue-tied,
In hat of antique shape, and cloak of gray,
The same the gypsies wore.
Shepherds had met him on the Hurst in spring;
At some lone alehouse in the Berkshire moors,
On the warm ingle-bench, the smock-frocked boors
Had found him seated at their entering.

But, 'mid their drink and clatter, he would fly.
And I myself seem half to know thy looks,
And put the shepherds, wanderer! on thy trace;
And boys who in lone wheatfields scare the rooks
I ask if thou hast passed their quiet place;
Or in my boat I lie
Moored to the cool bank in the summer-heats,
'Mid wide grass meadows which the sunshine fills,
And watch the warm, green-muffled Cumner hills,
And wonder if thou haunt'st their shy retreats.

For most, I know, thou lov'st retired ground!
Thee at the ferry Oxford riders blithe,
Returning home on summer-nights, have met
Crossing the stripling Thames at Bab-lock-hithe,
Trailing in the cool stream thy fingers wet,
As the punt's rope chops round;
And leaning backward in a pensive dream,
And fostering in thy lap a heap of flowers
Plucked in shy fields and distant Wychwood bowers,
And thine eyes resting on the moonlit stream.

And then they land, and thou art seen no more!—
Maidens, who from the distant hamlets come
To dance around the Fyfield elm in May,
Oft through the darkening fields have seen thee roam,
Or cross a stile into the public way.
Oft thou hast given them store
Of flowers—the frail-leafed, white anemone,
Dark bluebells drenched with dews of summer eves,
And purple orchises with spotted leaves—
But none hath words she can report of thee.

And, above Godstow Bridge, when hay-time's here
In June, and many a scythe in sunshine flames,
Men who through those wide fields of breezy grass

Where black-winged swallows haunt the glittering Thames,
To bathe in the abandoned lasher pass,
Have often passed thee near
Sitting upon the river bank o'ergrown;
Marked thine outlandish garb, thy figure spare,
Thy dark vague eyes, and soft abstracted air—
But, when they came from bathing, thou wast gone!

At some lone homestead in the Cumner hills,
Where at her open door the housewife darns,
Thou hast been seen, or hanging on a gate
To watch the threshers in the mossy barns.
Children, who early range these slopes and late
For cresses from the rills,
Have known thee eying, all an April-day,
The springing pastures and the feeding kine;
And marked thee, when the stars come out and shine,
Through the long dewy grass move slow away.

In autumn, on the skirts of Bagley Wood—
Where most the gypsies by the turf-edged way
Pitch their smoked tents, and every bush you see
With scarlet patches tagged and shreds of gray,
Above the forest-ground called Thessaly—
The blackbird, picking food,
Sees thee, nor stops his meal, nor fears at all;
So often has he known thee past him stray,
Rapt, twirling in thy hand a withered spray,
And waiting for the spark from heaven to fall.

And once, in winter, on the causeway chill
Where home through flooded fields foot-travelers go,
Have I not passed thee on the wooden bridge,
Wrapped in thy cloak and battling with the snow,
Thy face tow'rd Hinksey and its wintry ridge?

And thou hast climbed the hill,
And gained the white brow of the Cumner range;
Turned once to watch, while thick the snowflakes fall,
The line of festal light in Christ-Church hall—
Then sought thy straw in some sequestered grange.

But what—I dream! Two hundred years are flown
Since first thy story ran through Oxford halls,
And the grave Glanvil did the tale inscribe
That thou wert wandered from the studious walls
To learn strange arts, and join a gypsy tribe;
And thou from earth art gone
Long since, and in some quiet churchyard laid—
Some country-nook, where o'er thy unknown grave
Tall grasses and white flowering nettles wave,
Under a dark, red-fruited yew-tree's shade.

—No, no, thou hast not felt the lapse of hours!
For what wears out the life of mortal men?
'Tis that from change to change their being rolls;
'Tis that repeated shocks, again, again,
Exhaust the energy of strongest souls
And numb the elastic powers,
Till having used our nerves with bliss and teen,
And tired upon a thousand schemes our wit,
To the just-pausing Genius we remit
Our worn-out life, and are—what we have been.

Thou hast not lived, why should'st thou perish, so?
Thou hadst *one* aim, *one* business, *one* desire;
Else wert thou long since numbered with the dead!
Else hadst thou spent, like other men, thy fire!
The generations of thy peers are fled,
And we ourselves shall go;
But thou possessest an immortal lot,

And we imagine thee exempt from age
And living as thou liv'st on Glanvil's page,
Because thou hadst—what we, alas! have not.

For early didst thou leave the world, with powers
Fresh, undiverted to the world without,
Firm to their mark, not spent on other things;
Free from the sick fatigue, the languid doubt,
Which much to have tried, in much been baffled, brings.
O life unlike to ours!
Who fluctuate idly without term or scope,
Of whom each strives, nor knows for what he strives,
And each half lives a hundred different lives;
Who wait like thee, but not, like thee, in hope.

Thou waitest for the spark from heaven! and we,
Light half-believers of our casual creeds,
Who never deeply felt, nor clearly willed,
Whose insight never has borne fruit in deeds,
Whose vague resolves never have been fulfilled;
For whom each year we see
Breeds new beginnings, disappointments new;
Who hesitate and falter life away,
And lose tomorrow the ground won today—
Ah! do not we, wanderer! await it too?

Yes, we await it!—but it still delays,
And then we suffer! and amongst us one,
Who most hast suffered, takes dejectedly
His seat upon the intellectual throne;
And all his store of sad experience he
Lays bare of wretched days;
Tells us his misery's birth and growth and signs,
And how the dying spark of hope was fed,
And how the breast was soothed, and how the head,
And all his hourly varied anodynes.

This for our wisest! and we others pine,
And wish the long unhappy dream would end,
And waive all claim to bliss, and try to bear;
With close-lipped patience for our only friend,
Sad patience, too near neighbor to despair—
But none has hope like thine!
Thou through the fields and through the woods dost stray,
Roaming the country-side, a truant boy,
Nursing thy project in unclouded joy,
And every doubt long blown by time away.

O born in days when wits were fresh and clear,
And life ran gayly as the sparkling Thames;
Before this strange disease of modern life,
With its sick hurry, its divided aims,
Its head o'ertaxed, its palsied hearts, was rife—
Fly hence, our contact fear!
Still fly, plunge deeper in the bowering wood!
Averse, as Dido did with gesture stern
From her false friend's approach in Hades turn,
Wave us away, and keep thy solitude!

Still nursing the unconquerable hope,
Still clutching the inviolable shade,
With a free, onward impulse brushing through,
By night, the silvered branches of the glade—
Far on the forest-skirts, where none pursue,
On some mild pastoral slope
Emerge, and resting on the moonlit pales
Freshen thy flowers as in former years
With dew, or listen with enchanted ears,
From the dark dingles, to the nightingales!

But fly our paths, our feverish contact fly!
For strong the infection of our mental strife,

Which, though it gives no bliss, yet spoils for rest;
And we should win thee from thy own fair life,
Like us distracted, and like us unblest.
Soon, soon thy cheer would die,
Thy hopes grow timorous, and unfixed thy powers,
And thy clear aims be cross and shifting made;
And then thy glad perennial youth would fade,
Fade, and grow old at last, and die like ours.

Then fly our greetings, fly our speech and smiles!
—As some grave Tyrian trader, from the sea,
Descried at sunrise an emerging prow
Lifting the cool-haired creepers stealthily,
The fringes of a southward-facing brow
Among the Ægæan isles;
And saw the merry Grecian coaster come,
Freighted with amber grapes, and Chian wine,
Green, bursting figs, and tunnies steeped in brine—
And knew the intruders on his ancient home,

The young light-hearted masters of the waves—
And snatched his rudder, and shook out more sail;
And day and night held on indignantly
O'er the blue Midland waters with the gale,
Betwixt the Syrtes and soft Sicily,
To where the Atlantic raves
Outside the western straits; and unbent sails
There, where down cloudy cliffs, through sheets of foam,
Shy traffickers, the dark Iberians come;
And on the beach undid his corded bales.

Critical Analysis

ARNOLD'S POEM is famous for various virtues, and it may impress different readers in different ways, but a good critical analysis will see to it that all the major elements in the poem are considered and that the relationship between Arnold's method and the total effect of the poem is adequately accounted for.

It is perhaps most obviously a pastoral poem celebrating the quiet beauties of the countryside around Oxford, and it is so faithful to the locality that it can be used as a kind of guidebook for walks among the Cumner Hills and Berkshire moors. Arnold's scenes which convey the feeling of the countryside are precise and specific: the shaded top of the half-reaped field (stanzas 2–3), the punt which serves as a ferry over the "stripling Thames" at Bablockhithe, the housewife darning at the open door of some homestead, the gypsies camped on the edge of Bagley Wood, the blackbird undisturbed by the familiar figure going by. They are rich in suggestion, they are chosen in a very satisfying way from that area halfway between the ideal and the actual, and they exhibit wide variety and compass, consciously reflecting different seasons of the year—May, harvest-time, autumn, winter.

To give this descriptive poetry life we have a figure moving through it—the scholar gypsy whose story is told in a seventeenth-century book, Joseph Glanvill's *The Vanity of Dogmatizing.* Arnold introduces the source directly into the poem. Stanza 4 summarizes it, and stanza 5 describes the lesson the scholar was trying to learn from the gypsies. For the most part, the scholar's relationship to the countryside is emphasized as one of shy familiarity, and it is only toward the end of the first thirteen stanzas, which fill out the description, that the more general and significant meaning of the scholar's search is mentioned:

> And waiting for the spark from heaven to fall. (line 120)

The transition to the next section is strongly marked by rhetorical devices: "But what—I dream!" and the exclamation and question of the first lines of the succeeding stanzas.

Arnold now begins the development of his theme, for this is not a mere celebration of the Oxford countryside or a narrative from Oxford folklore, but a serious criticism of contemporary life. The essence of the scholar gypsy was unity of purpose, the poet says, and because of this unity of purpose he has gained immortality and youth, though perhaps he never succeeded in his search. A strong and explicit contrast is drawn between the scholar and us moderns, including the poet, who also wait for the spark from heaven, but "hesitate and falter life away." In fact, modern life is called a disease, "with its sick hurry, its divided aims," and the shy retiring avoidance of the world practiced by the scholar is now commended, for the quarrels ("mental strife"), indecision, and pessimism of the modern world are like an infection which it is only prudent to avoid. If he did not escape from life, in its modern form at any rate, the scholar would become "like us distracted, and like us unblest."

Here is a structural link between the first, descriptive section of the poem and the didactic second part. The justification for rejecting and escaping from modern life, or Arnold's interpretation of the nineteenth century, rests now upon the beauty of the pastoral Oxford countryside as given in the first section and the arguments of the second section. They reinforce each other.

Finally, since the scholar gypsy is something of a legend anyhow, now dead two hundred years and probably buried in some quiet country churchyard but still alive and youthful in the pages of Glanvill's book (and indeed much more so in Arnold's poem), he is associated with, or transformed into, a figure even farther back and more remote, an anonymous figure of the classical world. The "grave Tyrian trader" simile at the end of the poem is extended, in the epic manner; but its artistic significance is not that it shows Arnold's mastery of Greek material and his ability to handle it romantically without distortion; it is rather that the Tyrian, with his bold independence and his avoidance of the competition with Greek intruders, sails to the west across the Mediterranean. He is a symbol of the youth, optimism, independence which Arnold admired in the scholar gypsy. When we recover from the captivating intensity of the little narrative we see that it is a satisfying and consistent conclusion to the poem.

It returns our response to the level of beauty, where it started; it subsumes the critical didacticism of the second section, and it provides us with a remarkable example of the great range of Arnold's style—from the exotic richness of Keats to the simple, stark effectiveness of Wordsworth:

> There, where down cloudy cliffs, through sheets of foam,
> Shy traffickers, the dark Iberians come;
> And on the beach undid his corded bales.

Hymn to Earth

ELINOR WYLIE (1886–1929)

Farewell, incomparable element,
Whence man arose, where he shall not return;
And hail, imperfect urn
Of his last ashes, and his firstborn fruit;
Farewell, the long pursuit,
And all the adventures of his discontent;
The voyages which sent
His heart averse from home:
Metal of clay, permit him that he come
To thy slow-burning fire as to a hearth;
Accept him as a particle of earth.

Fire, being divided from the other three,
It lives removed, or secret at the core;
Most subtle of the four,
When air flies not, nor water flows,

It disembodied goes,
Being light, elixir of the first decree,
More volatile than he;
With strength and power to pass
Through space, where never his least atom was:
He has no part in it, save as his eyes
Have drawn its emanation from the skies.

A wingless creature heavier than air,
He is rejected of its quintessence;
Coming and going hence,
In the twin minutes of his birth and death,
He may inhale as breath,
As breath relinquish heaven's atmosphere,
Yet in it have no share,
Nor can survive therein
Where its outer edge is filtered pure and thin:
It doth but lend its crystal to his lungs
For his early crying, and his final songs.

The element of water has denied
Its child; it is no more his element;
It never will relent;
Its silver harvests are more sparsely given
Than the rewards of heaven,
And he shall drink cold comfort at its side:
The water is too wide:
The seamew and the gull
Feather a nest made soft and pitiful
Upon its foam; he has not any part
In the long swell of sorrow at its heart.

Hail and farewell, beloved element,
Whence he departed, and his parent once;
See where thy spirit runs

Which for so long hath had the moon to wife;
Shall this support his life
Until the arches of the waves be bent
And grow shallow and spent?
Wisely it cast him forth
With his dead weight of burdens nothing worth,
Leaving him, for the universal years,
A little seawater to make his tears.

Hail, element of earth, receive thy own,
And cherish, at thy charitable breast,
This man, this mongrel beast:
He plows the sand, and, at his hardest need,
He sows himself for seed;
He plows the furrow, and in this lies down
Before the corn is grown;
Between the apple bloom
And the ripe apple is sufficient room
In time, and matter, to consume his love
And make him parcel of a cypress grove.

Receive him as thy lover for an hour
Who will not weary, by a longer stay,
The kind embrace of clay;
Even within thine arms he is dispersed
To nothing, as at first;
The air flings downward from its four-quartered tower
Him whom the flames devour;
At the full tide, at the flood,
The sea is mingled with his salty blood:
The traveller dust, although the dust be vile,
Sleeps as thy lover for a little while.

Spring and Winter

WILLIAM SHAKESPEARE (1564–1616)

Spring

When daisies pied and violets blue
   And lady-smocks all silver-white
And cuckoo-buds of yellow hue
   Do paint the meadows with delight,
The cuckoo then, on every tree,
Mocks married men; for thus sings he,
                                        Cuckoo;
Cuckoo, cuckoo: O, word of fear,
Unpleasing to a married ear!

When shepherds pipe on oaten straws,
   And merry larks are ploughmen's clocks,
When turtles tread, and rooks, and daws,
   And maidens bleach their summer smocks,
The cuckoo then, on every tree,
Mocks married men; for thus sings he,
                                        Cuckoo;
Cuckoo, cuckoo: O, word of fear,
Unpleasing to a married ear!

Winter

When icicles hang by the wall,
   And Dick the shepherd blows his nail,
And Tom bears logs into the hall,
   And milk comes frozen home in pail,
When blood is nipp'd, and ways be foul,
Then nightly sings the staring owl,

Tu-who;
Tu-whit, tu-who—a merry note,
While greasy Joan doth keel the pot.

When all aloud the wind doth blow,
  And coughing drowns the parson's saw,
And birds sit brooding in the snow,
  And Marian's nose looks red and raw,
When roasted crabs hiss in the bowl,
Then nightly sings the staring owl,
Tu-who;
Tu-whit, tu-who—a merry note,
While greasy Joan doth keel the pot.

(*Love's Labour's Lost*, V, iii)

Full Fathom Five

WILLIAM SHAKESPEARE (1564–1616)

Full fathom five thy father lies;
    Of his bones are coral made;
Those are pearls that were his eyes:
    Nothing of him that doth fade,
But doth suffer a sea change
Into something rich and strange.
Sea nymphs hourly ring his knell:
Burthen. Ding-dong.
Hark! now I hear them,—Ding-dong, bell.

(*The Tempest*, I, ii)

Call for the Robin Redbreast and the Wren

JOHN WEBSTER (circa 1580–1634)

Call for the robin redbreast and the wren,
Since o'er shady groves they hover,
And with leaves and flowers do cover
The friendless bodies of unburied men.
Call unto his funeral dole
The ant, the field mouse, and the mole,
To rear him hillocks that shall keep him warm,
And, when gay tombs are robbed, sustain no harm;
But keep the wolf far thence, that's foe to men,
For with his nails he'll dig them up again.

(*The White Devil*, V, iv)

To Althea, from Prison

RICHARD LOVELACE (1618–1658)

When Love with unconfined wings
  Hovers within my gates,
And my divine Althea brings
  To whisper at the grates;
When I lie tangled in her hair
  And fettered to her eye,
The birds that wanton in the air
  Know no such liberty.

When flowing cups run swiftly round,
  With no allaying Thames,
Our careless heads with roses bound,
  Our hearts with loyal flames;
When thirsty grief in wine we steep,
  When healths and draughts go free,
Fishes that tipple in the deep
  Know no such liberty.

When, like committed linnets, I
  With shriller throat shall sing
The sweetness, mercy, majesty,
  And glories of my king;
When I shall voice aloud how good
  He is, how great should be,
Enlarged winds that curl the flood
  Know no such liberty.

Stone walls do not a prison make,
  Nor iron bars a cage:
Minds innocent and quiet take
  That for an hermitage.
If I have freedom in my love,
  And in my soul am free,
Angels alone, that soar above,
  Enjoy such liberty.

Like as the Waves Make towards the Pebbled Shore

WILLIAM SHAKESPEARE (1564–1616)

Like as the waves make towards the pebbled shore,
So do our minutes hasten to their end;
Each changing place with that which goes before,
In sequent toil all forwards do contend.
Nativity, once in the main of light,
Crawls to maturity, wherewith being crown'd,
Crooked eclipses 'gainst his glory fight,
And Time that gave doth now his gift confound.
Time doth transfix the flourish set on youth
And delves the parallels in beauty's brow,
Feeds on the rarities of nature's truth,
And nothing stands but for his scythe to mow:
  And yet to times in hope my verse shall stand,
  Praising thy worth, despite his cruel hand.

Critical Analysis

THIS SONNET seems to be a conventional poem on the well-worn theme of the passage of time and the ability of poetry to survive when other things are destroyed. Its subject matter offers nothing novel or unexpected; it is one of the most commonplace of themes. Yet the sonnet is one of the greatest, even among Shakespeare's. Why?

To answer this question we must respond first of all to the metaphorical language in the poem and take it seriously, for the essence of the poem lies in its metaphorical thinking. Because a

Shakespearean sonnet is composed of three quatrains and a couplet, it is natural to look first to see if the metaphors are adapted to this structure.

The first quatrain presents a clear image of "our minutes" (that is, time allotted to us, considered in particles) represented as waves of the sea, each succeeding another in steady, rapid, incessant progression. The movement is rapid ("hasten") but labored ("toil" and "contend"). "Make towards" is a nautical expression, used of a ship. (See Shakespeare's *Comedy of Errors* I, i, 93 for another example.) The fourth line, a summary of time considered as the sea, is full of abstract words ("sequent toil," "forwards," which Shakespeare here uses as a noun, etc.), and it stresses the verbal ideas heavily, as indeed the whole quatrain does. See how many of the words are verbs or near-verbs: "make towards," "do," "hasten," "end" (near-verb), "changing place," "goes," "sequent" (near-verb, especially if the Latin *sequor* is recalled), "toil" (near-verb), "forwards" (near-verb), "contend." All this motion and action in the space of four lines! The first quatrain, then, adopts the basic image of minutes as waves and then reinforces it by conveying to the reader a powerful sense of surging and continuing motion.

The metaphor of the second quatrain is not so clear, because the thing acting is an abstract, "nativity." To the modern reader this word has associations from religion, or from religious painting, but in the time of Shakespeare it had a much more common reference —that of any person's birth, a time at which it was usual to cast a horoscope and tell the infant's fortune from the situation of the stars at the moment of "nativity." In the fifth line nativity is said to have been once in the "main" or sea of light (the word is used as in the expression "the Spanish Main"), and then in the sixth line, he "crawls" to maturity. The image here is a curious but not illogical one, of a baby. But as the quatrain develops, we see more clearly that it is also the sun. Expanding the quatrain very crudely, we might say something like this: "Our time passes by as a baby grows to be a man, or as the sun climbs up the sky, *or as both*, because the birth, growth, and decline of the sun every day is merely a model of what happens to all of us." "Crooked eclipses," which blot out part of the sun's perfect circle and are therefore crooked, are said to come after noon, or maturity. (We will not bother with the astronomical accuracy of this, because what is important is the metaphor, the image.) The eighth line, the last of this quatrain, is again more general and summary in nature: Time, that gave (the gift was "glory" and "maturity") now confounds his own gift, that is, mars or destroys it.

The third quatrain is tied closely to the second by a repetition of the statement about time, and the first three lines of this quatrain are all declarations of time's actions. He transfixes the flourish set on youth, a general statement equivalent to line 8 but more positive and direct. Then he "delves the parallels" or digs the furrows in beauty's brow, feeds on the rarities, mows with his scythe. The metaphor is agricultural, and time has become not only the grim reaper with his scythe, but the plowman and the consumer of the rarities of the garden as well. (Some readers may be too squeamish to accept Shakespeare's image of the wrinkles in the brow of a beautiful person as the furrows dug by time's plow; the poet does not force the image very hard, but because of the next two lines he clearly intends it.) In abstract terms, Youth, Beauty and Nature all perish in time.

The progression of the general images in the three quatrains is full of interest: first the sea, then the sky, and finally the earth; this gives a sense of the whole world's being involved and serves as a background to the final statement. Moreover, there is *dramatic* progression: in the first quatrain time exerts no action on us; they are "our" minutes, to be sure, but the struggle seems one merely of movement, not of opposition. In the second quatrain the struggle is more active, but directed against nativity, or the sun, and does not directly implicate the reader. But cruelty is already apparent as a characteristic of time, in fighting against glory and in confounding the gift given. In the third quatrain the victims are, respectively, youth, beauty, and nature's truth, so the conclusion that nothing escapes the scythe is justified, and it includes us.

This feeling is so marked that the turn in the couplet must be very strong: *And yet!* Granting everything the three quatrains have established, still poetry will survive. "Shall" is strongly emphasized by the *s* sounds surrounding it, and the word order is carefully arranged to give the "despite" statement after the declaration, not before it. The couplet is tied to the last quatrain by the repetition of "stands—stand."

If we glance back through the quatrains we may also notice a fleeting suggestion here and there of riches, jewelry, magnificence —a suggestion coming from relationships between "crowned," "glory," "flourish," "rarities." The full purpose of these words cannot be seen until the couplet is reached. Then we become conscious of how fully prepared for is the word "worth" in the last line.

The metaphors in this poem fit the structure beautifully, they build up the strength of feeling which the sonnet reaches at its conclusion, and they illuminate the subject of time and change by converting them from abstract conceptions into realized imaginative experience. On these grounds one may assert that Shakespeare's sonnet is a great poem.

That Time of Year Thou Mayst in Me Behold

WILLIAM SHAKESPEARE (1564–1616)

That time of year thou mayst in me behold
When yellow leaves, or none, or few, do hang
Upon those boughs which shake against the cold,
Bare ruin'd choirs, where late the sweet birds sang.

In me thou see'st the twilight of such day,
As after sunset fadeth in the west,
Which by and by black night doth take away,
Death's second self, that seals up all in rest.
In me thou see'st the glowing of such fire,
That on the ashes of his youth doth lie,
As the death-bed whereon it must expire,
Consum'd with that which it was nourish'd by.
  This thou perceiv'st, which makes thy love more strong,
  To love that well which thou must leave ere long.

Let Me Not to the Marriage of True Minds

WILLIAM SHAKESPEARE (1564–1616)

Let me not to the marriage of true minds
Admit impediments. Love is not love
Which alters when it alteration finds,
Or bends with the remover to remove:
O, no! it is an ever-fixed mark,
That looks on tempests and is never shaken;
It is the star to every wandering bark,
Whose worth's unknown, although his height be taken.
Love's not Time's fool, though rosy lips and cheeks
Within his bending sickle's compass come;
Love alters not with his brief hours and weeks,
But bears it out even to the edge of doom.
  If this be error, and upon me prov'd,
  I never writ, nor no man ever lov'd.

When in the Chronicle of Wasted Time

WILLIAM SHAKESPEARE (1564–1616)

When in the chronicle of wasted time
I see descriptions of the fairest wights,
And beauty making beautiful old rime,
In praise of ladies dead and lovely knights;
Then, in the blazon of sweet beauty's best,
Of hand, of foot, of lip, of eye, of brow,
I see their antique pen would have express'd
Even such a beauty as you master now.
So all their praises are but prophecies
Of this our time, all you prefiguring;
And, for they look'd but with divining eyes,
They had not skill enough your worth to sing:
   For we, which now behold these present days,
   Have eyes to wonder, but lack tongues to praise.

Tired with All These

WILLIAM SHAKESPEARE (1564–1616)

Tired with all these, for restful death I cry,
As, to behold desert a beggar born,
And needy nothing trimmed in jollity,
And purest faith unhappily forsworn,
And gilded honor shamefully misplaced,
And maiden virtue rudely strumpeted,

And right perfection wrongfully disgraced,
And strength by limping sway disabled,
And art made tongue-tied by authority,
And folly, doctorlike, controlling skill,
And simple truth miscalled simplicity,
And captive good attending captain ill.
  Tired with all these, from these would I be gone,
  Save that, to die I leave my love alone.

A Valediction Forbidding Mourning

JOHN DONNE (1572–1631)

As virtuous men pass mildly away,
  And whisper to their souls to go,
Whilst some of their sad friends do say,
  "The breath goes now," and some say, "No";

So let us melt, and make no noise,
  No tear-floods nor sigh-tempests move;
'Twere profanation of our joys
  To tell the laity our love.

Moving of the earth brings harms and fears;
  Men reckon what it did and meant;
But trepidation of the spheres,
  Though greater far, is innocent.

Dull sublunary lovers' love,
  Whose soul is sense, cannot admit
Absence, because it doth remove
  Those things which elemented it.

But we, by a love so much refined
  That ourselves know not what it is,
Inter-assured of the mind,
  Care less eyes, lips, and hands to miss.

Our two souls, therefore, which are one,
  Though I must go, endure not yet
A breach, but an expansion,
  Like gold to airy thinness beat.

If they be two, they are two so
  As stiff twin compasses are two;
Thy soul, the fixed foot, makes no show
  To move, but doth if the other do.

And though it in the center sit,
  Yet when the other far doth roam,
It leans, and hearkens after it,
  And grows erect as that comes home.

Such wilt thou be to me, who must,
  Like the other foot, obliquely run;
Thy firmness makes my circle just,
  And makes me end where I begun.

When Our Two Souls Stand Up Erect and Strong

ELIZABETH BARRETT BROWNING (1806–1861)

When our two souls stand up erect and strong,
Face to face, silent, drawing nigh and nigher,
Until the lengthening wings break into fire
At either curved point,—what bitter wrong

Can the earth do to us, that we should not long
Be here contented? Think! In mounting higher,
The angels would press on us and aspire
To drop some golden orb of perfect song
Into our deep, dear silence. Let us stay
Rather on earth, Beloved,—where the unfit,
Contrarious moods of men recoil away
And isolate pure spirits, and permit
A place to stand and love in for a day,
With darkness and the death-hour rounding it.

To Autumn

JOHN KEATS (1795–1821)

Season of mists and mellow fruitfulness,
  Close bosom-friend of the maturing sun;
Conspiring with him how to load and bless
  With fruit the vines that round the thatch-eaves run;
To bend with apples the mossed cottage-trees,
  And fill all fruit with ripeness to the core;
  To swell the gourd, and plump the hazel shells
With a sweet kernel; to set budding more,
  And still more, later flowers for the bees,
  Until they think warm days will never cease,
    For Summer has o'er-brimmed their clammy cells.

Who hath not seen thee oft amid thy store?
  Sometimes whoever seeks abroad may find

Thee sitting careless on a granary floor,
Thy hair soft-lifted by the winnowing wind;
Or on a half-reaped furrow sound asleep,
Drowsed with the fume of poppies, while thy hook
Spares the next swath and all its twinèd flowers:
And sometimes like a gleaner thou dost keep
Steady thy laden head across a brook;
Or by a cider-press, with patient look,
Thou watchest the last oozings hours by hours.

Where are the songs of Spring? Ay, where are they?
Think not of them, thou hast thy music too,—
While barrèd clouds bloom the soft-dying day,
And touch the stubble-plains with rosy hue;
Then in a wailful choir the small gnats mourn
Among the river shallows, borne aloft
Or sinking as the light wind lives or dies;
And full-grown lambs loud bleat from hilly bourn;
Hedge-crickets sing; and now with treble soft
The red-breast whistles from a garden-croft;
And gathering swallows twitter in the skies.

The Garden

ANDREW MARVELL (1621–1678)

How vainly men themselves amaze
To win the palm, the oak, or bays,
And their incessant labors see
Crowned from some single herb, or tree,
Whose short and narrow-verged shade
Does prudently their toils upbraid;

While all flowers and all trees do close
To weave the garlands of repose!

Fair Quiet, have I found thee here,
And Innocence, thy sister dear?
Mistaken long, I sought you then
In busy companies of men.
Your sacred plants, if here below,
Only among the plants will grow;
Society is all but rude
To this delicious solitude.

No white nor red was ever seen
So amorous as this lovely green.
Fond lovers, cruel as their flame,
Cut in these trees their mistress' name:
Little, alas, they know or heed
How far these beauties hers exceed!
Fair trees, wheresoe'er your barks I wound,
No name shall but your own be found.

When we have run our passion's heat,
Love hither makes his best retreat.
The gods, that mortal beauty chase,
Still in a tree did end their race:
Apollo hunted Daphne so,
Only that she might laurel grow;
And Pan did after Syrinx speed,
Not as a nymph, but for a reed.

What wondrous life is this I lead!
Ripe apples drop about my head;
The luscious clusters of the vine
Upon my mouth do crush their wine;
The nectarine and curious peach

Into my hands themselves do reach;
Stumbling on melons, as I pass,
Insnared with flowers, I fall on grass.

Meanwhile the mind, from pleasure less
Withdraws into its happiness;
The mind, that ocean where each kind
Does straight its own resemblance find;
Yet it creates, transcending these,
Far other worlds and other seas,
Annihilating all that's made
To a green thought in a green shade.

Here at the fountain's sliding foot,
Or at some fruit-tree's mossy root,
Casting the body's vest aside,
My soul into the boughs does glide:
There, like a bird, it sits and sings,
Then whets and combs its silver wings,
And, till prepared for longer flight,
Waves in its plumes the various light.

Such was that happy garden-state,
While man there walked without a mate:
After a place so pure and sweet,
What other help could yet be meet!
But 'twas beyond a mortal's share
To wander solitary there:
Two paradises 'twere in one
To live in paradise alone.

How well the skilful gardener drew
Of flowers and herbs this dial new,
Where, from above, the milder sun
Does through a fragrant zodiac run;
And as it works, the industrious bee

Computes its time as well as we!
How could such sweet and wholesome hours
Be reckoned but with herbs and flowers?

Critical Analysis

THE TITLE of Marvell's poem might lead a reader to expect a description of flowers, fruits, and the contents of a garden. But the opening lines come as a shock to any such expectation. Nevertheless, the most cursory reading will reveal the central conceit: the garden is all experience; it is time. The experience of the speaker is the experience of the world (stanzas 1 and 2), and of love and passion (stanzas 3 and 4). Stanza 5, which is pivotal in the poem, continues with the experience of the physical sensation of the garden; stanzas 6 and 7 with the experience of intellectual and spiritual contemplation. The last stanza abstracts all experience in terms of time and the garden. Yet the poem is actually well named; for throughout, the scene is either before the speaker's eye or in his mind, and the imagery is centered on the selected aspects of this garden.

The first four stanzas develop skillfully and are almost a tour de force of wit. Actually, Marvell keeps presenting us with a series of apparent reversals of our common ideas and justifies each one by the logic of the poem. The paradoxes make our process of readjusting to Marvell's harmony a continual one, not a thing done once and for all, as in Keats' ode, "To Autumn," where the readers' presuppositions are attacked only once. (We expect spring to be glorified, and Keats glorifies autumn, but once we make that shift, everything is in harmony.) Marvell asks us to accept such apparently outrageous propositions as:

Stanza 1. Ambition is less well rewarded than laziness.

Stanza 2. Society, usually thought of as refined and polished, is really *ruder* (rougher, more uncouth) than solitude.

Stanza 3. Red and white, the colors of female beauty, are less *amorous* than green, and a tree is a more suitable object of a lover's ecstasies than a lady.

Stanza 4. The myths of Apollo and Pan mean the opposite of what they seem to. Apollo and Pan were not disappointed when their nymphs turned into plants. They were delighted; that is why they chased them.

Once he has made the reader swallow these reversals, he shifts his strategy. In stanzas 5–7, Marvell sweeps the reader into the ecstasy of the garden, first physical, then mental, then spiritual. Yet even these mental and spiritual ecstasies are conveyed by garden-images—by "green thought," and by the image of the soul as a bird. The shift to mental and spiritual ecstasy contains the only complicated imagery of the poem, but the shift is not abrupt. It has been prepared for in the imaginative treatment of the garden in previous stanzas, especially 2 and 3. The garden, even where it appears to be most physical (stanza 5), is a world of imagination.

The mind (stanza 6) moving from the lesser pleasures (line 41) withdraws into its own happiness, since (as we learn from the succeeding image) it is the essence or idea of happiness. The speaker then introduces a vast metaphor (lines 43–48). The mind is an ocean. The mind is to the body as the ocean is to the land, an idea based on the notion that for every kind or genus on land there is a parallel in marine life. The mind has all the counterparts of the body, but extending from these ("transcending" not in the sense of "separation" but of "extension") creates new essences ("Far other worlds and other seas") and reduces all ordinary creation in a material world to pure thought in solitude ("To a *green* thought in a *green* shade") which has all the basic color symbolism of the garden as well as the color of the transforming sea. In perfect solitude, the mind can transcend even vast reality. To a believer in only what he sees before him, this proposition is a difficult one; it is an abstraction of reality.

The seventh stanza considers the projection—almost the transfiguration—of the speaker from the body to the state of the soul in the form of a bird. The scene of the mind's or soul's power to do this is the fountain, the source of growth in the garden, or the foot of the fruit tree. The soul leaves the body, glides like a bird into the tree. The bird is not delineated beyond its silver wings, although its action is described ("sits and sings," "whets [preens] and combs its silver wings," "Waves in its plumes the various light"). There is no need to give the bird individual quality. It is simply a new form of the soul, liberated from the body under the influence of the garden—the state of solitude.

The two final paradoxes could not be sustained without the preparatory rhapsody. They are the great ones—that solitude in a garden out-paradises paradise (for perfect paradise, which is *solitude* in the Garden of Eden, existed only when Adam was alone and was lost with the advent of Eve) and that time, usually thought of as the great destroyer of pastoral, idyllic life (cf. Ralegh's "The Nymph's Reply to the Shepherd," page 73) is really not inimical to it at all, but is suitably measured and ordered *only* by herbs, flowers, and insects.

The last stanza, which draws attention to one part of the garden in the form of a sundial, gives Marvell opportunity to display the benevolence of the largest aspect of nature, the sun. The conclusive effect of the stanza is seen in the speaker's return to the world. He has had an imaginative, almost mystical vision of escape, but his place in the world remains, and he understands through the garden his own position in time.

The whole treatment of the garden is contemplative and imaginative and, in several cases, intellectual. Although the tone is complex, the imagery and form are not complicated. In a poem of this sort one might have expected to find the verses more loaded with imagery. In fact, the images, although occasionally extended (as in stanzas 6–7), are few. The floral rewards for civic achievement (palm), military achievement (oak), and literary prowess (bays) are striking symbols in contrast to men's deeds (stanza 1). Quiet and Innocence are personified in stanza 2 and Love in stanza 4. The mind as an ocean and the soul like a bird constitute the imagery of stanzas 6–7, already discussed, but it should be noted that the most fanciful stanzas of the poem contain the most concrete imagery.

Effects akin to those of imagery are obtained by literary allusion—to the Apollo-Daphne and Pan-Syrinx legends (stanza 4). The allusions are in keeping with a classical quality which the poem has and give it a sense of timelessness. The eighth stanza, which culminates what might be called the Christian or philosophical imagery begun in stanzas 6 and 7, is a witty treatment of the Garden of Eden legend in a way well suited to the movement and tone of the poem already established.

As the reader looks back over the poem, he can see that its structure is governed by the experience of the speaker. The speaker ends where he begins, in the garden, but he has sounded joys, real and imaginative, in his contact with the garden and with his view of his own soul, temporarily freed by the situation of the garden.

The stanzas (eight-line tetrameter couplets) form individual paragraphs, but their relation to each other and the idea of the world is clear. Stanzas 1 and 2 deal with the themes of ambition and solitude and are verbally connected by lines 8 and 9. The last lines of both stanzas have similar pictorial quality: "garlands of repose" and "delicious solitude." Stanzas 3 and 4 are closely related and deal with love and physical beauty. Stanza 5 concentrates on the physical effects of the garden on the speaker. The next two stanzas form a unit in content; the eighth, powerful in its paradox, is allusive and transitional. The last stanza returns to the garden itself, which becomes a symbol for the final contraction of all experience. In addition to the clarity provided by the paragraphing of the poem, the versification itself gives the effect of simplicity and directness which encourages the reader to move through the complications of the thought and the imagery.

Further analysis of the poem, in the light of seventeenth-century thought and of stanzas 6 and 7, particularly, in their relation to Neo-Platonic ideas, would be valuable and interesting. But even without such study the poem is rich in meaning. Skillful and controlled, it presents through a series of paradoxes, through imagination and symbolic action, a view of all experience, of time itself, from the vantage point of solitude—the garden. This analysis, though extensive, is obviously an incomplete record of the total effect of "The Garden."

The Passionate Shepherd to His Love

CHRISTOPHER MARLOWE (1564–1593)

Come live with me and be my love,
And we will all the pleasures prove
That valleys, groves, hills, and fields,
Woods, or steepy mountain yields.

And we will sit upon the rocks,
Seeing the shepherds feed their flocks,
By shallow rivers to whose falls
Melodious birds sing madrigals.

And I will make thee beds of roses
And a thousand fragrant posies,
A cap of flowers, and a kirtle
Embroidered all with leaves of myrtle;

A gown made of the finest wool
Which from our pretty lambs we pull;
Fair linèd slippers for the cold,
With buckles of the purest gold;

A belt of straw and ivy buds,
With coral clasps and amber studs:
And if these pleasures may thee move,
Come live with me and be my love.

The shepherds' swains shall dance and sing
For thy delight each May morning:
If these delights thy mind may move,
Then live with me and be my love.

The Nymph's Reply to the Shepherd

SIR WALTER RALEGH (1552–1618)

If all the world and love were young,
And truth in every shepherd's tongue,
These pretty pleasures might me move
To live with thee and be thy love.

Time drives the flocks from field to fold
When rivers rage and rocks grow cold,
And Philomel becometh dumb;
The rest complains of cares to come.

The flowers do fade, and wanton fields
To wayward winter reckoning yields;
A honey tongue, a heart of gall,
Is fancy's spring, but sorrow's fall.

Thy gowns, thy shoes, thy beds of roses,
Thy cap, thy kirtle, and thy posies

Soon break, soon wither, soon forgotten,—
In folly ripe, in reason rotten.

Thy belt of straw and ivy buds,
Thy coral clasps and amber studs,
All these in me no means can move
To come to thee and be thy love.

But could youth last and love still breed,
Had joys no date nor age no need,
Then these delights my mind might move
To live with thee and be thy love.

Rose Aylmer

WALTER SAVAGE LANDOR (1775–1864)

Ah, what avails the sceptred race,
  Ah, what the form divine!
What every virtue, every grace!
  Rose Aylmer, all were thine.

Rose Aylmer, whom these wakeful eyes
  May weep, but never see,
A night of memories and sighs
  I consecrate to thee.

Here Lies a Lady

JOHN CROWE RANSOM (1888-   )

Here lies a lady of beauty and high degree.
Of chills and fever she died, of fever and chills,
The delight of her husband, her aunts, an infant of three,
And of medicos marvelling sweetly on her ills.

For either she burned, and her confident eyes would blaze,
And her fingers fly in a manner to puzzle their heads—
What was she making? Why, nothing; she sat in a maze
Of old scraps of laces, snipped into curious shreds—

Or this would pass, and the light of her fire decline
Till she lay discouraged and cold as a thin stalk white and blown,
And would not open her eyes, to kisses, to wine;
The sixth of these states was her last; the cold settled down.

Sweet ladies, long may ye bloom, and toughly I hope ye may thole,
But was she not lucky? In flowers and lace and mourning,
In love and great honour we bade God rest her soul
After six little spaces of chill, and six of burning.

The Exequy

HENRY KING (1592–1669)

Accept, thou shrine of my dead saint,
Instead of dirges, this complaint;
And for sweet flowers to crown thy hearse,
Receive a strew of weeping verse
From thy grieved friend, whom thou might'st see
Quite melted into tears for thee.

Dear loss! since thy untimely fate
My task hath been to meditate
On thee, on thee; thou art the book,
The library whereon I look,
Though almost blind. For thee, loved clay,
I languish out, not live, the day,
Using no other exercise
But what I practise with mine eyes;
By which wet glasses I find out
How lazily time creeps about
To one that mourns; this, only this,
My exercise and business is.
So I compute the weary hours
With sighs dissolved into showers.

Nor wonder if my time go thus
Backward and most preposterous;
Thou hast benighted me; thy set
This eve of blackness did beget,
Who wast my day, though overcast
Before thou hadst thy noon-tide passed;
And I remember must in tears,

Thou scarce hadst seen so many years
As day tells hours. By thy clear sun
My love and fortune first did run;
But thou wilt never more appear
Folded within my hemisphere,
Since both thy light and motion
Like a fled star is fallen and gone;
And 'twixt me and my soul's dear wish
An earth now interposed is,
Which such a strange eclipse doth make
As ne'er was read in almanac.

I could allow thee for a time
To darken me and my sad clime;
Were it a month, a year, or ten,
I would thy exile live till then,
And all that space my mirth adjourn,
So thou wouldst promise to return,
And putting off thy ashy shroud,
At length disperse this sorrow's cloud.

But woe is me! the longest date
Too narrow is to calculate
These empty hopes; never shall I
Be so much blest as to descry
A glimpse of thee, till that day come
Which shall the earth to cinders doom,
And a fierce fever must calcine
The body of this world—like thine,
My little world. That fit of fire
Once off, our bodies shall aspire
To our souls' bliss; then we shall rise
And view ourselves with clearer eyes
In that calm region where no night
Can hide us from each other's sight.

Meantime, thou hast her, earth; much good
May my harm do thee. Since it stood
With heaven's will I might not call
Her longer mine, I give thee all
My short-lived right and interest
In her whom living I loved best;
With a most free and bounteous grief
I give thee what I could not keep.
Be kind to her, and prithee look
Thou write into thy doomsday book
Each parcel of this rarity
Which in thy casket shrined doth lie.
See that thou make thy reckoning straight,
And yield her back again by weight;
For thou must audit on thy trust
Each grain and atom of this dust,
As thou wilt answer Him that lent,
Not gave thee, my dear monument.
So close the ground, and 'bout her shade
Black curtains draw; my bride is laid.

Sleep on, my love, in thy cold bed,
Never to be disquieted!
My last good-night! Thou wilt not wake
Till I thy fate shall overtake;
Till age, or grief, or sickness must
Marry my body to that dust
It so much loves, and fill the room
My heart keeps empty in thy tomb.
Stay for me there; I will not fail
To meet thee in that hollow vale.
And think not much of my delay;
I am already on the way,
And follow thee with all the speed
Desire can make, or sorrows breed.

Each minute is a short degree,
And every hour a step towards thee.
At night when I betake to rest,
Next morn I rise nearer my west
Of life, almost by eight hours' sail,
Than when sleep breathed his drowsy gale.

Thus from the sun my bottom steers,
And my day's compass downward bears;
Nor labor I to stem the tide
Through which to thee I swiftly glide.

'Tis true, with shame and grief I yield,
Thou like the van first took'st the field,
And gotten hath the victory
In thus adventuring to die
Before me, whose more years might crave
A just precedence in the grave.
But hark! my pulse like a soft drum
Beats my approach, tells thee I come;
And slow howe'er my marches be,
I shall at last sit down by thee.

The thought of this bids me go on,
And wait my dissolution
With hope and comfort. Dear (forgive
The crime) I am content to live
Divided, with but half a heart,
Till we shall meet and never part.

On His Blindness

JOHN MILTON (1608–1674)

When I consider how my light is spent
Ere half my days in this dark world and wide,
And that one talent which is death to hide
Lodged with me useless, though my soul more bent
To serve therewith my Maker, and present
My true account, lest He returning chide,
"Doth God exact day-labor, light denied?"
I fondly ask. But Patience, to prevent
That murmur, soon replies, "God doth not need
Either man's work or his own gifts. Who best
Bear his mild yoke, they serve him best. His state
Is kingly: thousands at his bidding speed,
And post o'er land and ocean without rest;
They also serve who only stand and wait."

An Irish Airman Foresees His Death

WILLIAM BUTLER YEATS (1865–1939)

I know that I shall meet my fate
Somewhere among the clouds above;
Those that I fight I do not hate,
Those that I guard I do not love;

My country is Kiltartan Cross,
My countrymen Kiltartan's poor,
No likely end could bring them loss
Or leave them happier than before.
Nor law, nor duty bade me fight,
Nor public men, nor cheering crowds,
A lonely impulse of delight
Drove to this tumult in the clouds;
I balanced all, brought all to mind,
The years to come seemed waste of breath,
A waste of breath the years behind
In balance with this life, this death.

Ode

Written in the Beginning of the Year 1746

WILLIAM COLLINS (1721–1759)

I

How sleep the brave, who sink to rest,
By all their country's wishes blest!
When Spring, with dewy fingers cold,
Returns to deck their hallow'd mold,
She there shall dress a sweeter sod,
Than Fancy's feet have ever trod.

II

By fairy hands their knell is rung,
By forms unseen their dirge is sung;
There Honour comes, a pilgrim grey,
To bless the turf that wraps their clay,
And Freedom shall a while repair,
To dwell a weeping hermit there!

The Night Piece, to Julia

ROBERT HERRICK (1591–1674)

Her eyes the glowworm lend thee;
The shooting stars attend thee;
And the elves also,
Whose little eyes glow
Like the sparks of fire, befriend thee.

No will-o'-the-wisp mislight thee;
Nor snake or slowworm bite thee;
But on, on thy way,
Not making a stay,
Since ghost there's none to affright thee.

Let not the dark thee cumber;
What though the moon does slumber?
The stars of the night
Will lend thee their light,
Like tapers clear without number.

Then, Julia, let me woo thee,
Thus, thus to come unto me;
And when I shall meet
Thy silvery feet,
My soul I'll pour into thee.

Critical Analysis

HERRICK'S "Night Piece, to Julia" is a poem of invitation, addressed to a lady. It asks her, in the fourth stanza, to come to the poet, who will, he says, pour his soul into her. Nothing is said directly about the poet's feeling for Julia, and no arguments are given to overcome her possible reluctance to meet him. Instead, the first three stanzas develop a description of the night. The poem is a "Night Piece."

But the reader soon perceives that not much is told specifically about the night except that it is dark, with no moon shining, and only glowworms and stars for light. The first two stanzas, and perhaps also the third, take the form of a charm—something spoken to ward off danger, as one knocks on wood to avert bad luck. In the first stanza, the poet invokes guardians and friends for the lady—the glowworm, the shooting stars, and the elves. Both natural and supernatural things are thus in the picture, but the identity of the guardians suggests that the superstitious fears are not to be taken too seriously. But it *is* dark, and there are elves, so possibly there may be other inhabitants of the night who are rather to be feared than trusted. The second stanza is a conjuring of these dangers not to harm the lady—either will-o'-the-wisp, snake, or slowworm. And ghosts, perhaps the greatest terror of the night, are declared not to exist—at least not here.

By this time the poem has turned from a charm into a more direct appeal to the lady. The effect of the first two stanzas has been to give a curious mixed feeling, of awareness of the soft and tender beauties of the night with a slight nervousness and fear, somewhat feminine in quality. We seem to share the lady's apprehensions even as we hear the charm, for after all, will-o'-the-wisps, snakes, and ghosts are brought into the picture, even if only to be exorcised. In the middle of stanza 2 we even feel the hesitation of her step in the repetition of "But on, on thy way."

Therefore the third stanza is more urgent, more confident. We are led out of the atmosphere of elves and will-o'-the-wisps to starlight that is just as secure as indoors—"like tapers clear without number." The final stanza is most direct, with the urging repetition "thus, thus" and the promise of the last line.

If all this is so, there remains a question about the nature of the lady's timidity. Is it really simple fear of the dark? The delicacy and intimacy of the first two stanzas suggest something else. (Notice the feminine rhymes of lines 1, 2 and 5. How does this feature of versification affect the tone?) Finally, the wooing and the promise of the last line suggest that the feeling even in the first part of the poem is more personal, and has perhaps more to do with her waiting lover than with the night.

The tenderness and delicacy of the poem suggest that what appears to be said about the night is really said about the lady. This is then an oblique poem, meaning a good deal more than it says and concentrating that meaning in a specific direction—that of Julia's coyness. Julia is surrounded by intimate, tender feelings, yet in the midst of them there is still a sense of mild alarm and excitement. The poem woos her.

If the poem is primarily a wooing poem, why talk about the night? The qualities of the night have somehow become identified with those of Julia herself. So it is no shock, for example, to encounter her *silvery* feet in the next to the last line. In the context of the night the word is perfect, but one can think of other contexts in which the effect of this word's connotations would be unpleasant.

The last line of the poem is prepared for metrically. In the corresponding line of each of the previous stanzas, an anapestic foot is substituted for one of the normal iambs, giving a tripping effect. But the final line is simple, strong iambic throughout: "My soul I'll pour into thee." This might be interpreted as suggesting the stability of her arrival as contrasted with the light-footed skipping of her journey to her lover. But it has also another effect. The reader wonders about an innuendo in the last line, and begins to translate it into something else, but its straightforward simplicity (aided perhaps by the assonance of *soul* and *pour*) pulls him back into the statement of the line itself. The movement here might be said to give an air of sincerity.

The physical and sensual impressions in the poem are carefully controlled. The poet is not saying one thing and leering at the reader to show he means something else; this is no vulgar exercise in *double entendre*. The quality of "The Night Piece, to Julia" depends upon the fine balance between statement and suggestion, the complete integration of feelings about the girl and the night, and the firm control the poet maintains over sensations and suggestions vividly called up in the reader's mind.

Much of value could be learned from an analysis of the metrical elements of the poem—scansion, line length, and sound effects. This poem is especially interesting to study because Herrick took the verse form, the rhetorical device of the charm, and even an image or two from one of Ben Jonson's gypsy songs in *The Gipsies Metamorphosed;* it is sung just before the fortune-telling begins:

> The faery beam upon you,
> The stars to-glister on you,
> A moon of light
> In the noon of night
> Till the fire-drake hath o'ergone you!
>
> The wheel of fortune guide you,
> The boy with the bow beside you
> Run aye in the way,
> Till the bird of day
> And the luckier lot betide you!

("To-glister" in line 2 means "glitter brightly." The "fire-drake" in line 5 is a meteor—presumably the original of Herrick's shooting stars.)

In what ways has Herrick changed the poem? What are the

purposes and effect of these changes? What did he see in Jonson's poem that prompted him to use it as a model? What should be our final verdict about Herrick's originality?

Never Love unless You Can

THOMAS CAMPION (*1567–1620*)

Never love unless you can
Bear with all the faults of man;
Men sometimes will jealous be,
Though but little cause they see,
And hang the head, as discontent,
And speak what straight they will repent.

Men that but one saint adore
Make a show of love to more;
Beauty must be scorned in none,
Though but truly served in one;
For what is courtship but disguise?
True hearts may have dissembling eyes.

Men when their affairs require
Must a while themselves retire,
Sometimes hunt, and sometimes hawk,
And not ever sit and talk.
If these and such like you can bear,
Then like, and love, and never fear.

Still to Be Neat

BEN JONSON (1572–1637)

Still to be neat, still to be dressed,
As you were going to a feast;
Still to be powdered, still perfumed:
Lady, it is to be presumed,
Though art's hid causes are not found,
All is not sweet, all is not sound.

Give me a look, give me a face,
That makes simplicity a grace;
Robes loosely flowing, hair as free:
Such sweet neglect more taketh me
Than all the adulteries of art;
They strike mine eyes, but not my heart.

Delight in Disorder

ROBERT HERRICK (1591–1674)

A sweet disorder in the dress
Kindles in clothes a wantonness;
A lawn about the shoulders thrown
Into a fine distractiòn;
An erring lace, which here and there
Enthralls the crimson stomacher;
A cuff neglectful, and thereby

Ribands to flow confusèdly;
A winning wave (deserving note)
In the tempestuous petticoat;
A careless shoe-string, in whose tie
I see a wild civility:
Do more bewitch me, than when art
Is too precise in every part.

A Pretty a Day

E. E. CUMMINGS (1894–)

a pretty a day
(and every fades)
is here and away
(but born are maids
to flower an hour
in all,all)

o yes to flower
until so blithe
a doer a wooer
some limber and lithe
some very fine mower
a tall;tall

some jerry so very
(and nellie and fan)
some handsomest harry

(and sally and nan
they tremble and cower
so pale: pale)

for betty was born
to never say nay
but lucy could learn
and lily could pray
and fewer were shyer
than doll. doll

Song

WILLIAM BLAKE (1757–1827)

My silks and fine array,
My smiles and languished air,
By love are driven away;
And mournful lean Despair
Brings me yew to deck my grave:
Such end true lovers have.

His face is fair as heaven,
When springing buds unfold;
O why to him was't given
Whose heart is wintry cold?
His breast is love's all-worshiped tomb,
Where all love's pilgrims come.

Bring me an axe and spade,
Bring me a winding-sheet;

When I my grave have made
Let winds and tempests beat:
Then down I'll lie as cold as clay.
True love doth pass away!

The Great Lover

RUPERT BROOKE (1887–1915)

I have been so great a lover: filled my days
So proudly with the splendor of Love's praise,
The pain, the calm, and the astonishment,
Desire illimitable, and still content,
And all dear names men use, to cheat despair,
For the perplexed and viewless streams that bear
Our hearts at random down the dark of life.
Now, ere the unthinking silence on that strife
Steals down, I would cheat drowsy Death so far,
My night shall be remembered for a star
That outshone all the suns of all men's days.
Shall I not crown them with immortal praise
Whom I have loved, who have given me, dared with me
High secrets, and in darkness knelt to see
The inenarrable godhead of delight?
Love is a flame;—we have beaconed the world's night.
A city:—and we have built it, these and I.
An emperor:—we have taught the world to die.
So, for their sakes I loved, ere I go hence,
And the high cause of Love's magnificence,
And to keep loyalties young, I'll write those names

Golden for ever, eagles, crying flames,
And set them as a banner, that men may know,
To dare the generations, burn, and blow
Out on the wind of Time, shining and streaming . . .
These I have loved:
        White plates and cups, clean-gleaming,
Ringed with blue lines; and feathery, faery dust;
Wet roofs, beneath the lamp-light; the strong crust
Of friendly bread; and many-tasting food;
Rainbows; and the blue bitter smoke of wood;
And radiant raindrops couching in cool flowers;
And flowers themselves, that sway through sunny hours,
Dreaming of moths that drink them under the moon;
Then, the cool kindliness of sheets, that soon
Smooth away trouble; and the rough male kiss
Of blankets; grainy wood; live hair that is
Shining and free; blue-massing clouds; the keen
Unpassioned beauty of a great machine;
The benison of hot water; furs to touch;
The good smell of old clothes; and other such—
The comfortable smell of friendly fingers,
Hair's fragrance, and the musty reek that lingers
About dead leaves and last year's ferns . . .
                                        Dear names,
And thousand others throng to me! Royal flames;
Sweet water's dimpling laugh from tap or spring;
Holes in the ground; and voices that do sing;
Voices in laughter, too; and body's pain,
Soon turned to peace; and the deep-panting train;
Firm sands; the little dulling edge of foam
That browns and dwindles as the wave goes home;
And washen stones, gay for an hour; the cold
Graveness of iron; moist black earthen mould;
Sleep; and high places; footprints in the dew;
And oaks; and brown horse-chestnuts, glossy-new;

And new-peeled sticks; and shining pools on grass;—
All these have been my loves. And these shall pass,
Whatever passes not, in the great hour,
Nor all my passion, all my prayers, have power
To hold them with me through the gate of Death.
They'll play deserter, turn with the traitor breath,
Break the high bond we made, and sell Love's trust
And sacramented covenant to the dust.
—Oh, never a doubt but, somewhere, I shall wake,
And give what's left of love again, and make
New friends, now strangers. . . .
                                        But the best I've known,
Stays here, and changes, breaks, grows old, is blown
About the winds of the world, and fades from brains
Of living men and dies.
                                        Nothing remains.
O dear my loves, O faithless, once again
This one last gift I give: that after men
Shall know, and later lovers, far-removed,
Praise you, "All these were lovely"; say, "He loved."

To His Coy Mistress

ANDREW MARVELL (1621–1678)

Had we but world enough, and time,
This coyness, Lady, were no crime.
We would sit down, and think which way
To walk, and pass our long love's day.
Thou by the Indian Ganges' side
Shouldst rubies find; I by the tide

Of Humber would complain. I would
Love you ten years before the Flood,
And you should, if you please, refuse
Till the conversion of the Jews.
My vegetable love should grow
Vaster than empires and more slow;
An hundred years should go to praise
Thine eyes, and on thy forehead gaze;
Two hundred to adore each breast,
But thirty thousand to the rest;
An age at least to every part,
And the last age should show your heart.
For, Lady, you deserve this state,
Nor would I love at lower rate.
  But at my back I always hear
Time's wingèd chariot hurrying near;
And yonder all before us lie
Deserts of vast eternity.
Thy beauty shall no more be found,
Nor, in thy marble vault, shall sound
My echoing song; then worms shall try
That long-preserved virginity,
And your quaint honor turn to dust,
And into ashes all my lust:
The grave's a fine and private place,
But none, I think, do there embrace.
  Now therefore, while the youthful hue
Sits on thy skin like morning dew,
And while thy willing soul transpires
At every pore with instant fires,
Now let us sport us while we may.
And now, like amorous birds of prey,
Rather at once our time devour
Than languish in his slow-chapped power.
Let us roll all our strength and all

Our sweetness up into one ball,
And tear our pleasures with rough strife
Thorough the iron gates of life;
Thus, though we cannot make our sun
Stand still, yet we will make him run.

Tithonus

ALFRED, LORD TENNYSON (1809–1892)

The woods decay, the woods decay and fall,
The vapors weep their burthen to the ground;
Man comes and tills the field and lies beneath,
And after many a summer dies the swan.
Me only cruel immortality
Consumes; I wither slowly in thine arms,
Here at the quiet limit of the world,
A white-haired shadow roaming like a dream
The ever-silent spaces of the East,
Far-folded mists, and gleaming halls of morn.
  Alas! for this gray shadow, once a man—
So glorious in his beauty and thy choice,
Who madest him thy chosen, that he seemed
To his great heart none other than a god!
I asked thee, "Give me immortality."
Then didst thou grant mine asking with a smile,
Like wealthy men who care not how they give.
But thy strong Hours indignant worked their wills,
And beat me down and marred and wasted me,
And though they could not end me, left me maimed
To dwell in presence of immortal youth,

Immortal age beside immortal youth,
And all I was in ashes. Can thy love,
Thy beauty, make amends, though even now,
Close over us, the silver star, thy guide,
Shines in those tremulous eyes that fill with tears
To hear me? Let me go; take back thy gift.
Why should a man desire in any way
To vary from the kindly race of men,
Or pass beyond the goal of ordinance
Where all should pause, as is most meet for all?
  A soft air fans the cloud apart; there comes
A glimpse of that dark world where I was born.
Once more the old mysterious glimmer steals
From thy pure brows, and from thy shoulders pure,
And bosom beating with a heart renewed.
Thy cheek begins to redden through the gloom,
Thy sweet eyes brighten slowly close to mine,
Ere yet they blind the stars, and the wild team
Which love thee, yearning for thy yoke, arise,
And shake the darkness from their loosened manes,
And beat the twilight into flakes of fire.
  Lo! ever thus thou growest beautiful
In silence; then, before thine answer given,
Departest, and thy tears are on my cheek.
  Why wilt thou ever scare me with thy tears,
And make me tremble lest a saying learnt,
In days far-off, on that dark earth, be true?
"The gods themselves cannot recall their gifts."
  Ay me! ay me! with what another heart
In days far-off, and with what other eyes
I used to watch—if I be he that watched—
The lucid outline forming round thee; saw
The dim curls kindle into sunny rings;
Changed with thy mystic change, and felt my blood
Glow with the glow that slowly crimsoned all

Thy presence and thy portals, while I lay,
Mouth, forehead, eyelids, growing dewy-warm
With kisses balmier than half-opening buds
Of April, and could hear the lips that kissed
Whispering I knew not what of wild and sweet,
Like that strange song I heard Apollo sing,
While Ilion like a mist rose into towers.
 Yet hold me not forever in thine East;
How can my nature longer mix with thine?
Coldly thy rosy shadows bathe me, cold
Are all thy lights, and cold my wrinkled feet
Upon thy glimmering thresholds, when the steam
Floats up from those dim fields about the homes
Of happy men that have the power to die,
And grassy barrows of the happier dead.
Release me, and restore me to the ground.
Thou seest all things, thou wilt see my grave;
Thou wilt renew thy beauty morn by morn,
I earth in earth forget these empty courts,
And thee returning on thy silver wheels.

Critical Analysis

"Tithonus" presents a simple theme: the apparent glory of being apart from men and the ordinary course of human life, even in a state of immortality, does not yield happiness. The theme is dramatized in a monologue by Tithonus, a figure in Greek legend, on whom the goddess of dawn has bestowed immortal life. From the barest incidents of the legend Tennyson has developed a moving lament. The lament is not just a gasp and a sigh; the interjections (Alas! Ay me! Ay me!) are few. Tithonus pictures himself in a cycle of decay through age, recalls his bright days of youth and love, and makes a plea for release from the burdens of living forever. In one place only does the theme stand out from the texture and movement of the poem, and even here the lines are dramatically consistent with the character of Tithonus.

> Why should a man desire in any way
> To vary from the kindly race of men,
> Or pass beyond the goal of ordinance
> Where all should pause, as is most meet for all?

Through these direct and simple lines Tennyson voices in general terms a late Victorian sentiment: the worship of conformity. Immortal life, such as Tithonus has been granted, is simply an aberration from normal human existence: it is outside the ordered grooves of society. The theme offers nothing searching or new, but through the sheer magical effect of most of the verse the poem is a satisfying artistic experience.

Although the legend itself, when known to the reader, helps to establish the background of the poem, it contributes only a small part to the total effect of the poem. "Tithonus," though using figures in the legend, is purely a work of dramatic imagination. The legend concerns Tithonus, the son of Laodemon, King of Troy, who was beloved for his beauty by Aurora, the goddess of dawn. Aurora prevailed on Jupiter to grant Tithonus immortality but forgot to ask for perpetual youth. Tithonus grew old and feeble and finally asked to be allowed to die. Unable to retract the gift, Aurora changed Tithonus into a grasshopper.

The poem is not a reworking of the legend, but is a selected dramatic plea in the life of Tithonus. What distinguishes "Tithonus" is that in movement, diction, and the controlled richness of its imagery the verse is in almost perfect accord with the dramatic situation and the theme. The result is a tone poem, at once rich and hymn-like in quality.

The emotional effect of the contrasts of color (gray and silver) and contrasts of time and action (youth and age; love and death) is produced mainly through the imagery. The poem opens with the imagery of death: the decaying woods, weeping vapors, dying swan. The contrast to the cycle of death is in Tithonus' paradoxical statement: "Me only cruel immortality consumes." Immortality, not death, is personified as a devouring creature. Tithonus characterizes himself through images: "white-hair'd shadow roaming like a dream," and sets himself against the brilliant background of dawn with its "ever-silent spaces of the East," "far-folded mists," "gleaming halls of morn." The poem continues the contrasting images of brightness of dawn and youth and the gray of wornout life. Tithonus is "a white-hair'd shadow," a "gray shadow," "in ashes." Dawn is "gleaming," shining, soft, pure, of sweet eyes, glowing. The event of dawn as seen in sections III, V, and VII is packed with imagery which gives a strong impressionistic effect: "old mysterious glimmer," "dim curls kindle into sunny rings."

All the imagery is bound into the dramatic situation of "Tithonus." In not a single section is the "I" or "me" lost. Furthermore, there is little abstract conception of age and youth in the poem. Consequently the texture of the poem, though opulent, is not a profusion of extraneous imagery to dazzle the reader but a conscious, controlled development of the theme and situation through all the poetic devices and rich materials used. The poem follows a pattern which alternates reflection or contemplation and expression of immediate feeling. The irony of the dramatic situation is emphasized by the fact that the poem is addressed to Aurora, goddess of dawn, and hence of rebirth. Tithonus' strong final plea is a startling example of this irony:

> Release me, and restore me to the ground.
> Thou seest all things, thou wilt see my grave;
> Thou wilt renew thy beauty morn by morn,
> I earth in earth forget these empty courts,
> And thee returning on thy silver wheels.

It is interesting also to see how Tennyson can enhance what otherwise might be a rather pedestrian line by putting it into juxtaposition with a striking line. Read outside the poem, the line, "Man comes and tills the field and lies beneath," for all its effective conciseness, could have been written by the imitators of Thomas Gray, but the next line gives brilliance to the idea:

> And after many a summer dies the swan.

The importance of imagery in the impression the poem creates is great, but it has a splendid concomitant in the use of rhythm and sound. The movement of the blank verse is slow and regular, but not monotonous. The impression of reflection is created by the regular iambic movement of the first four lines:

> The woods | decay, || | the woods | decay | and fall, || |
>
> The va|pors weep | their bur|then to | the ground; || |
>
> Man comes | and tills | the field | and lies | beneath, || |
>
> And af|ter ma|ny a sum|mer dies | the swan. || |

The fifth line comes with a shock because of the inversion:

> Me on|ly cru|el im|mortal|ity |
>
> Consumes; || |

and the spondaic opening of the line; and Tithonus' feeling as he sees the glow of dawn is intensified in the verse by devices of sound: by alliteration, assonance and onomatopoetic effects in the last two lines of the first section:

> The ever-*s*ilent *s*paces of the *Ea*st,
> *F*ar-*f*olded *m*ists, and gl*eam*ing halls of *m*orn.

The stately tone of the second section is created by diction which has strong reminiscences of Virgil and the English Bible:

> Who madest him thy chosen, that he seemed
> To his great heart none other than a god!

and by the prominence of spondees in the rhythm. Rhythm, sound, diction, and imagery, working in perfect harmony, produce section VI, which, although it comes close to over-sweetness and lushness in tone and pictorial quality, is highly effective. The pace of the section is characterized by a continuously forward drive because of run-on lines. In lines 55–58 intensity is achieved through repetition of open *o* sounds and by the skillful piling up of caesuras.

> Changed with thy mystic change, and felt my blood
> Gl*o*w with the gl*o*w that sl*o*wly crimsoned all
> Thy presence and thy portals, while I lay,
> Mouth,||forehead,||eyelids,||growing dewy-warm

The preceding remarks—by no means a complete analysis of the poem—merely indicate how an awareness of the values of rhythm, sound, and imagery can increase the critical reader's appreciation of the poem, provided, of course, that the analysis of any of the elements is made with regard to the total emotional effect.

The reader who dwells on the theme might well ask, "Why all this elaboration? Why use a legend and all this consciously artistic imagery and decoration to say such a simple thing?" The answer is that the poem is not simply a communication of the theme we have stated at the beginning of this analysis. It is, like a symphony, a dramatic expression of theme, and the theme *and* the whole poem, not the theme alone, are the artistic experience of value.

The reader who seeks a record of Tennyson's personal feelings in the poem would need corroborative biographical information outside the poem. To attempt to read "Tithonus" simply as a personal record would be to read at a level below the very demands of the poem as a work of art. "Tithonus" is not just a footnote to biography. Its theme is simple—an observation accepted by poets and non-poets alike for many generations—and it does stem from Tennyson's own personal feelings. But the poem has become more than any record; it is a carefully wrought, studied, artistic accomplishment.

Ozymandias

PERCY BYSSHE SHELLEY (1792–1822)

I met a traveller from an antique land
Who said: Two vast and trunkless legs of stone
Stand in the desert. Near them, on the sand,
Half sunk, a shattered visage lies, whose frown,
And wrinkled lip, and sneer of cold command,
Tell that its sculptor well those passions read
Which yet survive, (stamped on these lifeless things,)
The hand that mocked them and the heart that fed:
And on the pedestal these words appear:
"My name is Ozymandias, king of kings:
Look on my works, ye Mighty, and despair!"
Nothing beside remains. Round the decay
Of that colossal wreck, boundless and bare
The lone and level sands stretch far away.

The Secular Masque

JOHN DRYDEN (1631–1700)

Enter JANUS.

JANUS.

Chronos, Chronos, mend thy pace,
A hundred times the rolling sun
Around the radiant belt has run

In his revolving race.
Behold, behold, the goal in sight,
Spread thy fans, and wing thy flight.

Enter CHRONOS, *with a scythe in his hand, and a globe on his back, which he sets down at his entrance.*

CHRONOS.

Weary, weary of my weight,
Let me, let me drop my freight,
And leave the world behind.
I could not bear,
Another year,
The load of humankind.

Enter MOMUS *laughing.*

MOMUS.

Ha! ha! ha! ha! ha! ha! well hast thou done
To lay down thy pack,
And lighten thy back,
The world was a fool, e'er since it begun,
And since neither Janus, nor Chronos, nor I
Can hinder the crimes,
Or mend the bad times,
'Tis better to laugh than to cry.

CHORUS OF ALL THREE.

'Tis better to laugh than to cry.

JANUS.

Since Momus comes to laugh below,
Old Time begin the show,
That he may see, in every scene,
What changes in this age have been.

CHRONOS.

Then goddess of the silver bow begin.
[*Horns, or hunting music within.*

Enter DIANA.

DIANA.

With horns and with hounds I waken the day;
And hie to the woodland-walks away:
I tuck up my robe, and am buskin'd soon,
And tie to my forehead a wexing moon.
I course the fleet stag, unkennel the fox,
And chase the wild goats o'er summits of rocks,
With shouting and hooting we pierce through the sky,
And Echo turns hunter, and doubles the cry.

CHORUS OF ALL.

With shouting and hooting we pierce thro' the sky,
And Echo turns hunter, and doubles the cry.

JANUS.

Then our age was in its prime:

CHRONOS.

Free from rage:

DIANA.

And free from crime:

MOMUS.

A very merry, dancing, drinking,
Laughing, quaffing, and unthinking time.

CHORUS OF ALL.

Then our age was in its prime,
Free from rage, and free from crime,
A very merry, dancing, drinking,
Laughing, quaffing, and unthinking time.

[*Dance of Diana's attendants.*

Enter MARS.

MARS.

Inspire the vocal brass, inspire;
The world is past its infant age:

  Arms and honour,
  Arms and honour,
Set the martial mind on fire,
And kindle manly rage.
Mars has look'd the sky to red;
And Peace, the lazy god, is fled.
Plenty, peace, and pleasure fly;
  The sprightly green,
In woodland-walks, no more is seen;
The sprightly green has drunk the Tyrian dye.

CHORUS OF ALL.

Plenty, peace, &c.

MARS.

Sound the trumpet, beat the drum;
Through all the world around,
Sound a reveillé, sound, sound,
The warrior god is come.

CHORUS OF ALL.

Sound the trumpet, &c.

MOMUS.

Thy sword within the scabbard keep,
  And let mankind agree;
Better the world were fast asleep,
Than kept awake by thee.
The fools are only thinner,
  With all our cost and care;
But neither side a winner,
  For things are as they were.

CHORUS OF ALL.

The fools are only, &c.

Enter VENUS.

VENUS.

Calms appear when storms are past;

Love will have his hour at last:
Nature is my kindly care;
Mars destroys, and I repair;
Take me, take me, while you may,
Venus comes not every day.

CHORUS OF ALL.

Take her, take her, &c.

CHRONOS.

The world was then so light,
I scarcely felt the weight;
Joy rul'd the day, and Love the night.
But, since the queen of pleasure left the ground,
  I faint, I lag,
  And feebly drag
The ponderous orb around.

MOMUS.

All, all of a piece throughout:
Thy chase had a beast in view;
[*Pointing to Diana.*
Thy wars brought nothing about; [*To Mars.*
Thy lovers were all untrue. [*To Venus.*

JANUS.

'Tis well an old age is out.

CHRONOS.

And time to begin a new.

CHORUS OF ALL.

All, all of a piece throughout;
Thy chase had a beast in view:
Thy wars brought nothing about;
Thy lovers were all untrue.
'Tis well an old age is out,
And time to begin a new.

[*Dance of huntsmen, nymphs, warriors, and lovers.*

Kubla Khan

SAMUEL TAYLOR COLERIDGE (1772–1834)

In Xanadu did Kubla Khan
A stately pleasure-dome decree:
Where Alph, the sacred river, ran
Through caverns measureless to man
  Down to a sunless sea.
So twice five miles of fertile ground
With walls and towers were girdled round:
And there were gardens bright with sinuous rills,
Where blossomed many an incense-bearing tree;
And here were forests ancient as the hills,
Enfolding sunny spots of greenery.

But oh! that deep romantic chasm which slanted
Down the green hill athwart a cedarn cover!
A savage place! as holy and enchanted
As e'er beneath a waning moon was haunted
By woman wailing for her demon-lover!
And from this chasm, with ceaseless turmoil seething,
As if this earth in fast thick pants were breathing,
A mighty fountain momently was forced:
Amid whose swift half-intermitted burst
Huge fragments vaulted like rebounding hail,
Or chaffy grain beneath the thresher's flail:
And 'mid these dancing rocks at once and ever
It flung up momently the sacred river.
Five miles meandering with a mazy motion
Through wood and dale the sacred river ran,
Then reached the caverns measureless to man,
And sank in tumult to a lifeless ocean:

And 'mid this tumult Kubla heard from far
Ancestral voices prophesying war!
The shadow of the dome of pleasure
Floated midway on the waves;
Where was heard the mingled measure
From the fountain and the caves.
It was a miracle of rare device,
A sunny pleasure-dome with caves of ice!

A damsel with a dulcimer
In a vision once I saw:
It was an Abyssinian maid,
And on her dulcimer she played,
Singing of Mount Abora.
Could I revive within me
Her symphony and song,
To such a deep delight 'twould win me,
That with music loud and long,
I would build that dome in air,
That sunny dome! those caves of ice!
And all who heard should see them there,
And all should cry, Beware! Beware!
His flashing eyes, his floating hair!
Weave a circle round him thrice,
And close your eyes with holy dread,
For he on honey-dew hath fed,
And drunk the milk of Paradise.

Ode on a Grecian Urn

JOHN KEATS (1795–1821)

Thou still unravish'd bride of quietness,
  Thou foster-child of silence and slow time,
Sylvan historian, who canst thus express
  A flowery tale more sweetly than our rhyme:
What leaf-fring'd legend haunts about thy shape
  Of deities or mortals, or of both,
    In Tempe or the dales of Arcady?
  What men or gods are these? What maidens loth?
What mad pursuit? What struggle to escape?
    What pipes and timbrels? What wild ecstasy?

Heard melodies are sweet, but those unheard
  Are sweeter; therefore, ye soft pipes, play on;
Not to the sensual ear, but, more endear'd,
  Pipe to the spirit ditties of no tone:
Fair youth, beneath the trees, thou canst not leave
  Thy song, nor ever can those trees be bare;
    Bold lover, never, never canst thou kiss,
Though winning near the goal—yet, do not grieve;
    She cannot fade, though thou hast not thy bliss,
  Forever wilt thou love, and she be fair!

Ah, happy, happy boughs! that cannot shed
  Your leaves, nor ever bid the spring adieu;
And, happy melodist, unwearied,
  Forever piping songs forever new;
More happy love! more happy, happy love!
  Forever warm and still to be enjoy'd,
    Forever panting, and forever young;

All breathing human passion far above,
That leaves a heart high-sorrowful and cloy'd,
A burning forehead, and a parching tongue.

Who are these coming to the sacrifice?
To what green altar, O mysterious priest,
Lead'st thou that heifer lowing at the skies,
And all her silken flanks with garlands drest?
What little town by river or sea-shore,
Or mountain-built with peaceful citadel,
Is emptied of this folk, this pious morn?
And, little town, thy streets forevermore
Will silent be; and not a soul to tell
Why thou art desolate, can e'er return.

O Attic shape! fair attitude! with brede
Of marble men and maidens overwrought,
With forest branches and the trodden weed;
Thou, silent form! dost tease us out of thought
As doth eternity. Cold Pastoral!
When old age shall this generation waste,
Thou shalt remain, in midst of other woe
Than ours, a friend to man, to whom thou say'st,
'Beauty is truth, truth beauty,' that is all
Ye know on earth, and all ye need to know.

Euclid Alone Has Looked on Beauty Bare

EDNA ST. VINCENT MILLAY (1892-)

Euclid alone has looked on Beauty bare.
Let all who prate of Beauty hold their peace,
And lay them prone upon the earth and cease
To ponder on themselves, the while they stare
At nothing, intricately drawn nowhere
In shapes of shifting lineage; let geese
Gabble and hiss, but heroes seek release
From dusty bondage into luminous air.

O blinding hour, O holy, terrible day,
When first the shaft into his vision shone
Of light anatomized! Euclid alone
Has looked on Beauty bare. Fortunate they
Who, though once only and then but far away,
Have heard her massive sandal set on stone.

Critical Analysis

THE following analysis of "Euclid Alone Has Looked on Beauty Bare" appears in *Directions in Modern Poetry*, by Elizabeth Drew and John L. Sweeney.

Here the poet's condition of heightened sensibility arises from the realization of that moment of pure intellectual beauty

> When first the shaft into his vision shone
> Of light anatomized!

The tone should be that of a sudden emotional apprehension of the awe and loveliness of pure naked abstractions; but neither the substance nor the shaping of the poem creates any feeling of emotional or intellectual *intensity* at all. There is a general emotional excitement, but it is not focused to a point. The author attempts to supply it by a pseudo-poetic vocabulary—"prate," "lay them prone," "the while"—which is intended to remove us from the atmosphere of every day into the realm of Beauty; and by a group of high-sounding phrases and images which are, however, loose and general, and in no living relationship with her central moment. They will not bear analysis; they create no sweep or flow in the mind; they are empty, splashy, exclamatory. The responses of the poet to the idea of Beauty are stock responses, immediately evoking the reaction of facile epithets like "blinding," "holy," "terrible" (compare Yeats' precise use in "a terrible beauty is born" in *Easter, 1916*). Nor is there any significance generated in the mind by the opposition of geese and heroes, nor in the symbolizing of the intellectual beauty of "light anatomized" as the *sound* of a massive sandal set on stone. The rhythm and language thus become inactive and irresponsible; they lose all precision of outline, straining for sublimity, and falling upwards into vacuity: the light becomes a blur, the anatomy shifting shapes of nothing.

This analysis attacks the poem very severely, especially with regard to the language used and its function, and to the suitability of the images and symbols chosen. Finally, and perhaps most destructive, the suggestion is made that the responses to the poem are not legitimately within the poem, but come from vague associations outside it—that any emotional effect the poem may produce upon the reader is probably phony.

With these criteria in mind, write a comparative analysis of Rupert Brooke's *The Great Lover* and Gerard Manley Hopkins' *Pied Beauty*.

Pied Beauty

GERARD MANLEY HOPKINS (1844–1889)

Glory be to God for dappled things—
For skies of couple-color as a brinded cow;
For rose-moles all in stipple upon trout that swim;
Fresh-firecoal chestnut-falls; finches' wings;
Landscape plotted and pieced—fold, fallow, and plough;
And all trades, their gear and tackle and trim.
All things counter, original, spare, strange;
Whatever is fickle, freckled (who knows how?)
With swift, slow; sweet, sour; adazzle, dim;
He fathers-forth whose beauty is past change:
Praise him.

The Windhover—To Christ Our Lord

GERARD MANLEY HOPKINS (1844–1889)

I caught this morning morning's minion, king-
dom of daylight's dauphin, dapple-dawn-drawn Falcon, in his riding
Of the rolling level underneath him steady air, and striding
High there, how he rung upon the rein of a wimpling wing

In his ecstasy! then off, off forth on swing,
As a skate's heel sweeps smooth on a bow-bend: the hurl and gliding
Rebuffed the big wind. My heart in hiding
Stirred for a bird,—the achieve of, the mastery of the thing!

Brute beauty and valor and act, oh, air, pride, plume, here
Buckle! And the fire that breaks from thee then, a billion
Times told lovelier, more dangerous, O my chevalier!

No wonder of it: sheer plod makes plough down sillion
Shine, and blue-bleak embers, ah my dear,
Fall, gall themselves, and gash gold-vermilion.

To Homer

JOHN KEATS (1795–1821)

Standing aloof in giant ignorance,
Of thee I hear and of the Cyclades,
As one who sits ashore and longs perchance
To visit dolphin-coral in deep seas.
So thou wast blind!—but then the veil was rent,
For Jove uncurtain'd Heaven to let thee live,
And Neptune made for thee a spumy tent,
And Pan made sing for thee his forest-hive;
Aye, on the shores of darkness there is light,
And precipices show untrodden green;
There is a budding morrow in midnight;
There is a triple sight in blindness keen;
Such seeing hadst thou, as it once befel
To Dian, Queen of Earth, and Heaven, and Hell.

Sailing to Byzantium

WILLIAM BUTLER YEATS (1865–1939)

That is no country for old men. The young
In one another's arms, birds in the trees
(Those dying generations) at their song,
The salmon-falls, the mackerel-crowded seas,
Fish, flesh, or fowl, commend all summer long
Whatever is begotten, born, and dies.
Caught in that sensual music, all neglect
Monuments of unaging intellect.

An aged man is but a paltry thing,
A tattered coat upon a stick, unless
Soul clap its hands and sing, and louder sing
For every tatter in its mortal dress;
Nor is there singing school but studying
Monuments of its own magnificence;
And therefore I have sailed the seas and come
To the holy city of Byzantium.

O sages, standing in God's holy fire
As in the gold mosaic of a wall,
Come from the holy fire, perne in a gyre,
And be the singing-masters of my soul.
Consume my heart away—sick with desire
And fastened to a dying animal
It knows not what it is—and gather me
Into the artifice of eternity.

Once out of nature I shall never take
My bodily form from any natural thing,
But such a form as Grecian goldsmiths make
Of hammered gold and gold enamelling
To keep a drowsy emperor awake;
Or set upon a golden bough to sing
To lords and ladies of Byzantium
Of what is past, or passing, or to come.

Critical Analysis

THIS POEM presents striking contrasts between two themes: the curse of old age and the "artifice of eternity" or an ageless existence of beauty and art, as opposed to nature. Its method is that of symbols, a method more easily illustrated than defined.

In the first stanza, for example, old men are said to be out of place in a country which is represented by the flesh—young lovers, birds singing in the trees, fish in the seas and rivers. These three kinds, fish, flesh, and fowl, represent all nature, and they are so intent upon life (celebrating "whatever is begotten, born, and dies") that they neglect monuments of unaging intellect. Their concern is with "that sensual music." So, starting with the abstraction of "youth," we have progressed to concrete examples, people, birds and fish, and they in turn have somehow come to be represented by what they are interested in—"that sensual music." This last phrase is then a symbol, standing not only for a meaning or denotation, but also for an attitude which is large enough to be a view of life.

Stanza 2 picks up the symbol and applies it to the old man. He can sing, but not with the body, only with the soul; there is no way to learn this singing except by studying "monuments of its own magnificence," the same monuments referred to in the last line of stanza 1. Therefore, the speaker says, he has come to Byzantium, the holy city of the Eastern empire in the early Middle Ages. Byzantium represents a degree of balance, of achievement and perfection in art. Byzantine art is conventionalized, not "natural" or representational, and it seems free from the more modern obsession with time and its passage, wholly devoted to the permanent and immortal. Byzantium is also a symbol, of course. It does not mean merely "Constantinople in earlier times."

The third stanza is a prayer, addressed to the saints in a Byzantine mosaic, to come from the wall and "perne in a gyre" (move upward in a spiral) and teach the speaker this singing, or in other words to gather him into the artifice of eternity.

Finally, in the last stanza, the speaker finds a form for himself when he is "once out of nature," beyond this dying animal life; it will be an artificial form, that of a golden bird, skillfully made so that it can sing. The music, which was introduced in the first stanza, has now gone through three phases—the flesh, the old man, and the golden bird. There are contrasts between the golden bird and those natural birds of the first stanza, and with the scarecrow in the second stanza. The gold of the mosaic wall ("God's holy fire") is also associated with the gold of the artificial bird at the end. The "monuments" of the first two stanzas are also related by contrast to the scarecrow and by similarity to the golden bird.

Many other relationships in the poem can be discovered by the attentive and sensitive reader. After he has explored the poem further, he should turn to the early drafts of the first two stanzas, to see how this magnificent imagery developed in Yeats' mind. The first draft of the first stanza is as follows:

All in this land—my Maker that is play
Or else asleep upon His Mother's knees,
Others that as the mountain people say
Are at their hunting and their gallantries
Under the hills, as in our fathers' day
The changing colours of the hills and seas
All that men know or think they know, being young,
Cry that my tale is told, my story sung.

This is a much more plaintive and personal wail of an old man. Even religion portrays Christ as a child, and all the popular folk tales and nature itself suggest that the old man is through. The tone of the stanza might almost be called that of a whimper. Yeats revised the stanza in a second draft:

> Here all is young; the chapel walls display
> An infant sleeping on his Mother's knees,
> Weary with toil Teig sleeps till break of day
> This other wearied with night's gallantries
> Sleeps the morning and the noon away
> And I have toiled and loved until I slept
> A slumbering labyrinth and leaves a snail
> Scrawl upon the mirror of the soul.

Here the speaker is less sentimental; he has objectified himself by making use of two invented characters, Teig the worker and "this other," the lover. He combines in himself the activities of the two, but his resulting sleep, however "poetically" it is described, is somewhat obscure and he has got off the track of the youth-age contrast. So in the third and published version, Yeats returns to the picture of youth and the sensual music. By now he has succeeded in avoiding the whining tone of the first draft and the irrelevances of the second. Notice what he has been willing to sacrifice of his original idea.

The second stanza has a similar history. At first it was direct, and again personal:

> I therefore travel towards Byzantium
> Among these sun-brown pleasant mariners
> Another dozen days and we shall come
> Under the jetty and the marble stair

But he revised it to give a more complete picture of Byzantium:

> But now these pleasant dark-skinned mariners
> Carry me towards that great Byzantium
> Where all is ancient, singing at the oars
> That I may look in the great church's dome
> On gold-embedded saints and emperors

After the mirroring waters and the foam
Where the dark drowsy fins a moment rise
Of fish that carry souls to paradise.

Finally, however (perhaps after the creation of the "sensual music" in the first stanza), the poet saw that what was needed was a principle of contrast and, rhetorically, another declarative statement like that with which the first stanza begins. The lovely description of Byzantium could be postponed. So the published draft of the second stanza begins

An aged man is but a paltry thing,
A tattered coat upon a stick, unless
Soul clap its hands and sing . . .

Again the reader is astonished at what Yeats has been willing to cut out. The rejected lines of these early drafts would be enough to make the reputation of a lesser poet.

A study of the successive stages of the poem (from which much more could be learned than is indicated here) makes clear that Yeats did not start with the symbols—he arrived at them. What constitutes the poem, then, changes in the process of writing it. Some of the details of the poem may be regarded as the happy results of direct inspiration: the surprising parenthesis of "those dying generations" in the first stanza, for example, or the continuance of the scarecrow image into the passage "and louder sing / For every tatter in its mortal dress" in the third. But the essential quality of the poem, its marvelous richness and compression, its rhetorical variety and its great compass in diction, from the plainest prose of "a tattered coat upon a stick" to the serene music of "And therefore I have sailed the seas and come / To the holy city of Byzantium" all derive from architecture and craftsmanship, like the "hammered gold and gold enamelling" of the Grecian goldsmiths. In fact the poem, surely one of the greatest of modern works of the imagination, continues to satisfy the reader because of its perfect fusion of subject and form; "Sailing to Byzantium" is itself an "artifice of eternity."

Street Song

EDITH SITWELL (1887-   )

"Love my heart for an hour, but my bone for a day—
At least the skeleton smiles, for it has a morrow:
But the hearts of the young are now the dark treasure of Death,
And summer is lonely.

Comfort the lonely light and the sun in its sorrow,
Come like the night, for terrible is the sun
As truth, and the dying light shows only the skeleton's hunger
For peace, under the flesh like the summer rose.

Come through the darkness of death, as once through the branches
Of youth you came, through the shade like the flowering door
That leads into Paradise, far from the street,—you, the unborn
City seen by the homeless, the night of the poor.

You walk in the city ways, where Man's threatening shadow
Red-edged by the sun like Cain, has a changing shape—
Elegant like the Skeleton, crouched like the Tiger,
With the age-old wisdom and aptness of the Ape.

The pulse that beats in the heart is changed to the hammer
That sounds in the Potter's Field where they build a new world
From our Bone, and the carrion-bird days' foul droppings and clamour—
But you are my night, and my peace,—

The holy night of conception, of rest, the consoling
Darkness when all men are equal,—the wrong and the right,

And the rich and the poor are no longer separate nations,—
They are brothers in night."

This was the song I heard; but the Bone is silent!
Who knows if the sound was that of the dead light calling,—
Of Caesar rolling onward his heart, that stone,
Or the burden of Atlas falling.

The Hand That Signed the Paper Felled a City

DYLAN THOMAS (1914–)

The hand that signed the paper felled a city;
Five sovereign fingers taxed the breath,
Doubled the globe of dead and halved a country;
These five kings did a king to death.

The mighty hand leads to a sloping shoulder,
The finger joints are cramped with chalk;
A goose's quill has put an end to murder
That put an end to talk.

The hand that signed the treaty bred a fever,
And famine grew, and locusts came;
Great is the hand that holds dominion over
Man by a scribbled name.

The five kings count the dead but do not soften
The crusted wound nor pat the brow;
A hand rules pity as a hand rules heaven;
Hands have no tears to flow.

If I Were Tickled by the Rub of Love

DYLAN THOMAS (1914–   )

If I were tickled by the rub of love,
A rooking girl who stole me for her side,
Broke through her straws, breaking my bandaged string,
If the red tickle as the cattle calve
Still set to scratch a laughter from my lung,
I would not fear the apple nor the flood
Nor the bad blood of spring.

Shall it be male or female? say the cells,
And drop the plum like fire from the flesh.
If I were tickled by the hatching hair,
The winging bone that sprouted in the heels,
The itch of man upon the baby's thigh,
I would not fear the gallows nor the axe
Nor the crossed sticks of war.

Shall it be male or female? say the fingers
That chalk the walls with green girls and their men.
I would not fear the muscling-in of love
If I were tickled by the urchin hungers
Rehearsing heat upon a raw-edged nerve.
I would not fear the devil in the loin
Nor the outspoken grave.

If I were tickled by the lovers' rub
That wipes away not crow's-foot nor the lock
Of sick old manhood on the fallen jaws,

Time and the crabs and the sweethearting crib
Would leave me cold as butter for the flies,
The sea of scums could drown me as it broke
Dead on the sweethearts' toes.

This world is half the devil's and my own,
Daft with the drug that's smoking in a girl
And curling round the bud that forks her eye.
An old man's shank one-marrowed with my bone,
And all the herrings smelling in the sea,
I sit and watch the worm beneath my nail
Wearing the quick away.

And that's the rub, the only rub that tickles.
The knobbly ape that swings along his sex
From damp love-darkness and the nurse's twist
Can never raise the midnight of a chuckle,
Nor when he finds a beauty in the breast
Of lover, mother, lovers, or his six
Feet in the rubbing dust.

And what's the rub? Death's feather on the nerve?
Your mouth, my love, the thistle in the kiss?
My Jack of Christ born thorny on the tree?
The words of death are dryer than his stiff,
My wordy wounds are printed with your hair.
I would be tickled by the rub that is:
Man be my metaphor.

Gerontion

T. S. ELIOT (1888–   )

Thou hast nor youth nor age
But as it were an after dinner sleep
Dreaming of both.

Here I am, an old man in a dry month,
Being read to by a boy, waiting for rain.
I was neither at the hot gates
Nor fought in the warm rain
Nor knee deep in the salt marsh, heaving a cutlass,
Bitten by flies, fought.
My house is a decayed house,
And the jew squats on the window sill, the owner,
Spawned in some estaminet of Antwerp,
Blistered in Brussels, patched and peeled in London.
The goat coughs at night in the field overhead;
Rocks, moss, stonecrop, iron, merds.
The woman keeps the kitchen, makes tea,
Sneezes at evening, poking the peevish gutter.
I an old man,
A dull head among windy spaces.

Signs are taken for wonders. "We would see a sign!"
The word within a word, unable to speak a word,
Swaddled with darkness. In the juvescence of the year
Came Christ the tiger

In depraved May, dogwood and chestnut, flowering judas,
To be eaten, to be divided, to be drunk
Among whispers; by Mr. Silvero

With caressing hands, at Limoges
Who walked all night in the next room:

By Hakagawa, bowing among the Titians;
By Madame de Tornquist, in the dark room
Shifting the candles: Fräulein von Kulp
Who turned in the hall, one hand on the door.
        Vacant shuttles
Weave the wind. I have no ghosts,
An old man in a draughty house
Under a windy knob.

After such knowledge, what forgiveness? Think now
History has many cunning passages, contrived corridors
And issues, deceives with whispering ambitions,
Guides us by vanities. Think now
She gives when our attention is distracted
And what she gives, gives with such supple confusions
That the giving famishes the craving. Gives too late
What's not believed in, or if still believed,
In memory only, reconsidered passion. Gives too soon
Into weak hands, what's thought can be dispensed with
Till the refusal propagates a fear. Think
Neither fear nor courage saves us. Unnatural vices
Are fathered by our heroism. Virtues
Are forced upon us by our impudent crimes.
These tears are shaken from the wrath-bearing tree.

The tiger springs in the new year. Us he devours.
        Think at last
We have not reached conclusion, when I
Stiffen in a rented house. Think at last
I have not made this show purposelessly
And it is not by any concitation
Of the backward devils.

I would meet you upon this honestly.
I that was near your heart was removed therefrom
To lose beauty in terror, terror in inquisition.
I have lost my passion: why should I need to keep it
Since what is kept must be adulterated?
I have lost my sight, smell, hearing, taste, and touch:
How should I use them for your closer contact?

These with a thousand small deliberations
Protract the profit of their chilled delirium,
Excite the membrane, when the sense has cooled,
With pungent sauces, multiply variety
In a wilderness of mirrors. What will the spider do,
Suspend its operations, will the weevil
Delay? De Bailhache, Fresca, Mrs. Cammel, whirled
Beyond the circuit of the shuddering Bear
In fractured atoms. Gull against the wind, in the windy straits
Of Belle Isle, or running on the Horn,
White feathers in the snow, the Gulf claims,
And an old man driven by the Trades
To a sleepy corner.
Tenants of the house,
Thoughts of a dry brain in a dry season.

Critical Analysis

DESPITE the fact that a good many of the references in this poem may seem to the reader erudite and obscure, it is possible to discover a good deal about the structure and meaning of "Gerontion" from within the poem itself. There are several themes in the poem which play against each other, and a reader who is at first puzzled might well begin by examining those themes and seeing what their implications are, in terms of imagery, attitude, tone and effect.

First of all, there is something about an old man. He is the speaker of the first lines of the poem proper, and he immediately identifies himself: "Here I am, an old man in a dry month." At the end of the first section, he repeats, "I an old man" and introduces a new image when he calls himself "A dull head among windy spaces." At the end of the second section the theme of the old man and the wind returns:

Vacant shuttles
Weave the wind. I have no ghosts,
An old man in a draughty house
Under a windy knob.

And near the end of the poem, a more extended and explicit passage begins to throw some light on the connection between the old man and the wind. We are given a picture of a sea gull, hovering against the wind, finally "claimed" by the Gulf, a picture of natural beauty and grace, in sharp contrast to the unattractive or even disgusting picture of the old man's environment in the beginning. But he too is affected by the wind: he is "driven by the Trades / To a sleepy corner." The "sleepy corner" reminds the attentive reader of the epigraph for the poem, three lines from Shakespeare's *Measure for Measure* (III, i, 32–34):

Thou hast nor youth nor age
But as it were an after dinner sleep
Dreaming of both.

Perhaps all the comment on old age in the poem is then a dream; perhaps old age is used figuratively or symbolically rather than literally. The title is a coinage from the Greek word meaning "old," so the concept rendered here by the figure of old age must be central in the poem.

Before proceeding further in the attempt to identify the old man, we might inquire into the other characteristics of the speaker. He is desiccated and has lost the use of his natural faculties:

I have lost my sight, smell, hearing, touch:
How should I use them for your closer contact?

The whole poem is described in the last line as "Thoughts of a dry brain in a dry season." The failure of the senses, and of passion, means that the old man can see in himself only vacancy and emptiness.

The old man mentions his house several times; it is "a decayed house," it is a rented house in which he stiffens, it is described indirectly by the description of the owner, "Blistered in Brussels, patched and peeled in London." (What is the value of these transferred epithets?) Finally, the thoughts of the dry brain which constitute the poem are "tenants of the house," so in some way the house and the brain of the old man are the same thing.

In fact, the impression is strongly conveyed to the reader that the brain and the house really stand for larger and more abstract matters—that they might be translated roughly as "our awareness of life" and "our environment." If this is so, much else in the poem is illuminated. The old man, who might stand for any of us or all of us, is aware in the first few lines that his life has not been heroic:

> I was neither at the hot gates
> Nor fought in the warm rain
> Nor knee deep in the salt marsh, heaving a cutlass,
> Bitten by flies, fought.

The "hot gates" is a mere translation into English of the Greek name Thermopylae, the scene of the great battle, and the salt marsh may refer to Hannibal at Trasimene. At any rate, here is a reference to heroic events in the classical world; the date of the poem is 1920, just after the first World War, and the feeling of sordid disillusionment instead of glory in heroic achievements may owe something to the mood of that time. History is no comfort to our consciousness; it has "many contrived passages," it "deceives," it often seems to work in reverse, by producing unnatural vices from what virtues we have, and by evolving virtues from "impudent crimes."

In the consciousness, and in the environment too, there is the greatest of these distortions—Christianity. The meaning of Christianity is expressed in a series of paradoxes: Christ is the incarnation of the Word, yet in a memorable passage in one of the sermons of Lancelot Andrewes, the seventeenth-century English divine, He is pictured before birth, silent in the womb: "What, *verbum infans,* the Word an infant? The Word and not able to speak a word?" In Eliot's appropriation of the passage there is the suggestion also that the silence of the Word means something about us and our sterile consciousness. In another paradox, Christ is the tiger; "us he devours." Yet in the contemporary world He is devoured; contemporary civilization does not submit itself to Him, and in another sense He is eaten, as in the celebration of Holy Communion, by the aesthete or collector Mr. Silvero, who spent the night at Limoges, famous for its enamels; by the Japanese Hakagawa, a culturally displaced person who bows to famous examples of western art and espouses Christianity as the correct thing to do; by Madame de Tornquist, who may be a medium of some sort; and by Fräulein von Kulp, who suggests by her name (from Latin *culpa,* sin or blame) that she worships only in her sin.

The extreme concreteness and precision of the poem is a barrier to some readers; they are looking for the vague and general statement and are thrown off when the poet confronts them with specific characters or situations to which they have not been introduced. Who are De Bailhache, Fresca, Mrs. Cammel, for example, who are "whirled beyond the circuit of the shuddering Bear in fractured atoms"? Are they anyone we know? The reader is left finally in ignorance, with a suspicion that they may be himself and his friends, unrecognizable perhaps because of the failure of the whole consciousness and of the whole civilization of which we are a part.

Though the final memorable images are those of the spider and the weevil at their work, destroying what we are so proud of as our civilization because it is dead and has lost meaning, and the image of the gull in the snow in comparison with the old man in a sleepy corner, the final effect and the general mood of the poem is not one of Spenglerian pessimism. The poem is a "dream" or "show," yet within its limits it is as concrete as an experience of tangible things.

> Think at last
> I have not made this show purposelessly
> And it is not by any concitation
> Of the backward devils.
> I would meet you upon this honestly.

The "honesty" of *Gerontion* depends upon the integration of the imagery, the transformation of what might have been a mere description of the decay of western civilization into an actual experience of the dryness and sterility produced by such decay. F. O. Matthiessen describes the theme of "Gerontion" as "the horror of a life without faith, its disillusioned weariness of knowledge, its agonized slow drying up of the springs of emotion." How could such a subject be treated differently? If it were merely described, the effect would be satirical, and the reader would be outside the situation, looking down on it, rather than inside it. Nor can the theme be treated directly and lyrically without sounding like the mere mood of the poet.

Eliot has used a supple and fluid verse, rhythmical and varied, which he learned from his reading of the Jacobean dramatists. This kind of verse allows for differences in tone of voice, it is dramatic, it is capable of carrying intense emotion and articulate thought with the same ease. Compare, for example, such passages as

> Who turned in the hall, one hand on the door.
> Vacant shuttles
> Weave the wind. I have no ghosts

with

> I have lost my passion: why should I need to keep it
> Since what is kept must be adulterated?

In fact, the nature of the verse makes possible the most striking effect of the poem and the one that is usually first felt: the extraordinary way in which a series of impressions is made to work together in a kind of unity. Thoughts, acutely specific details of description, melancholy memories and reflections, vivid pictorial images and almost hopelessly abstract statements are fused together into a whole.

The actual movement of the poem, the progression from passage to passage, is effected by rhetorical means. Each section ends in a kind of summary which returns the reader's attention to the figure of the old man, and to the poem itself rather than the statements of which it is composed. The use of commands ("Think now . . . think . . . Think at last") and of rhetorical questions ("After such knowledge, what forgiveness?" ". . . why should I need to keep it . . . ?" "How should I use them for your closer contact? . . ." "What will the spider do, / Suspend its operations, will the weevil delay?") vitalizes the discourse and exploits the fluid dramatic quality inherent in this particular kind of verse.

As the reading progresses, the reader sheds his expectation of narrative or logical structure, abandoning himself to the connections made by imagery, to the dramatic shifts of tone and to the extremely persuasive sound-texture of the verse. He may then feel that the apparent obscurity of the poem is disappearing and that in the great complexity of image, thought, and feeling he is able to find a unity which is his reward for a more than usual attention to a poem.

The Eye

ROBINSON JEFFERS (1887-   )

The Atlantic is a stormy moat, and the Mediterranean,
The blue pool in the old garden,
More than five thousand years has drunk sacrifice
Of ships and blood and shines in the sun; but here the Pacific:
The ships, planes, wars are perfectly irrelevant.
Neither our present blood-feud with the brave dwarfs
Nor any future world-quarrel of westering
And eastering man, the bloody migrations, greed of power, battle-falcons,
Are a mote of dust in the great scale-pan.
Here from this mountain shore, headland beyond stormy headland plunging like dolphins through the gray sea-smoke
Into pale sea, look west at the hill of water: it is half the planet: this dome, this half-globe, this bulging
Eyeball of water, arched over to Asia,
Australia and white Antarctica: those are the eyelids that never close; this is the staring unsleeping
Eye of the earth, and what it watches is not our wars.

Petition

W. H. AUDEN (1907-   )

Sir, no man's enemy, forgiving all
But will his negative inversion, be prodigal:
Send to us power and light, a sovereign touch
Curing the intolerable neural itch,
The exhaustion of weaning, the liar's quinsy,
And the distortions of ingrown virginity.
Prohibit sharply the rehearsed response
And gradually correct the coward's stance;
Cover in time with beams those in retreat
That, spotted, they turn though the reverse were great;
Publish each healer that in city lives
Or country houses at the end of drives;
Harrow the house of the dead; look shining at
New styles of architecture, a change of heart.

I Think Continually of Those

STEPHEN SPENDER (1909-   )

I think continually of those who were truly great.
Who, from the womb, remembered the soul's history
Through corridors of light where the hours are suns
Endless and singing. Whose lovely ambition

Was that their lips, still touched with fire,
Should tell of the Spirit clothed from head to foot in song.
And who hoarded from the Spring branches
The desires falling across their bodies like blossoms.

What is precious is never to forget
The essential delight of the blood drawn from ageless springs
Breaking through rocks in worlds before our earth.
Never to deny its pleasure in the morning simple light
Nor its grave evening demand for love.
Never to allow gradually the traffic to smother
With noise and fog the flowering of the spirit.

Near the snow, near the sun, in the highest fields
See how these names are feted by the waving grass
And by the streamers of white cloud
And whispers of wind in the listening sky.
The names of those who in their lives fought for life
Who wore at their hearts the fire's center.
Born of the sun they travelled a short while towards the sun,
And left the vivid air signed with their honor.

The Express

STEPHEN SPENDER (1909–)

After the first powerful plain manifesto
The black statement of pistons, without more fuss
But gliding like a queen, she leaves the station.
Without bowing and with restrained unconcern

She passes the houses which humbly crowd outside,
The gasworks and at last the heavy page
Of death, printed by gravestones in the cemetery.
Beyond the town there lies the open country
Where, gathering speed, she acquires mystery,
The luminous self-possession of ships on ocean.
It is now she begins to sing—at first quite low
Then loud, and at last with a jazzy madness—
The song of her whistle screaming at curves,
Of deafening tunnels, brakes, innumerable bolts.
And always light, aerial, underneath
Goes the elate meter of her wheels.
Steaming through metal landscape on her lines
She plunges new eras of wild happiness
Where speed throws up strange shapes, broad curves
And parallels clean like the steel of guns.
At last, further than Edinburgh or Rome,
Beyond the crest of the world, she reaches night
Where only a low streamline brightness
Of phosphorus on the tossing hills is white.
Ah, like a comet through flames she moves entranced
Wrapt in her music no bird song, no, nor bough
Breaking with honey buds, shall ever equal.

Critical Analysis

SPENDER's poem presents few difficulties, and the reader may miss something by thinking he has absorbed all of it at a first reading. The main effect of *The Express* is descriptive, with vivid evocation of the motion and sound of a train. The poem is an example of the celebration of an object of the machine age in terms as enthusiastic as any of those used by poets of the Romantic Movement for objects of nature. The real question for the critical reader of the poem is whether the heightened feeling at the end is really justified:

> Ah, like a comet through flame she moves entranced
> Wrapt in her music no bird song, no, nor bough
> Breaking with honey buds, shall ever equal.

The exclamation, "Ah," the repetition of "no," and the extremely romantic atmosphere of the comparison between the train and the "bough breaking with honey buds," the positive form of the future tense, "*shall* ever equal," all mark a high and unusual state of excitement about the train. And it is of course no justification to say, "Well, that is the way the poet felt. He likes trains more than most people do." For the poem to succeed, it is necessary to have this excitement prepared for and justified within the poem itself.

What are the attributes of the express train in which the poet shows us meaning and significance? There is first the authority of the engine: it issues a "manifesto"; the action of its pistons is a "black statement." Then the train, in motion, becomes a queen, gliding gracefully, without bowing, receiving with regal dignity the homage of the humbler houses which crowd outside. After ten lines the elements of dignity and majesty are dropped and the train in its speed becomes a thing of mystery. The poet plays with the contrast between the train's lightness and speed and its fierceness, its noise. It is, after all, an iron monster, but it has the cleanness and value of speed. The gradually amplifying song of the train, interpreted as it is, makes the mood heighten also, and the "jazzy madness" is perhaps an attribute of the style of the poem as well as of the express. Finally, since the train in her song has been made a thing of mystery, that mystery can best be apprehended by the concept of distance, of the leaving of lesser things behind. Therefore the poet moves from literal landscape, which he had only allegorized slightly and in details such as the "heavy page of death printed by gravestones in the cemetery" to a landscape which is "new eras of wild happiness," and the train moves "beyond the crest of the world" where the unseen and imagined country, dark except for a white line on the hills, is far enough away to be romantic. This is further than Edinburgh and Rome in the sense that now the train has moved out of our world of common recognition into a world of the imagination. Then, finally, the poet passes judgment on her, and we are prepared to share with him in the extravagance of the feeling at the end, without being aware that it is extravagant.

For all of his romantic treatment, Spender uses a diction which is disarming because of its easy colloquial quality. "Without more fuss," for example, or the frank description of "a jazzy madness," holds us back from a too serious or "poetic" attitude toward the subject until we are ready for it.

The poem is not a very ambitious one; the experience contained in it is not complex, and the subject and its attributes are easy to apprehend. But failure in such a limited effort is very easy, and a less sure sense of pace or control of the reader's response would have made it a bad minor poem instead of a good one. The importance of the right epithet, the exact adjective, can often better be illustrated in a poem of this sort than in a more complicated one. Consider, for example, the word "elate" to describe the "meter of her wheels." It is of some interest that Spender did not arrive at this word until the fourth draft of his poem. He at first wrote "tapping meter," changed it to "raving" when he wanted the word "tapping" for another line, which he later canceled, and then finally arrived at "elate" for the right description of the meter of the wheels. Consider the adjectives in the line preceding this, and comment on the poet's changes. (The various drafts of this poem, in a workbook of the poet's in the Lockwood Library at the University of Buffalo, are printed in Thomas and Brown, *Reading Poems*, pp. 624–629.)

The Emperor of Ice-Cream

WALLACE STEVENS (1879–   )

Call the roller of big cigars,
The muscular one, and bid him whip
In kitchen cups concupiscent curds.
Let the wenches dawdle in such dress
As they are used to wear, and let the boys
Bring flowers in last month's newspapers.
Let be be finale of seem.
The only emperor is the emperor of ice-cream.

Take from the dresser of deal,
Lacking the three glass knobs, that sheet
On which she embroidered fantails once
And spread it so as to cover her face.
If her horny feet protrude, they come
To show how cold she is, and dumb.
Let the lamp affix its beam.
The only emperor is the emperor of ice-cream.

The Love Song of J. Alfred Prufrock

T. S. ELIOT (1888–   )

Let us go then, you and I,
When the evening is spread out against the sky
Like a patient etherised upon a table;
Let us go, through certain half-deserted streets,
The muttering retreats
Of restless nights in one-night cheap hotels
And sawdust restaurants with oyster-shells:
Streets that follow like a tedious argument
Of insidious intent
To lead you to an overwhelming question . . .
Oh, do not ask, "What is it?"
Let us go and make our visit.

In the room the women come and go
Talking of Michelangelo.

The yellow fog that rubs its back upon the window-panes,
The yellow smoke that rubs its muzzle on the window-panes
Licked its tongue into the corners of the evening,
Lingered upon the pools that stand in drains,
Let fall upon its back the soot that falls from chimneys,
Slipped by the terrace, made a sudden leap,
And seeing that it was a soft October night,
Curled once about the house, and fell asleep.

And indeed there will be time
For the yellow smoke that slides along the street,
Rubbing its back upon the window-panes;
There will be time, there will be time

To prepare a face to meet the faces that you meet;
There will be time to murder and create,
And time for all the works and days of hands
That lift and drop a question on your plate;
Time for you and time for me,
And time yet for a hundred indecisions,
And for a hundred visions and revisions,
Before the taking of a toast and tea.

In the room the women come and go
Talking of Michelangelo.

And indeed there will be time
To wonder, "Do I dare?" and, "Do I dare?"
Time to turn back and descend the stair,
With a bald spot in the middle of my hair—
(They will say: "How his hair is growing thin!")
My morning coat, my collar mounting firmly to the chin,
My necktie rich and modest, but asserted by a simple pin—
(They will say: "But how his arms and legs are thin!")
Do I dare
Disturb the universe?
In a minute there is time
For decisions and revisions which a minute will reverse.

For I have known them all already, known them all:
Have known the evenings, mornings, afternoons,
I have measured out my life with coffee spoons;
I know the voices dying with a dying fall
Beneath the music from a farther room.
  So how should I presume?

And I have known the eyes already, known them all—
The eyes that fix you in a formulated phrase,
And when I am formulated, sprawling on a pin,

When I am pinned and wriggling on the wall,
Then how should I begin
To spit out all the butt-ends of my days and ways?
  And how should I presume?

And I have known the arms already, known them all—
Arms that are braceleted and white and bare
(But in the lamplight, downed with light brown hair!)
Is it perfume from a dress
That makes me so digress?
Arms that lie along a table, or wrap about a shawl.
  And should I then presume?
  And how should I begin?

* * * * *

Shall I say, I have gone at dusk through narrow streets
And watched the smoke that rises from the pipes
Of lonely men in shirt-sleeves, leaning out of windows? . . .

I should have been a pair of ragged claws
Scuttling across the floors of silent seas.

* * * * *

And the afternoon, the evening, sleeps so peacefully!
Smoothed by long fingers,
Asleep . . . tired . . . or it malingers,
Stretched on the floor, here beside you and me.
Should I, after tea and cakes and ices,
Have the strength to force the moment to its crisis?
But though I have wept and fasted, wept and prayed,
Though I have seen my head (grown slightly bald) brought in
    upon a platter,
I am no prophet—and here's no great matter;
I have seen the moment of my greatness flicker,

And I have seen the eternal Footman hold my coat, and snicker,
And in short, I was afraid.

And would it have been worth it, after all,
After the cups, the marmalade, the tea,
Among the porcelain, among some talk of you and me,
Would it have been worth while,
To have bitten off the matter with a smile,
To have squeezed the universe into a ball
To roll it toward some overwhelming question,
To say: "I am Lazarus, come from the dead,
Come back to tell you all, I shall tell you all"—
If one, settling a pillow by her head,
  Should say: "That is not what I meant at all;
  That is not it, at all."

And would it have been worth it, after all,
Would it have been worth while,
After the sunsets and the dooryards and the sprinkled streets,
After the novels, after the teacups, after the skirts that trail along
    the floor—
And this, and so much more?—
It is impossible to say just what I mean!
But as if a magic lantern threw the nerves in patterns on a screen:
Would it have been worth while
If one, settling a pillow or throwing off a shawl,
And turning toward the window, should say:
  "That is not it at all,
  That is not what I meant, at all."

* * * * *

No! I am not Prince Hamlet, nor was meant to be;
Am an attendant lord, one that will do
To swell a progress, start a scene or two,

Advise the prince; no doubt, an easy tool,
Deferential, glad to be of use,
Politic, cautious, and meticulous;
Full of high sentence, but a bit obtuse;
At times, indeed, almost ridiculous—
Almost, at times, the Fool.

I grow old . . . I grow old . . .
I shall wear the bottoms of my trousers rolled.

Shall I part my hair behind? Do I dare to eat a peach?
I shall wear white flannel trousers, and walk upon the beach.
I have heard the mermaids singing, each to each.

I do not think that they will sing to me.

I have seen them riding seaward on the waves
Combing the white hair of the waves blown back
When the wind blows the water white and black.

We have lingered in the chambers of the sea
By sea-girls wreathed with seaweed red and brown
Till human voices wake us, and we drown.

On First Looking into Chapman's Homer

JOHN KEATS (1795–1821)

Much have I travelled in the realms of gold,
  And many goodly states and kingdoms seen;
  Round many western islands have I been
Which bards in fealty to Apollo hold.

Oft of one wide expanse had I been told
That deep-browed Homer ruled as his demesne;
Yet did I never breathe its pure serene
Till I heard Chapman speak out loud and bold:
Then felt I like some watcher of the skies
When a new planet swims into his ken;
Or like stout Cortez when with eagle eyes
He stared at the Pacific—and all his men
Looked at each other with a wild surmise—
Silent, upon a peak in Darien.

Poetry

MARIANNE MOORE (1887-)

I too, dislike it: there are things that are important
beyond all this fiddle.
Reading it, however, with a perfect contempt for it,
one discovers in
it after all, a place for the genuine.
Hands that can grasp, eyes
that can dilate, hair that can rise
if it must, these things are important not because a

high sounding interpretation can be put upon them
but because they are
useful. When they become so derivative
as to become unintelligible,
the same thing may be said for all of us, that we

do not admire what
we cannot understand: the bat,
holding on upside down or in quest of something to

eat, elephants pushing, a wild horse taking a roll,
a tireless wolf under
a tree, the immovable critic twitching his skin
like a horse that feels a flea, the base-
ball fan, the statistician—
nor is it valid
to discriminate against "business documents and

school-books"; all these phenomena are important.
One must make a distinction
however: when dragged into prominence by half poets,
the result is not poetry,
nor till the poets among us can be
"literalists of
the imagination"—above
insolence and triviality and can present

for inspection, imaginary gardens with real toads in them,
shall we have
it. In the meantime, if you demand on the one hand,
the raw material of poetry in
all its rawness and
that which is on the other hand
genuine, then you are interested in poetry.

The Stories

The short story does not suffer from the prejudices so often directed at poetry. "I just don't understand poetry, but I like short stories and novels," is a familiar cry. True, the short story is a less concentrated form of art; it is written in a medium less highly arranged and systematized. It will probably communicate more readily to the average reader than most poetry. Whether the story be one of action or character or theme, the dramatic situation and the thread of narrative are often enough to keep the reader interested by the simple attraction of "What happens next?" But short stories, like poems, are too often read superficially, simply at the surface of the narrative level. A few years ago a large part of the stories which appeared in magazines of big circulation depended almost solely on the "what happens next?" pattern. Characters, motives, action, and content in general were developed according to rigid formulas. Yet in the hands of thoughtful writers the limits of the short story as an art form have not been confined to patterned plots and stock characters, and the variety of subject matter and treatment within the form is well illustrated in the fifteen stories selected for this volume.

The reader who seeks a yardstick for critical judgment might ask, "What is the ideal short story?" hoping for a definition and a guide in the answer. There is no simple answer, for indeed there is no "ideal short story." At the risk of incompleteness and vagueness but for the sake of discussion, one might say that a good short story is built around a theme or on interesting content, expressed through valid characters, and developed in fitting language—all proportioned to provide a calculated and understandable effect.

The core of the short story, then, is some kind of relatable experience of existence. It is obvious that the themes and substance of short stories are as many as life and imagination itself. Within a reasonable compass the writer selects those which will create and sustain interest and develop some desired effect. The story may deal with the tensions of men and women and the ultimate issues of the human lot, as does Joyce's "The Dead." It may concern nothing more profound than the entertaining history of Harold Peavey's wondrous cow. It may be based on the most painful and pressing of realities, the injustice of "Dry September," the waste and loss of "Babylon Revisited," and yet contain flashes of the fantastic—the nightmare idiocy of the lynching party, the feverish dream of Paris in the Jazz Age—which lead one to question the nature of reality. The very theme itself may be fantastic, as in "The Celestial Omnibus" and "The Rocking-Horse Winner," and yet render cogent comment on the verities of existence, such as the inviolability of art, the need for love.

Some of the stories are primarily stories of character and not of theme. "The Short Happy Life of Francis Macomber" and "Noon Wine" are examples. Francis Macomber, his wife, and the English hunter are first portrayed rather fully; then their characters develop in action and the action is developed through their characters; almost nothing, not even the adventure background of the story, interferes with the gradual revelation of character, which leads subtly and painfully to an apparently inevitable end. "Noon Wine," rather than tracing the effect of character on event, shows the effect of event on character. It stems not from the observation that if people are thus, they must act so, but rather that if events are thus, they must have these results on these people. It moves toward its final effect with pace fully controlled and calculated.

There is no "ideal" theme; there is also no "ideal" style. Each theme or group of characters demands in its conception a treatment suitable to it, and the ability of the artist is tested in meeting that demand. The structure of a story may be very simple and yet afford great opportunity for complexity and subtlety in characterization, as in "The Dead." The story may remain virtually stationary, as does "The Secret Life of Walter Mitty," which, through the clever description of one man's dreams, comments obliquely on the pitiful impotence and drab confined existence of an average man in our times, while, delightfully, it mocks the curious consolations and aspirations of humanity. Or it may move swiftly and inconspicuously through act after act of a highly personal and eventful drama as it focuses the reader's final attention on the eternal, philosophical joke of human littleness, as does "The Gioconda Smile." Or it may drag and digress as does "Gunner's Passage," reflecting the physical, inconsecutive, nostalgic qualities and the tedium of some kinds of army life, or, indeed, of any life.

The treatment of "The Lumber-Room" is slight and delicate as the child it concerns, cool, remote, and contemptuous as he is; yet the story sparkles with the secret joy of a boy's triumph over the coarse, obtuse adult world. The language of "A Song Writer in the Family" is choppy and colloquial, suitable to the story of one boy's adolescence. "Keela, the Outcast Indian Maiden" deals with two men's memory of a cruelty; it is told for the most part by these two men themselves, one in words, the other in expressed, though unspoken, thoughts. The tale as such is not the important thing; told objectively it would be nothing. What is skillfully pointed up is the difference in attitude between the tellers, and it is pointed up by the technique of a story within a story.

The critical reader will not be satisfied with the "what happens next?" level of reading alone, nor should he be content simply with an analysis of technique. Again, as in the reading of poetry, the total effect and how it is accomplished should be the broad outline for study. With this in mind the reader will come to see the degrees of artistry represented in the stories. He will look upon the short-story writer as one who faces the problems of selection, emphasis, and medium in his art, as do poets, painters, and composers. He will understand that a good story is always under the complete control of the writer, and that suggestion rather than statement (here he might contrast stories such as Halper's "A Song Writer in the Family" and Joyce's "The Dead") is a master tool of the short-story writer.

More specifically, the understanding of style and method involves a study of several technical aspects of the art of the short story, some of which have been mentioned already. The critical reader should be aware of and eventually be able to evaluate such important things as narrative method and point of view. Who tells the story? Is it a character in the story or is it the author with an omniscient view of characters and action? Is the author or the narrator close to the events or at a distance, and for what reasons? What are the advantages of the narrative method and point of view selected?

Other questions of how the story is told follow readily. How does the story begin? What means are used to introduce characters and establish setting? If the story is one in which mood is of major importance, how is that mood or atmosphere created?

The scope and the emphasis of the story deserve careful attention, for herein the writer practices the difficult arts of selection and suggestion. How much in time, space, and idea does the story encompass? Does it place emphasis on character, on theme, on atmosphere, or on plot? Where and how has the author centered the reader's interest and attention within the story? What is the key moment in the story, and where is it placed? How has the author developed event, action, conflict, and character to build toward a key moment? Where and how has the author presented the climax of the story? How does the story end, and to what effect? Other elements such as pace or speed of the narrative and the disposition of details also fall under any critical view of the scope and emphasis of the story. Pace is perhaps one of the more difficult elements to understand and evaluate, but it is an important factor by which an author exercises control over the story and the reader's reactions. Ultimately, the study of scope and emphasis will reveal the structure, the pattern or design of a story. The question for the critical reader is the value of that total arrangement.

Of other elements which might be studied, the reader should not fail to look closely at dialogue and monologue. How do characters talk to each other and to themselves? What are the characteristics of their language, and how much of the narrative is carried by dialogue? What is the nature and effectiveness of monologue, both external and internal? What psychological aspects of the story are expressed through internal (or interior) monologue? The kind and use of symbols in a story also demand attention. Every story does not have to use symbols, of course, but if they are used, what is their function and what do they contribute?

If the critical reader is not already bowed low with the previous paragraphs of questions, he might accept one more. What is the nature of "knowledge" in the story? How convincingly has the author presented both the general and detailed qualities of character, setting, and atmosphere? Does the sheer force of *recognition* provided by realistic detail serve the story well or stand apart as an almost separate interest for the reader? How does the author gain the reader's acceptance of realistic or fantastic detail?

The editors do not mean to say that every short-story writer asks himself all these questions. The questions are for the critical reader. It is a commonplace observation about literary authorship that an author may be aware of all the elements of interest to the student or critic without ever bothering to analyze what he has consciously or unconsciously chosen in every instance. The important thing for the user of this book is that he *see* thoroughly and understandingly what the author has done and how he has done it. To that end the questions raised should be useful; they are not offered, however, as the only approach to analysis.

In the introduction to the poems the editors have tried to lay one ghost of prejudice against the analysis of poetry. Perhaps the reader should be reminded that intelligent analysis does not destroy the short story either; it is a step toward greater appreciation and understanding of an art.

The order of the stories loosely represents an effort to move from the less difficult to the more difficult, but the editors have no intention of setting up a critical obstacle course of increasingly complex traps and pitfalls. They would prefer to have the reader begin where he will but to read at the level that the stories themselves demand.

The Lumber-Room

"SAKI" (H. H. MUNRO, 1870–1916)

THE CHILDREN were to be driven, as a special treat, to the sands at Jagborough. Nicholas was not to be of the party; he was in disgrace. Only that morning he had refused to eat his wholesome bread-and-milk on the seemingly frivolous ground that there was a frog in it. Older and wiser and better people had told him that there could not possibly be a frog in his bread-and-milk and that he was not to talk nonsense; he continued, nevertheless, to talk what seemed the veriest nonsense, and described with much detail the colouration and markings of the alleged frog. The dramatic part of the incident was that there really was a frog in Nicholas' basin of bread-and-milk; he had put it there himself, so he felt entitled to know something about it. The sin of taking a frog from the garden and putting it into a bowl of wholesome bread-and-milk was enlarged on at great length, but the fact that stood out clearest in the whole affair, as it presented itself to the mind of Nicholas, was that the older, wiser, and better people had been proved to be profoundly in error in matters about which they had expressed the utmost assurance.

"You said there couldn't possibly be a frog in my bread-and-milk; there *was* a frog in my bread-and-milk," he repeated, with the insistence of a skilled tactician who does not intend to shift from favourable ground.

So his boy-cousin and girl-cousin and his quite uninteresting younger brother were to be taken to Jagborough sands that afternoon and he was to stay at home. His cousins' aunt, who insisted, by an unwarranted stretch of imagination, in styling herself his aunt also, had hastily invented the Jagborough expedition in order to impress on Nicholas the delights that he had justly forfeited by his disgraceful conduct at the breakfast table. It was her habit, whenever one of the children fell from grace, to improvise something of a festival nature from which the offender would be rigorously debarred; if all the children sinned collectively they were suddenly informed of a circus in a neighbouring town, a circus of unrivalled merit and uncounted elephants, to which, but for their depravity, they would have been taken that very day.

A few decent tears were looked for on the part of Nicholas when the moment for the departure of the expedition arrived. As a matter of fact, however, all the crying was done by his girl-cousin, who scraped her knee rather painfully against the step of the carriage as she was scrambling in.

"How she did howl," said Nicholas cheerfully, as the party drove off without any of the elation of high spirits that should have characterized it.

"She'll soon get over that," said the *soi-disant* aunt; "it will be a glorious afternoon for racing about over those beautiful sands. How they will enjoy themselves!"

"Bobby won't enjoy himself much, and he won't race much either," said Nicholas with a grim chuckle; "his boots are hurting him. They're too tight."

"Why didn't he tell me they were hurting?" asked the aunt with some asperity.

"He told you twice, but you weren't listening. You often don't listen when we tell you important things."

"You are not to go into the gooseberry garden," said the aunt, changing the subject.

"Why not?" demanded Nicholas.

"Because you are in disgrace," said the aunt loftily.

Nicholas did not admit the flawlessness of the reasoning; he felt perfectly capable of being in disgrace and in a gooseberry garden at the same moment. His face took on an expression of considerable obstinacy. It was clear to his aunt that he was determined to get into the gooseberry garden, "only," as she remarked to herself, "because I have told him he is not to."

Now the gooseberry garden had two doors by which it might be entered, and once a small person like Nicholas could slip in there he could effectually disappear from view amid the masking growth of artichokes, raspberry canes, and fruit bushes. The aunt had many other things to do that afternoon, but she spent an hour or two in trivial gardening operations among flower beds and shrubberies, whence she could keep a watchful eye on the two doors that led to the forbidden paradise. She was a woman of few ideas, with immense powers of concentration.

Nicholas made one or two sorties into the front garden, wriggling his way with obvious stealth of purpose towards one or other of the doors, but never able for a moment to evade the aunt's watchful eye. As a matter of fact, he had no intention of trying to get into the gooseberry garden, but it was extremely convenient for him that his aunt should believe that he had; it was a belief that would keep her on self-imposed sentry-duty for the greater part of the afternoon. Having thoroughly confirmed and fortified her suspicions, Nicholas slipped back into the house and rapidly put into execution a plan of action that had long germinated in his brain. By standing on a chair in the library one could reach a shelf on which reposed a fat, important-looking key. The key was as important as it looked; it was the instrument which kept the mysteries of the lumber-room secure from unauthorized intrusion, which opened a way only for aunts and such-like privileged persons. Nicholas had not had much experience of the art of fitting keys into keyholes and turning locks, but for some days past he had practised with the key of the schoolroom door; he did not believe in trusting too much to luck and accident. The key turned stiffly in the lock, but it turned. The door opened, and Nicholas was in an unknown land, compared with which the gooseberry garden was a stale delight, a mere material pleasure.

Often and often Nicholas had pictured to himself what the lumber-room might be like, that region that was so carefully sealed from youthful eyes and concerning which no questions were ever answered. It came up to his expectations. In the first place it was large and dimly lit, one high window opening on to the forbidden garden being its only source of illumination. In the second place it was a storehouse of unimagined treasures. The aunt-by-assertion was one of those people who think that things spoil by use and consign them to dust and damp by way of preserving them. Such parts of the house as Nicholas knew best were rather bare and cheerless, but here there were wonderful things for the eye to feast on. First and foremost there was a piece of framed tapestry that was evidently meant to be a fire-screen. To Nicholas it was a living, breathing story; he sat down on a roll of Indian hangings, glowing in wonderful colours beneath a layer of dust, and took in all the details of the tapestry picture. A man, dressed in the hunting costume of some remote period, had just transfixed a stag with an arrow; it could not have been a difficult shot because the stag was only one or two paces away from him; in the thickly growing vegetation that the picture suggested it would not have been difficult to creep up to a feeding stag, and the two spotted dogs that were springing forward to join in the chase had evidently been trained to keep to heel till the arrow was discharged. That part of the picture was simple, if interesting, but did the huntsman see, what Nicholas saw, that four galloping wolves were coming in his direction through the wood? There might be more than four of them hidden behind the trees, and in any case would the man and his dogs be able to cope with the four wolves if they made an attack? The man had only two arrows left in his quiver, and he might miss with one or both of them; all one knew about his skill in shooting was that he could hit a large stag at a ridiculously short range. Nicholas sat for many golden minutes revolving the possibilities of the scene; he was inclined to think that there were more than four wolves and that the man and his dogs were in a tight corner.

But there were other objects of delight and interest claiming his instant attention: there were quaint twisted candlesticks in the shape of snakes, and a teapot fashioned like a china duck, out of whose open beak the tea was supposed to come. How dull and shapeless the nursery teapot seemed in comparison! And there was a carved sandal-wood box packed tight with aromatic cotton-wool, and between the layers of cotton-wool were little brass figures, hump-necked bulls, and peacocks and goblins, delightful to see and to handle. Less promising in appearance was a large square book with plain black covers; Nicholas peeped into it, and, behold, it was full of coloured pictures of birds. And such birds! In the garden, and in the lanes when he went for a walk, Nicholas came across a few birds, of which the largest were an occasional magpie or wood-pigeon; here were herons and bustards, kites, toucans, tiger-bitterns, brush turkeys, ibises, golden pheasants, a whole portrait gallery of undreamed-of creatures. And as he was admiring the colouring of the mandarin duck and assigning a life-history to it, the voice of his aunt in shrill vociferation of his name came from the gooseberry garden without. She had grown suspicious at his long disappearance, and had leapt to the conclusion that he had climbed over the wall behind the sheltering screen of the lilac bushes; she was now engaged in energetic and rather hopeless search for him among the artichokes and raspberry canes.

"Nicholas, Nicholas!" she screamed, "you are to come out of this at once. It's no use trying to hide there; I can see you all the time."

It was probably the first time for twenty years that any one had smiled in that lumber-room.

Presently the angry repetitions of Nicholas' name gave way to a shriek, and a cry for somebody to come quickly. Nicholas shut the book, restored it carefully to its place in a corner, and shook some dust from a neighbouring pile of newspapers over it. Then he crept from the room, locked the door, and replaced the key exactly where he had found it. His aunt was still calling his name when he sauntered into the front garden.

"Who's calling?" he asked.

"Me," came the answer from the other side of the wall; "didn't you hear me? I've been looking for you in the gooseberry garden, and I've slipped into the rain-water tank. Luckily there's no water in it, but the sides are slippery and I can't get out. Fetch the little ladder from under the cherry tree—"

"I was told I wasn't to go into the gooseberry garden," said Nicholas promptly.

"I told you not to, and now I tell you that you may," came the voice from the rain-water tank, rather impatiently.

"Your voice doesn't sound like aunt's," objected Nicholas; "you may be the Evil One tempting me to be disobedient. Aunt often tells me that the Evil One tempts me and that I always yield. This time I'm not going to yield."

"Don't talk nonsense," said the prisoner in the tank; "go and fetch the ladder."

"Will there be strawberry jam for tea?" asked Nicholas innocently.

"Certainly there will be," said the aunt, privately resolving that Nicholas should have none of it.

"Now I know that you are the Evil One and not aunt," shouted Nicholas gleefully; "when we asked aunt for strawberry jam yesterday she said there wasn't any. I know there are four jars of it in the store cupboard, because I looked, and of course you know it's there, but *she* doesn't, because she said there wasn't any. Oh, Devil, you *have* sold yourself!"

There was an unusual sense of luxury in being able to talk to an aunt as though one was talking to the Evil One, but Nicholas knew, with childish discernment, that such luxuries were not to be over-indulged in. He walked noisily away, and it was a kitchen-maid, in search of parsley, who eventually rescued the aunt from the rain-water tank.

Tea that evening was partaken of in a fearsome silence. The tide had been at its highest when the children had arrived at Jagborough Cove, so there had been no sands to play on—a circumstance that the aunt had overlooked in the haste of organizing her punitive expedition. The tightness of Bobby's boots had had disastrous effect on his temper the whole of the afternoon, and altogether the children could not have been said to have enjoyed themselves. The aunt maintained the frozen muteness of one who has suffered undignified and unmerited detention in a rain-water tank for thirty-five minutes. As for Nicholas, he, too, was silent, in the absorption of one who has much to think about; it was just possible, he considered, that the huntsman would escape with his hounds while the wolves feasted on the stricken stag.

The Secret Life of Walter Mitty

JAMES THURBER (1894–)

"WE'RE GOING through!" The Commander's voice was like thin ice breaking. He wore his full-dress uniform, with the heavily braided white cap pulled down rakishly over one cold gray eye. "We can't make it, sir. It's spoiling for a hurricane, if you ask me." "I'm not asking you, Lieutenant Berg," said the Commander. "Throw on the power light! Rev her up to 8,500! We're going through!" The pounding of the cylinders increased: ta-pocketa-pocketa-pocketa-*pocketa-pocketa*. The Commander stared at the ice forming on the pilot window. He walked over and twisted a row of complicated dials. "Switch on No. 8 auxiliary!" he shouted. "Switch on No. 8 auxiliary!" repeated Lieutenant Berg. "Full strength in No. 3 turret!" shouted the Commander. "Full strength in No. 3 turret!" The crew, bending to their various tasks in the huge, hurtling eight-engined Navy hydroplane, looked at each other and grinned. "The Old Man'll get us through," they said to one another. "The Old Man ain't afraid of Hell!" . . .

"Not so fast! You're driving too fast!" said Mrs. Mitty. "What are you driving so fast for?"

"Hmm?" said Walter Mitty. He looked at his wife, in the seat beside him, with shocked astonishment. She seemed grossly unfamiliar, like a strange woman who had yelled at him in a crowd. "You were up to fifty-five," she said. "You know I don't like to go more than forty. You were up to fifty-five." Walter Mitty drove on toward Waterbury in silence, the roaring of the SN202 through the worst storm in twenty years of Navy flying fading in the remote, intimate airways of his mind. "You're tensed up again," said Mrs. Mitty. "It's one of your days. I wish you'd let Dr. Renshaw look you over."

Walter Mitty stopped the car in front of the building where his wife went to have her hair done. "Remember to get those overshoes while I'm having my hair done," she said. "I don't need overshoes," said Mitty. She put her mirror back into her bag. "We've been all through that," she said, getting out of the car. "You're not a young man any longer." He raced the engine a little. "Why don't you wear your gloves? Have you lost your gloves?" Walter Mitty reached in a pocket and brought out the gloves. He put them on, but after she had turned and gone into the building and he had driven on to a red light, he took them off again. "Pick it up, brother!" snapped a cop as the light changed, and

Mitty hastily pulled on his gloves and lurched ahead. He drove around the streets aimlessly for a time, and then he drove past the hospital on his way to the parking lot.

. . . "It's the millionaire banker, Wellington McMillan," said the pretty nurse. "Yes?" said Walter Mitty, removing his gloves slowly. "Who has the case?" "Dr. Renshaw and Dr. Benbow, but there are two specialists here, Dr. Remington from New York and Mr. Pritchard-Mitford from London. He flew over." A door opened down a long, cool corridor and Dr. Renshaw came out. He looked distraught and haggard. "Hello, Mitty," he said. "We're having the devil's own time with McMillan, the millionaire banker and close personal friend of Roosevelt. Obstreosis of the ductal tract. Tertiary. Wish you'd take a look at him." "Glad to," said Mitty.

In the operating room there were whispered introductions: "Dr. Remington, Dr. Mitty. Mr. Pritchard-Mitford, Dr. Mitty." "I've read your book on streptothricosis," said Pritchard-Mitford, shaking hands. "A brilliant performance, sir." "Thank you," said Walter Mitty. "Didn't know you were in the States, Mitty," grumbled Remington. "Coals to Newcastle, bringing Mitford and me up here for a tertiary." "You are very kind," said Mitty. A huge, complicated machine, connected to the operating table, with many tubes and wires, began at this moment to go pocketa-pocketa-pocketa. "The new anesthetizer is giving way!" shouted an interne. "There is no one in the East who knows how to fix it!" "Quiet, man!" said Mitty, in a low, cool voice. He sprang to the machine, which was now going pocketa-pocketa-queep-pocketa-queep. He began fingering delicately a row of glistening dials. "Give me a fountain pen!" he snapped. Someone handed him a fountain pen. He pulled a faulty piston out of the machine and inserted the pen in its place. "That will hold for ten minutes," he said. "Get on with the operation." A nurse hurried over and whispered to Renshaw, and Mitty saw the man turn pale. "Coreopsis has set in," said Renshaw nervously. "If you would take over, Mitty?" Mitty looked at him and at the craven figure of

Benbow, who drank, and at the grave, uncertain faces of the two great specialists. "If you wish," he said. They slipped a white gown on him; he adjusted a mask and drew on thin gloves; nurses handed him shining . . .

"Back it up, Mac! Look out for that Buick!" Walter Mitty jammed on the brakes. "Wrong lane, Mac," said the parking-lot attendant, looking at Mitty closely. "Gee. Yeh," muttered Mitty. He began cautiously to back out of the lane marked "Exit Only." "Leave her sit there," said the attendant. "I'll put her away." Mitty got out of the car. "Hey, better leave the key." "Oh," said Mitty, handing the man the ignition key. The attendant vaulted into the car, backed it up with insolent skill, and put it where it belonged.

They're so damn cocky, thought Walter Mitty, walking along Main Street; they think they know everything. Once he had tried to take his chains off, outside New Milford, and he had got them wound around the axles. A man had had to come out in a wrecking car and unwind them, a young, grinning garageman. Since then Mrs. Mitty always made him drive to a garage to have the chains taken off. The next time, he thought, I'll wear my right arm in a sling; they won't grin at me then. I'll have my right arm in a sling and they'll see I couldn't possibly take the chains off myself. He kicked at the slush on the sidewalk. "Overshoes," he said to himself, and he began looking for a shoe store.

When he came out into the street again, with the overshoes in a box under his arm, Walter Mitty began to wonder what the other thing was his wife had told him to get. She had told him twice, before they set out from their house for Waterbury. In a way he hated these weekly trips to town—he was always getting something wrong. Kleenex, he thought, Squibb's, razor blades? No. Toothpaste, toothbrush, bicarbonate, carborundum, initiative and referendum? He gave it up. But she would remember it. "Where's the what's-its-name?" she would ask. "Don't tell me you forgot the what's-its-name." A newsboy went by shouting something about the Waterbury trial.

. . . "Perhaps this will refresh your memory." The District

Attorney suddenly thrust a heavy automatic at the quiet figure on the witness stand. "Have you ever seen this before?" Walter Mitty took the gun and examined it expertly. "This is my Webley-Vickers 50.80," he said calmly. An excited buzz ran around the courtroom. The judge rapped for order. "You are a crack shot with any sort of firearms, I believe?" said the District Attorney, insinuatingly. "Objection!" shouted Mitty's attorney. "We have shown that the defendant could not have fired the shot. We have shown that he wore his right arm in a sling on the night of the fourteenth of July." Walter Mitty raised his hand briefly and the bickering attorneys were stilled. "With any known make of gun," he said evenly, "I could have killed Gregory Fitzhurst at three hundred feet *with my left hand*." Pandemonium broke loose in the courtroom. A woman's scream rose above the bedlam and suddenly a lovely, dark-haired girl was in Walter Mitty's arms. The District Attorney struck at her savagely. Without rising from his chair, Mitty let the man have it on the point of the chin. "You miserable cur!" . . .

"Puppy biscuit," said Walter Mitty. He stopped walking and the buildings of Waterbury rose up out of the misty courtroom and surrounded him again. A woman who was passing laughed. "He said 'Puppy biscuit,' " she said to her companion. "That man said 'Puppy biscuit' to himself." Walter Mitty hurried on. He went into an A. & P., not the first one he came to but a smaller one farther up the street. "I want some biscuit for small, young dogs," he said to the clerk. "Any special brand, sir?" The greatest pistol shot in the world thought a moment. "It says 'Puppies Bark for It' on the box," said Walter Mitty.

His wife would be through at the hairdresser's in fifteen minutes, Mitty saw in looking at his watch, unless they had trouble drying it; sometimes they had trouble drying it. She didn't like to get to the hotel first; she would want him to be there waiting for her as usual. He found a big leather chair in the lobby, facing a window, and he put the overshoes and the puppy biscuit on the floor beside it. He picked up an old copy of *Liberty* and sank down into the chair. "Can Germany Conquer the World Through the Air?" Walter Mitty looked at the pictures of bombing planes and of ruined streets.

. . . "The cannonading has got the wind up in young Raleigh, sir," said the sergeant. Captain Mitty looked up at him through tousled hair. "Get him to bed," he said wearily. "With the others. I'll fly alone." "But you can't, sir," said the sergeant anxiously. "It takes two men to handle that bomber and the Archies are pounding hell out of the air. Von Richtman's circus is between here and Saulier." "Somebody's got to get that ammunition dump," said Mitty. "I'm going over. Spot of brandy?" He poured a drink for the sergeant and one for himself. War thundered and whined around the dugout and battered at the door. There was a rending of wood and splinters flew through the room. "A bit of a near thing," said Captain Mitty carelessly. "The box barrage is closing in," said the sergeant. "We only live once, Sergeant," said Mitty, with his faint, fleeting smile. "Or do we?" He poured another brandy and tossed it off. "I never see a man could hold his brandy like you, sir," said the sergeant. "Begging your pardon, sir." Captain Mitty stood up and strapped on his huge Webley-Vickers automatic. "It's forty kilometers through hell, sir," said the sergeant. Mitty finished one last brandy. "After all," he said softly, "what isn't?" The pounding of the cannon increased; there was the rat-tat-tatting of machine guns, and from somewhere came the menacing pocketa-pocketa-pocketa of the new flame-throwers. Walter Mitty walked to the door of the dugout humming "Auprès de Ma Blonde." He turned and waved to the sergeant. "Cheerio!" he said. . . .

Something struck his shoulder. "I've been looking all over this hotel for you," said Mrs. Mitty. "Why do you have to hide in this old chair? How did you expect me to find you?" "Things close in," said Walter Mitty vaguely. "What?" Mrs. Mitty said. "Did you get the what's-its-name? The puppy biscuit? What's in that box?" "Overshoes," said Mitty. "Couldn't you have put them on in the store?" "I was thinking," said Walter Mitty. "Does it ever occur to you that I am sometimes thinking?" She looked at him. "I'm going to take your temperature when I get you home," she said.

They went out through the revolving doors that made a faintly derisive whistling sound when you pushed them. It was two blocks to the parking lot. At the drugstore on the corner she said, "Wait here for me. I forgot something. I won't be a minute." She was more than a minute. Walter Mitty lighted a cigarette. It began to rain, rain with sleet in it. He stood up against the wall of the drugstore, smoking. . . . He put his shoulders back and his heels together. "To hell with the handkerchief," said Walter Mitty scornfully. He took one last drag on his cigarette and snapped it away. Then, with that faint, fleeting smile playing about his lips, he faced the firing squad; erect and motionless, proud and disdainful, Walter Mitty the Undefeated, inscrutable to the last.

Spindleberries

JOHN GALSWORTHY (1867–1933)

THE celebrated painter, Scudamore—whose studies of Nature had been hung on the line for so many years that he had forgotten the days when, not yet in the Scudamore manner, they depended from the sky—stood where his cousin had left him so abruptly. His lips, between comely grey moustache and comely pointed beard, wore a mortified smile, and he gazed rather dazedly at the spindleberries fallen on to the flagged courtyard from the branch she had brought to show him. Why had she thrown up her head as if he had struck her, and whisked round so that those dull-pink berries quivered and lost their rain-drops, and four had fallen? He had but said: "Charming! I'd like to use them!" And she had answered: "God!" and rushed away. Alicia really was crazed; who would have thought that once she had been so adorable? He stooped and picked up the four berries—a beautiful colour, that dull pink! And from below the coatings of success and the Scudamore manner a little thrill came up; the stir of emotional vision. Paint! What good? How express? He went across to the low wall which divided the courtyard of his expensively restored and beautiful old house from the first flood of the River Arun wandering silvery in pale winter sunlight. Yes, indeed! How express Nature, its translucence and mysterious unities, its mood never the same from hour to hour? Those brown-tufted rushes over there against the gold grey of light and water—those restless, hovering, white gulls. A kind of disgust at his own celebrated manner welled up within him—the disgust expressed in Alicia's "God!" Beauty! What use—how express it? Had she been thinking the same thing?

He looked at the four pink berries glistening on the grey stone of the wall and memory stirred. What a lovely girl she had been, with her grey-green eyes shining under long lashes, the rose-petal colour in her cheeks and the too-fine dark hair—now so very grey—always blowing a little wild. An enchanting, enthusiastic creature! He remembered, as if it had been but last week, that day when they started from Arundel Station by the road to Burpham, when he was twenty-nine and she twenty-five, both of them painters and neither of them famed—a day of showers and sunlight in the middle of March, and Nature preparing for full spring! How they had chattered at first; and when their arms touched, how he had thrilled, and the colour had deepened in her rain-wet cheeks; and then, gradually, they had grown silent; a wonderful walk, which seemed leading so surely to a more wonderful end. They had wandered round through the village and down past the chalk-pit and Jacob's ladder, into the field path and so to the river bank. And he had taken her ever so gently round the waist, still silent, waiting for that moment when his heart would leap out of him in words and hers—he was sure—would leap to meet it. The path entered a thicket of blackthorn with a few primroses close to the little river running full and gentle. The last drops of a shower were falling, but the sun had burst through, and the sky above the thicket was cleared to the blue of speedwell flowers. Suddenly she had stopped and cried: "Look, Dick! Oh, look! It's heaven!" A high bush of blackthorn was lifted there, starry white against the blue and that bright cloud. It seemed to sing, it was so lovely; the whole of spring was in it. But the sight of her ecstatic face had broken down all his restraint, and tightening his arm round her he had kissed her lips. He remembered still the expression of her face, like a child's startled out of sleep. She had gone rigid, gasped, started away from him, quivered and gulped, and broken suddenly into sobs. Then, slipping from his arm, she had fled. He had stood at first, amazed and hurt, utterly bewildered; then, recovering a little, had hunted for her full half an hour before at last he found her sitting on wet grass, with a stony look on her face. He had said nothing, and she nothing, except to murmur: "Let's go on; we shall miss our train!" And all the rest of that day and the day after, until they parted, he had suffered from the feeling of having tumbled down off some high perch in her estimation. He had not liked it at all; it had made him very angry. Never from that day to this had he thought of it as anything but a piece of wanton prudery. Had it—had it been something else?

He looked at the four pink berries, and, as if they had uncanny power to turn the wheel of memory, he saw another vision of his cousin five years later. He was married by then, and already hung on the line. With his wife he had gone down to Alicia's country cottage. A summer night, just dark and very warm. After many exhortations she had brought into the little drawing-room her last finished picture. He could see her now placing it where the light fell, her tall, slight form already rather sharp and meagre, as the figures of some women grow at thirty, if they are not married; the nervous, fluttering look on her charming face, as though she could hardly bear this inspection; the way she raised her shoulder just a little as if to ward off an expected blow of condemnation. No need! It had been a beautiful thing, a quite surprisingly beautiful study of night. He remembered with what a really jealous ache he had gazed at it—a better thing than he had ever done himself. And, frankly, he had said so. Her eyes had shone with pleasure.

"Do you really like it? I tried so hard!"

"The day you show that, my dear," he had said, "your name's made!" She had clasped her hands and simply sighed: "Oh, Dick!" He had felt quite happy in her happiness, and presently the three of them had taken their chairs out, beyond the curtains, on to the dark verandah, had talked a little, then somehow fallen silent. A wonderful warm, black, grape-bloom night, exquisitely gracious and inviting; the stars very high and white, the flowers glimmering in the garden-beds, and against the deep, dark blue, roses hanging, unearthly, stained with beauty. There was a scent of honeysuckle, he remembered, and many moths came fluttering by toward the tall, narrow chink of light between the curtains. Alicia had sat leaning forward, elbows on knees, ears buried in her hands. Probably they were silent because she sat like that. Once he heard her whisper to herself: "Lovely, lovely! Oh, God! How lovely!" His wife, feeling the dew, had gone in, and he had followed; Alicia had not seemed to notice. But when she too came in, her eyes were glistening with tears. She said something about bed in a queer voice; they had taken candles and gone up. Next morning, going to her little studio to give her advice about that picture, he had been literally horrified to see it streaked with lines of white—Alicia, standing before it, was dashing her brush in broad smears across and across. She heard him and turned round. There was a hard red spot in either cheek, and she said in a quivering voice: "It was blasphemy. That's all!"

And turning her back on him she had gone on smearing it with white. Without a word, he had turned tail in simple disgust. Indeed, so deep had been his vexation at that wanton destruction of the best thing she had ever done or was ever likely to do, that he had avoided her for years. He had always had a horror of eccentricity. To have planted her foot firmly on the ladder of fame and then deliberately kicked it away; to have wantonly foregone this chance of making money—for she had but a mere pittance! It had seemed to him really too exasperating, a thing only to be explained by tapping one's forehead. Every now and then he still heard of her, living down there, spending her days out in the woods and fields, and sometimes even her nights, they said, and steadily growing poorer and thinner and more eccentric; becoming, in short, impossibly difficult, as only Englishwomen can. People would speak of her as "such a dear," and talk of her charm, but always with that shrug which is hard to bear when applied to one's relations. What she did with the productions of her brush he never inquired, too disillusioned by that experience. Poor Alicia!

The pink berries glowed on the grey stone, and he had yet another memory. A family occasion when Uncle Martin Scudamore departed this life, and they all went up to bury him and hear his will. The old chap, whom they had looked on as a bit of a disgrace, money-grubbing up in the little grey Yorkshire town which owed its rise to his factory, was expected to make amends by his death, for he had never married—too sunk in industry, apparently, to have the time. By tacit agreement, his nephews and nieces had selected the Inn at Bolton Abbey, nearest beauty spot, for their stay. They had driven six miles to the funeral, in three carriages. Alicia had gone with him and his brother, the solicitor. In her plain black clothes she looked quite charming, in spite of the silver threads already thick in her fine dark hair, loosened by the moor wind. She had talked of painting to him with all her old enthusiasm, and her eyes had seemed to linger on his face as if she still had a little weakness for him. He had quite enjoyed that drive. They had come rather abruptly on the small grimy town clinging to the river banks, with old Martin's long, yellow-brick house dominating it, about two hundred yards above the mills. Suddenly, under the rug, he felt Alicia's hand seize his with a sort of desperation, for all the world as if she were clinging to something to support her. Indeed, he was sure she did not know it was his hand she squeezed. The cobbled streets, the muddy-looking water, the dingy, staring factories, the yellow, staring house, the little dark-clothed, dreadfully plain work-people, all turned out to do a last honour to their creator; the hideous new grey church, the dismal service, the brand-new tombstones—and all of a glorious autumn day! It was inexpressibly sordid—too ugly for words! Afterwards the will was read to them seated decorously on bright mahogany chairs in the yellow mansion, a very satisfactory will, distributing in perfectly adjusted portions, to his own kinsfolk and nobody else, a very considerable wealth. Scudamore had listened to it dreamily, with his eyes fixed on an oily picture, thinking, "My God! What a thing!" and longing to be back in the carriage smoking a cigar to take the reek of black clothes and sherry—sherry!—out of his nostrils. He happened to look at Alicia. Her eyes were closed; her lips, always sweet-looking, quivered amusedly. And at that very moment the will came to her name. He saw those eyes open wide, and marked a beautiful pink flush, quite like that of old days, come into her thin cheeks. "Splendid!" he had thought; "it's really jolly for her. I *am* glad! Now she won't have to pinch. Splendid!" He shared with her to the full the surprised relief showing in her still beautiful face.

All the way home in the carriage he felt at least as happy over her good fortune as over his own, which had been substantial. He took her hand under the rug and squeezed it, and she answered with a long, gentle pressure, quite unlike the clutch when they were driving in. That same evening he strolled out to where the river curved below the Abbey. The sun had not quite set, and its last smoky radiance slanted into the burnished autumn woods.

Some white-faced Herefords were grazing in lush grass, the river rippled and gleamed all over golden scales. About that scene was the magic which had so often startled the hearts of painters, the wistful gold—the enchantment of a dream. For some minutes he had gazed with delight which had in it a sort of despair. A little crisp rustle ran along the bushes; the leaves fluttered, then hung quite still. And he heard a voice—Alicia's—speaking. "The lovely, lovely world!" And moving forward a step, he saw her standing on the river bank, braced against the trunk of a birch tree, her head thrown back, and her arms stretched wide apart as though to clasp the lovely world she had apostrophised. To have gone up to her would have been like breaking up a lovers' interview, and he turned round instead and went away.

A week later he heard from his brother that Alicia had refused her legacy. "I don't want it," her letter had said simply; "I couldn't bear to take it. Give it to those poor people who live in that awful place." Really eccentricity could go no further! They decided to go down and see her. Such mad neglect of her own good must not be permitted without some effort to prevent it. They found her very thin and charming, humble, but quite obstinate in her refusal. "Oh! I couldn't really! I should be so unhappy. Those poor little stunted people who made it all for him! That little, awful town! I simply couldn't be reminded. Don't talk about it, please. I'm quite all right as I am." They had threatened her with lurid pictures of the workhouse and a destitute old age. To no purpose; she would not take the money. She had been forty when she refused that aid from heaven—forty, and already past any hope of marriage. For though Scudamore had never known for certain that she had ever wished or hoped for marriage, he had his theory—that all her eccentricity came from wasted sexual instinct. This last folly had seemed to him monstrous enough to be pathetic, and he no longer avoided her. Indeed, he would often walk over to tea in her little hermitage. With Uncle Martin's money he had bought and restored the beautiful old house over the River Arun, and was now only five miles from Alicia's, across country. She, too, would come tramping over at all hours, floating in with wild flowers or ferns, which she would put into water the moment she arrived. She had ceased to wear hats, and had by now a very doubtful reputation for sanity about the countryside. This was the period when Watts was on every painter's tongue, and he seldom saw Alicia without a disputation concerning that famous symbolist. Personally, he had no use for Watts, resenting his faulty drawing and crude allegories, but Alicia always maintained with her extravagant fervour that he was great because he tried to paint the soul of things. She especially loved a painting called "Iris"—a female symbol of the rainbow, which indeed, in its floating eccentricity, had a certain resemblance to herself. "Of course he failed," she would say; "he tried for the impossible and went on trying all his life. Oh! I can't bear your tales and catchwords, Dick; what's the good of them! Beauty's too big, too deep!" Poor Alicia! She was sometimes very wearing.

He never knew quite how it came about that she went abroad with them to Dauphiné in the autumn of 1904—a rather disastrous business. Never again would he take anyone travelling who did not know how to come in out of the cold. It was a painter's country, and he had hired a little *château* in front of Glandaz mountain—himself, his wife, their eldest girl, and Alicia. The adaptation of his famous manner to that strange scenery, its browns and French greys and filmy blues, so preoccupied him that he had scant time for becoming intimate with these hills and valleys. From the little gravelled terrace in front of the annexe, out of which he had made a studio, there was an absorbing view over the pantiled old town of Die. It glistened below in the early or late sunlight, flat-roofed and of pinkish yellow, with the dim, blue River Drôme circling one side, and cut, dark cypress trees dotting the vineyarded slopes. And he painted it continually. What Alicia did with herself they none of them very much knew, except that she would come in and talk ecstatically of things and beasts and people she had seen. One favourite haunt of hers they did visit—a ruined monastery high up in the amphitheatre of the Glandaz mountain. They had their lunch up there, a very charming and remote spot, where the watercourses and ponds and chapel of the old monks were still visible, though converted by the farmer to his use. Alicia left them abruptly in the middle of their praises, and they had not seen her again till they found her at home when they got back. It was almost as if she had resented laudation of her favourite haunt. She had brought in with her a great bunch of golden berries, of which none of them knew the name; berries almost as beautiful as these spindleberries glowing on the stone of the wall. And a fourth memory of Alicia came.

Christmas Eve, a sparkling frost, and every tree round the little *château* rimed so that they shone in the starlight as though dowered with cherry blossom. Never were more stars in clear black sky above the whitened earth. Down in the little town a few faint points of yellow light twinkled in the mountain wind keen as a razor's edge. A fantastically lovely night—quite "Japanese," but cruelly cold. Five minutes on the terrace had been enough for all of them except Alicia. She—unaccountable, crazy creature—would not come in. Twice he had gone out to her, with commands, entreaties, and extra wraps; the third time he could not find her. She had deliberately avoided his onslaught and slid off somewhere to keep this mad vigil by frozen starlight. When at last she did come in she reeled as if drunk. They tried to make her really drunk, to put warmth back into her. No good! In two days she was down with double pneumonia; it was two months before she was up again—a very shadow of herself. There had never been much health in her since then. She floated like a ghost through life, a crazy ghost, who would steal away, goodness knew where, and come in with a flush in her withered cheeks, and her grey hair wild blown, carrying her spoil—some flower, some leaf, some tiny bird or little soft rabbit. She never painted now, never even talked of it. They had made her give up her cottage and come to live with them, literally afraid that she would starve herself to death in her forgetfulness of everything. These spindleberries even! Why probably, she had been right up this morning to that sunny chalk-pit in the lew of the Downs to get them, seven miles there and back, when you wouldn't think she could walk seven hundred yards, and as likely as not had lain there on the dewy grass looking up at the sky, as he had come on her sometimes. Poor Alicia! And once he had been within an ace of marrying her! A life spoiled! By what, if not by love of beauty? But who would have ever thought that the intangible could wreck a woman, deprive her of love, marriage, motherhood, of fame, of wealth, of health? And yet—by George!—it had!

Scudamore flipped the four pink berries off the wall. The radiance and the meandering milky waters; that swan against the brown tufted rushes; those far, filmy Downs—there was beauty! *Beauty!* But, damn it all—moderation! Moderation! And, turning his back on that prospect, which he had painted so many times, in his celebrated manner, he went in, and up the expensively restored staircase to his studio. It had great windows on three sides, and perfect means for regulating light. Unfinished studies melted into walls so subdued that they looked like atmosphere. There were no completed pictures—they sold too fast. As he walked over to his easel his eye was caught by a spray of colour—the branch of spindleberries set in water, ready for him to use, just where the pale sunlight fell so that their delicate colour might glow and the few tiny drops of moisture still clinging to them shine. For a second he saw Alicia herself as she must have looked, setting them there, her transparent hands hovering, her eyes shining, that grey hair of hers all fine and loose. The vision vanished! But what had made her bring them after that horrified "God!" when he spoke of using them? Was it her way of saying: "Forgive me for being rude"? Really she was pathetic, that poor devotee! The spindleberries glowed in their silver-lustre jug, sprayed up against the sunlight. They looked triumphant—as well they might, who stood for that which had ruined—or was it saved?—a life! Alicia! She had made a pretty mess of it, and yet who knew what secret raptures she had felt with her subtle lover, Beauty, by starlight and sunlight and moonlight, in the fields and woods, on the hilltops, and by riverside? Flowers, and the flight of birds, and the ripple of the wind, and all the shifting play of light and colour which made a man despair when he wanted to use them; she had taken them, hugged them to her with no afterthought, and been happy! Who could say that she had missed the prize of life? Who could say it? . . . Spindleberries! A bunch of spindleberries to set such doubts astir in him! Why, what was beauty but just the extra value which certain forms and colours, blended, gave to things—just the extra value in the human market! Nothing else on earth, nothing! And the spindleberries glowed against the sunlight, delicate, remote!

Taking his palette, he mixed crimson lake, white, and ultramarine. What was that? Who sighed, away out there behind him? Nothing!

"Damn it all!" he thought; "this is childish. This is as bad as Alicia!" And he set to work to paint in his celebrated manner—spindleberries.

A Song Writer in the Family

ALBERT HALPER (1904–)

When I was a kid of seventeen, in those good old days right after the First World War when there were no juke boxes, rationing, or man-power commissions, I wanted to be a song writer. But terrific! I used to come home from work around six o'clock in the evening, eat supper, and monkey around my sister's upright piano. My sister, like most girls, had taken a couple years' piano

A Song Writer in the Family is from *The Yale Review*, copyright Yale University Press, 1943, and reprinted by arrangement with Maxim Lieber.

lessons when she had been a kid and then, growing older, had dropped the business. Therefore I was king of the family keyboard.

My family got an ear ache listening to my playing, but they had to stand it. After all, where else could they go? We didn't live in Charlie Schwab's mansion on Riverside Drive, New York. We lived on the West Side, near Kedzie Avenue, Chicago, the whole eight of us. My father didn't come home from his grocery until eight-thirty; so he missed most of my creative banging. But my mother, poor woman, got it going and coming.

"Dave," she said, tactfully, "are you sure you don't have to take lessons first?"

"Nah. Listen, Ma, does a guy have to take lessons to write poetry? Does a guy have to pay a teacher to learn how to breathe?"

"Yes, but you don't seem to know what notes to strike with your left hand—" she interposed, worried.

"Aw, Ma, it's like rolling off a log. You don't want me to get balled up with technique, do you? Geez, I'm a composer!" And I resumed banging out the opening chords of "I Miss You, Corrine," my forty-third composition. I wanged the bass, giving it all I had—not that tinkling Zez Confrey stuff like "Kitten on the Keys," but the real McCoy from off Madison Street, the new Chicago style. Holding her ears when she thought I wasn't looking, my mother went out onto the back porch, to talk to Mrs. Sandal. When I took a breather after the second chorus, I could hear them.

"I never had a genius in the family before—" my mother said, worried.

Mrs. Sandal, a short fat woman married to a butcher's helper, answered in her German accent. "Ach, don't vorry aboud him.—My older boy, Otto, is a genius, too. He sometimes drrrums on der kitchen table with some soup bones."

I banged on the bass harder than ever, shouting, "Oh, I miss you Corrine, my heart yearns for you—" On the back porch my mother's voice sounded more worried than ever.

I played almost two hours, then looked at the clock. Almost eight-thirty, almost time for my old man to come home. I put my scribbled composition notes under the lid of the piano bench, washed my face and hands, combed my hair and sailed out into the summer night to meet my pal Joey Mutsek, to talk about Paul Whiteman, women, and the new striped shirts the Washington Shirt Shoppe was featuring. Half way down the block I saw my father, short, heavy and tired, coming home from the store, and I hurried faster, cutting off Kedzie into Ohio Street. For some reason or other I didn't want to meet him. He had the habit lately of giving me a heavy silent stare which always crushed me. His stare said, "I'm getting old and tired standing on my feet fifteen hours a day in my grocery. You and your piano banging, your dreams—" No, I didn't want to meet him, even if he was my old man. He was growing bitter. When I had cut east into Ohio Street I breathed easier.

I saw Joey Mutsek sitting on the front stoop of his home half way down the block.

"What's tickling?" I asked him.

"The old cat's pickling," he answered.

This was our nightly password, and it hadn't changed for the past two months. Previous to this one, our password had been—Me: "What's with you?" Him: "I'm roiled with boils." That one had lasted only a week. I could repeat some of the older ones, but what's the use?

I sat down beside Joey on the front steps, and we stared out into the night, thinking of the shortness of summer, love, women, beauty, and death. Finally we began thinking of Rosa Picollini, both of us at the same time. I knew it because we sighed together.

"I saw her this evening," Joey opened.

"Where?" My mouth was dry.

"Walking north on Kedzie towards Madison."

"Was she alone?"

"No, Susie Pikowski was with her. Why do you think she goes with such a homely cow like Susie Pikowski?"

"I don't know," I said. "I can't ever dope it out why most pretty girls go with homely girl friends."

"I guess it's the mystery of the feminine sex," Joey said, wrinkling his brow. "It's something profound. I read it once in a book."

I didn't know what to say; so I said, "I guess it is."

While I sat on the stoop with Joey, the lyrics of my forty-third composition pounded in my head.

Corrine, I love you,
I love your hair, your eyes—

Corrine was my secret name for Rosa Picollini. It was my secret name because if my song got accepted by a New York publisher and became a smash hit and made a million dollars, no one would know who the real Corrine was until I rode up to her door in a long swell car and told Rosa Picollini myself.

"I really don't like girls," I stated.

"I don't either," Joey said. He threw a stone at the curb. "They're too unpredictable. The truth is, I don't really like Rosa Picollini. I like her cousin Grace—"

"Yes, but I thought you just said you didn't like—"

Joey laughed. "Well, the truth is I like Grace. Grace is small and isn't half as pretty as Rosa and hasn't got Rosa's queenly way of walking down a street, but I feel something singing inside me every time I see her. Aw, nuts." He pushed me.

My own blood was secretly singing. I really wasn't jealous of Joey, knowing that Rosa loved only me, but the less competition the better as I saw it.

"Well," I said, throwing the bull around, "I really don't like Rosa either. I guess I felt I had to moon and fall for her because she's so beautiful and wonderful, and everything she does is so perfect, but I really don't like her. Hell, I don't need girls."

Joey gave me a funny look, then turned away. At that minute I stared up the street and saw the subject of our conversation,

My heart plopped into my throat, then sank down into my stomach.

She wasn't alone. She wasn't walking with Susie Pikowski, either. She was walking with a young man.

They were coming our way. I sat turned into stone as they approached, and when she smiled and said, "Hello, Dave," I remained dumb as a post but finally blurted, "Hello—" The young man she was walking with was older than myself; he looked about nineteen or twenty, and not only did he own a good-looking blue suit but he wore a straw hat. They passed Joey and me and walked west, towards the park.

I sat there feeling a little sick to my stomach. I had never taken Rosa Picollini out on a date, in fact, I had never even asked her to go for a walk or to a movie. I was so much in love with her I never had had the nerve. Joey Mutsek stared at me again, then looked away.

"Aw, nuts," he finally said, understandingly. "Come on, let's go over to Goldmark's drug store and see who's there."

I got off the stairs, still feeling a little sick, and we went down the street.

Two hours later, when I got home, my father and mother weren't sleeping.

My Uncle Sam, who was in the pickle business on Taylor Street, had paid us an unexpected visit. With his dramatic hands waving in the air he was declaiming about art, literature, and politics. My mother, slightly ashamed of her "crazy" brother, kept looking first at the carpet, then at her lap. Sam always smelled of pickles, even when he had washed and changed into his best suit.

"Politics will never be clean," he was shouting, "until the men mixed up in politics are clean! Politics should be as fine and as beautiful as art, or music! And why not?"

My mother had no answer, and as for my father he suppressed a yawn behind his hand. It was half-past ten, long past his bedtime, and he was due to get up at five in the morning to open his store.

"Everything should be clean and beautiful," my uncle shouted. "Then life would be like a song, would be worth living!"

At that moment my mother saw me standing near the door. I was supposed to take after her crazy brother. On her face was a look of pain. The look said, "Isn't one in the family enough?" My father, turning his head, also noticed me. He frowned. Sam was the last to catch sight of me.

"My boy," he cried, "I was just explaining to your parents why everything is wrong in the world! Life is a rag for most of us, when it should be a banner!"

"Don't talk like an anarchist," my mother murmured, frightened.

Her brother ignored her. "Dave," he said to me, "never grow old! Let the years pile on top of you, let your hair fall out, let your shoulders stoop, but never grow old!"

My father, sitting patiently, coughed quietly behind his hand. "Why, how is that to be done?" he inquired. "When a person accumulates a lot of years he grows old, doesn't he?"

My uncle's face, turned towards me, lit up. "See? They don't understand. Not a word. No one in this room understands, Dave, except you and me."

My three older brothers came in from outside. They stood around listening for a while, until two of them yawned and excused themselves. Irving stood it a bit longer, then said he had to go wash his teeth. My mother was sitting on pins and needles worrying about the sleep my father was losing, but she couldn't bring herself to tell Sam to go home. Sam had already eaten the company cake my mother had set out and had drunk three glasses of tea, but he had just got started. My mother should have known better. Tea was like liquor to Sam; after two or three glasses he was good for all night.

"I still can't understand," my father put in quietly, "how you can fool nature. If nature gives you wrinkles and rheumatism, you can't laugh it off."

My uncle threw his magnificent smile of triumph at me. "See? They still don't understand, do they?"

They didn't. But I did. I wasn't crazy like my uncle for nothing.

"You take Dave here, take your boy," Sam said.

"You take him," my kid brother Sidney snickered, standing near the wall. He had just come in from the street.

"You shut up," my father told him, "or I'll lay my hand on you."

"I was only kidding," Sidney said in a hurry.

"You take your boy Dave here," said Sam. "He knows what I'm talking about. A couple of years ago he won the West Side roller-skating championship in Garfield Park, which he celebrated by writing a poem that got accepted by the Quaker Nut people in Battle Creek, Michigan, in a contest, and now he writes music. He wants people to sing, to be happy. He knows what I'm talking about."

This last statement aroused my father's curiosity. Though tired and slightly red-eyed from being up since five o'clock in the morning, he leaned forward attentively to find out why only his crazy son knew what Sam was talking about.

"Excuse me," he said, "but I don't get the connection."

"The line is busy," said my sister. She had just come in from a walk with her girl friend and was smiling.

"You shut up," said my father, "or I'll lay my hand on you."

My sister, smiling, excused herself for the evening. My old man then leaned forward more attentively than ever. "I repeat, excuse me, but about Dave and you—I don't get the connection."

Sam threw me another magnificent smile of triumph, his gold tooth shining.

"Mr. Bergman, sometimes people talk the same language but can't understand each other. It's not the fault of our educational system. It's the magnificent tragedy of the human race."

My mother looked more worried and uneasy than ever. She knew Sam had never graduated even from grammar school, and here he was using such big words.

"I think you're mixed up," my father said to Sam. "It's true Dave here won the West Side roller-skating championship; it's also true that he got two dollars for a poem sent to Battle Creek, Michigan, and that he writes something called music. So what? He now is an order-picker on roller skates for the Gold Bond Mail-Order House, and as for his songs he can't get his music published by anybody. He spends almost fifty cents a week on stamps."

Sam waved his dramatic hands again. "Makes no difference. The boy is all right. The main thing, he's full of music, he wants people to be happy!"

My parents looked at me. Had they missed something? Was I really full of music for the whole damned human race? My face turned as red as a fireman's flannel. My father finally shook his head.

"No, the boy wants to make a little money writing his songs."

Sam waved his hands again. "A little money won't do him any harm. It'll give him his freedom. No, a little money will never harm anybody. But he's not writing for money. He's writing to make people sing, to be happy."

My father stared at me again. Was Sam right? His brow furrowed. Had he failed to understand his next-to-youngest son?

"You take him," Sidney snickered.

"You shut up," my father said, "or I'll lay my hand on you."

My kid brother turned a little white, then went to sit quietly on a chair in a corner. "I was only kidding," he mumbled.

My mother continued to look worried. She had that uneasy look she always wore when I was being discussed.

"Dave is a good boy," she murmured.

"Right," said Sam. "He is *good*. That's the word. *Good*. Even if his music doesn't make him a millionaire, isn't it wonderful that he makes people sing, that he makes millions happy?"

"He hasn't had any of his songs published," my father reminded his brother-in-law.

"Makes no difference. This year, next year, makes no difference. Isn't it better than politics? Isn't it better than public trickery, better than playing with false words?"

"I don't know," said my father. "Maybe Dave's words are false, too. He's always writing songs about love. He's just seventeen—what does he know about love?"

Uncle Sam began shouting louder than ever. "Know? Why he knows *everything* about love! He's at the age when his whole life is full of love. His body is full of all the love in the world. Why, it's leaking out of him!"

My father looked at me again, at my red face. "I don't see a drop of it," he said cryptically. "Even his cheeks are dry."

I was glad my older brothers and my sister had gone to bed. My old man was sure going good tonight. How they would have enjoyed it! My mother's hands stirred nervously in her lap.

"Dave is a good boy," she repeated, worried.

My Uncle Sam kept talking about me. In his mind I was mixed up with love, music, goodness, and the hunger of the world. His wonderful words were like white fire to me, as they always were whenever he visited us, which was two or three times a year. I didn't mind the smell of pickles which came from him; I didn't care what my family thought about him. "He's cracked," my oldest brothers said every time his name was mentioned. "Why, he had a patent on a tarragon vinegar, and he gave it away—he let every manufacturer use it when he could have cleaned up a million. He's screwy." They sort of despised him. Even Sis did. Though he wore good clothes, even his best suit was baggy at the knees when he came to visit us. And why hadn't he ever gotten married? In our family a bachelor was looked upon with suspicion. Another uncle of mine with five kids, Uncle Harry, who lived on Harrison Street, had said Uncle Sam was too goddamn hard to please. He referred to the days when Uncle Sam was young and handsome and all the girls were wild about him.

But now my bachelor uncle was fifty, with a gold tooth in his mouth. His hair was getting gray, and he was growing stoop-shouldered from bending over pickle barrels in his two-by-four plant over on Taylor Street. My mother, worried about him as she was worried about me, stared at him with pity.

Finally my father got up from his chair and prepared to retire to his room.

"You may be right," he yawned, "but tomorrow is another day, and my customers, curse them, will be banging on the door of my store at five o'clock if I'm not there." Without saying good-night to Sam, he went into his bedroom, closing the door down the hall.

My mother, my kid brother, Uncle Sam, and I sat in silence for a few minutes. Sam's eyes were wet. Finally he pressed my mother's hand, looked at me, and left. Later on, when I was taking off my shirt in the hot night and getting ready to go to bed, I asked my mother what had been wrong with Uncle Sam towards the end of his visit tonight. She didn't want to answer at first, but I kept asking her. Finally she told me.

"You know," she said in a compassionate voice, "when he talks about you before us he's really talking about himself, about his lost youth. His tragedy is that he never met the right girl. He's the loneliest man in the world. That's why he's always talking about clean politics and music and making people happy. That's why he's always taking your side. He once fell in love with a beautiful girl, but she married somebody else."

"Why, I thought all the girls were crazy about him," I exclaimed.

"They were. But he hardly spoke to this girl, and she never suspected he loved her—so she married somebody else. And that's why—"

But I wasn't listening to the rest. My mother's words burned themselves into my mind. My God!

Finally I heard my mother's voice again. She was talking about the heat.

"Dave, take a shower before you go to bed tonight. It's so warm—"

I sat down in a chair, my eyes blurring, and started taking off my shoes while my mother went into her bedroom down the hall. In a few seconds I could hear her talking to my father.

"Why did you pick on Sam tonight? He's unhappy as it is—"

She must have awakened my father, for his voice sounded testy and thick.

"Why shouldn't I pick on him once in a while? Isn't one in the family enough? Eh?—"

Critical Questions

"A Song Writer in the Family" reads like a short piece of autobiography. The narrator, Dave Bergman, "a kid of seventeen," tells of himself and the attitudes of his family toward him from the distance of some twenty-five years. He dwells particularly on his Uncle Sam, whom he resembles in character in the eyes of his father and mother. The denouement of the story comes with Dave's mother's revelation of Uncle Sam's "true story." In her remarks Dave sees his love for Rosa Picollini in a new light.

The story, though apparently simple, raises many interesting problems of values and of craftsmanship. The following questions may be useful to a critical reader.

How is the distance of the narrator from the events established? What values does the distance have for the story? Is the distance consistently preserved and made full use of?

How is the story given a feeling of authenticity in background, time, and language?

What means are used to depict character?

What attitudes toward life are represented by Dave's father, mother, and Uncle Sam, and what do these attitudes contribute to the story?

What advantages or disadvantages to the story does Dave's mother's account of Uncle Sam have?

"You know," she said in a compassionate voice, "when he talks about you before us he's really talking about himself, about his lost youth. His tragedy is that he never met the right girl. He's the loneliest man in the world. That's why he's always talking about clean politics and music and making people happy. That's why he's always taking your side. He once fell in love with a beautiful girl, but she married somebody else."

"Why, I thought all the girls were crazy about him," I exclaimed.

"They were. But he hardly spoke to this girl, and she never suspected he loved her—so she married somebody else. And that's why—"

What place does the account of Rosa Picollini have in the story and what effect does it have on Dave's final feeling?

What do the last two sentences contribute to the story?

Harold Peavey's Fast Cow

GEORGE CRONYN (1889–)

WHEN HAROLD PEAVEY graduated from the State Agricultural College and won a prize in oratory on "The Plow is Mightier Than the Pen," we all thought he was a pretty smart boy, but when he leased the Eppingwell place on shares we changed our mind. The last family that took it worked five years and then they owed Old Lady Eppingwell five hundred and the bank another odd thousand. Parks, the man's name was, told me all he got out of it was a lame back and three more kids to raise.

So, when I saw smoke coming out of the chimney after two years when there wasn't any, I went over to call on my nearest neighbor. He was just carrying in a load of apple wood as I came in the front gate and, seeing me, he put it down.

"Hello, Bud," I says, "how's tricks?"

"Oke," he says, grinning. He was a nice-looking kid, standing over six feet, with a good set of teeth and hair that needed pruning. "Are you Pete Crumm?"

"Same," I says. "I used to know your folks at Medford. Your dad did me on a lumber deal, but I guess he's got you well educated."

"I don't know," he says thoughtfully. "I know all the spray formulas and the life history of the Woolly Aphis but I guess I've got plenty to learn."

"You have," I says, looking out over the twenty-seven acres of Eppingwell's Folly that was called an apple ranch. "Plenty. Your trees will stand a little pruning."

"Yes," he says. "They're pretty brushy. I've been working a couple of days and I've got twelve trees pruned."

"Not bad," I says. "You've only got two months' work ahead of you pruning at that rate, and it's the middle of March now. And there's another three weeks repairing the irrigation flumes that are all shot to hell. And maybe a week or two clearing the meadow patch—"

"You mean, I've got work ahead of me?"

"Not more'n fifteen hours a day. Have you got a good plow team?"

"None better. I've made a deal with Morrison to work his team and plow one day a week in return for helping him three days."

"I see. That leaves you four days for your own work, counting Sundays."

"Sundays I got a job driving the Sunday school bus."

"Well then," I says, "everything's jake. You can just sit down and take it easy the rest of the time. When are you getting a wife to do the house chores and cooking?"

"Not till I've saved about three hundred dollars," he says.

"I see," I says. "You'd as leave stay a bachelor."

"No, I wouldn't. I'd like to start a family." He looked out over the place in a sort of dreamy way. "And I'd like to have a cow." He picked up his chunks of apple wood and said, "It's a good view from the house here, with old Mount Sherman and Pine Butte and—"

"I see you've painted your hen house," I says.

"Yes," he says. "It matches up with the scenery. Morrison says he's got a good cow, a heifer. Black Jersey. I never heard of a black Jersey before. There can't be many of 'em."

"I've heard of *that* black Jersey," I says. "Her name is Mabel, but I don't know if I'd call her a cow."

"Why not?" he asks in surprise.

"Well," I says, "I don't know. It just never struck me that way. When are you getting her?"

"Tomorrow."

"I'll drive you over in my gas wagon," I says. "It's a mile and a half to Morrison's—quite a piece to lead Mabel."

So the next day about seven in the morning, after about a dozen flap-jacks, I tuned up the old bus and drove over to pick up Harold. There was a lot of smoke coming out of the kitchen door and when I stepped inside at first I couldn't see nothing but I could hear Harold coughing and choking around the wood stove.

"Morning," I says. "How's tricks?"

"It's the prunes," he sort of gasped. "I left 'em to cook while I started running a ditch through the meadow. I guess there wasn't enough water."

"Maybe there was too much prunes," I suggested. "Can you salvage any?"

"Sure!" he says. "The top layer is only burnt on one side. Would you care for any?"

"No," I says. "Prunes is a fruit that just spoils in me. I swell all up."

"Well," he says, scraping off half a dozen from the top, "they're full of vitamins."

"I know," I says. "That's why we always buy 'em in the package. The vitamins don't get into the packages."

After he ate as much as he could stand of the prunes and drunk what he said was coffee we climbed in the bus and drove over to Morrison's. On the way over I asked him how much Morrison was asking for the heifer.

"Only $35.50," he said, "and she's just coming fresh."

"What's the fifty cents for?"

"That's for the rope, and a dollar for the halter, so she really only comes to $34."

"Cheap enough," I says, "if she milks."

"She'll milk all right," he says hopefully. "Morrison guarantees that."

"Morrison guaranteed me a Poland China sow once," I says. "She wasn't no good raising pigs but she made fair to middling bacon. Old man Morrison's girl Sadie has got considerable of a shape."

"I met her at the Grange dance," the kid sort of stammered, "and I noticed she had blue eyes."

"Blue as a new pair of jumpers," I says. "And them lips of hers are just made for pecking at. She acts sort of stand-offish but if a fellow would just grab her—"

"Look at the sun," he says, "on Mount Sherman. The way it hits that glacier is something pretty!"

Old man Morrison was standing in the front yard with his two boys and the extra hand. The older boy, Perley, was coiling a rope and the young one, Sid, was mending an old halter with a piece of bailing wire. Old man Morrison looked as mean as ever but when he saw us drive in he brightened up like a winter sunset.

"Hello, Mr. Peavey," he says. "Hello, Pete. You're up bright and early."

"The early buzzard catches the snake," I says. "How's all the lawsuits?"

"Them lawyers," he says, "keep ahounding me. In the end they take all. But what's a poor man to do?"

"Keep out of court," I says. "Where's the heifer?"

"Down in the pasture," he says. "We're all fixed to bring her in."

"I mean Sadie," I says.

"Oh she!" he grunts. "She stays abed 'till 'most noontime. Says the morning air is bad for her complexion. If I thought tanning her hide would do any good—"

"Here's ten dollars down," says Harold stiffly, "and I'll pay the rest at the beginning of next month."

"You wouldn't need a receipt, I take it, Mr. Peavey?"

He was starting to say no when I says, "You bet. Business is business. You just write out the receipt while we go down and fetch the heifer."

"The boys'll do that for you," he says, scowling at me. "They know her better."

We went on in the kitchen where Mrs. Morrison was cooking up a mess of apples. The kitchen was full of the week's wash, the tables was heaped with dirty dishes, and a couple of kids was crawling on the floor playing with the butcher knife and a meat chopper.

"You men must be hungry," she says. "Set down and have some apple sauce."

"I'm not hungry," I says, looking around the kitchen, "but maybe Harold here is. He's batching."

"Poor man! He must be starved," she says, and began to ladle apple sauce into a soup bowl that you could see just had oatmeal in it. Mrs. Morrison is good hearted even if she has got a figure like a female walrus.

Harold made a noise in his throat, meaning "No, thank you," but hunger got the best of him and he began wolfing down the sauce.

"Sadie has been speaking of you, Mr. Peavey," says Mrs. Morrison, throwing a bunch of diapers into the washtub. "She heard all about your taking the prize for that speech on 'The Club is Mightier than the Pen,' and she thinks you dance real graceful. She'll be sorry to miss you. Maybe if I give her a call, she might come down."

"Oh," says Harold, gurgling into the apple sauce. "Don't—please don't disturb her!"

"It's all right," she says. "Sadie was going to town today anyhow." And rolling over to the upstairs door, she calls out, "Sa-die!"

After a few minutes, while I was trying to keep one of the kids from untying my shoelace, a voice like a sick cat calls down, "What do you want, ma? Can't you ever let me be when I'm trying to get a little rest?"

"There's a young man here to see you," says the Missus. "And he ain't got long to stay."

"Who is it? What does he want to see me for so early in the morning? Can't he come back in the afternoon? Who is it, anyway?"

"It's Mr. Penney and he's taking his cow home."

"Oh!" said the voice, sweet as honey. "Tell him to stop a while and I'll be right down!"

I look at Harold. He had his spoon full of apple sauce half way to his mouth and he'd forgotten about the next bit. His expression was like a calf when it hears the milk pail rattle—sort of eager and vacant.

"Gorry!" I thinks to myself. "The boy is caught! Hope Sadie don't fill out like her ma!"

Just then old man Morrison stuck his head in the outside door.

"The heifer's come up. You better take her right along. She's kind of restive."

Harold looked like he'd as lief stay there till moonrise but I took him by the elbow and he got up, pushing back the wobbly kitchen chair. I stooped down to tie the shoelace one of the brats had been playing with and when I looked up again Sadie was standing at the foot of the stairs. I will say, she looked pretty, if a man could stand her ways. Her hair was tousled but she'd thrown it up in a coil like a bundle of corn silk, and she had a pink kimono with yellow dots that set off her figure. There aren't many girls that look good just out of bed, but Sadie could get away with it, rubbing her eyes and half smiling at Harold.

"I'm so glad you came over to see me, Harold," she says, holding out her hand. "It was nice of you!"

"Well," says Harold, turning red, "I don't usually come around when people are in bed but I had to get my cow—"

"Oh," she says coolly, "the cow, of course! I hope you like her! Some day when your mind isn't taken up with your cow you might call around, if I'm home. Anyway, ma'll be here."

That's the way with the female, always trying to knock the pins out from under a man.

Harold gulped and I says, "He'll be back, missie, don't you worry. He don't give all his time to cows, he's—"

Right then we heard a commotion in the yard and old man Morrison hollering, "Hold her, dod blast it! Keep her out'n them lilies!"

"Well, goodbye, Mr. Penney," says Mrs. Morrison, wiping her sudsy hands on a dish cloth. "I suppose we can call you Harry?"

"Sure, you could!" says Harold. "I'll be around—"

Old man Morrison stuck his head in the door. He looked sort of red-purple and his eyes was bugged out. "Better take the heifer right along home," he says. "She's feelin' skittish this mornin'."

Harold looked calfish again at Sadie, we shook hands all around, and stepped out into the yard. The heifer was there waiting for us, and at first I couldn't make out exactly what they was doing with her. They had slung a hitch in the rope around her horns. One of the Morrison boys had a hold of one end and the other boy had a hold of the other end, and the extra hand was holding onto her halter rope. But what struck me as curious was the cow herself. The Morrisons had one of these rope swings hung from a big oak tree, that the three middle-size Morrison youngsters played in, and the cow was in the swing. I don't mean setting.

She had got her front legs and forepart through it so that the rope was under her belly, and she would take a run, dragging the two Morrisons and the extra hand, until the rope brought her up sharp, then she'd back up, kicking like a steer.

Harold looked at her like he was sort of puzzled and says, "She's pretty active for a cow, ain't she?"

"If it was the deer season," I says, "she'd pass for a young buck."

The fact is, Mabel did look more like a deer than anything. She was small, shiny black, and built lean and slender. Pretty, yes. But I couldn't see her as a milker.

"She's all right," old man Morrison mutters. "She'll give milk that's more'n half cream."

"I'd say she'd give butter, the way she's churning," I says.

Mabel put her head down and stood quiet. Perley Morrison yells, "Pa! Slip the swing out from under! She's all tuckered out!"

Before the old man could get to her, though, she made a lunge and brought the swing down out of the tree. Off she went, headed for the road, with the three boys hanging on for dear life. Luckily, the rope swing hooked onto the gate post as she went through and that held her.

"Well," I says to old man Morrison, "she seems to be stopped at the thirty-yard line. Guess we might as well amble along with her. Would you think maybe she'd go better in front or behind the bus?"

"Back up your car and we'll tie her on behind," he says, sort of gruff. "I'll put a half hitch around her muzzle."

I backed up the Ford, Harold climbed in, and they tied her up to the rear springs, with only about three feet of lead rope. Then they got the swing rope out from under her and untied the other one from her horns. All the while she stood quiet as a lamb, like she was meditating.

"Take it easy," says the extra hand. "You don't want to strain her."

"No," I says, putting the bus into low, "I don't want to—"

Right then she made a dive for the car and tried to climb into the rumble seat where I had two sacks of lime, a peck of oats, and a job lot of tools I had lately bought in town. She had got her front hoofs onto the rumble seat and it looked bad for the car, which is an old sport model and none too strong.

"Keep her out," I says to Harold. "We don't want her riding with us."

There was a cant hook in the rumble seat and Harold managed to yank it out. He shoved the end of it against her chest and she got off the car and tried to climb over the right fender. When she found she couldn't make it she headed off the other way, and the car nearly went into the ditch. I put the machine into second and for the next two minutes she did 'most everything an animal can do without twisting itself into knots. She reared, she bucked, side-stepped, swung from side to side, and played the devil with both fenders. Finally she fell down on her knees and I dragged her a dozen feet before I could stop.

"What this heifer seems to want is exercise," I says to Harold, who was beginning to look grim.

"I'll give it to her!" he says between his teeth, starting to get out.

"What the hell are you doing, Harold?"

"Going to lead her!"

"Don't be a fool! We'll borrow a horse off Jake Lentz down the road a piece and you can herd her back home. It'll be less wear and tear."

"I was fullback on the Ag. eleven and captain of the track team," he says with a stubborn look, "and I'm going to lead my cow home."

"Oke!" I says. "It's your cow."

While he was walking around the car I untied her halter rope, and thinking he would need some extra line to pay out in case of trouble, I tied onto it a length of stout hemp rope, about thirty feet, that was tucked away in the rumble seat. Mabel never made a move. She was still on her knees, like she was praying.

"I'll stay behind you, Harold," I says as I passed over the rope to him, "and if she starts any monkey business, I'll be right there to help out."

Harold went over and gave her a kick and she scrambled to her feet sort of dazed. He began to pull her and she followed along like all the spirit had left her.

"See?" he calls out. "All she needs is the right handling."

He hadn't no more than got the words out of his mouth when that cow got into motion, and she had only one speed, which was high. She spun Harold around and the line started running through his hand like a hawser on a big boat but he had sense enough to wrap the end of it twice around his fist. Or maybe it wasn't such good sense either, for when the line was all paid out he started traveling. I guess he must have been a pretty good runner at college for he sure made tracks, sometimes not hitting the ground for a yard or so. When I caught up with them, my speedometer showed they was going exactly fifteen miles an hour. The road here ran straight for a half a mile before turning off to our places and for the first quarter Mabel didn't slacken a mite. Then she eased up a bit, to about twelve.

"Whoopee!" I yells. "Stick to her, kid! She's a good pacemaker!"

Harold must have begun to lose some of his wind because I noticed he was maneuvering. The orchards came down close to the road at this point, so that some of the trees hung over it. Harold was trying to pick up enough speed on the heifer so's he could swing off and take a turn around a tree with the line and bring her hard to. But every time he'd make for a tree and get part way around, the cow would be so much ahead that he'd be jerked back around and have to try for another tree further down. I saw he wasn't going to make it that way and for fear he'd go on past the turn I stepped on the gas and shot around them, and at the turn I swung the bus sideways, blocking the road. For a minute I thought Mabel was going to jump right over the car, but I yelled bloody Moses and she swerved off down the home stretch. At Harold's gate I pulled the same trick, and so headed her into his barnyard. In another five minutes the two of us had hauled her into the barn and had her tied tight to a post. Then Harold sat down on the manure pile, looking all in.

"Well, boy," I says, "she's beginning to know her master."

After breathing hard for a few minutes he managed to gasp out, "And believe me, she's going to!"

When he had rested a while we came back on up to my place to get some liniment for Mabel's knees that had been badly skinned and Minnie, my old woman, thinking he looked hungry, passed him out a platter of doughnuts and a bowl of applesauce. He ate them with relish and drank three cups of strong coffee while he explained a new spray formula for Woolly Aphis. About half-past ten we came back down, as I had volunteered to hold Mabel while he bandaged the knees. I wasn't sure but that we would have to hobble her if she was anything like she had been. He was talking about planting nasturtiums in the front yard when we got to the barn.

"Nasturtiums in a center bed and patches of Golden Glow and maybe phlox—"

"It looks to me as if your barn door got kicked off its hinges, Harold," I says.

The barn was pretty old, a good ten years older than the house, and the barn door was lying flat and one plank had been knocked out of it. We looked inside but there was no Mabel. No cow and no post, either. The post she had been tied to was not a part of the frame; it was just a brace and probably not even toe-nailed. Anyway, it was gone. We looked down the wagon road that led to the meadow and we could see a furrow where she had dragged the post.

"She's a mighty strong and vigorous heifer you got, Harold," I says, "but she won't get far with that post. It's as good as a man could do to lift it, let alone a cow. Maybe it's just as well she took the post, she'll learn what it is to go pulling a man's barn apart. About the time she hits a stump or a ditch with that post, she's going to want to come back and be a nice cow."

Harold snorted. "I'll teach her to be a nice cow!" he growled.

"Is that your 'phone ringing?" I asked. Harold listened.

"Three rings—that's mine! Maybe somebody has caught her. Jake Lentz's place comes down to mine on the other side of the meadow. Maybe Jake has caught her and wants me to come and get her."

"I expect anybody that got her *would* want you to come and fetch her," I suggested.

"I'll go find out," he says.

He was gone quite a spell so I had time to smoke a pipeful, setting on the manure pile. I was thinking about the nature of cows in general, and how if they get off on the wrong hoof they are likely to run wild, like this one, same as some women folks, when he come running down, looking sort of wild-eyed and troubled.

"What's up?" I asks.

"Well! I don't know—damned funny! I can't make head nor tail of it. I guess I'm going nuts or else I didn't hear right."

"Has Jake got the cow?"

"No, but he saw her passing through his orchard. She took down a whole row of young Winter Bananas."

"That's no loss, Harold. The Winter Banana is mighty poor apple. It won't keep and it's losing out in the open market. Now, I had a patch of Winter Bananas that I yanked out—"

"He saw her and ran out of his house and started after her, yelling. She stopped and he thought he had her. He says she couldn't budge that post, walking. But then she made a run and got going with it again at a dead gallop, smashing a row of Delicious—"

"That's too bad! The Delicious is a first-rate fruit. Now, I took down a load—"

"And then she disappeared into the Larson place next to his."

"Well, now that's good! She'll never get across the Larson place. Too much barb-wire fences. They'll stop her! Did you call Larson?"

"Yes, I called Larson, and he said he'd go right out and take a look to see what she'd damaged, and—" Again that queer look came over him and he sort of choked out, "after a few minutes Larson rang me back and said—and said . . . that she was up in one of his trees!"

"Aw now, Harold! Larson was just kidding you. Larson is a great kidder."

"He didn't sound like he was kidding. He sounded mad. He said, 'You come quick and take your goddamn cow out of my tree before she spoil him!' "

"So he was mad, eh? He shouldn't get mad about a thing like that! It couldn't be a very big tree if she was up in it."

" 'But that's it!' Larson said. 'That cow she's up in my biggest, best walnut tree. Up clear in the top!' "

I got up off the manure pile. "Look here, Harold," I says, "I don't know which of you is lying or is nuts, but we might as well go and find out. I can swallow anything but about a cow in a walnut tree. Why, I know those walnut trees of Larson and nary one is less than thirty feet tall, and it ain't easy to climb a walnut tree, even for a man, without a ladder. And I *know* that cow didn't go up no ladder—not with that post tied to her! Come on, let's go!"

The trail of Mabel was easy enough to follow. It went down into the meadow and then across the meadow to where she'd taken a panel out of the snake fence on the other side. Then we came into Lentz's orchard and we could see where she'd laid down a row of young Winter Bananas, just as if she'd planned to do it—which, no doubt, she had.

"They're not hurt bad," I says, "just scraped on one side, and they'll all have to be staked again."

We also saw where she'd barked the row of Delicious. She had run straight down the row, figuring, I guess that she couldn't turn a corner with that post. Right at the end of the row Lentz's orchard stopped, and all at once I had a hunch about the walnut tree. The orchards in our valley are all laid out on "benches," and some of them mark the boundary lines. Now Jake's place was on a bench lying about thirty feet on the average above Larson's place. It dropped off so sudden that there was just a narrow fringe of alder thicket between the upper orchard and the lower one. Larson was an economical Swede and he had planted right up to the line. Apples wouldn't do any good so close to a high bank so he had put in a row of walnuts and they generally brought in a paying crop.

When we pushed through the thicket we saw Mabel. She was astraddle of a crotch in the walnut tree and for once her head was hanging low, for the halter rope was still attached to the post; it was let out as far as it would go, and the end of the post just barely touched the ground. If the rope had been six inches shorter, Mabel would have broke her neck.

Larson was standing under the tree and when he saw us he began to yell, "Take her out! Do you think I want a cow in my best walnut tree? Do you want to make a fool of me, letting a cow in my tree?"

"Shut up!" I yells back. "You'll make her nervous!"

Jake Lentz had come up and no sooner saw what a fix Mabel was in than he said, "Why, that's nothing! I got a hog out of my sixty-foot well once! Don't cut her halter rope till I get back or she'll start to flounder."

He ambled off and after a while came back with his tractor and a lot of heavy ropes and straps. I climbed into the tree and rigged her out in a sort of harness, slung a strand over a higher limb to hold her from hitting against the bank, then Harold cut the halter rope and Lentz drew her out with his tractor. It took a couple of hours and didn't bother nobody much except Larson, who kept dancing around and cursing underneath the tree.

When Harold unhitched her finally and began to lead her home, she followed along as meek and subdued as any cow.

"How about them trees, and the hire of my tractor, and my own time?" Jake asked.

"Don't worry," says Harold, "I'll come over and work it all out."

"Looks to me, Harold," I says, "as if you was doing more work for that cow than she is for you."

"Never mind," he says, stubborn again, "I'll work it out of her!"

He began working it out of her the next morning and kept it up every day for the next three weeks. I was so busy with bud spraying I didn't have a chance to get over for about a week but I would see him go past with her around 6 A.M. and come back nearly an hour later. The first three mornings she led him, but after he got into training form he led her. And I'm saying, they *traveled!* There was a stretch of road the opposite way from Morrison's, about two mile and a quarter. He told me afterward he'd let her hit her stride the whole way down, then give her five minutes to catch her wind, turn her around and head her back. He didn't get much milk—about a quart a day—but he got plenty of exercise. You'd think Mabel would tire of it. If she did, she didn't give any sign, and he would have to hobble her hind legs when he turned her out in the meadow.

At that, she learned to manage her hind quarters so she could get around, with a motion something like a hobby horse. The funny thing was, so far as milking went, she was docile enough. Just as soon as Harold would set down on the old wobbly milking stool, she'd turn and look at him, contented and satisfied, and if she had been a cat she would have purred.

It came Sunday so I ambled over to see how Harold was making out. He was stirring up something in a big bowl that he said was going to be corn fritters but I told him my stomach was delicate and we fell to talking.

"How's the heifer, Harold?" I says.

"I don't give her any rest in the morning. First thing, I go down and give her a kick—"

"I mean Sadie. How are you and Sadie hitting it off?"

"Oh, Sadie's too high-toned for me. I called her up three times and she said she had a date each time. It's that lawyer, Murfree, from Portland. He's handling a couple of her dad's lawsuits and he's got a Cadillac. I was coming back from Lentz's Wednesday when they passed me, going lickety-split. Sadie didn't even wave. Well, if she gets him I guess she'll be coming into a little piece of jack. It's jake with me. I guess when I've put in three or four years on this place, I'll pick me a girl who doesn't set too much store by mere wealth."

"If Sadie's set her cap for Murfree, she's not going to win no prize studhorse. He's slicker 'n a whistle and slipperier than a greased pig. Wait till he puts in his bill to the old man. Maybe she won't fancy him so well."

"It makes no difference to me who she fancies," he says. I could see he didn't want to talk about Sadie so I changed the subject to water coring and dry rot. After he had stowed away his mess of corn fritters, or whatever they was, he said, "I want you to come down and see a little contrivance I've rigged up for Mabel. I found something in the barn that's going to improve her disposition a lot."

"A goad?"

"No, I don't believe in using harsh methods in handling a cow. They're like human beings, you have to analyze 'em psychologically, then treat their complexes."

"I've always used Glover's Horse Tonic," I says. "It works for cows the same as horses."

"I don't mean that sort of remedy, Pete. It's for what is wrong in their heads. Now take Mabel. She's got a complex on running. Maybe she was repressed when she was a calf and couldn't run. Now she just *has* to run. Well to treat that, you have to let her run as much as she wants, but you have to direct her running, 'channel' it, as they say."

"I don't know," I says, "about channeling a cow to run. I'd rather channel her to milk."

"That will come later," he says.

We got to the barn and he showed me what he had fixed up for Mabel. It was a racing sulky, all painted bright and new, in green, with red trimming on the wheels.

"By gorry!" I says. "You ain't going to hitch the heifer onto that rig, are you?"

"Sure as shooting!" he says. "And I've greased the wheels and oiled up the harness. I had to adjust the harness. The belly band had to be lengthened, and of course there's no bit. You can't drive a cow like you can a horse—no use trying! And she doesn't need a check rein. She runs with her head up." It was plain that he was mighty proud of his work.

"I'm not throwing a wet blanket on your project, Harold," I says, "but how do you aim to stop her or turn her?"

"I won't have to. If I'm right about this, she'll stop herself and turn around. She does it every morning now. I've conditioned her to do it and she'll keep on."

"I hope you're right, Harold," I says, "but you had better be ready to jump—in case she don't stay in condition."

"I'll tell you, Pete, I intend to try her out tomorrow. I'm pretty sure she'll work into it all right, but I'd like to have you down at the end of the stretch, and if she starts to go through the fence where the road turns, you could stop her with a pitchfork."

"I don't know about stopping her, but I'll be mighty glad to be there and tell you when to jump."

So the next morning I told Minnie I had to have an early breakfast on account of going up to the head-gate to see about the irrigation, and at quarter to six I was driving down to the turn. I hadn't been there five minutes and was just taking the first puff on the corncob when I saw them coming over the rise about a mile away. I will say this for Mabel, she had lots of style and no end of speed as a racer. She had as pretty a pace as any gelding that ever come down a track and she never broke her gait in the whole two miles. When they got nearer it was a fine sight, with the rising sun making the new-painted wheels all a glitter of whizzing spokes and Harold holding onto the reins, which was more for decoration than use as they was fastened onto the halter.

I had jumped from the car and had my pitchfork ready. For a minute I thought I'd have to go into action and was just getting ready to holler to Harold to jump when she pulled up so sudden that Harold went right out of his little seat and landed plumb on her back. He fell off as Mabel came to a dead halt. Then, without his saying a word, she turned around. Off she went again, quick as lightning, and Harold, being taken by surprise, stood there with his mouth open.

"Oh well," he says, "it's no use my trying to catch her. She'll run right to the barn."

"Harold," I says, "you sure have got confidence in that cow!"

"It isn't confidence in her," he says. "I just know my psychology."

"Harold," I says, "I hope Larson isn't getting home from one of his all-night jags. If that cow passes him the way she's going, he's going right into d.t.'s!"

You might think that Harold Peavey's fast cow would get noised about the neighborhood but there were several things in the way of it. For instance, the hour of day, which was either milking or breakfast time. Then, it was the season when everybody was in a rush to get the spring work done and the first spray on the trees. Mainly it was because Harold and I were the only ones on our road except a shack that hadn't been occupied in ten years, and then only partly, the owner having been a half-wit. I didn't see much of Harold myself except Sundays while Minnie was taking herself to the United Congregation Church and that would give me a little time to rest. I found out in May that he'd gone so far in his cow-training that he was able to cut down the morning workouts to three times a week without Mabel getting restless, and he was getting two quarts of rich milk a day. As for his orchard, I've seen worse. Considering the time he had to work out for his neighbors, training Mabel, and thinking about Sadie, he didn't do so bad for the first year. At any rate, he rubbed off a lot he'd learned down at the Ag.

Sadie I saw a couple of times when her old man and me was negotiating over a boar-pig. Once I says to her, "Sadie, that young Peavey sure is a hustler! He's getting his place into jim-dandy shape. Wouldn't surprise me none if he went wife-hunting one of these days."

"Well!" she said, tossing her mop of corn-silk hair. "Now that's news! I thought he was a born bachelor. I hope he gets one that likes to cook and scrub dirty clothes and tend chickens and garden, for I don't!"

"Oh I don't know," I says. "Some girls like it better working when there's a husky young buck on the place than riding with an old codger that's half mummy!"

"Are you telling *me?*" she says saucily. "Thanks for your kind advice, Mr. Crumm! I prefer roses!"

"Humph!" I says. "To me they looks prettier on the vine than wired up in a florist shop!"

Old man Morrison, while he was arguing over the boar-pig, said that Murfree had gone back to Portland but was coming down again in June when one of his cases came to trial.

By the time June come along Harold told me he had cut the driving to once a week. He said Mabel didn't like it but he had irrigation on his hands and was in the middle of cultivating the orchard and an acre of carrots. Besides he was deep in cookery, studying cookbooks, and trying his hand at Birds'-Nest Pudding, Aunty Phelps' Pie Crust, and such. I told Minnie he was looking peaked and she invited him to Sunday dinners.

One Sunday, the last week in June, Harold was at our place for dinner. While Minnie was putting the finishing touches to chicken with dumplings, he was pouring over the Sunday edition of the Tillamook Gazette.

"Say!" he said suddenly, sort of excited. "I see there's going to be big doings at Tillamook on Fourth of July."

"Always is. Parade and fireworks and speeches."

"And racing!"

"Yep! They open up the county fair grounds for some racing. But it ain't much. Just local talent. Still, there's some pretty fast horses in the county and sometimes you see quite a few fast heats. I remember last year—"

"Look here, Pete," he says, shoving the paper at me. "Read that and tell me what it says."

I took the paper and read, " 'Final Event. Free-for-all One Mile Race for Drivers. All classes of racers may be entered and any style gig. This classic event, for one heat only, takes a purse of $100. Entries accepted up to the last minute.' That," I says, "is the windup of the whole shebang. And what a sight it is! Plenty of fun, too. Usually a couple of wrecks and a few wheels lost. Now I remember the year the President stopped over—"

"Does it say anywhere in that announcement that the racers have got to be *horses?*"

I looked at Harold with my eyes bugged out. "Young feller," I says, "just what have you got on your mind?"

We kept the whole thing a dead secret. The rest was simple. I hooked the sulky on behind the Ford and drove over on July 3. We made a deal with Jake Lentz to take Mabel over in his truck the same day, telling him she had to be treated at the veterinary for milk fever. He was going over for a load of fertilizer anyway so he said he'd do it for $5, but we would have to get her back some other way.

It was a broiling hot day and Tillamook was jammed. There was a parade of Boy Scouts, firemen, and Knights of Pythias in uniforms that made them look sort of proud and desperate. There were plenty of speeches, ending up with a long one by Lawyer Murfree. He kept wiping his bald head with a silk handkerchief and talking about the Constitution till my throat went plumb dry and I had to find the nearest bar. We stayed there an hour or two drinking beers, then we ambled over to the fair grounds where

I'd parked the sulky in a shed off in a patch of fir near the track. Harold had brought Mabel over there and while they were running off the first heats he curry-combed her until she shone all over like a black silk purse.

"The only thing that worries me, Pete," he says, "is whether she'll stick to a circular road. She's used to a straightaway, but if I can get her next to the fence I know she'll follow it because there's a fence runs along our stretch back home, and she's conditioned to a fence. How long is the track?"

"It's an even mile. How'll you stop her when she passes the judges' stand?"

"Oh, that won't matter. If she runs beyond, it makes no difference. They can't disqualify her for going over the finish line a piece. Anyway, if she runs too far, I can make a jump from the seat and bull-dog her. I guess I could steer her by the horns if I had to."

"Well, Harold," I says, "I'll be rooting for you and her." I looked at my watch. It was a quarter to four and the free-for-all was scheduled at four sharp. "Guess we'd better hitch up," I says.

We hitched up, Harold took hold of the lead rope, and we pulled over toward the starting line. The grandstands were packed from top to bottom and about a thousand cars were parked around the track. The crowd was milling around so and raising such a hullabaloo over each entry, what with the various kinds of vehicles in the race, that they didn't hardly notice our entry till we pulled up before the judges' box. Then they busted loose plenty. Harold walked over, holding out a five-dollar bill, and says, "I'm entering my racer, Mabel."

One of the judges turned as red as a beet, like he was mad, and the other two began laughing fit to kill.

"You can't enter a cow!" says the red-faced one.

"Oh yes I can!" says Harold, cool as a cucumber. He had the announcement with him and handed it over to the judge. "Read that," he says, "and see if it says anything about disqualifying racing cows."

"I say, you can't enter that animal!" bellows Red-face. "This is no cattle show!"

Just then Judge Olney, whom I knew personal, pushed his way through and says, "What's the trouble?"

"This man," the other judge bawls, "is trying to enter a cow in the last race!"

"Well," says Olney politely, "why not?" He winked at the other two judges. "It's a free-for-all, isn't it?"

"That's right, judge," says one of the others. "I guess a good-looking cow like that one has as good a right to run as some of them nags out on the track, that look like they was ready for the bone-yard!"

The upshot was, that the judges voted, two to one, to allow Mabel to run. Harold filled out a card and led her over to the starting line. If you had looked at her then, you would have said she was just getting ready to be milked, she was that docile. The rest of the entries was snorting and neighing and prancing, and the drivers was all yelling "Whoa!" or "Git up, there!" but Harold climbed into his seat and said nothing, and Mabel stood with her front hoofs just touching the line, as if she had her mind on green fodder.

One of the judges took a megaphone and hollered, "Now, men, there won't be no false starts. When the gun goes, you just lick in to it, and the first one home wins!"

Then the starter fired his gun and they started off. Mabel was three places away from the inside fence and for a minute I didn't think she'd start at all. She took a few short steps, then she sort of ambled for about ten yards, and finally she settled down to her pace. By that time the rest of the field was a good twenty-five yards ahead of her and there was nobody between her and the fence. She turned right in and stuck to it from then on. At the first turn the other drivers was still a good bit ahead of Harold, but the crowd was yelling like mad, throwing up their hats and ice cream cones, and leaning on each other laughing. On the far side of the track she began to pick up on them. At the other turn she had passed all but three of the horses, one of them being a big gray mare, a trotter, and in the professional class. I heard that she belonged to Murfree. Her name was Peaches-and-Cream, and they said Murfree was trying her out here before sending her south to the big tracks. Harold told me afterward that at the turn Peaches-and-Cream either caught a whiff of Mabel or heard the sound she made, which was a sort of fierce "moo!" At any rate, Peaches-and-Cream suddenly broke. She reared and jumped sideways, and Mabel passed her in a cloud of dust while the crowd went mad.

They came down the home stretch, Mabel running neck and neck with a sorrel gelding. That made me feel pretty good for in the first two minutes of the race I had placed two five-dollar bets on Mabel at ten to one.

She pulled away from the gelding and came over the line with three yards to spare. I guess you never heard such a rumpus!

When the yelling died down a little, the man with the megaphone yelled, "Mabel wins first place! Grand Mogul, second! Peaches-and-Cream, third!"

But Mabel was still going. If anything, she picked up a little speed on the second lap. I'm telling you, that was a cow! Nobody on the track or in the grandstand thought she'd keep up more than half way around, but she did. The finish line was like it is after a race. There was still gigs and sulkies standing around and little crowds milling around them, all talking and arguing when somebody hollered, "Look out! Here comes that cow!"

She drove through them like a whirlwind, stopped dead just beyond the judges' stand, turned around, and started back. By that time there was wild horses all over the place. Drivers was tangled up every way, and the loafers on the track broke and ran for cover like a flock of quail. When she come around the reverse way, some misguided fool, thinking the cow had gone loco, ran out with a horse blanket and tried to stop her by waving the blanket.

She hit the blanket square and it settled down over her and

Harold but she kept right on going. I guess with the blanket over her head she must have lost her direction for she made a beeline straight off the track, taking out a section of guard rail, and headed for the cars that were parked all over the grounds. I heard a crash and started running.

When I got up where it happened there was a crowd standing around looking at Harold. He was sitting on top of a limousine, wrapped in a blanket; one of the shafts of the sulky had gone through the top and the other had busted off. Mabel wasn't nowhere.

He stuck his head up out of the blanket, looking sort of dazed, and asked, "Did we win?"

"Hands down!" I yelled, reaching up to help him down.

On the way back home, Harold was feeling pretty blue about losing Mabel. We had traced her as far as the edge of town but we couldn't get any word of her after that.

"Well, Harold," I says, to cheer him up, "she ain't a total loss! After all, you paid $34 for her and she brought in a hundred-buck prize, that leaves a good profit even deducting the damage to Jake Lentz's orchard."

"Yeah?" he says gloomily. "Didn't you hear that circus fellow offer me five hundred on the spot for her?"

About five o'clock in the afternoon of the fourth day after the race, Harold come running over to my place. I could see right off he was all steamed up about something.

"She's come home!" he panted. "Walked right into the barn and stood in her stall, waiting to be milked. She looks pretty worn down and she didn't give more than half a pint of milk, but hell! she's no milker, anyway; she's a racer! I'll fix up the old sulky, break her in again, and sell her for five hundred!"

Well, Harold went to work on her and I'll say he worked hard. He let her rest up two days, then he hitched her up, and took her out for a spin. But she wouldn't spin, no sir, not even a slow trot! She wouldn't do any more than an ordinary cow! He fooled around with her a while and I came out to help but it wasn't any good; she'd turn around and look at us, all meek and gentle, like she was asking what in the world we were up to, and then she'd start, the way cows do, at a walk so slow you could pick daisies and keep up with her! Just seemed like the old racing spirit was gone. After a week of trying, Harold gave up.

"I'm beaten," he said, "and plumb disgusted! She don't milk and she don't run; I guess I'll have to beef her!"

Luckily, while he was making up his mind and too busy to take her down to the butcher, she began to show signs of being in the family way. In another few weeks it was plain enough she was going to calve. Well, we talked it over and decided that on the way back from Tillamook she must have dawdled.

"I guess," said Harold, "her racing days are over!"

The piebald bull calf, when it came, was as pretty as a picture and built like a fawn. At first Harold thought of training it to be a racer like its mother and maybe breeding a strain of fast cows but I argued that after that race they'd never let another bovine enter a track with horses, so he gave the calf to Sadie, which was a good thing because Harold for all his studying hadn't really learned to cook.

He's got other cows now but they keep Mabel for sentiment.

The Short Happy Life of Francis Macomber

ERNEST HEMINGWAY (1898–)

IT WAS NOW lunch time and they were all sitting under the double green fly of the dining tent pretending that nothing had happened.

"Will you have lime juice or lemon squash?" Macomber asked.

"I'll have a gimlet," Robert Wilson told him.

"I'll have a gimlet too. I need something," Macomber's wife said.

"I suppose it's the thing to do," Macomber agreed. "Tell him to make three gimlets."

The mess boy had started them already, lifting the bottles out of the canvas cooling bags that sweated wet in the wind that blew through the trees that shaded the tents.

"What had I ought to give them?" Macomber asked.

"A quid would be plenty," Wilson told him. "You don't want to spoil them."

"Will the headman distribute it?"

"Absolutely."

Francis Macomber had, half an hour before, been carried to his tent from the edge of the camp in triumph on the arms and shoulders of the cook, the personal boys, the skinner and the porters. The gun-bearers had taken no part in the demonstration. When the native boys put him down at the door of his tent, he had shaken all their hands, received their congratulations, and then gone into the tent and sat on the bed until his wife came in.

She did not speak to him when she came in and he left the tent at once to wash his face and hands in the portable wash basin outside and go over to the dining tent to sit in a comfortable canvas chair in the breeze and the shade.

"You've got your lion," Robert Wilson said to him, "and a damned fine one too."

Mrs. Macomber looked at Wilson quickly. She was an extremely handsome and well-kept woman of the beauty and social position which had, five years before, commanded five thousand dollars as the price of endorsing, with photographs, a beauty product which she had never used. She had been married to Francis Macomber for eleven years.

"He is a good lion, isn't he?" Macomber said. His wife looked at him now. She looked at both these men as though she had never seen them before.

One, Wilson, the white hunter, she knew she had never truly seen before. He was about middle height with sandy hair, a stubby mustache, a very red face and extremely cold blue eyes with faint white wrinkles at the corners that grooved merrily when he smiled. He smiled at her now and she looked away from his face at the way his shoulders sloped in the loose tunic he wore with the four big cartridges held in loops where the left breast pocket should have been, at his big brown hands, his old slacks, his very dirty boots and back to his red face again. She noticed where the baked red of his face stopped in a white line that marked the circle left by his Stetson hat that hung now from one of the pegs of the tent pole.

"Well, here's to the lion," Robert Wilson said. He smiled at her again and, not smiling, she looked curiously at her husband.

Francis Macomber was very tall, very well built if you did not mind that length of bone, dark, his hair cropped like an oarsman, rather thin-lipped, and was considered handsome. He was dressed in the same sort of safari clothes that Wilson wore except that his were new, he was thirty-five years old, kept himself very fit, was good at court games, had a number of big-game fishing records, and had just shown himself, very publicly, to be a coward.

"Here's to the lion," he said. "I can't ever thank you for what you did."

Margaret, his wife, looked away from him and back to Wilson.

"Let's not talk about the lion," she said.

Wilson looked over at her without smiling and now she smiled at him.

"It's been a very strange day," she said. "Hadn't you ought to put your hat on even under the canvas at noon? You told me that, you know."

"Might put it on," said Wilson.

"You know you have a very red face, Mr. Wilson," she told him and smiled again.

"Drink," said Wilson.

"I don't think so," she said. "Francis drinks a great deal, but his face is never red."

"It's red today," Macomber tried a joke.

"No," said Margaret. "It's mine that's red today. But Mr. Wilson's is always red."

"Must be racial," said Wilson. "I say, you wouldn't like to drop my beauty as a topic, would you?"

"I've just started on it."

"Let's chuck it," said Wilson.

"Conversation is going to be so difficult," Margaret said.

"Don't be silly, Margot," her husband said.

"No difficulty," Wilson said. "Got a damn fine lion."

Margot looked at them both and they both saw that she was going to cry. Wilson had seen it coming for a long time and he dreaded it. Macomber was past dreading it.

"I wish it hadn't happened. Oh, I wish it hadn't happened," she said and started for her tent. She made no noise of crying but they could see that her shoulders were shaking under the rose-colored, sun-proofed shirt she wore.

"Women upset," said Wilson to the tall man. "Amounts to nothing. Strain on the nerves and one thing'n another."

"No," said Macomber. "I suppose that I rate that for the rest of my life now."

"Nonsense. Let's have a spot of the giant killer," said Wilson. "Forget the whole thing. Nothing to it anyway."

"We might try," said Macomber. "I won't forget what you did for me though."

"Nothing," said Wilson. "All nonsense."

So they sat there in the shade where the camp was pitched under some wide-topped acacia trees with a boulder-strewn cliff behind them, and a stretch of grass that ran to the bank of a boulder-filled stream in front with forest beyond it, and drank their just-cool lime drinks and avoided one another's eyes while the boys set the table for lunch. Wilson could tell that the boys all knew about it now and when he saw Macomber's personal boy looking curiously at his master while he was putting dishes on the table he snapped at him in Swahili. The boy turned away with his face blank.

"What were you telling him?" Macomber asked.

"Nothing. Told him to look alive or I'd see he got about fifteen of the best."

"What's that? Lashes?"

"It's quite illegal," Wilson said. "You're supposed to fine them."

"Do you still have them whipped?"

"Oh, yes. They could raise a row if they chose to complain. But they don't. They prefer it to the fines."

"How strange!" said Macomber.

"Not strange, really," Wilson said. "Which would you rather do? Take a good birching or lose your pay?"

Then he felt embarrassed at asking it and before Macomber could answer he went on, "We all take a beating every day, you know, one way or another."

This was no better. "Good God," he thought. "I am a diplomat, aren't I?"

"Yes, we take a beating," said Macomber, still not looking at him. "I'm awfully sorry about that lion business. It doesn't have to go any further, does it? I mean no one will hear about it, will they?"

"You mean will I tell it at the Mathaiga Club?" Wilson looked at him now coldly. He had not expected this. So he's a bloody four-letter man as well as a bloody coward, he thought. I rather liked him too until today. But how is one to know about an American?

"No," said Wilson. "I'm a professional hunter. We never talk about our clients. You can be quite easy on that. It's supposed to be bad form to ask us not to talk though."

He had decided now that to break would be much easier. He would eat, then, by himself and could read a book with his meals. They would eat by themselves. He would see them through the safari on a very formal basis—what was it the French called it? Distinguished consideration—and it would be a damn sight easier than having to go through this emotional trash. He'd insult him and make a good clean break. Then he could read a book with his meals and he'd still be drinking their whisky. That was the phrase for it when a safari went bad. You ran into another white hunter and you asked, "How is everything going?" and he answered, "Oh, I'm still drinking their whisky," and you knew everything had gone to pot.

"I'm sorry," Macomber said and looked at him with his American face that would stay adolescent until it became middle-aged, and Wilson noted his crew-cropped hair, fine eyes only faintly shifty, good nose, thin lips and handsome jaw. "I'm sorry I didn't realize that. There are lots of things I don't know."

So what could he do, Wilson thought. He was all ready to break it off quickly and neatly and here the beggar was apologizing after he had just insulted him. He made one more attempt. "Don't worry about me talking," he said. "I have a living to make. You know in Africa no woman ever misses her lion and no white man ever bolts."

"I bolted like a rabbit," Macomber said.

Now what in hell were you going to do about a man who talked like that, Wilson wondered.

Wilson looked at Macomber with his flat, blue, machine-gunner's eyes and the other smiled back at him. He had a pleasant smile if you did not notice how his eyes showed when he was hurt.

"Maybe I can fix it up on buffalo," he said. "We're after them next, aren't we?"

"In the morning if you like," Wilson told him. Perhaps he had been wrong. This was certainly the way to take it. You most certainly could not tell a damned thing about an American. He was all for Macomber again. If you could forget the morning. But, of course, you couldn't. The morning had been about as bad as they come.

"Here comes the Memsahib," he said. She was walking over from her tent looking refreshed and cheerful and quite lovely. She had a very perfect oval face, so perfect that you expected her to be stupid. But she wasn't stupid, Wilson thought, no, not stupid.

"How is the beautiful red-faced Mr. Wilson? Are you feeling better, Francis, my pearl?"

"Oh, much," said Macomber.

"I've dropped the whole thing," she said, sitting down at the table. "What importance is there to whether Francis is any good at killing lions? That's not his trade. That's Mr. Wilson's trade. Mr. Wilson is really very impressive killing anything. You do kill anything, don't you?"

"Oh, anything," said Wilson. "Simply anything." They are, he thought, the hardest in the world; the hardest, the cruelest, the most predatory and the most attractive and their men have softened or gone to pieces nervously as they have hardened. Or is it that they pick men they can handle? They can't know that much at the age they marry, he thought. He was grateful that he had gone through his education on American women before now because this was a very attractive one.

"We're going after buff in the morning," he told her.

"I'm coming," she said.

"No, you're not."

"Oh, yes, I am. Mayn't I, Francis?"

"Why not stay in camp?"

"Not for anything," she said. "I wouldn't miss something like today for anything."

When she left, Wilson was thinking, when she went off to cry, she seemed a hell of a fine woman. She seemed to understand, to realize, to be hurt for him and for herself and to know how things really stood. She is away for twenty minutes and now she is back, simply enamelled in that American female cruelty. They are the damnedest women. Really the damnedest.

"We'll put on another show for you tomorrow," Francis Macomber said.

"You're not coming," Wilson said.

"You're very mistaken," she told him. "And I want *so* to see you perform again. You were lovely this morning. That is if blowing things' heads off is lovely."

"Here's the lunch," said Wilson. "You're very merry, aren't you?"

"Why not? I didn't come out here to be dull."

"Well, it hasn't been dull," Wilson said. He could see the boulders in the river and the high bank beyond with the trees and he remembered the morning.

"Oh, no," she said. "It's been charming. And tomorrow. You don't know how I look forward to tomorrow."

"That's eland he's offering you," Wilson said.

"They're the big cowy things that jump like hares, aren't they?"

"I suppose that describes them," Wilson said.

"It's very good meat," Macomber said.

"Did you shoot it, Francis?" she asked.

"Yes."

"They're not dangerous, are they?"

"Only if they fall on you," Wilson told her.

"I'm so glad."

"Why not let up on the bitchery just a little, Margot," Macomber said, cutting the eland steak and putting some mashed potato, gravy and carrot on the down-turned fork that tined through the piece of meat.

"I suppose I could," she said, "since you put it so prettily."

"Tonight we'll have champagne for the lion," Wilson said. "It's a bit too hot at noon."

"Oh, the lion," Margot said. "I'd forgotten the lion!"

So, Robert Wilson thought to himself, she *is* giving him a ride, isn't she? Or do you suppose that's her idea of putting up a good show? How should a woman act when she discovers her husband is a bloody coward? She's damn cruel but they're all cruel. They govern, of course, and to govern one has to be cruel sometimes. Still, I've seen enough of their damn terrorism.

"Have some more eland," he said to her politely.

That afternoon, late, Wilson and Macomber went out in the motor car with the native driver and the two gun-bearers. Mrs. Macomber stayed in the camp. It was too hot to go out, she said, and she was going with them in the early morning. As they drove off Wilson saw her standing under the big tree, looking pretty rather than beautiful in her faintly rosy khaki, her dark hair drawn back off her forehead and gathered in a knot low on her neck, her face as fresh, he thought, as though she were in England. She waved to them as the car went off through the swale of high grass and curved around through the trees into the small hills of orchard bush.

In the orchard bush they found a herd of impala, and leaving the car they stalked one old ram with long, wide-spread horns and Macomber killed it with a very creditable shot that knocked the buck down at a good two hundred yards and sent the herd off bounding wildly and leaping over one another's backs in long, leg-drawn-up leaps as unbelievable and as floating as those one makes sometimes in dreams.

"That was a good shot," Wilson said. "They're a small target."

"Is it a worth-while head?" Macomber asked.

"It's excellent," Wilson told him. "You shoot like that and you'll have no trouble."

"Do you think we'll find buffalo tomorrow?"

"There's a good chance of it. They feed out early in the morning and with luck we may catch them in the open."

"I'd like to clear away that lion business," Macomber said. "It's not very pleasant to have your wife see you do something like that."

I should think it would be even more unpleasant to do it, Wilson thought, wife or no wife, or to talk about it having done it. But he said, "I wouldn't think about that any more. Any one could be upset by his first lion. That's all over."

But that night after dinner and a whisky and soda by the fire before going to bed, as Francis Macomber lay on his cot with the mosquito bar over him and listened to the night noises it was not all over. It was neither all over nor was it beginning. It was there exactly as it happened with some parts of it indelibly emphasized and he was miserably ashamed at it. But more than shame he felt cold, hollow fear in him. The fear was still there like a cold slimy hollow in all the emptiness where once his confidence had been and it made him feel sick. It was still there with him now.

It had started the night before when he had wakened and heard the lion roaring somewhere up along the river. It was a deep sound and at the end there were sort of coughing grunts that made him seem just outside the tent, and when Francis Macomber woke in the night to hear it he was afraid. He could hear his wife breathing quietly, asleep. There was no one to tell he was afraid, nor to be afraid with him, and, lying alone, he did not know the Somali proverb that says a brave man is always frightened three times by a lion; when he first sees his track, when he first hears him roar and when he first confronts him. Then while they were eating breakfast by lantern light out in the dining tent, before the sun was up, the lion roared again and Francis thought he was just at the edge of camp.

"Sounds like an old-timer," Robert Wilson said, looking up from his kippers and coffee. "Listen to him cough."

"Is he very close?"

"A mile or so up the stream."

"Will we see him?"

"We'll have a look."

"Does his roaring carry that far? It sounds as though he were right in camp."

"Carries a hell of a long way," said Robert Wilson. "It's strange the way it carries. Hope he's a shootable cat. The boys said there was a very big one about here."

"If I get a shot, where should I hit him," Macomber asked, "to stop him?"

"In the shoulders," Wilson said. "In the neck if you can make it. Shoot for bone. Break him down."

"I hope I can place it properly," Macomber said.

"You shoot very well," Wilson told him. "Take your time. Make sure of him. The first one in is the one that counts."

"What range will it be?"

"Can't tell. Lion has something to say about that. Won't shoot unless it's close enough so you can make sure."

"At under a hundred yards?" Macomber asked.

Wilson looked at him quickly.

"Hundred's about right. Might have to take him a bit under. Shouldn't chance a shot at much over that. A hundred's a decent range. You can hit him wherever you want at that. Here comes the Memsahib."

"Good morning," she said. "Are we going after that lion?"

"As soon as you deal with your breakfast," Wilson said. "How are you feeling?"

"Marvellous," she said. "I'm very excited."

"I'll just go and see that everything is ready," Wilson went off. As he left the lion roared again.

"Noisy beggar," Wilson said. "We'll put a stop to that."

"What's the matter, Francis?" his wife asked him.

"Nothing," Macomber said.

"Yes, there is," she said. "What are you upset about?"

"Nothing," he said.

"Tell me," she looked at him. "Don't you feel well?"

"It's that damned roaring," he said. "It's been going on all night, you know."

"Why didn't you wake me," she said. "I'd love to have heard it."

"I've got to kill the damned thing," Macomber said, miserably.

"Well, that's what you're out here for, isn't it?"

"Yes. But I'm nervous. Hearing the thing roar gets on my nerves."

"Well then, as Wilson said, kill him and stop his roaring."

"Yes, darling," said Francis Macomber. "It sounds easy, doesn't it?"

"You're not afraid, are you?"

"Of course not. But I'm nervous from hearing him roar all night."

"You'll kill him marvellously," she said. "I know you will. I'm awfully anxious to see it."

"Finish your breakfast and we'll be starting."

"It's not light yet," she said. "This is a ridiculous hour."

Just then the lion roared in a deep-chested moaning, suddenly guttural, ascending vibration that seemed to shake the air and ended in a sigh and a heavy, deep-chested grunt.

"He sounds almost here," Macomber's wife said.

"My God," said Macomber. "I hate that damned noise."

"It's very impressive."

"Impressive. It's frightful."

Robert Wilson came up then carrying his short, ugly, shockingly big-bored .505 Gibbs and grinning.

"Come on," he said. "Your gun-bearer has your Springfield and the big gun. Everything's in the car. Have you solids?"

"Yes."

"I'm ready," Mrs. Macomber said.

"Must make him stop that racket," Wilson said. "You get in front. The Memsahib can sit back here with me."

They climbed into the motor car and, in the gray first daylight, moved off up the river through the trees. Macomber opened the breech of his rifle and saw he had metal-cased bullets, shut the bolt and put the rifle on safety. He saw his hand was trembling. He felt in his pocket for more cartridges and moved his fingers over the cartridges in the loops of his tunic front. He turned back to where Wilson sat in the rear seat of the doorless, box-bodied motor car beside his wife, them both grinning with excitement, and Wilson leaned forward and whispered,

"See the birds dropping. Means the old boy has left his kill."

On the far bank of the stream Macomber could see, above the trees, vultures circling and plummeting down.

"Chances are he'll come to drink along here," Wilson whispered. "Before he goes to lay up. Keep an eye out."

They were driving slowly along the high bank of the stream which here cut deeply to its boulder-filled bed, and they wound in and out through big trees as they drove. Macomber was watching the opposite bank when he felt Wilson take hold of his arm. The car stopped.

"There he is," he heard the whisper. "Ahead and to the right. Get out and take him. He's a marvellous lion."

Macomber saw the lion now. He was standing almost broadside, his great head up and turned toward them. The early morning breeze that blew toward them was just stirring his dark mane, and the lion looked huge, silhouetted on the rise of bank in the gray morning light, his shoulders heavy, his barrel of a body bulking smoothly.

"How far is he?" asked Macomber, raising his rifle.

"About seventy-five. Get out and take him."

"Why not shoot from where I am?"

"You don't shoot them from cars," he heard Wilson saying in his ear. "Get out. He's not going to stay there all day."

Macomber stepped out of the curved opening at the side of the front seat, onto the step and down onto the ground. The lion still stood looking majestically and coolly toward this object that his eyes only showed in silhouette, bulking like some super-rhino. There was no man smell carried toward him and he watched the object, moving his great head a little from side to side. Then watching the object, not afraid, but hesitating before going down the bank to drink with such a thing opposite him, he saw a man figure detach itself from it and he turned his heavy head and swung away toward the cover of the trees as he heard a cracking crash and felt the slam of a .30–06 220-grain solid bullet that bit his flank and ripped in sudden hot scalding nausea through his stomach. He trotted, heavy, big-footed, swinging wounded full-bellied, through the trees toward the tall grass and cover, and the crash came again to go past him ripping the air apart. Then it crashed again and he felt the blow as it hit his lower ribs and ripped on through, blood sudden hot and frothy in his mouth, and he galloped toward the high grass where he could crouch and not be seen and make them bring the crashing thing close enough so he could make a rush and get the man that held it.

Macomber had not thought how the lion felt as he got out of the car. He only knew his hands were shaking and as he walked away from the car it was almost impossible for him to make his legs move. They were stiff in the thighs, but he could feel the muscles fluttering. He raised the rifle, sighted on the junction of the lion's head and shoulders and pulled the trigger. Nothing happened though he pulled until he thought his finger would break. Then he knew he had the safety on and as he lowered the rifle to move the safety over he moved another frozen pace forward, and the lion seeing his silhouette now clear of the silhouette of the car, turned and started off at a trot, and, as Macomber fired, he heard a whunk that meant that the bullet was home; but the lion kept on going. Macomber shot again and every one saw the bullet throw a spout of dirt beyond the trotting lion. He shot again, remembering to lower his aim, and they all heard the bullet hit, and the lion went into a gallop and was in the tall grass before he had the bolt pushed forward.

Macomber stood there feeling sick at his stomach, his hands that held the Springfield still cocked, shaking, and his wife and Robert Wilson were standing by him. Beside him too were the two gun-bearers chattering in Wakamba.

"I hit him," Macomber said. "I hit him twice."

"You gut-shot him and you hit him somewhere forward," Wilson said without enthusiasm. The gun-bearers looked very grave. They were silent now.

"You may have killed him," Wilson went on. "We'll have to wait a while before we go in to find out."

"What do you mean?"

"Let him get sick before we follow him up."

"Oh," said Macomber.

"He's a hell of a fine lion," Wilson said cheerfully. "He's gotten into a bad place though."

"Why is it bad?"

"Can't see him until you're on him."

"Oh," said Macomber.

"Come on," said Wilson. "The Memsahib can stay here in the car. We'll go to have a look at the blood spoor."

"Stay here, Margot," Macomber said to his wife. His mouth was very dry and it was hard for him to talk.

"Why?" she asked.

"Wilson says to."

"We're going to have a look," Wilson said. "You stay here. You can see even better from here."

"All right."

Wilson spoke in Swahili to the driver. He nodded and said, "Yes, Bwana."

Then they went down the steep bank and across the stream,

climbing over and around the boulders and up the other bank, pulling up by some projecting roots, and along it until they found where the lion had been trotting when Macomber first shot. There was dark blood on the short grass that the gun-bearers pointed out with grass stems, and that ran away behind the river bank trees.

"What do we do?" asked Macomber.

"Not much choice," said Wilson. "We can't bring the car over. Bank's too steep. We'll let him stiffen up a bit and then you and I'll go in and have a look for him."

"Can't we set the grass on fire?" Macomber asked.

"Too green."

"Can't we send beaters?"

Wilson looked at him appraisingly. "Of course we can," he said. "But it's just a touch murderous. You see we know the lion's wounded. You can drive an unwounded lion—he'll move on ahead of a noise—but a wounded lion's going to charge. You can't see him until you're right on him. He'll make himself perfectly flat in cover you wouldn't think would hide a hare. You can't very well send boys in there to that sort of a show. Somebody bound to get mauled."

"What about the gun-bearers?"

"Oh, they'll go with us. It's their *shauri*. You see, they signed on for it. They don't look too happy though, do they?"

"I don't want to go in there," said Macomber. It was out before he knew he'd said it.

"Neither do I," said Wilson very cheerily. "Really no choice though." Then, as an afterthought, he glanced at Macomber and saw suddenly how he was trembling and the pitiful look on his face.

"You don't have to go in, of course," he said. "That's what I'm hired for, you know. That's why I'm so expensive."

"You mean you'd go in by yourself? Why not leave him there?"

Robert Wilson, whose entire occupation had been with the lion and the problem he presented, and who had not been thinking about Macomber except to note that he was rather windy, suddenly felt as though he had opened the wrong door in a hotel and seen something shameful.

"What do you mean?"

"Why not just leave him?"

"You mean pretend to ourselves he hasn't been hit?"

"No. Just drop it."

"It isn't done."

"Why not?"

"For one thing, he's certain to be suffering. For another, some one else might run onto him."

"I see."

"But you don't have to have anything to do with it."

"I'd like to," Macomber said. "I'm just scared, you know."

"I'll go ahead when we go in," Wilson said, "with Kongoni tracking. You keep behind me and a little to one side. Chances are we'll hear him growl. If we see him we'll both shoot. Don't worry about anything. I'll keep you backed up. As a matter of fact, you know, perhaps you'd better not go. It might be much better. Why don't you go over and join the Memsahib while I just get it over with?"

"No, I want to go."

"All right," said Wilson. "But don't go in if you don't want to. This is my *shauri* now, you know."

"I want to go," said Macomber.

They sat under a tree and smoked.

"Want to go back and speak to the Memsahib while we're waiting?" Wilson asked.

"No."

"I'll just step back and tell her to be patient."

"Good," said Macomber. He sat there, sweating under his arms, his mouth dry, his stomach hollow feeling, wanting to find courage to tell Wilson to go on and finish off the lion without him. He could not know that Wilson was furious because he had not noticed the state he was in earlier and sent him back to his wife.

While he sat there Wilson came up. "I have your big gun," he said. "Take it. We've given him time, I think. Come on."

Macomber took the big gun and Wilson said:

"Keep behind me and about five yards to the right and do exactly as I tell you." Then he spoke in Swahili to the two gun-bearers who looked the picture of gloom.

"Let's go," he said.

"Could I have a drink of water?" Macomber asked. Wilson spoke to the older gun-bearer, who wore a canteen on his belt, and the man unbuckled, unscrewed the top and handed it to Macomber, who took it noticing how heavy it seemed and how hairy and shoddy the felt covering was in his hand. He raised it to drink and looked ahead at the high grass with the flat-topped trees behind it. A breeze was blowing toward them and the grass rippled gently in the wind. He looked at the gun-bearer and he could see the gun-bearer was suffering too with fear.

Thirty-five yards into the grass the big lion lay flattened out along the ground. His ears were back and his only movement was a slight twitching up and down of his long, black-tufted tail. He had turned at bay as soon as he had reached this cover and he was sick with the wound through his full belly, and weakening with the wound through his lungs that brought a thin foamy red to his mouth each time he breathed. His flanks were wet and hot and flies were on the little openings the solid bullets had made in his tawny hide, and his big yellow eyes, narrowed with hate, looked straight ahead, only blinking when the pain came as he breathed, and his claws dug in the soft baked earth. All of him, pain, sickness, hatred and all of his remaining strength, was tightening into an absolute concentration for a rush. He could hear the men talking and he waited, gathering all of himself into this preparation for a charge as soon as the men would come into the grass. As he heard their voices his tail stiffened to twitch up and down, and, as they came into the edge of the grass, he made a coughing grunt and charged.

Kongoni, the old gun-bearer, in the lead watching the blood

spoor, Wilson watching the grass for any movement, his big gun ready, the second gun-bearer looking ahead and listening, Macomber close to Wilson, his rifle cocked, they had just moved into the grass when Macomber heard the blood-choked coughing grunt, and saw the swishing rush in the grass. The next thing he knew he was running; running wildly, in panic in the open, running toward the stream.

He heard the *ca-ra-wong!* of Wilson's big rifle, and again in a second a crashing *carawong!* and turning saw the lion, horrible-looking now, with half his head seeming to be gone, crawling toward Wilson in the edge of the tall grass while the red-faced man worked the bolt on the short ugly rifle and aimed carefully as another blasting *carawong!* came from the muzzle, and the crawling, heavy, yellow bulk of the lion stiffened and the huge, mutilated head slid forward and Macomber, standing by himself in the clearing where he had run, holding a loaded rifle, while two black men and a white man looked back at him in contempt, knew the lion was dead. He came toward Wilson, his tallness all seeming a naked reproach, and Wilson looked at him and said:

"Want to take pictures?"

"No," he said.

That was all any one had said until they reached the motor car. Then Wilson had said:

"Hell of a fine lion. Boys will skin him out. We might as well stay here in the shade."

Macomber's wife had not looked at him nor he at her and he had sat by her in the back seat with Wilson sitting in the front seat. Once he had reached over and taken his wife's hand without looking at her and she had removed her hand from his. Looking across the stream to where the gun-bearers were skinning out the lion he could see that she had been able to see the whole thing. While they sat there his wife had reached forward and put her hand on Wilson's shoulder. He turned and she had leaned forward over the low seat and kissed him on the mouth.

"Oh, I say," said Wilson, going redder than his natural baked color.

"Mr. Robert Wilson," she said. "The beautiful red-faced Mr. Robert Wilson."

Then she sat down beside Macomber again and looked away across the stream to where the lion lay, with uplifted, white-muscled, tendon-marked naked forearms, and white bloating belly, as the black men fleshed away the skin. Finally the gun-bearers brought the skin over, wet and heavy, and climbed in behind with it, rolling it up before they got in, and the motor car started. No one had said anything more until they were back in camp.

That was the story of the lion. Macomber did not know how the lion had felt before he started his rush, nor during it when the unbelievable smash of the .505 with a muzzle velocity of two tons had hit him in the mouth, nor what kept him coming after that, when the second ripping crash had smashed his hind quarters and he had come crawling on toward the crashing, blasting thing that had destroyed him. Wilson knew something about it and only expressed it by saying, "Damned fine lion," but Macomber did not know how Wilson felt about things either. He did not know how his wife felt except that she was through with him.

His wife had been through with him before but it never lasted. He was very wealthy, and would be much wealthier, and he knew she would not leave him ever now. That was one of the few things that he really knew. He knew about that, about motor cycles—that was earliest—about motor cars, about duck-shooting, about fishing, trout, salmon and big-sea, about sex in books, many books, too many books, about all court games, about dogs, not much about horses, about hanging on to his money, about most of the other things his world dealt in, and about his wife not leaving him. His wife had been a great beauty and she was still a great beauty in Africa, but she was not a great enough beauty any more at home to be able to leave him and better herself and she knew it and he knew it. She had missed the chance to leave him and he knew it. If he had been better with women she would probably have started to worry about him getting another new, beautiful wife; but she knew too much about him to worry about him either. Also, he had always had a great tolerance which seemed the nicest thing about him if it were not the most sinister.

All in all they were known as a comparatively happily married couple, one of those whose disruption is often rumored but never occurs, and as the society columnist put it, they were adding more than a spice of *adventure* to their much envied and ever-enduring *Romance* by a *Safari* in what was known as *Darkest Africa* until the Martin Johnsons lighted it on so many silver screens where they were pursuing *Old Simba* the lion, the buffalo, *Tembo* and the elephant and as well collecting specimens for the Museum of Natural History. This same columnist had reported them *on the verge* at least three times in the past and they had been. But they always made it up. They had a sound basis of union. Margot was too beautiful for Macomber to divorce her and Macomber had too much money for Margot ever to leave him.

It was now about three o'clock in the morning and Francis Macomber, who had been asleep a little while after he had stopped thinking about the lion, wakened and then slept again, woke suddenly, frightened in a dream of the bloody-headed lion standing over him, and listening while his heart pounded, he realized that his wife was not in the other cot in the tent. He lay awake with that knowledge for two hours.

At the end of that time his wife came into the tent, lifted her mosquito bar and crawled cozily into bed.

"Where have you been?" Macomber asked in the darkness.

"Hello," she said. "Are you awake?"

"Where have you been?"

"I just went out to get a breath of air."

"You did, like hell."

"What do you want me to say, darling?"

"Where have you been?"

"Out to get a breath of air."

"That's a new name for it. You *are* a bitch."

"Well, you're a coward."

"All right," he said. "What of it?"

"Nothing as far as I'm concerned. But please let's not talk, darling, because I'm very sleepy."

"You think that I'll take anything."

"I know you will, sweet."

"Well, I won't."

"Please, darling, let's not talk. I'm so very sleepy."

"There wasn't going to be any of that. You promised there wouldn't be."

"Well, there is now," she said sweetly.

"You said if we made this trip that there would be none of that. You promised."

"Yes, darling. That's the way I meant it to be. But the trip was spoiled yesterday. We don't have to talk about it, do we?"

"You don't wait long when you have an advantage, do you?"

"Please let's not talk. I'm so sleepy, darling."

"I'm going to talk."

"Don't mind me then, because I'm going to sleep." And she did.

At breakfast they were all three at the table before daylight and Francis Macomber found that, of all the many men that he had hated, he hated Robert Wilson the most.

"Sleep well?" Wilson asked in his throaty voice, filling a pipe.

"Did you?"

"Topping," the white hunter told him.

You bastard, thought Macomber, you insolent bastard.

So she woke him when she came in, Wilson thought, looking at them both with his flat, cold eyes. Well, why doesn't he keep his wife where she belongs? What does he think I am, a bloody plaster saint? Let him keep her where she belongs. It's his own fault.

"Do you think we'll find buffalo?" Margot asked, pushing away a dish of apricots.

"Chance of it," Wilson said and smiled at her. "Why don't you stay in camp?"

"Not for anything," she told him.

"Why not order her to stay in camp?" Wilson said to Macomber.

"You order her," said Macomber coldly.

"Let's not have any ordering, nor," turning to Macomber, "any silliness, Francis," Margot said quite pleasantly.

"Are you ready to start?" Macomber asked.

"Any time," Wilson told him. "Do you want the Memsahib to go?"

"Does it make any difference whether I do or not?"

The hell with it, thought Robert Wilson. The utter complete hell with it. So this is what it's going to be like. Well, this is what it's going to be like, then.

"Makes no difference," he said.

"You're sure you wouldn't like to stay in camp with her yourself and let me go out and hunt the buffalo?" Macomber asked.

"Can't do that," said Wilson. "Wouldn't talk rot if I were you."

"I'm not talking rot. I'm disgusted."

"Bad word, disgusted."

"Francis, will you please try to speak sensibly?" his wife said.

"I speak too damned sensibly," Macomber said. "Did you ever eat such filthy food?"

"Something wrong with the food?" asked Wilson quietly.

"No more than with everything else."

"I'd pull yourself together, laddybuck," Wilson said very quietly. "There's a boy waits at table that understands a little English."

"The hell with him."

Wilson stood up and puffing on his pipe strolled away, speaking a few words in Swahili to one of the gun-bearers who was standing waiting for him. Macomber and his wife sat on at the table. He was staring at his coffee cup.

"If you make a scene I'll leave you, darling," Margot said quietly.

"No, you won't."

"You can try it and see."

"You won't leave me."

"No," she said. "I won't leave you and you'll behave yourself."

"Behave myself? That's a way to talk. Behave myself."

"Yes. Behave yourself."

"Why don't *you* try behaving?"

"I've tried it so long. So very long."

"I hate that red-faced swine," Macomber said. "I loathe the sight of him."

"He's really *very* nice."

"Oh, *shut up*," Macomber almost shouted. Just then the car came up and stopped in front of the dining tent and the driver and the two gun-bearers got out. Wilson walked over and looked at the husband and wife sitting there at the table.

"Going shooting?" he asked.

"Yes," said Macomber, standing up. "Yes."

"Better bring a woolly. It will be cool in the car," Wilson said.

"I'll get my leather jacket," Margot said.

"The boy has it," Wilson told her. He climbed into the front with the driver and Francis Macomber and his wife sat, not speaking, in the back seat.

Hope the silly beggar doesn't take a notion to blow the back of my head off, Wilson thought to himself. Women *are* a nuisance on safari.

The car was grinding down to cross the river at a pebbly ford in the gray daylight and then climbed, angling up the steep bank, where Wilson had ordered a way shovelled out the day before so they could reach the parklike wooded rolling country on the far side.

It was a good morning, Wilson thought. There was a heavy dew and as the wheels went through the grass and low bushes he could smell the odor of the crushed fronds. It was an odor like verbena and he liked this early morning smell of the dew, the crushed bracken and the look of the tree trunks showing black through the early morning mist, as the car made its way through the untracked, parklike country. He had put the two in the back seat out of his mind now and was thinking about buffalo. The buffalo that he was after stayed in the daytime in a thick swamp where it was impossible to get a shot, but in the night they fed out into an open stretch of country and if he could come between them and their swamp with the car, Macomber would have a good chance at them in the open. He did not want to hunt buff with Macomber in thick cover. He did not want to hunt buff or anything else with Macomber at all, but he was a professional hunter and he had hunted with some rare ones in his time. If they got buff today there would only be rhino to come and the poor man would have gone through his dangerous game and things might pick up. He'd have nothing more to do with the woman and Macomber would get over that too. He must have gone through plenty of that before by the look of things. Poor beggar. He must have a way of getting over it. Well, it was the poor sod's own bloody fault.

He, Robert Wilson, carried a double size cot on safari to accommodate any windfalls he might receive. He had hunted for a certain clientele, the international, fast, sporting set, where the women did not feel they were getting their money's worth unless they had shared that cot with the white hunter. He despised them when he was away from them although he liked some of them well enough at the time, but he made his living by them; and their standards were his standards as long as they were hiring him.

They were his standards in all except the shooting. He had his own standards about the killing and they could live up to them or get some one else to hunt them. He knew, too, that they all respected him for this. This Macomber was an odd one though. Damned if he wasn't. Now the wife. Well, the wife. Yes, the wife. Hm, the wife. Well he'd dropped all that. He looked around at them. Macomber sat grim and furious. Margot smiled at him. She looked younger today, more innocent and fresher and not so professionally beautiful. What's in her heart God knows, Wilson thought. She hadn't talked much last night. At that it was a pleasure to see her.

The motor car climbed up a slight rise and went on through the trees and then out into a grassy prairie-like opening and kept in the shelter of the trees along the edge, the driver going slowly and Wilson looking carefully out across the prairie and all along its far side. He stopped the car and studied the opening with his field glasses. Then he motioned to the driver to go on and the car moved slowly along, the driver avoiding wart-hog holes and driving around the mud castles ants had built. Then, looking across the opening, Wilson suddenly turned and said,

"By God, there they are!"

And looking where he pointed, while the car jumped forward and Wilson spoke in rapid Swahili to the driver, Macomber saw three huge, black animals looking almost cylindrical in their long heaviness, like big black tank cars, moving at a gallop across the far edge of the open prairie. They moved at a stiff-necked, stiff-bodied gallop and he could see the upswept wide black horns on their heads as they galloped heads out; the heads not moving.

"They're three old bulls," Wilson said. "We'll cut them off before they get to the swamp."

The car was going a wild forty-five miles an hour across the open and as Macomber watched, the buffalo got bigger and bigger until he could see the gray, hairless, scabby look of one huge bull and how his neck was a part of his shoulders and the shiny black of his horns as he galloped a little behind the others that were strung out in that steady plunging gait; and then, the car swaying as though it had just jumped a road, they drew up close and he could see the plunging hugeness of the bull, and the dust in his sparsely haired hide, the wide boss of horn and his outstretched, wide-nostrilled muzzle, and he was raising his rifle when Wilson shouted, "Not from the car, you fool!" and he had no fear, only hatred of Wilson, while the brakes clamped on and the car skidded, plowing sideways to an almost stop and Wilson was out on one side and he on the other, stumbling as his feet hit the still speeding-by of the earth, and then he was shooting at the bull as he moved away, hearing the bullets whunk into him, emptying his rifle at him as he moved steadily away, finally remembering to get his shots forward into the shoulder, and as he fumbled to re-load, he saw the bull was down. Down on his knees, his big head tossing, and seeing the other two still galloping he shot at the leader and hit him. He shot again and missed and he heard the *carawonging* roar as Wilson shot and saw the leading bull slide forward onto his nose.

"Get that other," Wilson said. "Now you're shooting!"

But the other bull was moving steadily at the same gallop and he missed, throwing a spout of dirt, and Wilson missed and the dust rose in a cloud and Wilson shouted, "Come on. He's too far!" and grabbed his arm and they were in the car again, Macomber and Wilson hanging on the sides and rocketing swayingly over the uneven ground, drawing up on the steady, plunging, heavy-necked, straight-moving gallop of the bull.

They were behind him and Macomber was filling his rifle, dropping shells onto the ground, jamming it, clearing the jam, then they were almost up with the bull when Wilson yelled "Stop," and the car skidded so that it almost swung over and Macomber fell forward onto his feet, slammed his bolt forward and fired as far forward as he could aim into the galloping, rounded black back, aimed and shot again, then again, then again, and the bullets, all of them hitting, had no effect on the buffalo that he could see. Then Wilson shot, the roar deafening him, and he could see the bull stagger. Macomber shot again, aiming carefully, and down he came, onto his knees.

"All right," Wilson said. "Nice work. That's three."

Macomber felt a drunken elation.

"How many times did you shoot?" he asked.

"Just three," Wilson said. "You killed the first bull. The biggest one. I helped you finish the other two. Afraid they might have got into cover. You had them killed. I was just mopping up a little. You shot damn well."

"Let's go to the car," said Macomber. "I want a drink."

"Got to finish off that buff first," Wilson told him. The buffalo was on his knees and he jerked his head furiously and bellowed in pig-eyed, roaring rage as they came toward him.

"Watch he doesn't get up," Wilson said. Then, "Get a little broadside and take him in the neck just behind the ear."

Macomber aimed carefully at the center of the huge, jerking, rage-driven neck and shot. At the shot the head dropped forward.

"That does it," said Wilson. "Got the spine. They're a hell of a looking thing, aren't they?"

"Let's get the drink," said Macomber. In his life he had never felt so good.

In the car Macomber's wife sat very white faced. "You were marvellous, darling," she said to Macomber. "What a ride."

"Was it rough?" Wilson asked.

"It was frightful. I've never been more frightened in my life."

"Let's all have a drink," Macomber said.

"By all means," said Wilson. "Give it to the Memsahib." She drank the neat whisky from the flask and shuddered a little when she swallowed. She handed the flask to Macomber who handed it to Wilson.

"It was frightfully exciting," she said. "It's given me a dreadful headache. I didn't know you were allowed to shoot them from cars though."

"No one shot from cars," said Wilson coldly.

"I mean chase them from cars."

"Wouldn't ordinarily," Wilson said. "Seemed sporting enough to me though while we were doing it. Taking more chance driving that way across the plain full of holes and one thing and another than hunting on foot. Buffalo could have charged us each time we shot if he liked. Gave him every chance. Wouldn't mention it to any one though. It's illegal if that's what you mean."

"It seemed very unfair to me," Margot said, "chasing those big helpless things in a motor car."

"Did it?" said Wilson.

"What would happen if they heard about it in Nairobi?"

"I'd lose my licence for one thing. Other unpleasantnesses," Wilson said, taking a drink from the flask. "I'd be out of business."

"Really?"

"Yes, really."

"Well," said Macomber, and he smiled for the first time all day. "Now she has something on you."

"You have such a pretty way of putting things, Francis," Margot Macomber said. Wilson looked at them both. If a four-letter man marries a five-letter woman, he was thinking, what number of letters would their children be? What he said was, "We lost a gun-bearer. Did you notice it?"

"My God, no," Macomber said.

"Here he comes," Wilson said. "He's all right. He must have fallen off when we left the first bull."

Approaching them was the middle-aged gun-bearer, limping along in his knitted cap, khaki tunic, shorts and rubber sandals, gloomy-faced and disgusted looking. As he came up he called out to Wilson in Swahili and they all saw the change in the white hunter's face.

"What does he say?" asked Margot.

"He says the first bull got up and went into the bush," Wilson said with no expression in his voice.

"Oh," said Macomber blankly.

"Then it's going to be just like the lion," said Margot, full of anticipation.

"It's not going to be a damned bit like the lion," Wilson told her. "Did you want another drink, Macomber?"

"Thanks, yes," Macomber said. He expected the feeling he had had about the lion to come back but it did not. For the first time in his life he really felt wholly without fear. Instead of fear he had a feeling of definite elation.

"We'll go and have a look at the second bull," Wilson said. "I'll tell the driver to put the car in the shade."

"What are you going to do?" asked Margaret Macomber.

"Take a look at the buff," Wilson said.

"I'll come."

"Come along."

The three of them walked over to where the second buffalo bulked blackly in the open, head forward on the grass, the massive horns swung wide.

"He's a very good head," Wilson said. "That's close to a fifty-inch spread."

Macomber was looking at him with delight.

"He's hateful looking," said Margot. "Can't we go into the shade?"

"Of course," Wilson said. "Look," he said to Macomber, and pointed. "See that patch of bush?"

"Yes."

"That's where the first bull went in. The gun-bearer said when he fell off the bull was down. He was watching us helling along and the other two buff galloping. When he looked up there was the bull up and looking at him. Gun-bearer ran like hell and the bull went off slowly into that bush."

"Can we go in after him now?" asked Macomber eagerly.

Wilson looked at him appraisingly. Damned if this isn't a strange one, he thought. Yesterday he's scared sick and today he's a ruddy fire eater.

"No, we'll give him a while."

"Let's please go into the shade," Margot said. Her face was white and she looked ill.

They made their way to the car where it stood under a single, wide-spreading tree and all climbed in.

"Chances are he's dead in there," Wilson remarked. "After a little we'll have a look."

Macomber felt a wild unreasonable happiness that he had never known before.

"By God, that was a chase," he said. "I've never felt any such feeling. Wasn't it marvellous, Margot?"

"I hated it."

"Why?"

"I hated it," she said bitterly. "I loathed it."

"You know I don't think I'd ever be afraid of anything again," Macomber said to Wilson. "Something happened in me after we first saw the buff and started after him. Like a dam bursting. It was pure excitement."

"Cleans out your liver," said Wilson. "Damn funny things happen to people."

Macomber's face was shining. "You know something did happen to me," he said. "I feel absolutely different."

His wife said nothing and eyed him strangely. She was sitting far back in the seat and Macomber was sitting forward talking to Wilson who turned sideways talking over the back of the front seat.

"You know, I'd like to try another lion," Macomber said. "I'm really not afraid of them now. After all, what can they do to you?"

"That's it," said Wilson. "Worst one can do is kill you. How does it go? Shakespeare. Damned good. See if I can remember. Oh, damned good. Used to quote it to myself at one time. Let's see. 'By my troth, I care not; a man can die but once; we owe God a death and let it go which way it will, he that dies this year is quit for the next.' Damned fine, eh?"

He was very embarrassed, having brought out this thing he had lived by, but he had seen men come of age before and it always moved him. It was not a matter of their twenty-first birthday.

It had taken a strange chance of hunting, a sudden precipitation into action without opportunity for worrying beforehand, to bring this about with Macomber, but regardless of how it had happened it had most certainly happened. Look at the beggar now, Wilson thought. It's that some of them stay little boys so long, Wilson thought. Sometimes all their lives. Their figures stay boyish when they're fifty. The great American boy-men.

Damned strange people. But he liked this Macomber now. Damned strange fellow. Probably meant the end of cuckoldry too. Well, that would be a damned good thing. Damned good thing. Beggar had probably been afraid all his life. Don't know what started it. But over now. Hadn't had time to be afraid with the buff. That and being angry too. Motor car too. Motor cars made it familiar. Be a damn fire eater now. He'd seen it in the war work the same way. More of a change than any loss of virginity. Fear gone like an operation. Something else grew in its place. Main thing a man had. Made him into a man. Women knew it too. No bloody fear.

From the far corner of the seat Margaret Macomber looked at the two of them. There was no change in Wilson. She saw Wilson as she had seen him the day before when she had first realized what his great talent was. But she saw the change in Francis Macomber now.

"Do you have that feeling of happiness about what's going to happen?" Macomber asked, still exploring his new wealth.

"You're not supposed to mention it," Wilson said, looking in the other's face. "Much more fashionable to say you're scared. Mind you, you'll be scared too, plenty of times."

"But you *have* a feeling of happiness about action to come?"

"Yes," said Wilson. "There's that. Doesn't do to talk too much about all this. Talk the whole thing away. No pleasure in anything if you mouth it up too much."

"You're both talking rot," said Margot. "Just because you've chased some helpless animals in a motor car you talk like heroes."

"Sorry," said Wilson. "I have been gassing too much." She's worried about it already, he thought.

"If you don't know what we're talking about why not keep out of it?" Macomber asked his wife.

"You've gotten awfully brave, awfully suddenly," his wife said contemptuously, but her contempt was not secure. She was very afraid of something.

Macomber laughed, a very natural hearty laugh. "You know I *have*," he said. "I really have."

"Isn't it sort of late?" Margot said bitterly. Because she had done the best she could for many years back and the way they were together now was no one person's fault.

"Not for me," said Macomber.

Margot said nothing but sat back in the corner of the seat.

"Do you think we've given him time enough?" Macomber asked Wilson cheerfully.

"We might have a look," Wilson said. "Have you any solids left?"

"The gun-bearer has some."

Wilson called in Swahili and the older gun-bearer, who was skinning out one of the heads, straightened up, pulled a box of solids out of his pocket and brought them over to Macomber, who filled his magazine and put the remaining shells in his pocket.

"You might as well shoot the Springfield," Wilson said. "You're used to it. We'll leave the Mannlicher in the car with the Memsahib. Your gun-bearer can carry your heavy gun. I've this damned cannon. Now let me tell you about them." He had saved this until the last because he did not want to worry Macomber. "When a buff comes he comes with his head high and thrust straight out. The boss of the horns covers any sort of a brain shot. The only shot is straight into the nose. The only other shot is into his chest or, if you're to one side, into the neck or the shoulders. After they've been hit once they take a hell of a lot of killing. Don't try anything fancy. Take the easiest shot there is. They've finished skinning out that head now. Should we get started?"

He called to the gun-bearers, who came up wiping their hands, and the older one got into the back.

"I'll only take Kongoni," Wilson said. "The other can watch to keep the birds away."

As the car moved slowly across the open space toward the island of brushy trees that ran in a tongue of foliage along a dry water course that cut the open swale, Macomber felt his heart pounding and his mouth was dry again, but it was excitement, not fear.

"Here's where he went in," Wilson said. Then to the gun-bearer in Swahili, "Take the blood spoor."

The car was parallel to the patch of bush. Macomber, Wilson and the gun-bearer got down. Macomber, looking back, saw his wife, with the rifle by her side, looking at him. He waved to her and she did not wave back.

The brush was very thick ahead and the ground was dry. The middle-aged gun-bearer was sweating heavily and Wilson had his hat down over his eyes and his red neck showed just ahead of Macomber. Suddenly the gun-bearer said something in Swahili to Wilson and ran forward.

"He's dead in there," Wilson said. "Good work," and he turned to grip Macomber's hand and as they shook hands, grinning at each other, the gun-bearer shouted wildly and they saw him coming out of the bush sideways, fast as a crab, and the bull coming, nose out, mouth tight closed, blood dripping, massive head straight out, coming in a charge, his little pig eyes bloodshot as he looked at them. Wilson, who was ahead, was kneeling shooting, and Macomber, as he fired, unhearing his shot in the roaring of Wilson's gun, saw fragments like slate burst from the huge boss of the horns, and the head jerked, he shot again at the wide nostrils and saw the horns jolt again and fragments fly, and he did not see Wilson now and, aiming carefully, shot again with the buffalo's huge bulk almost on him and his rifle almost level with the on-coming head, nose out, and he could see the little wicked eyes and the head started to lower and he felt a sudden white-hot, blinding flash explode inside his head and that was all he ever felt.

Wilson had ducked to one side to get in a shoulder shot. Macomber had stood solid and shot for the nose, shooting a touch high each time and hitting the heavy horns, splintering and chipping them like hitting a slate roof, and Mrs. Macomber, in the car, had shot at the buffalo with the 6.5 Mannlicher as it seemed about to gore Macomber and had hit her husband about two inches up and a little to one side of the base of his skull.

Francis Macomber lay now, face down, not two yards from where the buffalo lay on his side and his wife knelt over him with Wilson beside her.

"I wouldn't turn him over," Wilson said.

The woman was crying hysterically.

"I'd get back in the car," Wilson said. "Where's the rifle?"

She shook her head, her face contorted. The gun-bearer picked up the rifle.

"Leave it as it is," said Wilson. Then, "Go get Abdulla so that he may witness the manner of the accident."

He knelt down, took a handkerchief from his pocket, and spread it over Francis Macomber's crew-cropped head where it lay. The blood sank into the dry, loose earth.

Wilson stood up and saw the buffalo on his side, his legs out, his thinly-haired belly crawling with ticks. "Hell of a good bull," his brain registered automatically. "A good fifty inches, or better. Better." He called to the driver and told him to spread a blanket over the body and stay by it. Then he walked over to the motor car where the woman sat crying in the corner.

"That was a pretty thing to do," he said in a toneless voice. "He *would* have left you too."

"Stop it," she said.

"Of course it's an accident," he said. "I know that."

"Stop it," she said.

"Don't worry," he said. "There will be a certain amount of unpleasantness but I will have some photographs taken that will be very useful at the inquest. There's the testimony of the gun-bearers and the driver too. You're perfectly all right."

"Stop it," she said.

"There's a hell of a lot to be done," he said. "And I'll have to send a truck off to the lake to wireless for a plane to take the three of us into Nairobi. Why didn't you poison him? That's what they do in England."

"Stop it. Stop it. Stop it," the woman cried.

Wilson looked at her with his flat blue eyes.

"I'm through now," he said. "I was a little angry. I'd begun to like your husband."

"Oh, please stop it," she said. "Please, please stop it."

"That's better," Wilson said. "Please is much better. Now I'll stop."

The Gioconda Smile

ALDOUS HUXLEY (1894–)

"MISS SPENCE will be down directly, sir."

"Thank you," said Mr. Hutton, without turning round. Janet Spence's parlourmaid was so ugly—ugly on purpose, it always seemed to him, malignantly, criminally ugly—that he could not bear to look at her more than was necessary. The door closed. Left to himself, Mr. Hutton got up and began to wander round the room, looking with meditative eyes at the familiar objects it contained.

Photographs of Greek statuary, photographs of the Roman Forum, coloured prints of Italian masterpieces, all very safe and well known. Poor, dear Janet, what a prig—what an intellectual snob! Her real taste was illustrated in that water-colour by the pavement artist, the one she had paid half a crown for (and thirty-five shillings for the frame). How often he had heard her tell the story, how often expatiate on the beauties of that skilful imitation of an oleograph! "A real Artist in the streets," and you could hear the capital A in Artist as she spoke the words. She made you feel that part of his glory had entered into Janet Spence when she tendered him that half-crown for the copy of the oleograph. She was implying a compliment to her own taste and penetration. A genuine Old Master for half a crown. Poor, dear Janet!

Mr. Hutton came to a pause in front of a small oblong mirror. Stooping a little to get a full view of his face, he passed a white, well-manicured finger over his moustache. It was as curly, as freshly auburn as it had been twenty years ago. His hair still retained its colour, and there was no sign of baldness yet—only a certain elevation of the brow. "Shakespearean," thought Mr. Hutton, with a smile, as he surveyed the smooth and polished expanse of his forehead.

Others abide our question, thou art free. . . . Footsteps in the sea . . . Majesty . . . Shakespeare, thou shouldst be living at this hour. No, that was Milton, wasn't it? Milton, the Lady of Christ's. There was no lady about him. He was what the women would call a manly man. That was why they liked him—for the curly auburn moustache and the discreet redolence of tobacco. Mr. Hutton smiled again; he enjoyed making fun of himself. Lady of Christ's? No, no. He was the Christ of Ladies. Very pretty, very pretty. The Christ of Ladies. Mr. Hutton wished there were somebody he could tell the joke to. Poor, dear Janet wouldn't appreciate it, alas!

He straightened himself up, patted his hair, and resumed his peregrination. Damn the Roman Forum; he hated those dreary photographs.

Suddenly he became aware that Janet Spence was in the room, standing near the door. Mr. Hutton started, as though he had been taken in some felonious act. To make these silent and spectral appearances was one of Janet Spence's peculiar talents. Perhaps she had been there all the time, had seen him looking at himself in the mirror. Impossible! But, still, it was disquieting.

"Oh, you gave me such a surprise," said Mr. Hutton, recovering his smile and advancing with outstretched hand to meet her.

Miss Spence was smiling too: her Gioconda smile, he had once called it in a moment of half-ironical flattery. Miss Spence had taken the compliment seriously, and had always tried to live up to the Leonardo standard. She smiled on his silence while Mr. Hutton shook hands; that was part of the Gioconda business.

"I hope you're well," said Mr. Hutton. "You look it."

What a queer face she had! That small mouth pursed forward by the Gioconda expression into a little snout with a round hole in the middle as though for whistling—it was like a penholder seen from the front. Above the mouth a well-shaped nose, finely aquiline. Eyes large, lustrous, and dark, with the largeness, lustre, and darkness that seems to invite sties and an occasional bloodshot suffusion. They were fine eyes, but unchangingly grave. The penholder might do its Gioconda trick, but the eyes never altered in their earnestness. Above them, a pair of boldly arched, heavily pencilled black eyebrows lent a surprising air of power, as of a Roman matron, to the upper portion of the face. Her hair was dark and equally Roman; Agrippina from the brows upward.

"I thought I'd just look in on my way home," Mr. Hutton went on. "Ah, it's good to be back here"—he indicated with a wave of his hand the flowers in the vases, the sunshine and greenery beyond the windows—"it's good to be back in the country after a stuffy day of business in town."

Miss Spence, who had sat down, pointed to a chair at her side.

"No, really, I can't sit down," Mr. Hutton protested. "I must get back to see how poor Emily is. She was rather seedy this morning." He sat down, nevertheless. "It's these wretched liver chills. She's always getting them. Women—" He broke off and coughed, so as to hide the fact that he had uttered. He was about to say that women with weak digestions ought not to marry; but the remark was too cruel, and he didn't really believe it. Janet Spence, moreover, was a believer in eternal flames and spiritual attachments. "She hopes to be well enough," he added, "to see you at luncheon to-morrow. Can you come? Do!" He smiled persuasively. "It's my invitation too, you know."

She dropped her eyes, and Mr. Hutton almost thought that he

detected a certain reddening of the cheek. It was a tribute; he stroked his moustache.

"I should like to come if you think Emily's really well enough to have a visitor."

"Of course. You'll do her good. You'll do us both good. In married life three is often better company than two."

"Oh, you're cynical."

Mr. Hutton always had a desire to say "Bow-wow-wow" whenever that last word was spoken. It irritated him more than any other word in the language. But instead of barking he made haste to protest.

"No, no. I'm only speaking a melancholy truth. Reality doesn't always come up to the ideal, you know. But that doesn't make me believe any the less in the ideal. Indeed, I believe in it passionately—the ideal of a matrimony between two people in perfect accord. I think it's realisable. I'm sure it is."

He paused significantly and looked at her with an arch expression. A virgin of thirty-six, but still unwithered; she had her charms. And there was something really rather enigmatic about her. Miss Spence made no reply but continued to smile. There were times when Mr. Hutton got rather bored with the Gioconda. He stood up.

"I must really be going now. Farewell, mysterious Gioconda." The smile grew intenser, focused itself, as it were, in a narrower snout. Mr. Hutton made a Cinquecento gesture, and kissed her extended hand. It was the first time he had done such a thing; the action seemed not to be resented. "I look forward to to-morrow."

"Do you?"

For answer Mr. Hutton once more kissed her hand, then turned to go. Miss Spence accompanied him to the porch.

"Where's your car?" she asked.

"I left it at the gate of the drive."

"I'll come and see you off."

"No, no." Mr. Hutton was playful, but determined. "You must do no such thing. I simply forbid you."

"But I should like to come," Miss Spence protested, throwing a rapid Gioconda at him.

Mr. Hutton held up his hand. "No," he repeated, and then, with a gesture that was almost the blowing of a kiss, he started to run down the drive, lightly on his toes, with long, bounding strides like a boy's. He was proud of that run; it was quite marvellously youthful. Still, he was glad the drive was no longer. At the last bend, before passing out of sight of the house, he halted and turned round. Miss Spence was still standing on the steps, smiling her smile. He waved his hand, and this time quite definitely and overtly wafted a kiss in her direction. Then, breaking once more into his magnificent canter, he rounded the last dark promontory of trees. Once out of sight of the house he let his high paces decline to a trot, and finally to a walk. He took out his handkerchief and began wiping his neck inside his collar. What fools, what fools! Had there ever been such an ass as poor, dear Janet Spence? Never, unless it was himself. Decidedly he was the more malignant fool, since he, at least, was aware of his folly and still persisted in it. Why did he persist? Ah, the problem that was himself, the problem that was other people.

He had reached the gate. A large, prosperous-looking motor was standing at the side of the road.

"Home, M'Nab." The chauffeur touched his cap. "And stop at the cross-roads on the way, as usual," Mr. Hutton added, as he opened the door of the car. "Well?" he said, speaking into the obscurity that lurked within.

"Oh, Teddy Bear, what an age you've been!" It was a fresh and childish voice that spoke the words. There was the faintest hint of Cockney impurity about the vowel sounds.

Mr. Hutton bent his large form and darted into the car with the agility of an animal regaining its burrow.

"Have I?" he said, as he shut the door. The machine began to move. "You must have missed me a lot if you found the time so long." He sat back in the low seat; a cherishing warmth enveloped him.

"Teddy Bear . . ." and with a sigh of contentment a charming little head declined on to Mr. Hutton's shoulder. Ravished, he looked down sideways at the round, babyish face.

"Do you know, Doris, you look like the pictures of Louise de Kerouaille." He passed his fingers through a mass of curly hair.

"Who's Louise de Kera-whatever-it-is?" Doris spoke from remote distances.

"She was, alas! *Fuit*. We shall all be 'was' one of these days. Meanwhile . . ."

Mr. Hutton covered the babyish face with kisses. The car rushed smoothly along. M'Nab's back, through the front window, was stonily impassive, the back of a statue.

"Your hands," Doris whispered. "Oh, you mustn't touch me. They give me electric shocks."

Mr. Hutton adored her for the virgin imbecility of the words. How late in one's existence one makes the discovery of one's body!

"The electricity isn't in me, it's in you." He kissed her again, whispering her name several times: Doris, Doris, Doris. The scientific appellation of the sea-mouse, he was thinking as he kissed the throat, she offered him, white and extended like the throat of a victim awaiting the sacrificial knife. The sea-mouse was a sausage with iridescent fur: very peculiar. Or was Doris the sea cucumber, which turns itself inside out in moments of alarm? He would really have to go to Naples again, just to see the aquarium. These sea creatures were fabulous, unbelievably fantastic.

"Oh, Teddy Bear!" (More zoology; but he was only a land animal. His poor little jokes!) "Teddy Bear, I'm so happy."

"So am I," said Mr. Hutton. Was it true?

"But I wish I knew if it were right. Tell me, Teddy Bear, is it right or wrong?"

"Ah, my dear, that's just what I've been wondering for the last thirty years."

"Be serious, Teddy Bear. I want to know if this is right; if it's right that I should be here with you and that we should love one another, and that it should give me electric shocks when you touch me."

"Right? Well, it's certainly good that you should have electric shocks rather than sexual repressions. Read Freud; repressions are the devil."

"Oh, you don't help me. Why aren't you ever serious? If only you knew how miserable I am sometimes, thinking it's not right. Perhaps, you know, there is a hell, and all that. I don't know what to do. Sometimes I think I ought to stop loving you."

"But could you?" asked Mr. Hutton, confident in the powers of his seduction and his moustache.

"No, Teddy Bear, you know I couldn't. But I could run away, I could hide from you, I could lock myself up and force myself not to come to you."

"Silly little thing!" He tightened his embrace.

"Oh, dear, I hope it isn't wrong. And there are times when I don't care if it is."

Mr. Hutton was touched. He had a certain protective affection for this little creature. He laid his cheek against her hair and so, interlaced, they sat in silence, while the car, swaying and pitching a little as it hastened along, seemed to draw in the white road and the dusty hedges towards it devouringly.

"Good-bye, good-bye."

The car moved on, gathered speed, vanished round a curve, and Doris was left standing by the sign-post at the cross-roads, still dizzy and weak with the languor born of those kisses and the electrical touch of those gentle hands. She had to take a deep breath, to draw herself up deliberately, before she was strong enough to start her homeward walk. She had half a mile in which to invent the necessary lies.

Alone, Mr. Hutton suddenly found himself the prey of an appalling boredom.

II

Mrs. Hutton was lying on the sofa in her boudoir, playing Patience. In spite of the warmth of the July evening a wood fire was burning on the hearth. A black Pomeranian, extenuated by the heat and the fatigues of digestion, slept before the blaze.

"Phew! Isn't it rather hot in here?" Mr. Hutton asked as he entered the room.

"You know I have to keep warm, dear." The voice seemed breaking on the verge of tears. "I get so shivery."

"I hope you're better this evening."

"Not much, I'm afraid."

The conversation stagnated. Mr. Hutton stood leaning his back against the mantelpiece. He looked down at the Pomeranian lying at his feet, and with the toe of his right boot he rolled the little dog over and rubbed its white-flecked chest and belly. The creature lay in an inert ecstasy. Mrs. Hutton continued to play Patience. Arrived at an *impasse*, she altered the position of one card, took back another, and went on playing. Her Patiences always came out.

"Dr. Libbard thinks I ought to go to Llandrindod Wells this summer."

"Well—go, my dear—go, most certainly."

Mr. Hutton was thinking of the events of the afternoon: how they had driven, Doris and he, up to the hanging wood, had left the car to wait for them under the shade of the trees, and walked together out into the windless sunshine of the chalk down.

"I'm to drink the waters for my liver, and he thinks I ought to have massage and electric treatment, too."

Hat in hand, Doris had stalked four blue butterflies that were dancing together round a scabious flower with a motion that was like the flickering of blue fire. The blue fire burst and scattered into whirling sparks; she had given chase, laughing and shouting like a child.

"I'm sure it will do you good, my dear."

"I was wondering if you'd come with me, dear."

"But you know I'm going to Scotland at the end of the month."

Mrs. Hutton looked up at him entreatingly. "It's the journey," she said. "The thought of it is such a nightmare. I don't know if I can manage it. And you know I can't sleep in hotels. And then there's the luggage and all the worries. I can't go alone."

"But you won't be alone. You'll have your maid with you." He spoke impatiently. The sick woman was usurping the place of the healthy one. He was being dragged back from the memory of the sunlit down and the quick, laughing girl, back to this unhealthy, overheated room and its complaining occupant.

"I don't think I shall be able to go."

"But you must, my dear, if the doctor tells you to. And, besides, a change will do you good."

"I don't think so."

"But Libbard thinks so, and he knows what he's talking about."

"No, I can't face it. I'm too weak. I can't go alone." Mrs. Hutton pulled a handkerchief out of her black silk bag, and put it to her eyes.

"Nonsense, my dear, you must make the effort."

"I had rather be left in peace to die here." She was crying in earnest now.

"O Lord! Now do be reasonable. Listen now, please." Mrs. Hutton only sobbed more violently. "Oh, what is one to do?" He shrugged his shoulders and walked out of the room.

Mr. Hutton was aware that he had not behaved with proper patience; but he could not help it. Very early in his manhood he had discovered that not only did he not feel sympathy for the poor, the weak, the diseased, and deformed; he actually hated them. Once, as an undergraduate, he spent three days at a mission in the East End. He had returned, filled with a profound and ineradicable disgust. Instead of pitying, he loathed the unfortunate. It was not, he knew, a very comely emotion; and he had been ashamed of it at first. In the end he had decided that it was temperamental, inevitable, and had felt no further qualms. Emily had been healthy and beautiful when he married her. He had loved her then. But now—was it his fault that she was like this?

Mr. Hutton dined alone. Food and drink left him more benevolent than he had been before dinner. To make amends for his show of exasperation he went up to his wife's room and offered to read to her. She was touched, gratefully accepted the offer, and Mr. Hutton, who was particularly proud of his accent, suggested a little light reading in French.

"French? I am so fond of French." Mrs. Hutton spoke of the language of Racine as though it were a dish of green peas.

Mr. Hutton ran down to the library and returned with a yellow volume. He began reading. The effort of pronouncing perfectly absorbed his whole attention. But how good his accent was! The fact of its goodness seemed to improve the quality of the novel he was reading.

At the end of fifteen pages an unmistakable sound aroused him. He looked up; Mrs. Hutton had gone to sleep. He sat still for a little while, looking with a dispassionate curiosity at the sleeping face. Once it had been beautiful; once, long ago, the sight of it, the recollection of it, had moved him with an emotion profounder, perhaps, than any he had felt before or since. Now it was lined and cadaverous. The skin was stretched tightly over the cheekbones, across the bridge of the sharp, bird-like nose. The closed eyes were set in profound bone-rimmed sockets. The lamplight striking on the face from the side emphasized with light and shade its cavities and projections. It was the face of a dead Christ by Morales.

Le squelette était invisible
Au temps heureux de l'art païen.

He shivered a little, and tiptoed out of the room.

On the following day Mrs. Hutton came down to luncheon. She had had some unpleasant palpitations during the night, but she was feeling better now. Besides, she wanted to do honour to her guest. Miss Spence listened to her complaints about Llandrindod Wells, and was loud in sympathy, lavish with advice. Whatever she said was always said with intensity. She leaned forward, aimed, so to speak, like a gun, and fired her words. Bang! the charge in her soul was ignited, the words whizzed forth at the narrow barrel of her mouth. She was a machine-gun riddling her hostess with sympathy. Mr. Hutton had undergone similar bombardments, mostly of a literary or philosophic character—bombardments of Maeterlinck, of Mrs. Besant, of Bergson, of William James. To-day the missiles were medical. She talked about insomnia, she expatiated on the virtues of harmless drugs and beneficent specialists. Under the bombardment Mrs. Hutton opened out, like a flower in the sun.

Mr. Hutton looked on in silence. The spectacle of Janet Spence evoked in him an unfailing curiosity. He was not romantic enough to imagine that every face masked an interior physiognomy of beauty or strangeness, that every woman's small talk was like a vapour hanging over mysterious gulfs. His wife, for example, and Doris; they were nothing more than what they seemed to be. But with Janet Spence it was somehow different. Here one could be sure that there was some kind of a queer face behind the Gioconda smile and the Roman eyebrows. The only question was: What exactly was there? Mr. Hutton could never quite make out.

"But perhaps you won't have to go to Llandrindod after all," Miss Spence was saying. "If you get well quickly Dr. Libbard will let you off."

"I only hope so. Indeed, I do really feel rather better to-day."

Mr. Hutton felt ashamed. How much was it his own lack of sympathy that prevented her from feeling well every day? But he comforted himself by reflecting that it was only a case of feeling, not of being better. Sympathy does not mend a diseased liver or a weak heart.

"My dear, I wouldn't eat those red currants if I were you," he said, suddenly solicitous. "You know that Libbard has banned everything with skins and pips."

"But I am so fond of them," Mrs. Hutton protested, "and I feel so well to-day."

"Don't be a tyrant," said Miss Spence, looking first at him and then at his wife. "Let the poor invalid have what she fancies; it will do her good." She laid her hand on Mrs. Hutton's arm and patted it affectionately two or three times.

"Thank you, my dear." Mrs. Hutton helped herself to the stewed currants.

"Well, don't blame me if they make you ill again."

"Do I ever blame you, dear?"

"You have nothing to blame me for," Mr. Hutton answered playfully. "I am the perfect husband."

They sat in the garden after luncheon. From the island of shade under the old cypress tree they looked out across a flat expanse of lawn, in which the parterres of flowers shone with a metallic brilliance.

Mr. Hutton took a deep breath of the warm and fragrant air. "It's good to be alive," he said.

"Just to be alive," his wife echoed, stretching one pale, knot-jointed hand into the sunlight.

A maid brought the coffee; the silver pots and the little blue cups were set on a folding table near the group of chairs.

"Oh, my medicine!" exclaimed Mrs. Hutton. "Run in and fetch it, Clara, will you? The white bottle on the sideboard."

"I'll go," said Mr. Hutton. "I've got to go and fetch a cigar in any case."

He ran in towards the house. On the threshold he turned round for an instant. The maid was walking back across the lawn. His wife was sitting up in her deck-chair, engaged in opening her white parasol. Miss Spence was bending over the table, pouring out the coffee. He passed into the cool obscurity of the house.

"Do you like sugar in your coffee?" Miss Spence inquired.

"Yes, please. Give me rather a lot. I'll drink it after my medicine to take the taste away."

Mrs. Hutton leaned back in her chair, lowering the sunshade

over her eyes, so as to shut out from her vision the burning sky.

Behind her, Miss Spence was making a delicate clinking among the coffee-cups.

"I've given you three large spoonfuls. That ought to take the taste away. And here comes the medicine."

Mr. Hutton had reappeared, carrying a wine-glass, half full of a pale liquid.

"It smells delicious," he said, as he handed it to his wife.

"That's only the flavouring." She drank it off at a gulp, shuddered, and made a grimace. "Ugh, it's so nasty. Give me my coffee."

Miss Spence gave her the cup; she sipped at it. "You've made it like syrup. But it's very nice, after that atrocious medicine."

At half-past three Mrs. Hutton complained that she did not feel as well as she had done, and went indoors to lie down. Her husband would have said something about the red currants, but checked himself; the triumph of an "I told you so" was too cheaply won. Instead, he was sympathetic, and gave her his arm to the house.

"A rest will do you good," he said. "By the way, I shan't be back till after dinner."

"But why? Where are you going?"

"I promised to go to Johnson's this evening. We have to discuss the war memorial, you know."

"Oh, I wish you weren't going." Mrs. Hutton was almost in tears. "Can't you stay? I don't like being alone in the house."

"But, my dear, I promised—weeks ago." It was a bother having to lie like this. "And now I must get back and look after Miss Spence."

He kissed her on the forehead and went out again into the garden. Miss Spence received him aimed and intense.

"Your wife is dreadfully ill," she fired off at him.

"I thought she cheered up so much when you came."

"That was purely nervous, purely nervous. I was watching her closely. With a heart in that condition and her digestion wrecked—yes, wrecked—anything might happen."

"Libbard doesn't take so gloomy a view of poor Emily's health." Mr. Hutton held open the gate that led from the garden into the drive; Miss Spence's car was standing by the front door.

"Libbard is only a country doctor. You ought to see a specialist."

He could not refrain from laughing. "You have a macabre passion for specialists."

Miss Spence held up her hand in protest. "I am serious. I think poor Emily is in a very bad state. Anything might happen—at any moment."

He handed her into the car and shut the door. The chauffeur started the engine and climbed into his place, ready to drive off.

"Shall I tell him to start?" He had no desire to continue the conversation.

Miss Spence leaned forward and shot a Gioconda in his direction. "Remember, I expect you to come and see me again soon."

Mechanically he grinned, made a polite noise, and, as the car moved forward, waved his hand. He was happy to be alone.

A few minutes afterwards Mr. Hutton himself drove away. Doris was waiting at the cross-roads. They dined together twenty miles from home, at a roadside hotel. It was one of those bad, expensive meals which are only cooked in country hotels frequented by motorists. It revolted Mr. Hutton, but Doris enjoyed it. She always enjoyed things. Mr. Hutton ordered a not very good brand of champagne. He was wishing he had spent the evening in his library.

When they started homewards Doris was a little tipsy and extremely affectionate. It was very dark inside the car, but looking forward, past the motionless form of M'Nab, they could see a bright and narrow universe of forms and colours scooped out of the night by the electric head-lamps.

It was after eleven when Mr. Hutton reached home. Dr.

Libbard met him in the hall. He was a small man with delicate hands and well-formed features that were almost feminine. His brown eyes were large and melancholy. He used to waste a great deal of time sitting at the bedside of his patients, looking sadness through those eyes and talking in a sad, low voice about nothing in particular. His person exhaled a pleasing odour, decidedly antiseptic but at the same time suave and discreetly delicious.

"Libbard?" said Mr. Hutton in surprise. "You here? Is my wife ill?"

"We tried to fetch you earlier," the soft, melancholy voice replied. "It was thought you were at Mr. Johnson's, but they had no news of you there."

"No, I was detained. I had a breakdown," Mr. Hutton answered irritably. It was tiresome to be caught out in a lie.

"Your wife wanted to see you urgently."

"Well, I can go now." Mr. Hutton moved towards the stairs.

Dr. Libbard laid a hand on his arm. "I am afraid it's too late."

"Too late?" He began fumbling with his watch; it wouldn't come out of the pocket.

"Mrs. Hutton passed away half an hour ago."

The voice remained even in its softness, the melancholy of the eyes did not deepen. Dr. Libbard spoke of death as he would speak of a local cricket match. All things were equally vain and equally deplorable.

Mr. Hutton found himself thinking of Janet Spence's words. At any moment—at any moment. She had been extraordinarily right.

"What happened?" he asked. "What was the cause?"

Dr. Libbard explained. It was heart failure brought on by a violent attack of nausea, caused in its turn by the eating of something of an irritant nature. Red currants? Mr. Hutton suggested. Very likely. It had been too much for the heart. There was chronic valvular disease: something had collapsed under the strain. It was all over; she could not have suffered much.

III

"It's a pity they should have chosen the day of the Eton and Harrow match for the funeral," old General Grego was saying as he stood, his top hat in his hand, under the shadow of the lych gate, wiping his face with his handkerchief.

Mr. Hutton overheard the remark and with difficulty restrained a desire to inflict grievous bodily pain on the General. He would have liked to hit the old brute in the middle of his big red face. Monstrous great mulberry, spotted with meal! Was there no respect for the dead? Did nobody care? In theory he didn't much care; let the dead bury their dead. But here, at the graveside, he had found himself actually sobbing. Poor Emily, they had been pretty happy once. Now she was lying at the bottom of a seven-foot hole. And here was Grego complaining that he couldn't go to the Eton and Harrow match.

Mr. Hutton looked round at the groups of black figures that were drifting slowly out of the churchyard towards the fleet of cabs and motors assembled in the road outside. Against the brilliant background of the July grass and flowers and foliage, they had a horribly alien and unnatural appearance. It pleased him to think that all these people would soon be dead, too.

That evening Mr. Hutton sat up late in his library reading the life of Milton. There was no particular reason why he should have chosen Milton; it was the book that first came to hand, that was all. It was after midnight when he had finished. He got up from his armchair, unbolted the French windows, and stepped out on to the little paved terrace. The night was quiet and clear. Mr. Hutton looked at the stars and at the holes between them, dropped his eyes to the dim lawns and hueless flowers of the garden, and let them wander over the farther landscape, black and grey under the moon.

He began to think with a kind of confused violence. There were the stars, there was Milton. A man can be somehow the peer of stars and night. Greatness, nobility. But is there seriously a difference between the noble and the ignoble? Milton, the stars, death, and himself—himself. The soul, the body; the higher and the lower nature. Perhaps there was something in it, after all. Milton had a god on his side and righteousness. What had he? Nothing, nothing whatever. There were only Doris's little breasts. What was the point of it all? Milton, the stars, death, and Emily in her grave, Doris and himself—always himself . . .

Oh, he was a futile and disgusting being. Everything convinced him of it. It was a solemn moment. He spoke aloud: "I will, I will." The sound of his own voice in the darkness was appalling; it seemed to him that he had sworn that infernal oath which binds even the gods: "I will, I will." There had been New Year's days and solemn anniversaries in the past, when he had felt the same contritions and recorded similar resolutions. They had all thinned away, these resolutions, like smoke, into nothingness. But this was a greater moment and he had pronounced a more fearful oath. In the future it was to be different. Yes, he would live by reason, he would be industrious, he would curb his appetites, he would devote his life to some good purpose. It was resolved and it would be so.

In practice he saw himself spending his mornings in agricultural pursuits, riding round with the bailiff, seeing that his land was farmed in the best modern way—silos and artificial manures and continuous cropping, and all that. The remainder of the day should be devoted to serious study. There was that book he had been intending to write for so long—*The Effect of Diseases on Civilization.*

Mr. Hutton went to bed humble and contrite, but with a sense that grace had entered into him. He slept for seven and a half hours, and woke to find the sun brilliantly shining. The emotions of the evening before had been transformed by a good night's rest into his customary cheerfulness. It was not until a good many seconds after his return to conscious life that he remembered his resolution, his Stygian oath. Milton and death seemed somehow different in the sunlight. As for the stars, they were not there. But the resolutions were good; even in the daytime he could see that. He had his horse saddled after breakfast, and rode round the farm with the bailiff. After luncheon he read Thucydides on the plague at Athens. In the evening he made a few notes on malaria in Southern Italy. While he was undressing he remembered that there was a good anecdote in Skelton's jest-book about the Sweating Sickness. He would have made a note of it if only he could have found a pencil.

On the sixth morning of his new life Mr. Hutton found among his correspondence an envelope addressed in that peculiarly vulgar handwriting which he knew to be Doris's. He opened it, and began to read. She didn't know what to say; words were so inadequate. His wife dying like that, and so suddenly—it was too terrible. Mr. Hutton sighed, but his interest revived somewhat as he read on:

"Death is so frightening, I never think of it when I can help it. But when something like this happens, or when I am feeling ill or depressed, then I can't help remembering it is there so close, and I think about all the wicked things I have done and about you and me, and I wonder what will happen, and I am so frightened. I am so lonely, Teddy Bear, and so unhappy, and I don't know what to do. I can't get rid of the idea of dying, I am so wretched and helpless without you. I didn't mean to write to you; I meant to wait till you were out of mourning and could come and see me again, but I was so lonely and miserable, Teddy Bear, I had to write. I couldn't help it. Forgive me, I want you so much; I have nobody in the world but you. You are so good and gentle and understanding; there is nobody like you. I shall never forget how good and kind you have been to me, and you are so clever and know so much, I can't understand how you ever came to pay any attention to me, I am so dull and stupid, much less like me and love me, because you do love me a little, don't you, Teddy Bear?"

Mr. Hutton was touched with shame and remorse. To be thanked like this, worshipped for having seduced the girl—it was too much. It had just been a piece of imbecile wantonness. Imbecile, idiotic: there was no other way to describe it. For, when all was said, he had derived very little pleasure from it. Taking all things together, he had probably been more bored than amused. Once upon a time he had believed himself to be a hedonist. But to be a hedonist implies a certain process of reasoning, a deliberate choice of known pleasures, a rejection of known pains. This had been done without reason, against it. For he knew beforehand—so well, so well—that there was no interest or pleasure to be derived from these wretched affairs. And yet each time the vague itch came upon him he succumbed, involving himself once more in the old stupidity. There had been Maggie, his wife's maid, and Edith, the girl on the farm, and Mrs. Pringle, and the waitress in London, and others—there seemed to be dozens of them. It had all been so stale and boring. He knew it would be; he always knew. And yet, and yet . . . Experience doesn't teach.

Poor little Doris! He would write to her kindly, comfortingly, but he wouldn't see her again. A servant came to tell him that his horse was saddled and waiting. He mounted and rode off. That morning the old bailiff was more irritating than usual.

Five days later Doris and Mr. Hutton were sitting together on the pier at Southend; Doris, in white muslin with pink garnishings, radiated happiness; Mr. Hutton, legs outstretched and chair tilted, had pushed the panama back from his forehead, and was trying to feel like a tripper. That night, when Doris was asleep, breathing and warm by his side, he recaptured, in this moment of darkness and physical fatigue, the rather cosmic emotion which had possessed him that evening, not a fortnight ago, when he had made his great resolution. And so his solemn oath had already gone the way of so many other resolutions. Unreason had triumphed;

at the first itch of desire he had given way. He was hopeless, hopeless.

For a long time he lay with closed eyes, ruminating his humiliation. The girl stirred in her sleep. Mr. Hutton turned over and looked in her direction. Enough faint light crept in between the half-drawn curtains to show her bare arm and shoulder, her neck, and the dark tangle of hair on the pillow. She was beautiful, desirable. Why did he lie there moaning over his sins? What did it matter? If he were hopeless, then so be it; he would make the best of his hopelessness. A glorious sense of irresponsibility suddenly filled him. He was free, magnificently free. In a kind of exaltation he drew the girl towards him. She woke, bewildered, almost frightened under his rough kisses.

The storm of his desire subsided into a kind of serene merriment. The whole atmosphere seemed to be quivering with enormous silent laughter.

"Could anyone love you as much as I do, Teddy Bear?" The question came faintly from distant worlds of love.

"I think I know somebody who does," Mr. Hutton replied. The submarine laughter was swelling, rising, ready to break the surface of silence and resound.

"Who? Tell me. What do you mean?" The voice had come very close; charged with suspicion, anguish, indignation, it belonged to this immediate world.

"A—ah!"

"Who?"

"You'll never guess." Mr. Hutton kept up the joke until it began to grow tedious, and then pronounced the name "Janet Spence."

Doris was incredulous. "Miss Spence of the Manor? That old woman?" It was too ridiculous. Mr. Hutton laughed too.

"But it's quite true," he said. "She adores me." Oh, the vast joke. He would go and see her as soon as he returned—see and conquer. "I believe she wants to marry me," he added.

"But you wouldn't . . . you don't intend . . ."

The air was fairly crepitating with humour. Mr. Hutton laughed aloud. "I intend to marry you," he said. It seemed to him the best joke he had ever made in his life.

When Mr. Hutton left Southend he was once more a married man. It was agreed that, for the time being, the fact should be kept secret. In the autumn they would go abroad together, and the world should be informed. Meanwhile he was to go back to his own house and Doris to hers.

The day after his return he walked over in the afternoon to see Miss Spence. She received him with the old Gioconda.

"I was expecting you to come."

"I couldn't keep away," Mr. Hutton gallantly replied.

They sat in the summer-house. It was a pleasant place—a little old stucco temple bowered among dense bushes of evergreen. Miss Spence had left her mark on it by hanging up over the seat a blue-and-white Della Robbia plaque.

"I am thinking of going to Italy this autumn," said Mr. Hutton. He felt like a ginger-beer bottle, ready to pop with bubbling humorous excitement.

"Italy. . . ." Miss Spence closed her eyes ecstatically. "I feel drawn there too."

"Why not let yourself be drawn?"

"I don't know. One somehow hasn't the energy and initiative to set out alone."

"Alone. . . ." Ah, sound of guitars and throaty singing! "Yes, travelling alone isn't much fun."

Miss Spence lay back in her chair without speaking. Her eyes were still closed. Mr. Hutton stroked his moustache. The silence prolonged itself for what seemed a very long time.

Pressed to stay to dinner, Mr. Hutton did not refuse. The fun had hardly started. The table was laid in the loggia. Through its arches they looked out on to the sloping garden, to the valley below and the farther hills. Light ebbed away; the heat and silence were oppressive. A huge cloud was mounting up the sky, and there were distant breathings of thunder. The thunder drew nearer, a wind began to blow, and the first drops of rain fell. The table was cleared. Miss Spence and Mr. Hutton sat on in the growing darkness.

Miss Spence broke a long silence by saying meditatively:

"I think everyone has a right to a certain amount of happiness, don't you?"

"Most certainly." But what was she leading up to? Nobody makes generalisations about life unless they mean to talk about themselves. Happiness: he looked back on his own life, and saw a cheerful, placid existence disturbed by no great griefs or discomforts or alarms. He had always had money and freedom; he had been able to do very much as he wanted. Yes, he supposed he had been happy—happier than most men. And now he was not merely happy; he had discovered in irresponsibility the secret of gaiety. He was about to say something about his happiness when Miss Spence went on speaking.

"People like you and me have a right to be happy some time in our lives."

"Me?" said Mr. Hutton surprised.

"Poor Henry! Fate hasn't treated either of us very well."

"Oh, well, it might have treated me worse."

"You're being cheerful. That's brave of you. But don't think I can't see behind the mask."

Miss Spence spoke louder and louder as the rain came down more and more heavily. Periodically the thunder cut across her utterances. She talked on, shouting against the noise.

"I have understood you so well and for so long."

A flash revealed her, aimed and intent, leaning towards him. Her eyes were two profound and menacing gun-barrels. The darkness re-engulfed her.

"You were a lonely soul seeking a companion soul. I could sympathise with you in your solitude. Your marriage . . ."

The thunder cut short the sentence. Miss Spence's voice became audible once more with the words:

". . . could offer no companionship to a man of your stamp. You needed a soul mate."

A soul mate—he! a soul mate. It was incredibly fantastic. "Georgette Leblanc, the ex-soul mate of Maurice Maeterlinck." He had seen that in the paper a few days ago. So it was thus that Janet Spence had painted him in her imagination—a soul-mater. And for Doris he was a picture of goodness and the cleverest man in the world. And actually, really, he was what?—Who knows?

"My heart went out to you. I could understand; I was lonely, too." Miss Spence laid her hand on his knee. "You were so patient." Another flash. She was still aimed, dangerously. "You never complained. But I could guess—I could guess."

"How wonderful of you!" So he was an *âme incomprise*. "Only a woman's intuition . . ."

The thunder crashed and rumbled, died away, and only the sound of the rain was left. The thunder was his laughter, magnified, externalised. Flash and crash, there it was again, right on top of them.

"Don't you feel that you have within you something that is akin to this storm?" He could imagine her leaning forward as she uttered the words. "Passion makes one the equal of the elements."

What was his gambit now? Why, obviously, he should have said "Yes," and ventured on some unequivocal gesture. But Mr. Hutton suddenly took fright. The ginger beer in him had gone flat. The woman was serious—terribly serious. He was appalled.

Passion? "No," he desperately answered. "I am without passion."

But his remark was either unheard or unheeded, for Miss Spence went on with a growing exaltation, speaking so rapidly, however, and in such a burningly intimate whisper that Mr. Hutton found it very difficult to distinguish what she was saying. She was telling him, as far as he could make out, the story of her life. The lightning was less frequent now, and there were long intervals of darkness. But at each flash he saw her still aiming towards him, still yearning forward with a terrifying intensity. Darkness, the rain, and then flash! her face was there, close at hand. A pale mask, greenish white; the large eyes, the narrow barrel of the mouth, the heavy eyebrows. Agrippina, or wasn't it rather—yes, wasn't it rather George Robey?

He began devising absurd plans for escaping. He might suddenly jump up, pretending he had seen a burglar—Stop thief! stop thief!—and dash off into the night in pursuit. Or should he say that he felt faint, a heart attack? or that he had seen a ghost—Emily's ghost—in the garden? Absorbed in his childish plotting, he had ceased to pay any attention to Miss Spence's words. The spasmodic clutching of her hand recalled his thoughts.

"I honoured you for that, Henry," she was saying.

Honoured him for what?

"Marriage is a sacred tie, and your respect for it, even when the marriage was, as it was in your case, an unhappy one, made me respect you and admire you, and—shall I dare say the word?—"

Oh, the burglar, the ghost in the garden! But it was too late.

". . . yes, love you, Henry, all the more. But we're free now, Henry."

Free? There was a movement in the dark, and she was kneeling on the floor by his chair.

"Oh, Henry, Henry, I have been unhappy too."

Her arms embraced him, and by the shaking of her body he could feel that she was sobbing. She might have been a suppliant crying for mercy.

"You mustn't, Janet," he protested. Those tears were terrible, terrible. "Not now, not now! You must be calm; you must go to bed." He patted her shoulder, then got up, disengaging himself from her embrace. He left her still crouching on the floor beside the chair on which he had been sitting.

Groping his way into the hall, and without waiting to look for his hat, he went out of the house, taking infinite pains to close the front door noiselessly behind him. The clouds had blown over, and the moon was shining from a clear sky. There were puddles all along the road, and a noise of running water rose from the gutters and ditches. Mr. Hutton splashed along, not caring if he got wet.

How heartrendingly she had sobbed! With the emotions of pity and remorse that the recollection evoked in him there was a certain resentment: why couldn't she have played the game that he was playing—the heartless, amusing game? Yes, but he had known all the time that she wouldn't, she couldn't play that game; he had known and persisted.

What had she said about passion and the elements? Something absurdly stale, but true, true. There she was, a cloud black bosomed and charged with thunder, and he, like some absurd little Benjamin Franklin, had sent up a kite into the heart of the menace. Now he was complaining that his toy had drawn the lightning.

She was probably still kneeling by that chair in the loggia, crying.

But why hadn't he been able to keep up the game? Why had his irresponsibility deserted him, leaving him suddenly sober in a cold world? There were no answers to any of his questions. One idea burned steady and luminous in his mind—the idea of flight. He must get away at once.

IV

"What are you thinking about, Teddy Bear?"

"Nothing."

There was a silence. Mr. Hutton remained motionless, his elbows on the parapet of the terrace, his chin in his hands, looking down over Florence. He had taken a villa on one of the hilltops to the south of the city. From a little raised terrace at the end of the garden one looked down a long fertile valley on to the town and beyond it to the bleak mass of Monte Morello and, eastward of it, to the peopled hill of Fiesole, dotted with white houses. Everything was clear and luminous in the September sunshine.

"Are you worried about anything?"

"No, thank you."

"Tell me, Teddy Bear."

"But, my dear, there's nothing to tell." Mr. Hutton turned round, smiled, and patted the girl's hand. "I think you'd better go in and have your siesta. It's too hot for you here."

"Very well, Teddy Bear. Are you coming too?"

"When I've finished my cigar."

"All right. But do hurry up and finish it, Teddy Bear." Slowly, reluctantly, she descended the steps of the terrace and walked towards the house.

Mr. Hutton continued his contemplation of Florence. He had need to be alone. It was good sometimes to escape from Doris and the restless solicitude of her passion. He had never known the pains of loving hopelessly, but he was experiencing now the pains of being loved. These last weeks had been a period of growing discomfort. Doris was always with him, like an obsession, like a guilty conscience. Yes, it was good to be alone.

He pulled an envelope out of his pocket and opened it; not without reluctance. He hated letters; they always contained something unpleasant—nowadays, since his second marriage. This was from his sister. He began skimming through the insulting home-truths of which it was composed. The words "indecent haste," "social suicide," "scarcely cold in her grave," "person of the lower classes," all occurred. They were inevitable now in any communication from a well-meaning and right-thinking relative. Impatient, he was about to tear the stupid letter to pieces when his eye fell on a sentence at the bottom of the third page. His heart beat with uncomfortable violence as he read it. It was too monstrous! Janet Spence was going about telling everyone that he had poisoned his wife in order to marry Doris. What damnable malice! Ordinarily a man of the suavest temper, Mr. Hutton found himself trembling with rage. He took the childish satisfaction of calling names—he cursed the woman.

Then suddenly he saw the ridiculous side of the situation. The notion that he should have murdered anyone in order to marry Doris! If they only knew how miserably bored he was. Poor, dear Janet! She had tried to be malicious; she had only succeeded in being stupid.

A sound of footsteps aroused him; he looked round. In the garden below the little terrace the servant girl of the house was picking fruit. A Neapolitan, strayed somehow as far north as Florence, she was a specimen of the classical type—a little debased. Her profile might have been taken from a Sicilian coin of a bad period. Her features, carved floridly in the grand tradition, expressed an almost perfect stupidity. Her mouth was the most beautiful thing about her; the calligraphic hand of nature had richly curved it into an expression of mulish bad temper. . . . Under her hideous black clothes, Mr. Hutton divined a powerful body, firm and massive. He had looked at her before with a vague interest and curiosity. To-day the curiosity defined and focused itself into a desire. An idyll of Theocritus. Here was the woman; he, alas, was not precisely like a goatherd on the volcanic hills. He called to her.

"Armida!"

The smile with which she answered him was so provocative, attested so easy a virtue, that Mr. Hutton took fright. He was on the brink once more—on the brink. He must draw back, oh! quickly, quickly, before it was too late. The girl continued to look up at him.

"*Ha chiamato?*" she asked at last.

Stupidity or reason? Oh, there was no choice now. It was imbecility every time.

"*Scendo,*" he called back to her. Twelve steps led from the garden to the terrace. Mr. Hutton counted them. Down, down, down, down. . . . He saw a vision of himself descending from one circle of the inferno to the next—from a darkness full of wind and hail to an abyss of stinking mud.

V

For a good many days the Hutton case had a place on the front page of every newspaper. There had been no more popular murder trial since George Smith had temporarily eclipsed the European War by drowning in a warm bath his seventh bride. The public imagination was stirred by this tale of a murder brought to light months after the date of the crime. Here, it was felt, was one of those incidents in human life, so notable because they are so rare, which do definitely justify the ways of God to man. A wicked man had been moved by an illicit passion to kill his wife. For months he had lived in sin and fancied security—only to be dashed at last more horribly into the pit he had prepared for himself. Murder will out, and here was a case of it. The readers of the newspapers were in a position to follow every movement of the hand of God. There had been vague, but persistent, rumours in the neighbourhood; the police had taken action at last. Then came the exhumation order, the post-mortem examination, the inquest, the evidence of the experts, the verdict of the coroner's jury, the trial, the condemnation. For once Providence had done its duty, obviously, grossly, didactically, as in a melodrama. The newspapers were right in making of the case the staple intellectual food of a whole season.

Mr. Hutton's first emotion when he was summoned from Italy to give evidence at the inquest was one of indignation. It was a monstrous, a scandalous thing that the police should take such idle, malicious gossip seriously. When the inquest was over he would bring an action for malicious prosecution against the Chief Constable; he would sue the Spence woman for slander.

The inquest was opened; the astonishing evidence unrolled itself. The experts had examined the body, and had found traces of arsenic; they were of opinion that the late Mrs. Hutton had died of arsenic poisoning.

Arsenic poisoning. . . . Emily had died of arsenic poisoning?

After that, Mr. Hutton learned with surprise that there was enough arsenicated insecticide in his greenhouses to poison an army.

It was now, quite suddenly, that he saw it: there was a case against him. Fascinated, he watched it growing, growing, like some monstrous tropical plant. It was enveloping him, surrounding him; he was lost in a tangled forest.

When was the poison administered? The experts agreed that it must have been swallowed eight or nine hours before death. About lunch-time? Yes, about lunch-time. Clara, the parlourmaid, was called. Mrs. Hutton, she remembered, had asked her to go and fetch her medicine. Mr. Hutton had volunteered to go instead; he had gone alone. Miss Spence—ah, the memory of the storm, the white aimed face! the horror of it all!—Miss Spence confirmed Clara's statement, and added that Mr. Hutton had come back with the medicine already poured out in a wineglass, not in the bottle.

Mr. Hutton's indignation evaporated. He was dismayed, frightened. It was all too fantastic to be taken seriously, and yet this nightmare was a fact—it was actually happening.

M'Nab had seen them kissing, often. He had taken them for a drive on the day of Mrs. Hutton's death. He could see them reflected in the wind-screen, sometimes out of the tail of his eye.

The inquest was adjourned. That evening Doris went to bed with a headache. When he went to her room after dinner, Mr. Hutton found her crying.

"What's the matter?" He sat down on the edge of her bed and began to stroke her hair. For a long time she did not answer, and he went on stroking her hair mechanically, almost unconsciously; sometimes, even he bent down and kissed her bare shoulder. He had his own affairs, however, to think about. What had happened? How was it that the stupid gossip had actually come true? Emily had died of arsenic poisoning. It was absurd, impossible. The order of things had been broken, and he was at the mercy of an irresponsibility. What had happened, what was going to happen? He was interrupted in the midst of his thoughts.

"It's my fault—it's my fault!" Doris suddenly sobbed out. "I shouldn't have loved you; I oughtn't to have let you love me. Why was I ever born?"

Mr. Hutton didn't say anything, but looked down in silence at the abject figure of misery lying on the bed.

"If they do anything to you I shall kill myself."

She sat up, held him for a moment at arm's length, and looked at him with a kind of violence, as though she were never to see him again.

"I love you, I love you, I love you." She drew him, inert and passive, towards her, clasped him, pressed herself against him. "I didn't know you loved me as much as that, Teddy Bear. But why did you do it—why did you do it?"

Mr. Hutton undid her clasping arms and got up. His face became very red. "You seem to take it for granted that I murdered my wife," he said. "It's really too grotesque. What do you all take me for? A cinema hero?" He had begun to lose his temper. All the exasperation, all the fear and bewilderment of the day, was transformed into a violent anger against her. "It's all such damned stupidity. Haven't you any conception of a civilised man's mentality? Do I look the sort of man who'd go about slaughtering people? I suppose you imagined I was so insanely in love with you that I could commit any folly. When will you women understand that one isn't insanely in love? All one asks for is a quiet life, which you won't allow one to have. I don't know what the devil ever induced me to marry you. It was all a damned stupid, practical joke. And now you go about saying I'm a murderer. I won't stand it."

Mr. Hutton stamped towards the door. He had said horrible things, he knew—odious things that he ought speedily to unsay. But he wouldn't. He closed the door behind him.

"Teddy Bear!" He turned the handle; the latch clicked into place. "Teddy Bear!" The voice that came to him through the closed door was agonised. Should he go back? He ought to go back. He touched the handle, then withdrew his fingers and quickly walked away. When he was halfway down the stairs he halted. She might try to do something silly—throw herself out of the window or God knows what! He listened attentively; there was no sound. But he pictured her very clearly, tiptoeing across the room, lifting the sash as high as it would go, leaning out into the cold night air. It was raining a little. Under the window lay the paved terrace. How far below? Twenty-five or thirty feet? Once, when he was walking along Piccadilly, a dog had jumped out of a third-story window of the Ritz. He had seen it fall; he had heard it strike the pavement. Should he go back? He was damned if he would; he hated her.

He sat for a long time in the library. What had happened? What was happening? He turned the question over and over in his mind and could find no answer. Suppose the nightmare dreamed itself out to its horrible conclusion. Death was waiting for him. His eyes filled with tears; he wanted so passionately to live. "Just to be alive." Poor Emily had wished it too, he remembered: "Just to be alive." There were still so many places in this astonishing world unvisited, so many queer delightful people still unknown, so many lovely women never so much as seen. The huge white oxen would still be dragging their wains along the Tuscan roads, the cypresses would still go up, straight as pillars, to the blue heaven; but he would not be there to see them. And the sweet southern wines—Tear of Christ and Blood of Judas—others would drink them, not he. Others would walk down the obscure and narrow lanes between the bookshelves in the London Library, sniffing the dusty perfume of good literature, peering at strange titles, discovering unknown names, exploring the fringes of vast domains of knowledge. He would be lying in a hole in the ground. And why, why? Confusedly he felt that some extraordinary kind of justice was being done. In the past he had been wanton and imbecile and irresponsible. Now Fate was playing as wantonly, as irresponsibly, with him. It was tit for tat, and God existed after all.

He felt that he would like to pray. Forty years ago he used to kneel by his bed every evening. The nightly formula of his childhood came to him almost unsought from some long unopened chamber of the memory. "God bless Father and Mother, Tom and Cissie and the Baby, Mademoiselle and Nurse, and everyone that I love, and make me a good boy. Amen." They were all dead now—all except Cissie.

His mind seemed to soften and dissolve; a great calm descended upon his spirit. He went upstairs to ask Doris's forgiveness. He found her lying on the couch at the foot of the bed. On the floor beside her stood a blue bottle of liniment, marked "Not to be taken"; she seemed to have drunk about half of it.

"You didn't love me," was all she said when she opened her eyes to find him bending over her.

Dr. Libbard arrived in time to prevent any very serious consequences. "You mustn't do this again," he said while Mr. Hutton was out of the room.

"What's to prevent me?" she asked defiantly.

Dr. Libbard looked at her with his large, sad eyes. "There's nothing to prevent you," he said. "Only yourself and your baby. Isn't it rather bad luck on your baby, not allowing it to come into the world because you want to go out of it?"

Doris was silent for a time. "All right," she whispered. "I won't."

Mr. Hutton sat by her bedside for the rest of the night. He felt himself now to be indeed a murderer. For a time he persuaded himself that he loved this pitiable child. Dozing in his chair, he woke up, stiff and cold, to find himself drained dry, as it were, of every emotion. He had become nothing but a tired and suffering carcase. At six o'clock he undressed and went to bed for a couple of hours' sleep. In the course of the same afternoon the coroner's jury brought in a verdict of "Wilful Murder," and Mr. Hutton was committed for trial.

VI

Miss Spence was not at all well. She had found her public appearances in the witness-box very trying, and when it was all over she had something that was very nearly a breakdown. She slept badly, and suffered from nervous indigestion. Dr. Libbard used to call every other day. She talked to him a great deal—mostly about the Hutton case. . . . Her moral indignation was always on the boil. Wasn't it appalling to think that one had had a murderer in one's house. Wasn't it extraordinary that one could have been for so long mistaken about the man's character? (But she had had an inkling from the first.) And then the girl he had gone off with—so low class, so little better than a prostitute. The news that the second Mrs. Hutton was expecting a baby—the posthumous child of a condemned and executed criminal—revolted her; the thing was shocking—an obscenity. Dr. Libbard answered her gently and vaguely, and prescribed bromide.

One morning he interrupted her in the midst of her customary tirade. "By the way," he said in his soft, melancholy voice, "I suppose it was really you who poisoned Mrs. Hutton."

Miss Spence stared at him for two or three seconds with enormous eyes, and then quietly said, "Yes." After that she started to cry.

"In the coffee, I suppose."

She seemed to nod assent. Dr. Libbard took out his fountain-pen, and in his neat, meticulous calligraphy wrote out a prescription for a sleeping-draught.

Critical Analysis

At the outset it is important to consider the tone of "The Gioconda Smile." What might be a murder-mystery thriller becomes a vehicle for brilliant wit and satirical characterization, expressing a derisive view of human nature. Everyone is ridiculed. Huxley's characters live in a world where they either shun responsibility or step in arbitrarily to solve the problems of others. In either case they become fools, and eventually lose what they want. Mr. Hutton's and Janet Spence's views of themselves and others about them bring death and frustration. Huxley's attitude toward his characters and his manner of presenting that attitude provide the satirical and witty tone of "The Gioconda Smile."

The story is told in six parts, not to block out neatly the narrative of events but to provide episodes and incidents which give Huxley the best opportunity for satiric effects and ironical situations. Expected "big scenes" of action of the conventional type are usually merely stated in passing. What ordinary murder story, for example, would omit the trial of Mr. Hutton? The parts vary in range, intensity, and satiric force but all contribute to the total effect of irony and satire. The first part introduces Mr. Hutton and, mainly through his observation, Janet Spence. Notice how the story begins—with Mr. Hutton's monologue on Janet Spence and a reverie of self-admiration as he gazes into the mirror. Mr. Hutton's own proud approval of his long, bounding strides and his "youth" gives the reader a strong hint of his physical quality and his egocentricity. The ironic contrast between what Mr. Hutton protests: "I must get back to see how poor Emily is," and the truth of Doris, waiting in the "obscurity" of the back seat of the car for her "Teddy Bear," provides a humorous surprise—and a view of the true Mr. Hutton.

The section is primarily used to introduce character but not in a plain expository manner. Wit and satire supply the tone, especially in the description of Janet's taste in art and in Doris's baby talk. Actually, the only plot development is the invitation for Janet Spence, Mr. Hutton's "mysterious Gioconda," to come to luncheon. Part II might be called the life and death of sickly, though once pretty, Mrs. Hutton; now her cadaverous, lifeless mien is in strong contrast to Mr. Hutton and to the frolicsome

Doris, who even at this moment occupies his thoughts. To Mr. Hutton Janet Spence is an enigma, but, ironically, the probing of the riddle is to be his doom.

The irony of contrasting situation is again stressed in the activities of Mr. Hutton. Supposedly on a visit to the Johnsons "to discuss the war memorial, you know," he is actually with Doris, bored with his rendezvous at a roadside hotel, while at home his wife has died (poisoned by a woman in love with him!).

The penitence of Mr. Hutton opens the third section, but the penitence is not only short-lived; it is too late. His plan to take personal interest in his estate and also to write his great work on *The Effect of Diseases on Civilization* fails quickly. Reason is defeated; Doris wins. Mr. Hutton's intention of marrying Doris "seemed to him the best joke he had ever made in his life"; yet it is a joke which is to have ironic payment in Part IV. Janet Spence's confession of love allows him one more opportunity for grim "fun," but Mr. Hutton, "like some absurd little Benjamin Franklin, had sent up a kite in the heart of the menace. Now he was complaining that his toy had drawn lightning." The very simile is a good example of Huxley's witty laughter at the character.

It might be useful here to notice that Huxley up to this point has set up incidents and situations from which the story is to be completed. From the view of plot, the reader might well remember that Miss Spence had given Mrs. Hutton the fatal coffee at the luncheon (p. 254) and had remarked to Mr. Hutton:

> "I think Emily is in a very bad state. Anything might happen—at any moment."

Important both for plot and character are the actions and attitudes of Mr. Hutton, Doris, and Janet. The boredom which Doris can arouse in Mr. Hutton (page 248) is a mere sample of what married life with the lady was to be. Mr. Hutton's horror at the proposal to be Janet's "soul mate" has left a potential avenger in the story.

Part IV shifts the scene to Florence, to Mr. Hutton's life with Doris, and to his continued sensual drive. Bored with the lusty Doris, he sees Armida, the Neapolitan girl, standing enticingly before him, and he makes the decision for "imbecility." Huxley's wit in the treatment of character is carefully expressed in Mr. Hutton's intellectualized literary vision of his descent to Armida.

> "*Scendo*," he called back to her. Twelve steps led from the garden to the terrace. Mr. Hutton counted them. Down, down, down, down. . . . He saw a vision of himself descending from one circle of the inferno to the next—from a darkness full of wind and hail to an abyss of stinking mud.

The tone for the conclusion of the story is set by the second sentence of Section V: "There had been no more popular murder trial since George Smith had temporarily eclipsed the European War by drowning in a warm bath his seventh bride." Huxley handles the detail briskly and briefly. What he wishes to stress most in the chapter is the final irony, the real irony of the story. To Mr. Hutton's disgust, Doris looks upon him as a murderer of the cinema-hero type, but he is psychologically and morally a murderer as he realizes what action Doris might take. Yet then follows the confession of his desire to live: "His eyes filled with tears; he wanted so passionately to live." And note what Mr. Hutton wants to live for—travel, new scenes, rare wines, the old volumes, "so many lovely women never so much as seen." The derisive laughter of Huxley at Mr. Hutton is here at its height. The formula of penitence, late and absurd, is repeated. The plot, whose elements have been in secondary position, becomes important in the brevity of its expression: "In the course of the same afternoon the coroner's jury brought in a verdict of 'Wilful Murder,' and Mr. Hutton was committed for trial."

At the very end of Part VI is Janet's confession, briefly given, but this short section shows Huxley's skill in drawing the final ironic portrait of a ridiculous, revengeful woman. He does it simply by a short mocking display of her point of view.

Her moral indignation was always on the boil. Wasn't it appalling to think that one had had a murderer in one's house? Wasn't it extraordinary that one could have been for so long mistaken about the man's character? (But she had had an inkling from the first.) And then the girl he had gone off with—so low class, so little better than a prostitute. The news that the second Mrs. Hutton was expecting a baby—the posthumous child of a condemned and executed criminal—revolted her; the thing was shocking—an obscenity.

Dr. Libbard, an observer in the story, has seen Mr. Hutton and the three women who affected his life. He knows all; he has the true key to the mystery of the "murderer," Mr. Hutton, and to the mind and action of Janet Spence. But he is a scrupulously "professional" soul, apparently beyond positive moral action. The conventional narrative would not have ended with Janet Spence's confession to her doctor. Why does Huxley end the story in this way? He has accomplished all he set out to do—to show his people caught in their own actions and ideas of life. Mr. Hutton is his main interest, and in Mr. Hutton's career the irony of the story is concentrated.

Huxley has paraded his fools. Mr. Hutton is torn between passion and reason and always does the absurd thing. Janet is a self-centred romantic, volatile and revengeful. Through her action the title, "The Gioconda Smile," becomes clear. The enticing, enigmatic charm of the smile of the wife of Francesco del Giocondo captivated Leonardo da Vinci, who painted her portrait, known as the Mona Lisa. Janet Spence's studied Gioconda smile has led Mr. Hutton, the polite, playfully chivalric sensualist, to his death. Doris, who in Mr. Hutton's opinion resembles a mistress of Charles II, is the flesh, the glorifier of conventional melodramatic action. Mrs. Hutton is the rose faded, the self-indulgent invalid in mind and body.

The irony and comic satire of "The Gioconda Smile" are at once an expression of and a part of the wit with which the story is conceived and executed. Wit best serves character and idea rather than plot and creates the final comic ironic tone of the tale. Huxley has paid most attention to Mr. Hutton, both as Mr. Hutton reveals himself and as he sees others. Though self-revealed as a sensualist and an egocentric, he has a curious intellectualized imagination which occasionally expresses itself wittily in references to philology, marine biology, literature, and art. To Janet's remark that he is cynical, he has the desire to answer "Bow-wow-wow," a philological retort stemming from the literal meaning of "cynical," doglike (Greek, kynikos). When he tells Doris that the "electricity" is in *her*, he recalls her as the sea-mouse, a sea worm of the genus *Aphrodite* or as a sea-cucumber, "which turns itself inside out in moments of alarm." His remarks about Milton's being called the "Lady of Christ's" (i.e. Christ's College, Cambridge) give him a neat opportunity to call himself "Christ of Ladies." The ailing Mrs. Hutton has in Mr. Hutton's view "the face of a dead Christ by Morales." But many times Mr. Hutton's intellectual byplay and descriptive power seem more a product of Huxley's own style than anything developed from the established character of Mr. Hutton. In one case, although the reader is led to believe that he is observing Janet Spence through Mr. Hutton's consciousness, the witty description of the lady seems to be Huxley's own.

> What a queer face she had! That small mouth pursed forward by the Gioconda expression into a little snout with a round hole in the middle as though for whistling—it was like a penholder seen from the front. Above the mouth a well-shaped nose, finely aquiline. Eyes large, lustrous, and dark, with the largeness, lustre, and darkness that seems to invite sties and an occasional bloodshot suffusion. They were fine eyes, but unchangingly grave. The penholder might do its Gioconda trick, but the eyes never altered in their earnestness. Above them, a pair of boldly arched, heavily pencilled black eyebrows lent a surprising air of power, as of a Roman matron, to the upper portion of the face. Her hair was dark and equally Roman; Agrippina from the brows upward.

Huxley has other useful tricks. Mr. Hutton is always *Mr.* Hutton, except for the moments of his greatest emotional fervor in his scene with Janet—when he becomes "Henry," "Poor Henry." To Doris he is always "Teddy Bear," and she scarcely addresses a sentence to him without the nickname. By repetition these comic-satiric devices become very effective tags. Other examples are the "old Gioconda" which Janet throws at Mr. Hutton, and the characterization of Janet as Agrippina, or as Huxley devastatingly asks in the height of Janet's crisis, "Wasn't it rather George Robey?" The undertone of laughter runs through the description both of event and of character. The thunderstorm which rages during Janet's confession of love provides intensity, but of a comic-opera sort.

Huxley's brilliant verbal virtuosity, although it occasionally draws too much attention to itself, is derived from his whole approach to the story. This is not a story of plot. It is a skillfully ironic, brilliantly written portrait of an irresponsible sensualist, trying to live, but getting caught in a world which absurdly glorifies or condemns his actions. The characters in "The Gioconda Smile" are in mortal coils and Huxley laughs at each one of them.

Gunners' Passage

IRWIN SHAW (1913–)

"In Brazil," Whitejack was saying, "the problem was girls. American girls."

They were lying on the comfortable cots, with the mosquito netting looped gracefully over their heads and the barracks quiet and empty, except for the two of them, and shaded and cool, when you remembered that outside the full sun of Africa stared down.

"Three months in the jungle, on rice and monkey meat." Whitejack lit a large, long, nickel cigar and puffed deeply, squinting up at the tin roof. "When we got to Rio, we felt we deserved an American girl. So the lieutenant and Johnny Moffat and myself, we got the telephone directory of the American Embassy and we went down the list, calling up likely names—secretaries, typists, interpreters, filing clerks—" Whitejack grinned up at the ceiling. He had a large, sunburned, rough face that was broken into good looks by his smile, and his speech was Southern, but not the kind of Southern that puts a Northerner's teeth on edge.

"It was the lieutenant's idea, and by the time we got to the Q's, he was ready to give up. But we hit pay dirt on the S's." Slowly he blew out a long column of cigar smoke. "Uh-uh," he said, closing his eyes reflectively. "Two months and eleven days of honey and molasses. Three tender and affectionate American girls, as loving as the day is long, with their own flat. Beer in the icebox from Sunday to Sunday, steaks big enough to saddle a mule with, and nothing to do—just lie on the beach in the afternoon and go swimmin' when the mood seized yuh. On per diem."

"How were the girls?" Stais asked. "Pretty?"

"Well, Sergeant." Whitejack paused thoughtfully and pursed his lips. "To tell you the truth, Sergeant, the girls the lieutenant and Johnny had were as smart and pretty as chipmunks. Mine . . ." Once more he paused. "Ordinarily, my girl would find herself hard put to collect a man in the middle of a full division of infantry soldiers. She was small and runty and she had less curves than a rifle barrel and she wore glasses. But from the first time she looked at me, I could see she wasn't interested in Johnny or the lieutenant. She looked at me, and behind her glasses her eyes were soft and hopeful and humble and appealing." Whitejack flicked the cigar ash off into a little tin can which was resting on his bare chest. "Sometimes," he said slowly, "a man feels mighty small if he just thinks of himself and turns down an appeal like that. Let me tell you something, Sergeant. I was in Rio two months and eleven days and I didn't look at another woman. All those dark-brown women walkin' along the beach, three-quarters out of their bathing suits, just wavin' it in front of your face—I didn't look at them. This runty, skinny little thing with glasses was the most lovin' and satisfactory and decent little person a man could possibly conceive of and a man'd just have to be hog-greedy with sex to have winked an eye at another woman." Whitejack doused his cigar, took the tin can off his chest, and rolled over on his belly. "Now," he said, "I'm going to get myself a little sleep."

In a moment Whitejack was snoring gently, his tough mountaineer's face tucked childishly into the crook of one arm. Outside, on the shady side of the building, a native boy hummed low and wild to himself as he ironed a pair of suntan trousers. From the field, two hundred yards away, again and again came the sliding roar of engines climbing or descending the afternoon sky.

Stais closed his eyes wearily. Ever since he'd got into Accra, he had done nothing but sleep and lie on his cot daydreaming, listening to Whitejack talk.

"Hi," Whitejack had said as Stais had come slowly into the barracks two days before. "Which way you going?"

"Home," Stais had said, smiling wearily, as he did every time he said it. "Going home. Which way you going?"

"Not home." Whitejack had grinned a little. "Not home at all."

Stais liked to listen to Whitejack. Whitejack talked about America, about the woods of the Blue Ridge Mountains, where he had been in the forestry service, about his mother's cooking and how he had owned great dogs who had been extraordinary at finding a trail and holding it, about how they had tried hunting deer in the hills from the medium bomber (no good because of the swirling winds rising from the gorges), about pleasant, indiscriminate weekend parties in the woods with his friend Johnny Moffat and the girls from the mill in the next town. Stais had been away from America for nineteen months now, and Whitejack's talk made his native country seem present and pleasantly real to him.

"There was a man in my town by the name of Thomas Wolfe," Whitejack had said irrelevantly that morning. "He was a great big feller and he went away to New York to be an author. Maybe you heard of him?"

"Yes," said Stais. "I read two books of his."

"Well, I read that book of his," said Whitejack, "and the people in town were yellin' to lynch him for a while, but I read that book, and he got that town down fair and proper, and when they brought him back dead, I came down from the hills and I went to his funeral. There were a lot of important people from New York and over to Chapel Hill down for the funeral and it was a hot day, too, and I'd never met the feller, but I felt it was only right to go to his funeral after readin' his book. And the whole town was there, very quiet, although just five years before they were yellin' to lynch him, and it was a sad and impressive sight and I'm glad I went."

And another time, the slow, deep voice rolling between sleep and sleep in the shaded heat, "My mother takes a quail and bones it, and then she scoops out a great big sweet potato and lays some bacon on it, then she puts the quail in and cooks it slow for three hours, bastin' it with butter all the time. You got to try that sometime."

"Yes," said Stais, "I will."

Stais did not have a high-priority number and there seemed to be a flood of colonels surging toward America, taking all the seats on the C-54s setting out westward, so he'd had to wait. It hadn't been bad. Just to lie down, stretched full out, unbothered, these days, was holiday enough after Greece, and anyway he didn't want to arrive home, in front of his mother, until he'd stopped looking like a tired old man. And the barracks usually were empty and quiet and the chow good at the transient mess and you could get Coca-Cola and chocolate milk at the PX. The rest of the enlisted men in Whitejack's crew were young and ambitious and were out swimming all day and going to the movies or playing poker in another barracks all night, and Whitejack's talk was smooth and amusing in the periods between sleep and dreams. Whitejack was an aerial photographer and gunner in a mapping and survey squadron and he'd been in Alaska and Brazil and back to the States and now was on his way to India, full of conversation. He was in a Mitchell squadron and the whole squadron was supposed to be on its way together, but two of the Mitchells had crashed and burned on the takeoff at Natal as Whitejack's plane had circled the field, waiting to form up. The rest of the squadron had been held at Natal and Whitejack's plane had been sent on to Accra, across the ocean, by itself.

Vaguely and slowly, lying on the warm cot, with the wild song of the Negro boy outside the window, Stais thought of the two Mitchells burning between sea and jungle three thousand miles away, and of other planes burning elsewhere, and of what it was going to be like sitting down in the armchair of his own house and looking across the room at his mother, and the pretty Viennese girl in Jerusalem, and of the DC-3 coming down slowly, like an angel in the dusk, to the rough, secret pasture in the Peloponnesian hills.

He fell asleep. His bones knit gently into dreams on the soft cot, with the sheets, in the quiet barracks, and he was over Athens again, with the ruins pale and shining on the hills, and the fighters boring in, and Lathrop saying, over the intercom, as they persisted into a hundred, fifty yards, twisting, swift and shifty, in the bright Greek sky, "They grounded all the students today. They have the instructors up this afternoon." And, suddenly and wildly, fifty feet over Ploesti, with Liberators going down into the filth in dozens, flaming . . . Then swimming off the white beach at Benghasi, with the dead boys playing in the mild, tideless swell, then the parachute pulling at every muscle in his body, then the green and forest blue of Minnesota woods and his father, fat and small, sleeping on pine needles on his Sunday off, then Athens again, Athens . . .

"I don't know what's come over the lieutenant," a new voice was saying as Stais came out of his dream. "He passes us on the field and he just don't seem to see us."

Stais opened his eyes. Novak, a farm boy from Oklahoma, was sitting on the edge of Whitejack's bed, talking. "It has all the guys real worried." He had a high, shy, rather girlish voice. "I used to think they never came better than the lieutenant. Now—" Novak shrugged. "If he does see you, he snaps at you like he was General Ulysses S. Grant."

"Maybe," Whitejack said, "maybe seeing Lieutenant Brogan go down in Natal . . . He and Brogan were friends since they were ten years old. Like as if I saw Johnny Moffat go down."

"It's not that." Novak went over to his own cot and got out his writing pad. "It began back in Miami, four weeks ago. Didn't you notice it?"

"I noticed it," Whitejack said slowly.

"You ought to ask him about it." Novak started writing a letter. "You and him are good friends. After all, going into combat now, it's bad—the lieutenant just lookin' through us when he passes us on the field. You don't think he's drunk all the time, do you?"

"He's not drunk."

"You ought to ask him."

"Maybe I will." Whitejack sat up. "Maybe I will." He looked forlornly down at his stomach. "Since I got into the Army, I've turned pig-fat. On the day I took the oath, I was twenty-eight and one-half inches around the waist. Today I'm thirty-two and three-quarters if I'm an inch. The Army . . . Maybe I shouldn't've joined. I was in a reserved profession, and I was the sole support of an ailing mother."

"Why did you join?" Stais asked.

"Oh." Whitejack smiled at him. "You're awake. Feeling any better, Sergeant?"

"Feeling fine, thanks. Why did you join?"

"Well—" Whitejack rubbed the side of his jaw. "Well, I waited and I waited. I sat up in my cabin in the hills and I tried to avoid listenin' to the radio, and I waited and I waited, and finally I went downtown to my mother and I said, 'Ma'am, I just can't wait any longer,' and I joined up."

"When was that?" Stais asked.

"Eight days"—Whitejack lay down again, plumping the pillow under his head—"eight days after Pearl Harbor."

"Sergeant," Novak said, "Sergeant Stais, you don't mind if I tell my girl you're a Greek, do you?"

"No," Stais said gravely. "I don't mind. You know, I was born in Minnesota."

"I know," said Novak, writing industriously. "But your parents came from Greece. My girl'll be very interested, your parents coming from Greece and you bombing Greece and being shot down there."

"What do you mean, your girl?" Whitejack asked. "I thought you said she was going around with a technical sergeant in Flushing, Long Island."

"That's true," Novak said apologetically. "But I still like to think of her as my girl."

"It's the ones that stay at home," said Whitejack darkly, "that get all the stripes and all the girls. My motto is, don't write to a girl once you get out of pillowcase distance from her."

"I like to write to this girl in Flushing, Long Island," Novak said, his voice shy but stubborn. Then to Stais, "How many days were you in the hills before the Greek farmers found you?"

"Fourteen," said Stais.

"And how many of you were wounded?"

"Three. Out of seven. The others were dead."

"Maybe he doesn't like to talk about it, Charlie," Whitejack said.

"Oh, I'm sorry." Novak looked up, his young, unlined face crossed with concern.

"That's all right," Stais said. "I don't mind."

"Did you tell them you were a Greek, too?" Novak asked. "When one finally showed up who could speak English."

"That must be funny," Novak said reflectively. "Being a Greek, bombing Greece, not speaking the language. Can I tell my girl they had a radio and they radioed to Cairo?"

"It's the girl of a technical sergeant in Flushing, Long Island," Whitejack chanted. "Why don't you look facts in the face?"

"I prefer it this way," Novak said, with dignity.

"I guess you can tell about the radio," Stais said. "It was pretty long ago. Three days later, the DC-3 came down through a break in the clouds. It'd been raining all the time and it just stopped for about thirty minutes at dusk and that plane came down, throwin' water fifteen feet in the air. We cheered, but we couldn't get up from where we were sitting, any of us, because we were too weak to stand."

"I got to write that to my girl," Novak said. "Too weak to stand."

"Then it started to rain again and the field was hip-deep in mud and when we all got into the DC-3, we couldn't get it started." Stais spoke calmly and thoughtfully, as though he were alone, reciting to himself. "We were just bogged down in that Greek mud. Then the pilot got out—he was a captain—and he looked around, with the rain coming down and all those farmers just standing there, sympathizing with him, and nothing anyone could do, and he just cursed for ten minutes. He was from San Francisco and he really knew how to curse. Then everybody started breaking branches off the trees in the woods around that pasture, even those of us who couldn't stand an hour before, and we just covered that big DC-3 complete with branches and waited for the rain to stop. We just sat in the woods and prayed no German patrols would come out in weather like that. In those three days I learned five words of Greek."

"What are they?" Novak asked.

"*Vouno*," Stais said. "That means 'mountain.' *Vrohi:* rain. *Theos:* God. *Avrion:* tomorrow. And *yassou.* That means 'farewell.'"

"*Yassou*," Novak said. "Farewell."

"Then the sun came out and the field started to steam and nobody said anything. We just sat there, watching the water dry off the grass, then the puddles started to go, here and there, then the mud to cake a little. Then we got into the DC-3 and the Greeks pushed and hauled for a while and we broke loose and got out. And those farmers just standing below waving at us, as though they were seeing us off at Grand Central Station. Ten miles further on we went right over a German camp. They fired at us a couple of times, but they didn't come anywhere close. The best moment of my whole life was getting into that hospital bed in Cairo. I just stood there and looked at it for a whole minute, looking at the sheets. Then I got in, very slow."

"Did you ever find out what happened to those Greeks?" Novak asked.

"No," said Stais. "I guess they're still there, waiting for us to come back someday."

There was silence, broken only by the slow scratching of Novak's pen. Stais thought of the thin, dark mountain faces of the men he had last seen, fading away, waving, standing in the scrub and short silver grass of the hill pasture near the Aegean Sea. They had been cheerful and anxious to please, and there was a look on their faces that made you feel they expected to die.

"How many missions were you on?" Novak asked.

"Twenty-one and a half," Stais said. He smiled. "I count the last one as half."

"How old are you?" Novak was obviously keeping the technical sergeant's girl carefully posted on all points of interest.

"Nineteen."

"You look older," said Whitejack.

"Yes," said Stais.

"A lot older."

"Yes."

"Did you shoot down any planes?" Novak peered at him shyly, his red face uncertain and embarrassed, like a little boy asking a doubtful question about girls. "Personally?"

"Two," Stais said. "Personally."

"What did you feel?"

"Why don't you leave him alone?" Whitejack said. "He's too tired to keep his eyes open as it is."

"I felt—relieved," Stais said. He tried to think of what he'd really felt when the tracers went in and the Focke-Wulf started to smoke like a crazy smudge pot and the German pilot fought wildly for half a second with the cowling and then didn't fight wildly any more. There was no way of telling these men, no way of remembering, in words, himself. "You'll find out," he said. "Soon enough. The sky's full of Germans."

"Japs," Whitejack said. "We're going to India."

"The sky's full of Japs."

There was silence once more, with the echo of the word "Japs" rustling thinly in the long, quiet room, over the empty rows of cots. Stais felt the old waving dizziness starting behind his eyes that the doctor in Cairo had said came from shock or starvation or exposure or all of these things, and lay back, still keeping his eyes open, because it became worse and waved more violently when he closed his eyes.

"One more question," Novak said. "Are—are guys afraid?"

"You'll be afraid," Stais said.

"Do you want to send that back to your girl in Flushing?" Whitejack asked sardonically.

"No," said Novak quietly. "I wanted that for myself."

"If you want to sleep," said Whitejack, "I'll shut this farmer up."

"Oh, no," said Stais. "I'm pleased to talk."

"If you're not careful," Whitejack said, "he'll talk about his girl in Flushing."

"I'd be pleased to hear it," said Stais.

"It's only natural I should want to talk about her," Novak said. "She was the best girl I ever knew in my whole life. I'd've married her if I could."

"My motto," said Whitejack, "is never marry a girl who goes

to bed with you the first time out. The chances are she isn't pure. The second time—that, of course, is different." He winked at Stais.

"I was in Flushing, Long Island, taking a five-week course in aerial cameras," Novak said, "and I was living at the Y.M.C.A."

"This is where I leave." Whitejack got off the bed and put on his pants.

"The Y.M.C.A. was very nice. There were bathrooms for every two rooms, and the food was very good," said Novak, talking earnestly to Stais, "but I must confess, I was lonely in Flushing, Long Island."

"I'll be back"—Whitejack was buttoning up his shirt—"for the ninth installment."

"As long as you're going out," Novak said to him, "I wish you'd talk to the lieutenant. It really makes me feel queer, passing him and him just looking through me like I was a window pane."

"Maybe I'll talk to the lieutenant," Whitejack said. "And leave the Sergeant alone. Remember, he's a tired man who's been to the war and he needs his rest." He went out.

Novak stared after Whitejack. "There's something wrong with him, too," he said. "Just lying on his back here for ten days, reading and sleeping. He never did that before. He was the liveliest man in the United States Air Force. Seeing those two planes go down . . . It's a funny thing, you fly with fellers all over the world, over America, Brazil, Alaska, you watch them shoot porpoises and sharks in gunnery practice over the Gulf Stream, you get drunk with them, go to their weddings, talk to them over the radio with their planes maybe a hundred feet away, in the air, and after all that flying, in one minute, for no reason, two planes go down. Fourteen fellers you've been livin' with for over a year." Novak shook his head. "There was a particular friend of Whitejack's in one of those planes. Frank Sloan. Just before we left Miami, they had a big fight. Frank went off and married a girl that Whitejack'd been going with off and on for a year, every time we hit Miami. Whitejack told him he was crazy, half the squadron had slept with the lady, and that was true, too, and just to teach him a lesson he'd sleep with her himself after they'd been married. And he did, too." Novak sighed. "A lot of funny things happen in the Army when fellers've been together a long time and get to know each other real well. And then, one minute, the Mitchell goes down. I guess Whitejack must've felt sort of queer, watching Frankie burn." Novak had put his writing pad down and now he screwed the top on his fountain pen. "The truth is," he said, "I don't feel so solid myself. That's why I like to talk. Especially to you. You've been through it. You're young, but you've been through it. But if it's any bother to you, I'll keep quiet."

"No," said Stais, still lying back, abstractedly wondering whether the waving would get worse or better, "not at all."

"This girl in Flushing, Long Island," Novak said slowly. "It's easy for Whitejack to make fun of me. The girls fall all over themselves chasing after him. He has no real conception of what it's like to be a man like me. Not very good-looking. Not much money. Not an officer. Not humorous. Shy."

Stais couldn't help grinning. "You're going to have a tough time in India."

"I know," Novak said. "I've resigned myself to not having a girl until the armistice. How did you do with the girls in the Middle East?" he asked politely.

"There was a nice Viennese girl in Jerusalem," Stais said dreamily. "But otherwise zero. You have to be very good, unless you're an officer, in the Middle East."

"That's what I heard," Novak said sorrowfully. "Well, it won't be so different to me from Oklahoma. That was the nice thing about this girl in Flushing, Long Island. She saw me come into the jewelry store where she worked and I was in my fatigues and I was with a very smooth feller who made a date with her for the night. But she smiled at me and I knew if I had the guts I could ask her for a date, too. But of course I didn't. But then later that night I was sitting in my room in the Y.M.C.A. and my phone rang. It was this girl. The other feller had stood her up, she said, and would I take her out." Novak smiled dimly, thinking of that tremulous moment of glory in the small Y.M.C.A. room far away. "I got my fatigues off in one minute and shaved and showered and I picked her up. We went to Coney Island. It was the first time in my entire life I had ever seen Coney Island. It took three and a half weeks for me to finish my course and I went out with that girl every single night. Nothing like that ever happened to me before in my life—a girl who just wanted to see me every night of the week. Then, the night before I was due to leave to join my squadron, she told me she had got permission to take the afternoon off and she would like to see me down to the train, if I let her. I called at the jewelry shop at noon and her boss shook my hand and she had a package under her arm and we got into the subway and we rode to New York City. Then we went into a cafeteria and had a wonderful lunch and she saw me off and gave me the package. It was Schrafft's candy, and she was crying at the gate there, crying for me, and she said she would like me to write, no matter what." Novak paused and Stais could tell that the scene at the gate, the hurrying crowds, the package of Schrafft's chocolates, the weeping young girl, were as clear as the afternoon sunlight to Novak, there on the coast of Africa. "So I keep writing," Novak said. "She's written me she has a technical sergeant now, but I keep writing. I haven't seen her in a year and a half and what's a girl to do? Do you blame her?"

"No," said Stais. "I don't blame her."

"I hope I haven't bored you," Novak said.

"Not at all." Stais smiled at him. Suddenly the dizziness had gone and he could close his eyes. As he drifted down into that weird and ever-present pool of sleep in which he half lived these days, he heard Novak say, "Now I have to write my mother."

Outside, the Negro boy sang, and the planes grumbled down from the Atlantic and laboriously set out across the Sahara Desert.

Dreams again: Arabs, bundled in rags, driving camels along the perimeter of the field, outlined against the parked Liberators and waiting bombs; two Mitchells still burning on the shores of Brazil and Frank Sloan burning there and circling above him, Whitejack, who had told him he'd sleep with his wife and had; the hills around Jerusalem, gnarled, rocky, dusty, with the powdered green of olive groves set on slopes here and there, clinging against the desert wind; Mitchells slamming along the gorges of the Blue Ridge Mountains, bucking in the updrafts, their guns going, hunting deer; the Mediterranean, bluer than anything in America, below them on the way home from Italy, coming down below oxygen level, with the boys singing dirty songs over the intercom, and leave in Alexandria ahead of them. The girl from Flushing, Long Island, quietly going hand in hand with Novak to Coney Island on a summer's night.

It was Whitejack who awakened him. He woke slowly. It was dark outside and the electric light was shining in his eyes and Whitejack was standing over him, shaking him gently.

"I thought you'd like to know," Whitejack was saying, "your name's on the bulletin board. You're leaving tonight."

"Thanks," Stais said, dimly grateful at being shaken out of the broken and somehow sorrowful dreams.

"I took the liberty of initialling it for you, opposite your name," Whitejack said. "Save you a trip up to the field."

"Thanks," said Stais. "Very kind of you."

"Also," said Whitejack, "there's fried chicken for chow."

Stais pondered over the fried chicken. He was a little hungry, but the effort of getting up and putting on his shoes and walking the hundred yards to the mess hall had to be weighed in the balance. "Thanks. I'll just lie right here," he said. "Any news of your boys?" he asked.

"Yes," said Whitejack. "The squadron came in."

"That's good."

"All except one plane." Whitejack sat down on the end of Stais' cot. His voice was soft and expressionless. "Johnny Moffat's plane."

In all the months that Stais had been in the Air Forces, on fields to which planes had failed to return, he had learned that there was nothing to say. He was only nineteen years old, but he had learned that. So he lay quiet.

"They got separated in the clouds on the way out of Ascension, and they never picked them up again. There's still a chance," Whitejack said, "that they'll drop in any minute." He looked at his watch. "Still a chance for another hour and forty minutes."

There was still nothing to say, so Stais lay silent.

"Johnny Moffat," said Whitejack, "at one time looked as though he was going to marry my sister. In a way, it's a good thing he didn't. It'd be a little hard, being brothers-in-law, on some of the parties the Air Force goes on in one place and another." Whitejack fell silent and looked down at his belly. Deliberately, he let his belt out a notch, then pulled it to, with a severe little click. "That fried chicken was mighty good," he said. "You sure you want to pass it up?"

"I'm saving my appetite for my mother's cooking," Stais said.

"My sister was passing fond of Johnny," said Whitejack, "and I have a feeling when he gets home from the war and settles down, she's going to snag him. She came to me right before I left and she asked me if I would let her have ten acres on the north side of my property and three acres of timber to build their house. I said it was O.K. with me." He was silent again, thinking of the rolling ten acres of upland meadow in North Carolina and the three tall acres of standing timber, oak and pine, from which it would be possible to build a strong country house. "There's nobody in the whole world I'd rather have living on my property than Johnny Moffat. I've known him for twenty years and I've had six fist fights with him and won them all, and been alone with him in the woods for two months at a time, and I still say that." He got up and went over to his own cot, then turned and came back. "By the way," he said softly, "this is between you and me, Sergeant."

"Sure," said Stais.

"My sister said she'd murder me for my hide and taller if I ever let Johnny know what was in store for him." He grinned a little. "Women're very confident in certain fields," he said. "And I never did tell Johnny, not even when I was so drunk I was singing 'Casey Jones' naked in the middle of the city of Tampa at three o'clock in the morning." He went over to his musette bag and got out a cigar and lit it thoughtfully. "You'd be surprised," he said, "how fond you become of nickel cigars in the Army."

"I tried smoking," said Stais. "I think I'll wait until I get a little older." Whitejack sat heavily on his own cot. "Do you think they'll send you out to fight again?" he asked.

Stais stared up at the ceiling. "I wouldn't be surprised," he said. "There's nothing really wrong with me. I'm just tired."

Whitejack nodded, smoking slowly. "By the way," he said, "you heard us talking about the lieutenant, didn't you?"

"Yes."

"I went out to the field and had a little conversation with him. He's just been sittin' there all day and most of the night since we got here, outside the Operations room, just lookin' and starin' across at the planes comin' in. Him and me, we've been good friends for a long time and I asked him point-blank. I said, 'Freddie,' I said, 'there's a question the boys're askin' themselves these days about you.' And he said, 'What's the matter?' And I said, 'The boys're asking if you've turned bad. You pass 'em and you don't even look at them as though you recognize 'em. What is it, you turn G.I. after a year?' I said. He looked at me and then he looked at the ground and he didn't say anything for maybe a minute. Then he said, 'I beg your pardon, Arnold. It never occurred to me.' Then he told me what was on his mind." Whitejack looked at his watch, almost automatically, then lifted his head again. "Ever since we got the order to go overseas, he's been worrying. You know Simpson, in our crew. Well, he's worrying about him and his navigator."

"What's he worrying about?" For a moment a crazy list of all the thousand things you can worry about in the crew of one airplane flashed through Stais' head.

"They're not fighting men," Whitejack said slowly. "They're both good fellers, you wouldn't want better, but the lieutenant's been watchin' 'em for a long time on the ground, in the air, at their guns, and he's convinced they won't measure. And he feels he's responsible for taking the Mitchell in and getting it out with as many of us alive as possible and he feels Simpson and the navigator're dangerous to have in the plane. And he's makin' up his mind to put in a request for two new men when we get to India, and he can't bear to think of what it'll do to Simpson and the navigator when they find out he's asked to have 'em grounded. That's why he just sits there outside Operations, not even seein' us when we go by." Whitejack sighed. "He's twenty-two years old, the lieutenant. It's a strain, something like that, for a man twenty-two years old. If you see Simpson or Novak, you won't tell them anything, will you?"

"No," said Stais.

"I suppose things like this come up all the time in any army."

"All the time," said Stais.

Whitejack looked at his watch. Outside there was the growing and lapsing roar of engines that had been the constant sound of both their lives for so many months.

"Ah," said Whitejack, "they should've put me in the infantry. I can hit a rabbit at three hundred yards with a rifle. They put me in the Air Force and give me a camera. Well, Sergeant, I think it's about time you were movin'."

Slowly, Stais got up. He put on his shoes and put his shaving kit into his musette bag and slung it over one shoulder.

"You ready?" asked Whitejack.

"Yes," said Stais.

"That all the baggage you got, that little musette bag?"

"Yes," said Stais. "I was listed as missing, presumed dead, and they sent all my stuff into the supply room and all my personal belongings home to my mother."

Stais looked around the barracks. They shone in the harsh Army light of barracks at night all over the world, by now familiar, homelike, to all the men who passed through them. He had left nothing.

They walked out into the soft, engine-filled night. A beacon flashed nervously across the sky, dimming the enormous pale twinkle of southern stars for a moment.

As they passed the Operations room, Stais saw a young lieutenant slumped down in a wobbly old wicker chair, staring out across the field.

"They come yet?" Whitejack asked.

"No," said the lieutenant, without looking up.

Stais went into the building and into the room where they had the rubber raft and the patented radio and the cloth painted blue on one side and yellow on the other. A fat, middle-aged A.T.C. captain wearily told them about ditching procedure. There were more than thirty people in the room, all passengers on Stais' plane. There were two small, yellow Chinamen and five bouncing fat Red Cross women and three sergeants with a lot of Air Force medals, trying not to seem excited about going home, and two colonels in the Engineers, looking too old for this war. Stais only half listened as the fat captain explained how to inflate the raft, what strings to pull, what levers to move, where to find the water-proofed Bible.

Whitejack was standing outside when Stais started for his plane. He gave Stais a slip of paper. "It's my home address," he said. "After the war, just come down sometime in October and I'll take you hunting."

"Thank you very much," said Stais gravely. Over Whitejack's shoulder he saw the lieutenant, still slumped in the wicker chair, still staring fixedly out across the dark field.

Whitejack walked out to the great plane with Stais, along the oil-spattered concrete of the runway, among the Chinamen and loud Red Cross women and the sergeants. The two men stopped without a word at the steps going up to the doorway of the plane and the other passengers filed past them.

They stood there, silently, with the two days of random conversation behind them, and Brazil and Athens behind them, and five hundred flights behind them, and Jerusalem and Miami behind them, and the girls from Vienna and the American Embassy and Flushing, Long Island, behind them, and the Greek mountaineers behind them, and Thomas Wolfe's funeral, and friends burning like torches, and dogs under treed raccoons in the Blue Ridge Mountains behind them, and a desperate twenty-two-year-old lieutenant painfully staring across a dusty airfield for ten days behind them, and the Mediterranean and the hospital bed in Cairo and Johnny Moffat wandering that night over the southern Atlantic, with ten acres of meadow and three acres of timber for his house and Whitejack's sister waiting for him, all behind them. And, ahead of Stais, home, and a mother who had presumed him dead and wept over his personal belongings, and ahead of Whitejack the cold, bitter mountains of India and China, and the tearing dead sound of the fifties and the sky full of Japs.

"All right, Sergeant," the voice of the lieutenant checking the passengers said. "Get on."

Stais waved, a little broken wave, at Whitejack standing there. "See you," he said, "in North Carolina."

"Some October." Whitejack smiled a little, in the light of the flood lamps.

The door closed and Stais sat down in the seat in front of the two Chinamen.

"I think these planes are absolutely charming," one of the Red Cross women was saying loudly. "Don't you?"

The engines started and the big plane began to roll. Stais looked out of the window. A plane was landing. It came slowly into the light of the runway lamps and set down heavily, bumping wearily. Stais stared. It was a Mitchell. Stais sighed. As the big C-54 wheeled at the head of the runway, then started clumsily down, Stais put the slip of paper with "Arnold Whitejack" written on it, and the address, in scrawling, childlike handwriting, into his pocket. And as he saw the Mitchell pull to a stop near the Operations room, he felt for the moment a little less guilty for going home.

Dry September

WILLIAM FAULKNER (1897–)

THROUGH the bloody September twilight, aftermath of sixty-two rainless days, it had gone like a fire in dry grass—the rumor, the story, whatever it was. Something about Miss Minnie Cooper and a negro. Attacked, insulted, frightened: none of them, gathered in the barbershop on that Saturday evening where the ceiling fan stirred, without freshening it, the vitiated air, sending back upon them, in recurrent surges of stale pomade and lotion, their own stale breath and odors, knew exactly what had happened.

"Except it wasn't Will Mayes," a barber said. He was a man of middle age; a thin, sand-colored man with a mild face, who was shaving a client. "I know Will Mayes. He's a good nigger. And I know Miss Minnie Cooper, too."

"What do you know about her?" a second barber said.

"Who is she?" the client said. "A girl?"

"No," the barber said. "She's about forty, I reckon. She ain't married. That's why I don't believe—"

"Believe hell!" a hulking youth in a sweat-stained silk shirt said. "Won't you take a white woman's word before a nigger's?"

"I don't believe Will Mayes did it," the barber said. "I know Will Mayes."

"Maybe you know who did it, then. Maybe you already got him out of town, you damn nigger-lover."

"I don't believe anybody did anything. I don't believe anything happened. I leave it to you fellows if them ladies that gets old without getting married don't have notions that a man can't—"

"Then you're a hell of a white man," the client said. He moved under the cloth. The youth had sprung to his feet.

"You don't?" he said. "Do you accuse a white woman of telling a lie?"

The barber held the razor poised above the half-risen client. He did not look around.

"It's this durn weather," another said. "It's enough to make any man do anything. Even to her."

Nobody laughed. The barber said in his mild, stubborn tone: "I ain't accusing nobody of nothing. I just know and you fellows know how a woman that never—"

"You damn nigger-lover!" the youth said.

"Shut up, Butch," another said. "We'll get the facts in plenty of time to act."

"Who is? Who's getting them?" the youth said. "Facts, hell! I—"

"You're a fine white man," the client said. "Ain't you?" In his frothy beard he looked like a desert-rat in the moving pictures. "You tell them, Jack," he said to the youth. "If they ain't any white men in this town, you can count on me, even if I ain't only a drummer and a stranger."

"That's right, boys," the barber said. "Find out the truth first. I know Will Mayes."

"Well, by God!" the youth shouted. "To think that a white man in this town—"

"Shut up, Butch," the second speaker said. "We got plenty of time."

The client sat up. He looked at the speaker. "Do you claim that anything excuses a nigger attacking a white woman? Do you mean to tell me that you're a white man and you'll stand for it? You better go back North where you come from. The South don't want your kind here."

"North what?" the second said. "I was born and raised in this town."

"Well, by God!" the youth said. He looked about with a strained, baffled gaze, as if he was trying to remember what it was he wanted to say or do. He drew his sleeve across his sweating face. "Damn if I'm going to let a white woman—"

"You tell them, Jack," the drummer said. "By God, if they—"

The screen-door crashed open. A man stood in the floor, his feet apart and his heavy-set body poised easily. His white shirt was open at the throat; he wore a felt hat. His hot, bold glance swept the group. His name was Plunkett. He had commanded troops at the front in France and had been decorated for valor.

"Well," he said, "are you going to sit there and let a black son rape a white woman on the streets of Jefferson?"

Butch sprang up again. The silk of his shirt clung flat to his heavy shoulders. At each armpit was a dark half-moon. "That's what I been telling them! That's what I—"

"Did it really happen?" a third said. "This ain't the first man-scare she ever had, like Hawkshaw says. Wasn't there something about a man on the kitchen roof, watching her undress, about a year ago?"

"What?" the client said. "What's that?" The barber had been slowly forcing him back into the chair; he arrested himself reclining, his head lifted, the barber still pressing him down.

Plunkett whirled on the third speaker. "Happen? What the hell difference does it make? Are you going to let the black sons get away with it until one really does it?"

"That's what I'm telling them!" Butch shouted. He cursed, long and steady, pointless.

"Here, here," a fourth said. "Not so loud. Don't talk so loud."

"Sure," Plunkett said; "no talking necessary at all. I've done my talking. Who's with me?" He poised on the balls of his feet, roving his gaze.

The barber held the client's face down, the razor poised. "Find out the facts first, boys. I know Willy Mayes. It wasn't him. Let's get the sheriff and do this thing right."

Plunkett whirled upon him his furious, rigid face. The barber did not look away. They looked like men of different races. The other barbers had ceased also above their prone clients. "You mean to tell me," Plunkett said, "that you'd take a nigger's word before a white woman's? Why, you damn nigger-loving—"

The third rose and grasped Plunkett's arm; he too had been a soldier. "Now, now! Let's figure this thing out. Who knows anything about what really happened?"

"Figure out hell!" Plunkett jerked his arm free. "All that're with me get up from there. The ones that ain't—" He roved his gaze, dragging his sleeve across his face.

Three men rose. The client in the chair sat up. "Here," he said, jerking at the cloth around his neck; "get this rag off me. I'm with him. I don't live here, but, by God, if our mothers and wives and sisters—" He smeared the cloth over his face and flung it to the floor. Plunkett stood in the floor and cursed the others. Another rose and moved toward him. The remainder sat uncomfortably, not looking at one another, then one by one they rose and joined him.

The barber picked the cloth from the floor. He began to fold it neatly. "Boys, don't do that. Will Mayes never done it. I know."

"Come on," Plunkett said. He whirled. From his hip pocket protruded the butt of a heavy automatic pistol. They went out. The screen-door crashed behind them reverberant in the dead air.

The barber wiped the razor carefully and swiftly, and put it away, and ran to the rear, and took his hat from the wall. "I'll be back soon as I can," he said to the other barbers. "I can't let—" He went out, running. The two other barbers followed him to the door and caught it on the rebound, leaning out and looking up the street after him. The air was flat and dead. It had a metallic taste at the base of the tongue.

"What can he do?" the first said. The second one was saying "Jees Christ, Jees Christ" under his breath. "I'd just as lief be Will Mayes as Hawk, if he gets Plunkett riled."

"Jees Christ, Jees Christ," the second whispered.

"You reckon he really done it to her?" the first said.

II

She was thirty-eight or thirty-nine. She lived in a small frame house with her invalid mother and a thin, sallow, unflagging aunt, where each morning, between ten and eleven, she would appear on the porch in a lace-trimmed boudoir cap, to sit swinging in the porch swing until noon. After dinner she lay down for a while, until the afternoon began to cool. Then, in one of the three or four new voile dresses which she had each summer, she would go down-town to spend the afternoon in the stores with the other ladies, where they would handle the goods and haggle over prices in cold, immediate voices, without any intention of buying.

She was of comfortable people—not the best in Jefferson, but good people enough—and she was still on the slender side of ordinary-looking, with a bright, faintly haggard manner and dress. When she was young she had had a slender, nervous body and a sort of hard vivacity which had enabled her to ride for the time upon the crest of the town's social life as exemplified by the high-school party and church-social period of her contemporaries while still children enough to be un-classconscious.

She was the last to realize that she was losing ground; that those among whom she had been a little brighter and louder flame than any other were beginning to learn the pleasure of snobbery—male—and retaliation—female. That was when her face began to wear that bright, haggard look. She still carried it to parties on shadowy porticos and summer lawns, like a mask or a flag, with that bafflement and furious repudiation of truth in her eyes. One evening at a party she heard a boy and two girls, all schoolmates, talking. She never accepted another invitation.

She watched the girls with whom she had grown up as they married and got houses and children, but no man ever called on her steadily until the children of the other girls had been calling her "aunty" for several years, the while their mothers told them in bright voices about how popular Minnie had been as a girl. Then the town began to see her driving on Sunday afternoons with the cashier in the bank. He was a widower of about forty—a high-colored man, smelling always faintly of the barbershop or of whiskey. He owned the first automobile in town, a red runabout; Minnie had the first motoring bonnet and veil the town ever saw. Then the town began to say: "Poor Minnie!" "But she is old enough to take care of herself," others said. That was when she first asked her schoolmates that the children call her "cousin" instead of "aunty."

It was twelve years now since she had been relegated into adultery by public opinion, and eight years since the cashier had gone to a Memphis bank, returning for one day each Christmas, which he spent at an annual bachelors' party in a hunting-club on the river. From behind their curtains the neighbors would see him pass, and during the across-the-street Christmas-day visiting they would tell her about him, about how well he looked, and how they heard that he was prospering in the city, watching with bright, secret eyes her haggard, bright face. Usually by that hour there would be the scent of whiskey on her breath. It was supplied her by a youth, a clerk at the soda-fountain: "Sure; I buy it for the old gal. I reckon she's entitled to a little fun."

Her mother kept to her room altogether now; the gaunt aunt ran the house. Against that background Minnie's bright dresses, her idle and empty days, had a quality of furious unreality. She went out in the evenings only with women now, neighbors, to the moving pictures. Each afternoon she dressed in one of the new dresses and went down-town alone, where her young cousins were already strolling in the late afternoons with their delicate, silken heads and thin, awkward arms and conscious hips, clinging to one another or shrieking and giggling with paired boys in the soda-fountain when she passed and went on along the serried stores, in the doors of which sitting and lounging men did not even follow her with their eyes any more.

III

The barber went swiftly up the street where the sparse lights, insect-swirled, glared in rigid and violent suspension in the lifeless air. The day had died in a pall of dust; above the darkened square, shrouded by the spent dust, the sky was clear as the inside of a brass bell. Below the east was a rumor of the twice-waxed moon.

When he overtook them Plunkett and three others were getting into a car parked in an alley. Plunkett stooped his thick head, peering out beneath the top. "Changed your mind, did you?" he said. "Damn good thing; by God, to-morrow when this town hears about how you talked to-night—"

"Now, now," the other ex-soldier said. "Hawkshaw's all right. Come on, Hawk; jump in!"

"Will Mayes never done it, boys," the barber said. "If anybody done it. Why, you all know well as I do there ain't any town where they got better niggers than us. And you know how a lady will kind of think things about men when there ain't any reason to, and Miss Minnie anyway—"

"Sure, sure," the soldier said. "We're just going to talk to him a little; that's all."

"Talk hell!" Butch said. "When we're done with the—"

"Shut up, for God's sake!" the soldier said. "Do you want everybody in town—"

"Tell them, by God!" Plunkett said. "Tell every one of the sons that'll let a white woman—"

"Let's go; let's go: here's the other car." The second car slid squealing out of a cloud of dust at the alley-mouth. Plunkett started his car and backed out and took the lead. Dust lay like fog in the street. The street lights hung nimbused as in water. They drove on out of town.

A rutted lane turned at right angles. Dust hung above it too, and above all the land. The dark bulk of the ice-plant, where the negro Mayes was night-watchman, rose against the sky. "Better stop here, hadn't we?" the soldier said. Plunkett did not reply. He hurled the car up and slammed to a stop, the headlights glaring on the blank wall.

"Listen here, boys," the barber said; "if he's here, don't that prove he never done it? Don't it? If it was him, he would run. Don't you see he would?" The second car came up and stopped. Plunkett got down; Butch sprang down beside him. "Listen, boys," the barber said.

"Cut the lights off!" Plunkett said. The breathless darkness rushed down. There was no sound in it save their lungs as they sought air in the parched dust in which for two months they had lived; then the diminishing crunch of Plunkett's and Butch's feet, and a moment later Plunkett's voice:

"Will! . . . Will!"

Below the east the wan hemorrhage of the moon increased. It heaved above the ridge, silvering the air, the dust, so that they seemed to breathe, live, in a bowl of molten lead. There was no sound of night-bird nor insect, no sound save their breathing and a faint ticking of contracting metal about the cars. Where their bodies touched one another they seemed to sweat dryly, for no more moisture came. "Christ!" a voice said; "let's get out of here."

But they didn't move until vague noises began to grow out of the darkness ahead; then they got out and waited tensely in the breathless dark. There was another sound: a blow, a hissing expulsion of breath and Plunkett cursing in undertone. They stood a moment longer, then they ran forward. They ran in a stumbling clump, as though they were fleeing something. "Kill him, kill the son!" a voice whispered. Plunkett flung them back.

"Not here," he said. "Get him into the car." They hauled the negro up. "Kill him, kill the black son!" the voice murmured.

They dragged the negro to the car. The barber had waited beside the car. He could feel himself sweating and he knew he was going to be sick at the stomach.

"What is it, captains?" the negro said. "I ain't done nothing. 'Fore God, Mr. John." Some one produced handcuffs. They worked busily about him as though he were a post, quiet, intent, getting in one another's way. He submitted to the handcuffs, looking swiftly and constantly from dim face to face. "Who's here, captains?" he said, leaning to peer into the faces until they could feel his breath and smell his sweaty reek. He spoke a name or two. "What you-all say I done, Mr. John?"

Plunkett jerked the car-door open. "Get in!" he said.

The negro did not move. "What you-all going to do with me, Mr. John? I ain't done nothing. White folks, captains, I ain't done nothing: I swear 'fore God." He called another name.

"Get in!" Plunkett said. He struck the negro. The others expelled their breath in a dry hissing and struck him with random blows, and he whirled and cursed them, and swept his manacled hands across their faces and slashed the barber upon the mouth, and the barber struck him also. "Get him in there," Plunkett said. They pushed at him. He ceased struggling and got in, and sat quietly as the others took their places. He sat between the barber and the soldier, drawing his limbs in so as not to touch them, his eyes going swiftly and constantly from face to face. Butch clung to the running-board. The car moved on. The barber nursed his mouth in his handkerchief.

"What's the matter, Hawk?" the soldier said.

"Nothing," the barber said. They regained the high road and turned away from town. The second car dropped back out of the dust. They went on, gaining speed; the final fringe of houses dropped behind.

"Goddam, he stinks!" the soldier said.

"We'll fix that," the man in front beside Plunkett said. On the running-board Butch cursed into the hot rush of air. The barber leaned suddenly forward and touched Plunkett's shoulder.

"Let me out, John."

"Jump out, nigger-lover," Plunkett said without turning his head. He drove swiftly. Behind them the sourceless lights of the second car glared in the dust. Presently Plunkett turned into a narrow road. It too was rutted in disuse. It led back to an old brick-kiln—a series of reddish mounds and weed-and-vine-choked vats without bottom. It had been used for pasture once, until one day the owner missed one of his mules. Although he prodded carefully in the vats with a long pole, he could not even find the bottom of them.

"John," the barber said.

"Jump out, then," Plunkett said, hurling the car along the ruts. Beside the barber the negro spoke:

"Mr. Henry."

The barber sat forward. The narrow tunnel of the road rushed up and past. Their motion was like an extinct furnace blast: cooler, but utterly dead. The car bounded from rut to rut.

"Mr. Henry," the negro said.

The barber began to tug furiously at the door. "Look out, there!" the soldier said, but he had already kicked the door open and swung onto the running-board. The soldier leaned across the negro and grasped at him, but he had already jumped. The car went on without checking speed.

The impetus hurled him crashing, through dust-sheathed weeds, into the ditch. Dust puffed about him, and in a thin, vicious crackling of sapless stems he lay choking and retching until the second car passed and died away. Then he rose and limped on until he reached the high road and turned toward town, brushing at his clothes with his hands. The moon was higher, riding high and clear of the dust at last, and after a while the town began to glare beneath the dust. He went on, limping. Presently he heard the cars and the glow of them grew in the dust behind him and he left the road and crouched again in the weeds until they passed. Plunkett's car came last now. There were four people in it and Butch was not on the running-board.

They went on; the dust swallowed them; the glare and the sound died away. The dust of them hung for a while, but soon the eternal dust absorbed it again. The barber climbed back onto the road and limped on toward town.

IV

As she dressed after supper, on that Saturday evening, her own flesh felt like fever. Her hands trembled among the hooks and eyes, and her eyes had a feverish look, and her hair swirled crisp and crackling under the comb. While she was still dressing, the friends called for her and sat while she donned her sheerest underthings and stockings and a new voile dress. "Do you feel strong enough to go out?" they said, their eyes bright too, with a dark glitter. "When you have had time to get over the shock, you must tell us what happened. What he said and did; everything."

In the leafed darkness, as they walked toward the square, she began to breathe deeply, something like a swimmer preparing to dive, until she ceased trembling, the four of them walking slowly because of the terrible heat and out of solicitude for her. But as they neared the square she began to tremble again, walking with her head up, her hands clinched at her sides, their voices about her murmurous, also with that feverish, glittering quality of their eyes.

They entered the square, she in the centre of the group, fragile in her fresh dress. She was trembling worse. She walked slower and slower, as children eat ice-cream, her head up and her eyes bright in the haggard banner of her face, passing the hotel and the coatless drummers in chairs along the curb looking around at her: "That's the one: see? The one in pink in the middle." "Is that her? What did they do with the nigger? Did they—?" "Sure. He's all right." "All right, is he?" "Sure. He went on a little trip." Then the drug-store, where even the young men lounging in the doorway tipped their hats and followed with their eyes the motion of her hips and legs when she passed.

They went on, passing the lifted hats of the gentlemen, the

suddenly ceased voices, protective, deferent. "Do you see?" the friends said. Their voices sounded like long hovering sighs of hissing exultation. "There's not a negro on the square. Not one."

They reached the picture-show. It was like a miniature fairyland with its lighted lobby and colored lithographs of life caught in its terrible and beautiful mutations. Her lips began to tingle. In the dark, when the picture began, it would be all right; she could hold back the laughing so it would not waste away so fast and so soon. So she hurried on before the turning faces, the undertones of low astonishment, and they took their accustomed places where she could see the aisle against the silver glare and the young men and girls coming in two and two against it.

The lights flicked away; the screen glowed silver, and soon life began to unfold, beautiful and passionate and sad, while still the young men and girls entered, scented and sibilant in the half-dark, their paired backs in silhouette delicate and sleek, their slim, quick bodies awkward, divinely young, while beyond them the silver dream accumulated, inevitably on and on. She began to laugh. In trying to suppress it, it made more noise than ever; heads began to turn. Still laughing, her friends raised her and led her out, and she stood at the curb, laughing on a high, sustained note, until the taxi came up and they helped her in.

They removed the pink voile and the sheer underthings, and the stockings, and put her to bed, and cracked ice for her temples, and sent for the doctor. He was hard to locate, so they ministered to her with hushed ejaculations, renewing the ice and fanning her. While the ice was fresh and cold she stopped laughing and lay still for a time, moaning only a little. But soon the laughing welled again and her voice rose screaming.

"Shhhhhhhhhhh! Shhhhhhhhhhh!" they said, freshening the ice-pack, smoothing her hair, examining it for gray; "poor girl!" Then to one another: "Do you suppose anything really happened?" their eyes darkly aglitter, secret and passionate. "Shhhhhhhhhh! Poor girl! Poor Minnie!"

V

It was midnight when Plunkett drove up to his neat new house. It was trim and fresh as a bird-cage and almost as small, with its clean green-and-white paint. He locked the car and mounted the porch and entered. His wife rose from a chair beside the reading-lamp. Plunkett stopped in the floor and stared at her until she looked down.

"Look at that clock!" he said, lifting his arm, pointing. She stood before him, her face lowered, a magazine in her hands. Her face was pale, strained, and weary-looking. "Haven't I told you about sitting up like this, waiting to see when I come in?"

"John!" she said. She laid the magazine down. Poised on the balls of his feet, he glared at her with his hot eyes, his sweating face.

"Didn't I tell you?" He went toward her. She looked up then. He caught her shoulder. She stood passive, looking at him.

"Don't, John. I couldn't sleep. . . . The heat; something. Please, John. You're hurting me."

"Didn't I tell you?" He released her and half struck, half flung her across the chair, and she lay there and watched him quietly as he left the room.

He went on through the house, ripping off his shirt, and on the dark, screened porch at the rear he stood and mopped his head and shoulders with the shirt and flung it away. He took the pistol from his hip and laid it on the table beside the bed, and sat on the bed and removed his shoes, and rose and slipped his trousers off. He was sweating again already, and he stooped and hunted furiously for the shirt. At last he found it and wiped his body again, and, with his body pressed against the dusty screen, he stood panting. There was no movement, no sound, not even an insect. The dark world seemed to lie stricken beneath the cold moon and the lidless stars.

Babylon Revisited

F. SCOTT FITZGERALD (1896–1940)

"AND where's Mr. Campbell?" Charlie asked.

"Gone to Switzerland. Mr. Campbell's a pretty sick man, Mr. Wales."

"I'm sorry to hear that. And George Hardt?" Charlie inquired.

"Back in America, gone to work."

"And where is the Snow Bird?"

"He was in here last week. Anyway, his friend, Mr. Schaeffer, is in Paris."

Two familiar names from the long list of a year and a half ago. Charlie scribbled an address in his notebook and tore out the page.

"If you see Mr. Schaeffer, give him this," he said. "It's my brother-in-law's address. I haven't settled on a hotel yet."

He was not really disappointed to find Paris was so empty. But the stillness in the Ritz bar was strange and portentous. It was not an American bar any more—he felt polite in it, and not as if he owned it. It had gone back into France. He felt the stillness from the moment he got out of the taxi and saw the doorman, usually in a frenzy of activity at this hour, gossiping with a *chasseur* by the servants' entrance.

Passing through the corridor, he heard only a single, bored voice in the once-glamorous women's room. When he turned into the bar he travelled the twenty feet of green carpet with his eyes fixed straight ahead by old habit; and then, with his foot firmly on the rail, he turned and surveyed the room, encountering only a single pair of eyes that fluttered up from a newspaper in the corner. Charlie asked for the head barman, Paul, who in the latter days of the bull market had come to work in his own custom-built car—disembarking, however, with due nicety at the nearest corner. But Paul was at his country house today and Alix giving him information.

"No, no more," Charlie said, "I'm going slow these days."

Alix congratulated him: "You were going pretty strong a couple of years ago."

"I'll stick to it all right," Charlie assured him. "I've stuck to it for over a year and a half now."

"How do you find conditions in America?"

"I haven't been to America for months. I'm in business in Prague, representing a couple of concerns there. They don't know about me down there."

Alix smiled.

"Remember the night of George Hardt's bachelor dinner here?" said Charlie. "By the way, what's become of Claude Fessenden?"

Alix lowered his voice confidentially: "He's in Paris, but he doesn't come here any more. Paul doesn't allow it. He ran up a bill of thirty thousand francs, charging all his drinks and his lunches, and usually his dinner, for more than a year. And when Paul finally told him he had to pay, he gave him a bad check."

Alix shook his head sadly.

"I don't understand it, such a dandy fellow. Now he's all bloated up—" He made a plump apple of his hands.

Charlie watched a group of strident queens installing themselves in a corner.

"Nothing affects them," he thought. "Stocks rise and fall, people loaf or work, but they go on forever." The place oppressed him. He called for the dice and shook with Alix for the drink.

"Here for long, Mr. Wales?"

"I'm here for four or five days to see my little girl."

"Oh-h! You have a little girl?"

Outside, the fire-red, gas-blue, ghost-green signs shone smokily through the tranquil rain. It was late afternoon and the streets were in movement; the *bistros* gleamed. At the corner of the Boulevard des Capucines he took a taxi. The Place de la Concorde moved by in pink majesty; they crossed the logical Seine, and Charlie felt the sudden provincial quality of the Left Bank.

Charlie directed his taxi to the Avenue de l'Opera, which was out of his way. But he wanted to see the blue hour spread over the magnificent façade, and imagine that the cab horns, playing endlessly the first few bars of *Le Plus que Lent*, were the trumpets of the Second Empire. They were closing the iron grill in front of Brentano's Book-store, and people were already at dinner behind the trim little bourgeois hedge of Duval's. He had never eaten at a really cheap restaurant in Paris. Five-course dinner, four francs fifty, eighteen cents, wine included. For some odd reason he wished that he had.

As they rolled on to the Left Bank and he felt its sudden provincialism, he thought, "I spoiled this city for myself. I didn't realize it, but the days came along one after another, and then two years were gone, and everything was gone, and I was gone."

He was thirty-five, and good to look at. The Irish mobility of his face was sobered by a deep wrinkle between his eyes. As he rang his brother-in-law's bell in the Rue Palatine, the wrinkle deepened till it pulled down his brows; he felt a cramping sensation in his belly. From behind the maid who opened the .door darted a lovely little girl of nine who shrieked "Daddy!" and flew up, struggling like a fish, into his arms. She pulled his head around by one ear and set her cheek against his.

"My old pie," he said.

"Oh, daddy, daddy, daddy, daddy, dads, dads, dads!"

She drew him into the salon, where the family waited, a boy and girl his daughter's age, his sister-in-law and her husband. He greeted Marion with his voice pitched carefully to avoid either feigned enthusiasm or dislike, but her response was more frankly tepid, though she minimized her expression of unalterable distrust by directing her regard toward his child. The two men clasped hands in a friendly way and Lincoln Peters rested his for a moment on Charlie's shoulder.

The room was warm and comfortably American. The three children moved intimately about, playing through the yellow oblongs that led to other rooms; the cheer of six o'clock spoke in the eager smacks of the fire and the sounds of French activity in the kitchen. But Charlie did not relax; his heart sat up rigidly in his body and he drew confidence from his daughter, who from time to time came close to him, holding in her arms the doll he had brought.

"Really extremely well," he declared in answer to Lincoln's question. "There's a lot of business there that isn't moving at all, but we're doing even better than ever. In fact, damn well. I'm bringing my sister over from America next month to keep house for me. My income last year was bigger than it was when I had money. You see, the Czechs—"

His boasting was for a specific purpose; but after a moment, seeing a faint restiveness in Lincoln's eye, he changed the subject:

"Those are fine children of yours, well brought up, good manners."

"We think Honoria's a great little girl too."

Marion Peters came back from the kitchen. She was a tall woman with worried eyes, who had once possessed a fresh American loveliness. Charlie had never been sensitive to it and was always surprised when people spoke of how pretty she had been. From the first there had been an instinctive antipathy between them.

"Well, how do you find Honoria?" she asked.

"Wonderful. I was astonished how much she's grown in ten months. All the children are looking well."

"We haven't had a doctor for a year. How do you like being back in Paris?"

"It seems very funny to see so few Americans around."

"I'm delighted," Marion said vehemently. "Now at least you can go into a store without their assuming you're a millionaire.

We've suffered like everybody, but on the whole it's a good deal pleasanter."

"But it was nice while it lasted," Charlie said. "We were a sort of royalty, almost infallible, with a sort of magic around us. In the bar this afternoon"—he stumbled, seeing his mistake—"there wasn't a man I knew."

She looked at him keenly. "I should think you'd have had enough of bars."

"I only stayed a minute. I take one drink every afternoon, and no more."

"Don't you want a cocktail before dinner?" Lincoln asked.

"I take only one drink every afternoon, and I've had that."

"I hope you keep to it," said Marion.

Her dislike was evident in the coldness with which she spoke, but Charlie only smiled; he had larger plans. Her very aggressiveness gave him an advantage, and he knew enough to wait. He wanted them to initiate the discussion of what they knew had brought him to Paris.

At dinner he couldn't decide whether Honoria was most like him or her mother. Fortunate if she didn't combine the traits of both that had brought them to disaster. A great wave of protectiveness went over him. He thought he knew what to do for her. He believed in character; he wanted to jump back a whole generation and trust in character again as the eternally valuable element. Everything wore out.

He left soon after dinner, but not to go home. He was curious to see Paris by night with clearer and more judicious eyes than those of other days. He bought a *strapontin* for the Casino and watched Josephine Baker go through her chocolate arabesques.

After an hour he left and strolled toward Montmartre, up the Rue Pigalle into the Place Blanche. The rain had stopped and there were a few people in evening clothes disembarking from taxis in front of cabarets, and *cocottes* prowling singly or in pairs, and many Negroes. He passed a lighted door from which issued music, and stopped with the sense of familiarity; it was Bricktop's, where he had parted with so many hours and so much money. A few doors farther on he found another ancient rendezvous and incautiously put his head inside. Immediately an eager orchestra burst into sound, a pair of professional dancers leaped to their feet and a maître d'hôtel swooped toward him, crying, "Crowd just arriving, sir!" But he withdrew quickly.

"You have to be damn drunk," he thought.

Zelli's was closed, the bleak and sinister cheap hotels surrounding it were dark; up in the Rue Blanche there was more light and a local, colloquial French crowd. The Poet's Cave had disappeared, but the two great mouths of the Café of Heaven and the Café of Hell still yawned—even devoured, as he watched, the meagre contents of a tourist bus—a German, a Japanese, and an American couple who glanced at him with frightened eyes.

So much for the effort and ingenuity of Montmartre. All the catering to vice and waste was on an utterly childish scale, and he suddenly realized the meaning of the word "dissipate"—to dissipate into thin air; to make nothing out of something. In the little hours of the night every move from place to place was an enormous human jump, an increase of paying for the privilege of slower and slower motion.

He remembered thousand-franc notes given to an orchestra for playing a single number, hundred-franc notes tossed to a doorman for calling a cab.

But it hadn't been given for nothing.

It had been given, even the most wildly squandered sum, as an offering to destiny that he might not remember the things most worth remembering, the things that now he would always remember—his child taken from his control, his wife escaped to a grave in Vermont.

In the glare of a *brasserie* a woman spoke to him. He bought her some eggs and coffee, and then, eluding her encouraging stare, gave her a twenty-franc note and took a taxi to his hotel.

II

He woke upon a fine fall day—football weather. The depression of yesterday was gone and he liked the people on the streets. At noon he sat opposite Honoria at Le Grand Vatel, the only restaurant he could think of not reminiscent of champagne dinners and long luncheons that began at two and ended in a blurred and vague twilight.

"Now, how about vegetables? Oughtn't you to have some vegetables?"

"Well, yes."

"Here's *épinards* and *chou-fleur* and carrots and *haricots*."

"I'd like *chou-fleur*."

"Wouldn't you like to have two vegetables?"

"I usually only have one at lunch."

The waiter was pretending to be inordinately fond of children. "*Qu'elle est mignonne, la petite! Elle parle exactement comme une française.*"

"How about dessert? Shall we wait and see?"

The waiter disappeared. Honoria looked at her father expectantly.

"What are we going to do?"

"First, we're going to that toy store in the Rue Saint-Honoré and buy you anything you like. And then we're going to the vaudeville at the Empire."

She hesitated. "I like it about the vaudeville, but not the toy store."

"Why not?"

"Well, you brought me this doll." She had it with her. "And I've got lots of things. And we're not rich any more, are we?"

"We never were. But today you are to have anything you want."

"All right," she agreed resignedly.

When there had been her mother and a French nurse he had been inclined to be strict; now he extended himself, reached out for a new tolerance; he must be both parents to her and not shut any of her out of communication.

"I want to get to know you," he said gravely. "First let me introduce myself. My name is Charles J. Wales, of Prague."

"Oh, daddy!" her voice cracked with laughter.

"And who are you, please?" he persisted, and she accepted a rôle immediately: "Honoria Wales, Rue Palatine, Paris."

"Married or single?"

"No, not married. Single."

He indicated the doll. "But I see you have a child, madame."

Unwilling to disinherit it, she took it to her heart and thought quickly: "Yes, I've been married, but I'm not married now. My husband is dead."

He went on quickly, "And the child's name?"

"Simone. That's after my best friend at school."

"I'm very pleased that you're doing so well at school."

"I'm third this month," she boasted. "Elsie"—that was her cousin—"is only about eighteenth, and Richard is about at the bottom."

"You like Richard and Elsie, don't you?"

"Oh, yes. I like Richard quite well and I like her all right."

Cautiously and casually he asked: "And Aunt Marion and Uncle Lincoln—which do you like best?"

"Oh, Uncle Lincoln, I guess."

He was increasingly aware of her presence. As they came in, a murmur of ". . . adorable" followed them, and now the people at the next table bent all their silences upon her, staring as if she were something no more conscious than a flower.

"Why don't I live with you?" she asked suddenly. "Because mamma's dead?"

"You must stay here and learn more French. It would have been hard for daddy to take care of you so well."

"I don't really need much taking care of any more. I do everything for myself."

Going out of the restaurant, a man and a woman unexpectedly hailed him.

"Well, the old Wales!"

"Hello there, Lorraine. . . . Dunc."

Sudden ghosts out of the past: Duncan Schaeffer, a friend from college. Lorraine Quarrles, a lovely, pale blonde of thirty; one of a crowd who had helped them make months into days in the lavish times of three years ago.

"My husband couldn't come this year," she said, in answer to his question. "We're poor as hell. So he gave me two hundred a month and told me I could do my worst on that. . . . This your little girl?"

"What about coming back and sitting down?" Duncan asked.

"Can't do it." He was glad for an excuse. As always, he felt Lorraine's passionate, provocative attraction, but his own rhythm was different now.

"Well, how about dinner?" she asked.

"I'm not free. Give me your address and let me call you."

"Charlie, I believe you're sober," she said judicially. "I honestly believe he's sober, Dunc. Pinch him and see if he's sober."

Charlie indicated Honoria with his head. They both laughed.

"What's your address?" said Duncan sceptically.

He hesitated, unwilling to give the name of his hotel.

"I'm not settled yet. I'd better call you. We're going to see the vaudeville at the Empire."

"There! That's what I want to do," Lorraine said. "I want to see some clowns and acrobats and jugglers. That's just what we'll do, Dunc."

"We've got to do an errand first," said Charlie. "Perhaps we'll see you there."

"All right, you snob. . . . Good-by, beautiful little girl."

"Good-by."

Honoria bobbed politely.

Somehow, an unwelcome encounter. They liked him because he was functioning, because he was serious; they wanted to see him, because he was stronger than they were now, because they wanted to draw a certain sustenance from his strength.

At the Empire, Honoria proudly refused to sit upon her father's folded coat. She was already an individual with a code of her own, and Charlie was more and more absorbed by the desire of putting a little of himself into her before she crystallized utterly. It was hopeless to try to know her in so short a time.

Between the acts they came upon Duncan and Lorraine in the lobby where the band was playing.

"Have a drink?"

"All right, but not up at the bar. We'll take a table."

"The perfect father."

Listening abstractedly to Lorraine, Charlie watched Honoria's eyes leave their table, and he followed them wistfully about the room, wondering what they saw. He met her glance and she smiled.

"I liked that lemonade," she said.

What had she said? What had he expected? Going home in a taxi afterward, he pulled her over until her head rested against his chest.

"Darling, do you ever think about your mother?"

"Yes, sometimes," she answered vaguely.

"I don't want you to forget her. Have you got a picture of her?"

"Yes, I think so. Anyhow, Aunt Marion has. Why don't you want me to forget her?"

"She loved you very much."

"I loved her too."

They were silent for a moment.

"Daddy, I want to come and live with you," she said suddenly.

His heart leaped; he had wanted it to come like this.

"Aren't you perfectly happy?"

"Yes, but I love you better than anybody. And you love me better than anybody, don't you, now that mummy's dead?"

"Of course I do. But you won't always like me best, honey.

You'll grow up and meet somebody your own age and go marry him and forget you ever had a daddy."

"Yes, that's true," she agreed tranquilly.

He didn't go in. He was coming back at nine o'clock and he wanted to keep himself fresh and new for the thing he must say then.

"When you're safe inside, just show yourself in that window."

"All right. Good-by, dads, dads, dads, dads."

He waited in the dark street until she appeared, all warm and glowing, in the window above and kissed her fingers out into the night.

III

They were waiting. Marion sat behind the coffee service in a dignified black dinner dress that just faintly suggested mourning. Lincoln was walking up and down with the animation of one who had already been talking. They were as anxious as he was to get into the question. He opened it almost immediately:

"I suppose you know what I want to see you about—why I really came to Paris."

Marion played with the black stars on her necklace and frowned.

"I'm awfully anxious to have a home," he continued. "And I'm awfully anxious to have Honoria in it. I appreciate your taking in Honoria for her mother's sake, but things have changed now"—he hesitated and then continued more forcibly—"changed radically with me, and I want to ask you to reconsider the matter. It would be silly for me to deny that about three years ago I was acting badly—"

Marion looked up at him with hard eyes.

"—but all that's over. As I told you, I haven't had more than a drink a day for over a year, and I take that drink deliberately, so that the idea of alcohol won't get too big in my imagination. You see the idea?"

"No," said Marion succinctly.

"It's a sort of stint I set myself. It keeps the matter in proportion."

"I get you," said Lincoln. "You don't want to admit it's got any attraction for you."

"Something like that. Sometimes I forget and don't take it. But I try to take it. Anyhow, I couldn't afford to drink in my position. The people I represent are more than satisfied with what I've done, and I'm bringing my sister over from Burlington to keep house for me, and I want awfully to have Honoria too. You know that even when her mother and I weren't getting along well we never let anything that happened touch Honoria. I know she's fond of me and I know I'm able to take care of her and—well, there you are. How do you feel about it?"

He knew that now he would have to take a beating. It would last an hour or two hours, and it would be difficult, but if he modulated his inevitable resentment to the chastened attitude of the reformed sinner, he might win his point in the end.

Keep your temper, he told himself. You don't want to be justified. You want Honoria.

Lincoln spoke first: "We've been talking it over ever since we got your letter last month. We're happy to have Honoria here. She's a dear little thing, and we're glad to be able to help her, but of course that isn't the question—"

Marion interrupted suddenly. "How long are you going to stay sober, Charlie?" she asked.

"Permanently, I hope."

"How can anybody count on that?"

"You know I never did drink heavily until I gave up business and came over here with nothing to do. Then Helen and I began to run around with—"

"Please leave Helen out of it. I can't bear to hear you talk about her like that."

He stared at her grimly; he had never been certain how fond of each other the sisters were in life.

"My drinking only lasted about a year and a half—from the time we came over until I—collapsed."

"It was time enough."

"It was time enough," he agreed.

"My duty is entirely to Helen," she said. "I try to think what she would have wanted me to do. Frankly, from the night you did that terrible thing you haven't really existed for me. I can't help that. She was my sister."

"Yes."

"When she was dying she asked me to look out for Honoria. If you hadn't been in a sanitarium then, it might have helped matters."

He had no answer.

"I'll never in my life be able to forget the morning when Helen knocked at my door, soaked to the skin and shivering, and said you'd locked her out."

Charlie gripped the sides of the chair. This was more difficult than he expected; he wanted to launch out into a long expostulation and explanation, but he only said: "The night I locked her out—" and she interrupted, "I don't feel up to going over that again."

After a moment's silence Lincoln said: "We're getting off the subject. You want Marion to set aside her legal guardianship and give you Honoria. I think the main point for her is whether she has confidence in you or not."

"I don't blame Marion," Charlie said slowly, "but I think she can have entire confidence in me. I had a good record up to three years ago. Of course, it's within human possibilities I might go wrong any time. But if we wait much longer I'll lose Honoria's childhood and my chance for a home." He shook his head, "I'll simply lose her, don't you see?"

"Yes, I see," said Lincoln.

"Why didn't you think of all this before?" Marion asked.

"I suppose I did, from time to time, but Helen and I were getting along badly. When I consented to the guardianship, I was flat on my back in a sanitarium and the market had cleaned me out. I knew I'd acted badly, and I thought if it would bring any peace to Helen, I'd agree to anything. But now it's different. I'm functioning, I'm behaving damn well, so far as—"

"Please don't swear at me," Marion said.

He looked at her, startled. With each remark the force of her dislike became more and more apparent. She had built up all her fear of life into one wall and faced it toward him. This trivial reproof was possibly the result of some trouble with the cook several hours before. Charlie became increasingly alarmed at leaving Honoria in this atmosphere of hostility against himself; sooner or later it would come out, in a word here, a shake of the head there, and some of that distrust would be irrevocably implanted in Honoria. But he pulled his temper down out of his face and shut it up inside him; he had won a point, for Lincoln realized the absurdity of Marion's remark and asked her lightly since when she had objected to the word "damn."

"Another thing," Charlie said: "I'm able to give her certain advantages now. I'm going to take a French governess to Prague with me. I've got a lease on a new apartment—"

He stopped, realizing that he was blundering. They couldn't be expected to accept with equanimity the fact that his income was again twice as large as their own.

"I suppose you can give her more luxuries than we can," said Marion. "When you were throwing away money we were living along watching every ten francs. . . . I suppose you'll start doing it again."

"Oh, no," he said. "I've learned. I worked hard for ten years, you know—until I got lucky in the market, like so many people. Terribly lucky. It didn't seem any use working any more, so I quit. It won't happen again."

There was a long silence. All of them felt their nerves straining, and for the first time in a year Charlie wanted a drink. He was sure now that Lincoln Peters wanted him to have his child.

Marion shuddered suddenly; part of her saw that Charlie's feet were planted on the earth now, and her own maternal feeling recognized the naturalness of his desire; but she had lived for a long time with a prejudice—a prejudice founded on a curious disbelief in her sister's happiness, and which, in the shock of one terrible night, had turned to hatred for him. It had all happened at a point in her life where the discouragement of ill health and adverse circumstances made it necessary for her to believe in tangible villainy and a tangible villain.

"I can't help what I think!" she cried out suddenly. "How much you were responsible for Helen's death, I don't know. Its something you'll have to square with your own conscience."

An electric current of agony surged through him; for a moment he was almost on his feet, an unuttered sound echoing in his throat. He hung on to himself for a moment, another moment.

"Hold on there," said Lincoln uncomfortably. "I never thought you were responsible for that."

"Helen died of heart trouble," Charlie said dully.

"Yes, heart trouble." Marion spoke as if the phrase had another meaning for her.

Then, in the flatness that followed her outburst, she saw him plainly and she knew he had somehow arrived at control over the situation. Glancing at her husband, she found no help from him, and as abruptly as if it were a matter of no importance, she threw up the sponge.

"Do what you like!" she cried, springing up from her chair. "She's your child. I'm not the person to stand in your way. I think if it were my child I'd rather see her—" She managed to check herself. "You two decide it. I can't stand this. I'm sick. I'm going to bed."

She hurried from the room; after a moment Lincoln said:

"This has been a hard day for her. You know how strongly she feels—" His voice was almost apologetic: "When a woman gets an idea in her head."

"Of course."

"It's going to be all right. I think she sees now that you—can provide for the child, and so we can't very well stand in your way or Honoria's way."

"Thank you, Lincoln."

"I'd better go along and see how she is."

"I'm going."

He was still trembling when he reached the street, but a walk down the Rue Bonaparte to the quais set him up, and as he crossed the Seine, fresh and new by the quai lamps, he felt exultant. But back in his room he couldn't sleep. The image of Helen haunted him. Helen whom he had loved so until they had senselessly begun to abuse each other's love, tear it into shreds. On that terrible February night that Marion remembered so vividly, a slow quarrel had gone on for hours. There was a scene at the Florida, and then he attempted to take her home, and then she kissed young Webb at a table; after that there was what she had hysterically said. When he arrived home alone he turned the key in the lock in wild anger. How could he know she would arrive an hour later alone, that there would be a snowstorm in which she wandered about in slippers, too confused to find a taxi? Then the aftermath, her escaping pneumonia by a miracle, and all the attendant horror. They were "reconciled," but that was the beginning of the end, and Marion, who had seen with her own eyes and who imagined it to be one of many scenes from her sister's martyrdom, never forgot.

Going over it again brought Helen nearer, and in the white, soft light that steals upon half sleep near morning he found himself talking to her again. She said that he was perfectly right about Honoria and that she wanted Honoria to be with him. She said she was glad he was being good and doing better. She said a lot of other things—very friendly things—but she was in a swing in a white dress, and swinging faster and faster all the time, so that at the end he could not hear clearly all that she said.

IV

He woke up feeling happy. The door of the world was open again. He made plans, vistas, futures for Honoria and himself, but suddenly he grew sad, remembering all the plans he and Helen had made. She had not planned to die. The present was the thing—work to do and someone to love. But not to love too much, for he knew the injury that a father can do to a daughter or a mother to a son by attaching them too closely: afterward, out in the world, the child would seek in the marriage partner the same blind tenderness and, failing probably to find it, turn against love and life.

It was another bright, crisp day. He called Lincoln Peters at the bank where he worked and asked if he could count on taking Honoria when he left for Prague. Lincoln agreed that there was no reason for delay. One thing—the legal guardianship. Marion wanted to retain that a while longer. She was upset by the whole matter, and it would oil things if she felt that the situation was still in her control for another year. Charlie agreed, wanting only the tangible, visible child.

Then the question of a governess. Charlie sat in a gloomy agency and talked to a cross Bernaise and to a buxom Breton peasant, neither of whom he could have endured. There were others whom he would see tomorrow.

He lunched with Lincoln Peters at Griffons, trying to keep down his exultation.

"There's nothing quite like your own child," Lincoln said. "But you understand how Marion feels too."

"She's forgotten how hard I worked for seven years there," Charlie said. "She just remembers one night."

"There's another thing." Lincoln hesitated. "While you and Helen were tearing around Europe throwing money away, we were just getting along. I didn't touch any of the prosperity because I never got ahead enough to carry anything but my insurance. I think Marion felt there was some kind of injustice in it—you not even working toward the end, and getting richer and richer."

"It went just as quick as it came," said Charlie.

"Yes, a lot of it stayed in the hands of *chasseurs* and saxophone players and maîtres d'hôtel—well, the big party's over now. I just said that to explain Marion's feeling about those crazy years. If you drop in about six o'clock tonight before Marion's too tired, we'll settle the details on the spot."

Back at his hotel, Charlie found a *pneumatique* that had been redirected from the Ritz bar where Charlie had left his address for the purpose of finding a certain man.

DEAR CHARLIE: You were so strange when we saw you the other day that I wondered if I did something to offend you. If so, I'm not conscious of it. In fact, I have thought about you too much for the last year, and it's always been in the back of my mind that I might see you if I came over here. We *did* have such good times that crazy spring, like the night you and I stole the butcher's tricycle, and the time we tried to call on the president and you had the old derby rim and the wire cane. Everybody seems so old lately, but I don't feel old a bit. Couldn't we get together some time today for old time's sake? I've got a vile hang-over for the moment, but will be feeling better this afternoon and will look for you about five in the sweat-shop at the Ritz.

Always devotedly,

LORRAINE.

His first feeling was one of awe that he had actually, in his mature years, stolen a tricycle and pedalled Lorraine all over the Étoile between the small hours and dawn. In retrospect it was a nightmare. Locking out Helen didn't fit in with any other act of his life, but the tricycle incident did—it was one of many. How many weeks or months of dissipation to arrive at that condition of utter irresponsibility?

He tried to picture how Lorraine had appeared to him then—very attractive; Helen was unhappy about it, though she said nothing. Yesterday, in the restaurant, Lorraine had seemed trite, blurred, worn away. He emphatically did not want to see her, and he was glad Alix had not given away his hotel address. It was a relief to think, instead, of Honoria, to think of Sundays spent with her and of saying good morning to her and of knowing she was there in his house at night, drawing her breath in the darkness.

At five he took a taxi and bought presents for all the Peters—a piquant cloth doll, a box of Roman soldiers, flowers for Marion, big linen handkerchiefs for Lincoln.

He saw, when he arrived in the apartment, that Marion had accepted the inevitable. She greeted him now as though he were a recalcitrant member of the family, rather than a menacing outsider. Honoria had been told she was going; Charlie was glad to see that her tact made her conceal her excessive happiness. Only on his lap did she whisper her delight and the question "When?" before she slipped away with the other children.

He and Marion were alone for a minute in the room, and on an impulse he spoke out boldly:

"Family quarrels are bitter things. They don't go according to any rules. They're not like aches or wounds; they're more like splits in the skin that won't heal because there's not enough material. I wish you and I could be on better terms."

"Some things are hard to forget," she answered. "It's a question of confidence." There was no answer to this and presently she asked, "When do you propose to take her?"

"As soon as I can get a governess. I hoped the day after tomorrow."

"That's impossible. I've got to get her things in shape. Not before Saturday."

He yielded. Coming back into the room, Lincoln offered him a drink.

"I'll take my daily whisky," he said.

It was warm here, it was a home, people together by a fire. The children felt very safe and important; the mother and father were serious, watchful. They had things to do for the children more important than his visit here. A spoonful of medicine was, after all, more important than the strained relations between Marion and himself. They were not dull people, but they were very much in the grip of life and circumstances. He wondered if he couldn't do something to get Lincoln out of his rut at the bank.

A long peal at the door-bell; the *bonne de toute faire* passed through and went down the corridor. The door opened upon another long ring, and then voices, and the three in the salon looked up expectantly; Richard moved to bring the corridor within his range of vision, and Marion rose. Then the maid came back along the corridor, closely followed by the voices, which developed under the light into Duncan Schaeffer and Lorraine Quarrles.

They were gay, they were hilarious, they were roaring with laughter. For a moment Charlie was astounded; unable to understand how they ferreted out the Peters' address.

"Ah-h-h!" Duncan wagged his finger rougishly at Charlie. "Ah-h-h!"

They both slid down another cascade of laughter. Anxious and at a loss, Charlie shook hands with them quickly and presented them to Lincoln and Marion. Marion nodded, scarcely speaking. She had drawn back a step toward the fire; her little girl stood beside her, and Marion put an arm about her shoulder.

With growing annoyance at the intrusion, Charlie waited for them to explain themselves. After some concentration Duncan said:

"We came to invite you out to dinner. Lorraine and I insist that all this shishi, cagy business 'bout your address got to stop."

Charlie came closer to them, as if to force them backward down the corridor.

"Sorry, but I can't. Tell me where you'll be and I'll phone you in half an hour."

This made no impression. Lorraine sat down suddenly on the side of a chair, and focussing her eyes on Richard, cried, "Oh, what a nice little boy! Come here, little boy." Richard glanced at his mother, but did not move. With a perceptible shrug of her shoulders, Lorraine turned back to Charlie:

"Come and dine. Sure your cousins won' mine. See you so sel'om. Or solemn."

"I can't," said Charlie sharply. "You two have dinner and I'll phone you."

Her voice became suddenly unpleasant. "All right, we'll go. But I remember once when you hammered on my door at four A.M. I was enough of a good sport to give you a drink. Come on, Dunc."

Still in slow motion, with blurred, angry faces, with uncertain feet, they retired along the corridor.

"Good night," Charlie said.

"Good night!" responded Lorraine emphatically.

When he went back into the salon Marion had not moved, only now her son was standing in the circle of her other arm. Lincoln was still swinging Honoria back and forth like a pendulum from side to side.

"What an outrage!" Charlie broke out. "What an absolute outrage!"

Neither of them answered. Charlie dropped into an armchair, picked up his drink, set it down again and said:

"People I haven't seen for two years having the colossal nerve—"

He broke off. Marion had made the sound "Oh!" in one swift, furious breath, turned her body from him with a jerk and left the room.

Lincoln set down Honoria carefully.

"You children go in and start your soup," he said, and when they obeyed, he said to Charlie:

"Marion's not well and she can't stand shocks. That kind of people make her really physically sick."

"I didn't tell them to come here. They wormed your name out of somebody. They deliberately—"

"Well, it's too bad. It doesn't help matters. Excuse me a minute."

Left alone, Charlie sat tense in his chair. In the next room he could hear the children eating, talking in monosyllables, already oblivious to the scene between their elders. He heard a murmur of conversation from a farther room and then the ticking bell of a telephone receiver picked up, and in a panic he moved to the other side of the room and out of earshot.

In a minute Lincoln came back. "Look here, Charlie. I think we'd better call off dinner for tonight. Marion's in bad shape."

"Is she angry with me?"

"Sort of," he said, almost roughly. "She's not strong and—"

"You mean she's changed her mind about Honoria?"

"She's pretty bitter right now. I don't know. You phone me at the bank tomorrow."

"I wish you'd explain to her I never dreamed these people would come here. I'm just as sore as you are."

"I couldn't explain anything to her now."

Charlie got up. He took his coat and hat and started down the corridor. Then he opened the door of the dining room and said in a strange voice, "Good night, children."

Honoria rose and ran around the table to hug him.

"Good night, sweetheart," he said vaguely, and then trying to make his voice more tender, trying to conciliate something, "Good night, dear children."

V

Charlie went directly to the Ritz bar with the furious idea of finding Lorraine and Duncan, but they were not there, and he realized that in any case there was nothing he could do. He had not touched his drink at the Peters', and now he ordered a whisky-and-soda. Paul came over to say hello.

"It's a great change," he said sadly. "We do about half the business we did. So many fellows I hear about back in the States lost everything, maybe not in the first crash, but then in the second. Your friend George Hardt lost every cent, I hear. Are you back in the States?"

"No, I'm in business in Prague."

"I heard that you lost a lot in the crash."

"I did," and he added grimly, "but I lost everything I wanted in the boom."

"Selling short."

"Something like that."

Again the memory of those days swept over him like a nightmare—the people they had met travelling; the people who couldn't add a row of figures or speak a coherent sentence. The little man Helen had consented to dance with at the ship's party, who had insulted her ten feet from the table; the women and girls carried screaming with drink or drugs out of public places—

—The men who locked their wives out in the snow, because the snow of twenty-nine wasn't real snow. If you didn't want it to be snow, you just paid some money.

He went to the phone and called the Peters' apartment; Lincoln answered.

"I called up because this thing is on my mind. Has Marion said anything definite?"

"Marion's sick," Lincoln answered shortly. "I know this thing isn't altogether your fault, but I can't have her go to pieces about it. I'm afraid we'll have to let it slide for six months; I can't take the chance of working her up to this state again."

"I see."

"I'm sorry, Charlie."

He went back to his table. His whisky glass was empty, but he shook his head when Alix looked at it questioningly. There wasn't much he could do now except send Honoria some things; he would send her a lot of things tomorrow. He thought rather angrily that this was just money—he had given so many people money. . . .

"No, no more," he said to another waiter. "What do I owe you?"

He would come back some day; they couldn't make him pay forever. But he wanted his child, and nothing was much good now, beside that fact. He wasn't young any more, with a lot of nice thoughts and dreams to have by himself. He was absolutely sure Helen wouldn't have wanted him to be so alone.

Critical Questions

THE ACTION of the story takes place against the background of the prosperity of the twenties and the great depression of the thirties. But the interest of the story is focused on Charlie Wales' personal problem: will he get his daughter? To what extent does the success of the story depend on the reader's having lived through the period in which it is set? How much does Fitzgerald count on his reader's knowledge to recreate a period and an attitude, when stimulated by a few key references?

What connection does Fitzgerald make between the social framework of the story and Charlie Wales' problem? The answer to this question involves, of course, a definition of Wales' character, and an analysis of the causes of his failure. On this point consider the following passages:

> Charlie felt the sudden provincial quality of the Left Bank. [Page 314.]
>
> But he wanted to see the blue hour spread over the magnificent façade, and imagine that the cab horns . . . were the trumpets of the Second Empire. [Page 314.]
>
> He believed in character; he wanted to jump back a whole generation and trust in character again as the eternally valuable element. Everything else wore out. [Page 316.]
>
> "You know I never did drink heavily until I gave up business and came over here with nothing to do." [Page 323.]
>
> "I worked hard for ten years, you know—until I got lucky in the market, like so many people." [Page 325.]
>
> He was absolutely sure Helen wouldn't have wanted him to be so alone. [Page 335.]

Keela, the Outcast Indian Maiden

EUDORA WELTY (1909–   )

ONE MORNING in summertime, when all his sons and daughters were off picking plums and Little Lee Roy was all alone, sitting on the porch and only listening to the screech owls away down in the woods, he had a surprise.

First he heard white men talking. He heard two white men coming up the path from the highway. Little Lee Roy ducked his head and held his breath; then he patted all around back of him for his crutches. The chickens all came out from under the house and waited attentively on the steps.

The men came closer. It was the young man who was doing all of the talking. But when they got through the fence, Max, the older man, interrupted him. He tapped him on the arm and pointed his thumb toward Little Lee Roy.

He said, "Bud? Yonder he is."

But the younger man kept straight on talking, in an explanatory voice.

"Bud?" said Max again. "Look, Bud, yonder's the only little clubfooted nigger man was ever around Cane Springs. Is he the party?"

They came nearer and nearer to Little Lee Roy and then stopped and stood there in the middle of the yard. But the young man was so excited he did not seem to realize that they had arrived anywhere. He was only about twenty years old, very sunburned. He talked constantly, making only one gesture—raising his hand stiffly and then moving it a little to one side.

"They dressed it in a red dress, and it ate chickens alive," he said. "I sold tickets and I thought it was worth a dime, honest. They gimme a piece of paper with the thing wrote off I had to say. That was easy. 'Keela, the Outcast Indian Maiden!' I call it out through a pasteboard megaphone. Then ever' time it was fixin' to eat a live chicken, I blowed the sireen out front."

"Just tell me, Bud," said Max, resting back on the heels of his perforated tan-and-white sport shoes. "Is this nigger the one? Is that him sittin' there?"

Little Lee Roy sat huddled and blinking, a smile on his face. . . . But the young man did not look his way.

"Just took the job that time. I didn't mean to—I mean, I meant to go to Port Arthur because my brother was on a boat," he said. "My name is Steve, mister. But I worked with this show selling tickets for three months, and I never would of knowed it was like that if it hadn't been for that man." He arrested his gesture.

"Yeah, what man?" said Max in a hopeless voice.

Little Lee Roy was looking from one white man to the other, excited almost beyond respectful silence. He trembled all over, and a look of amazement and sudden life came into his eyes.

"Two years ago," Steve was saying impatiently. "And we was travelin' through Texas in those ole trucks.—See, the reason nobody ever come clost to it before was they give it a iron bar this long. And tole it if anybody come near, to shake the bar good at 'em, like this. But it couldn't say nothin'. Turned out they'd tole it it couldn't say nothin' to anybody ever, so it just kind of mumbled and growled, like a animal."

"Hee! hee!" This from Little Lee Roy, softly.

"Tell me again," said Max, and just from his look you could tell that everybody knew old Max. "Somehow I can't get it straight in my mind. Is this the boy? Is this little nigger boy the same as this Keela, the Outcast Indian Maiden?"

Up on the porch, above them, Little Lee Roy gave Max a glance full of hilarity, and then bent the other way to catch Steve's next words.

"Why, if anybody was to even come near it or even bresh their shoulder against the rope it'd growl and take on and shake its iron rod. When it would eat the live chickens it'd growl somethin' awful—you ought to heard it."

"Hee! hee!" It was a soft, almost incredulous laugh that began to escape from Little Lee Roy's tight lips, a little mew of delight.

"They'd throw it this chicken, and it would reach out an' grab it. Would sort of rub over the chicken's neck with its thumb an' press on it good, an' then it would bite its head off."

"O.K.," said Max.

"It skint back the feathers and stuff from the neck and sucked the blood. But ever'body said it was still alive." Steve drew closer to Max and fastened his light-colored, troubled eyes on his face.

"O.K."

"Then it would pull the feathers out easy and neat-like, awful fast, an' growl the whole time, kind of moan, an' then it would commence to eat all the white meat. I'd go in an' look at it. I reckon I seen it a thousand times."

"That was you, boy?" Max demanded of Little Lee Roy unexpectedly.

But Little Lee Roy could only say, "Hee! hee!" The little man at the head of the steps where the chickens sat, one on each step, and the two men facing each other below made a pyramid.

Steve stuck his hand out for silence. "They said—I mean, I said it, out front through the megaphone, I said it myself, that it wouldn't eat nothin' but only live meat. It was supposed to be a Indian woman, see, in this red dress an' stockin's. It didn't have on no shoes, so when it drug its foot ever'body could see. . . . When it come to the chicken's heart, it would eat that too, real fast, and the heart would still be jumpin'."

"Wait a second, Bud," said Max briefly. "Say, boy, is this white man here crazy?"

Little Lee Roy burst into hysterical, deprecatory giggles. He said, "Naw suh, don't think so." He tried to catch Steve's eye, seeking appreciation, crying, "Naw suh, don't think he crazy, mista."

Steve gripped Max's arm. "Wait! Wait!" he cried anxiously. "You ain't listenin'. I want to tell you about it. You didn't catch my name—Steve. You never did hear about that little nigger—all that happened to him? Lived in Cane Springs, Miss'ippi?"

"But," said Max, disengaging himself, "I don't hear anything. I got a juke box, see, so I don't have to listen."

"Look—I was really the one," said Steve more patiently, but nervously, as if he had been slowly breaking bad news. He walked up and down the bare-swept ground in front of Little Lee Roy's porch, along the row of princess feathers and snow-on-the-mountain. Little Lee Roy's turning head followed him. "I was the one—that's what I'm tellin' you."

"Suppose I was to listen to what every dope comes in Max's Place got to say, *I'd* be nuts," said Max.

"It's all me, see," said Steve. "I know that. I was the one was the cause for it goin' on an' on an' not bein' found out—such an awful thing. It was me, what I said out front through the megaphone."

He stopped still and stared at Max in despair.

"Look," said Max. He sat on the steps, and the chickens hopped off. "I know I ain't nobody but Max. I got Max's Place. I only run a place, understand, fifty yards down the highway. Liquor buried twenty feet from the premises, and no trouble yet. I ain't ever been up here before. I don't claim to been anywhere. People come to my place. Now. You're the hitchhiker. You're tellin' me, see. You claim a lot of information. If I don't get it I don't get it and I ain't complainin' about it, see. But I think you're nuts, and did from the first. I only come up here with you because I figured you's crazy."

"Maybe you don't believe I remember every word of it even now," Steve was saying gently. "I think about it at night—that an' drums on the midway. You ever hear drums on the midway?" He paused and stared politely at Max and Little Lee Roy.

"Yeh," said Max.

"Don't it make you feel sad? I remember how the drums was goin' and I was yellin', 'Ladies and gents! Do not try to touch Keela, the Outcast Indian Maiden—she will only beat your brains out with her iron rod, and eat them alive!'" Steve waved his arm gently in the air, and Little Lee Roy drew back and squealed. "'Do not go near her, ladies and gents! I'm warnin' you!' So nobody ever did. Nobody ever come near her. Until that man."

"Sure," said Max. "That fella." He shut his eyes.

"Afterwards when he come up so bold, I remembered seein' him walk up an' buy the ticket an' go in the tent. I'll never forget that man as long as I live. To me he's a sort of—well—"

"Hero," said Max.

"I wish I could remember what he looked like. Seem like he was a tallish man with a sort of white face. Seem like he had bad teeth, but I may be wrong. I remember he frowned a lot. Kept frownin'. Whenever he'd buy a ticket, why, he'd frown."

"Ever seen him since?" asked Max cautiously, still with his eyes closed. "Ever hunt him up?"

"No, never did," said Steve. Then he went on. "He'd frown an' buy a ticket ever' day we was in these two little smelly towns in Texas, sometimes three-four times a day, whether it was fixin' to eat a chicken or not."

"O.K., so he gets in the tent," said Max.

"Well, what the man finally done was, he walked right up to the little stand where it was tied up and laid his hand out open on the planks in the platform. He just laid his hand out open there and said, 'Come here,' real low and quick, that-a-way."

Steve laid his open hand on Little Lee Roy's porch and held it there, frowning in concentration.

"I get it," said Max. "He'd caught on it was a fake."

Steve straightened up. "So ever'body yelled to git away, git away," he continued, his voice rising, "because it was growlin' an' carryin' on an' shakin' its iron bar like they tole it. When I heard all that commotion—boy! I was scared."

"You didn't know it was a fake."

Steve was silent for a moment, and Little Lee Roy held his breath, for fear everything was all over.

"Look," said Steve finally, his voice trembling. "I guess I was supposed to feel bad like this, and you wasn't. I wasn't supposed to ship out on that boat from Port Arthur and all like that. This other had to happen to me—not you all. Feelin' responsible. You'll be O.K., mister, but I won't. I feel awful about it. That poor little old thing."

"Look, you got him right here," said Max quickly. "See him? Use your eyes. He's O.K., ain't he? Looks O.K. to me. It's just you. You're nuts, is all."

"You know—when that man laid out his open hand on the boards, why, it just let go the iron bar," continued Steve, "let it fall down like that—bang—and act like it didn't know what to do. Then it drug itself over to where the fella was standin' an' leaned down an' grabbed holt onto that white man's hand as tight as it could an' cried like a baby. It didn't want to hit him!"

"Hee! hee! hee!"

"No sir, it didn't want to hit him. You know what it wanted?"

Max shook his head.

"It wanted him to help it. So the man said, 'Do you wanta get out of this place, whoever you are?' An' it never answered—none of us knowed it could talk—but it just wouldn't let that man's hand a-loose. It hung on, cryin' like a baby. So the man says, 'Well, wait here till I come back.' "

"Uh-huh?" said Max.

"Went off an' come back with the sheriff. Took us all to jail. But just the man owned the show and his son got took to the pen. They said I could go free. I kep' tellin' 'em I didn't know it wouldn't hit me with the iron bar an' kep' tellin' 'em I didn't know it could tell what you was sayin' to it."

"Yeh, guess you told 'em," said Max.

"By that time I felt bad. Been feelin' bad ever since. Can't hold onto a job or stay in one place for nothin' in the world. They made it stay in jail to see if it could talk or not, and the first night it wouldn't say nothin'. Some time it cried. And they undressed it an' found out it wasn't no outcast Indian woman a-tall. It was a little clubfooted nigger man."

"Hee! hee!"

"You mean it was this boy here—yeh. It was him."

"Washed its face, and it was paint all over it made it look red. It all come off. And it could talk—as good as me or you. But they'd tole it not to, so it never did. They'd tole it if anybody was to come near it they was comin' to git it—and for it to hit 'em quick with that iron bar an' growl. So nobody ever come near it—until that man. I was yellin' outside, tellin' 'em to keep away, keep away. You could see where they'd whup it. They had to whup it some to make it eat all the chickens. It was awful dirty. They let it go back home free, to where they got it in the first place. They made them pay its ticket from Little Oil, Texas, to Cane Springs, Miss'ippi."

"You got a good memory," said Max.

"The way it *started* was," said Steve, in a wondering voice, "the show was just travelin' along in ole trucks through the country, and just seen this little deformed nigger man, sittin' on a fence, and just took it. It couldn't help it."

Little Lee Roy tossed his head back in a frenzy of amusement.

"I found it all out later. I was up on the Ferris wheel with one of the boys—got to talkin' up yonder in the peace an' quiet—an' said they just kind of happened up on it. Like a cyclone happens: it wasn't nothin' it could do. It was just took up." Steve suddenly paled through his sunburn. "An' they found out that back in Miss'ippi it had it a little bitty pair of crutches an' could just go runnin' on 'em!"

"And there they are," said Max.

Little Lee Roy held up a crutch and turned it about, and then snatched it back like a monkey.

"But if it hadn't been for that man, I wouldn't of knowed it till yet. If it wasn't for him bein' so bold. If he hadn't knowed what he was doin'."

"You remember that man this fella's talkin' about, boy?" asked Max, eying Little Lee Roy.

Little Lee Roy, in reluctance and shyness, shook his head gently.

"Naw suh, I can't say as I remembas that ve'y man, suh," he said softly, looking down where just then a sparrow alighted on his child's shoe. He added happily, as if on inspiration, "Now I remembas *this* man."

Steve did not look up, but when Max shook with silent laughter, alarm seemed to seize him like a spasm in his side. He walked painfully over and stood in the shade for a few minutes, leaning his head on a sycamore tree.

"Seemed like that man just studied it out an' knowed it was somethin' wrong," he said presently, his voice coming more remotely than ever. "But I didn't know. I can't look at nothin' an' be sure what it is. Then afterwards I know. Then I see how it was."

"Yeh, but you're nuts," said Max affably.

"You wouldn't of knowed it either!" cried Steve in sudden boyish, defensive anger. Then he came out from under the tree and stood again almost pleadingly in the sun, facing Max where he was sitting below Little Lee Roy on the steps. "You'd of let it go on an' on when they made it do those things—just like I did."

"Bet I could tell a man from a woman and an Indian from a nigger though," said Max.

Steve scuffed the dust into little puffs with his worn shoe. The chickens scattered, alarmed at last.

Little Lee Roy looked from one man to the other radiantly, his hands pressed over his grinning gums.

Then Steve sighed, and as if he did not know what else he

could do, he reached out and without any warning hit Max in the jaw with his fist. Max fell off the steps.

Little Lee Roy suddenly sat as still and dark as a statue, looking on.

"Say! Say!" cried Steve. He pulled shyly at Max where he lay on the ground, with his lips pursed up like a whistler, and then stepped back. He looked horrified. "How you feel?"

"Lousy," said Max thoughtfully. "Let me alone." He raised up on one elbow and lay there looking all around, at the cabin, at Little Lee Roy sitting cross-legged on the porch, and at Steve with his hand out. Finally he got up.

"I can't figure out how I could of ever knocked down an athaletic guy like you. I had to do it," said Steve. "But I guess you don't understand. I had to hit you. First you didn't believe me, and then it didn't bother you."

"That's all O.K., only hush," said Max, and added, "Some dope is always giving me the lowdown on something, but this is the first time one of 'em ever got away with a thing like this. I got to watch out."

"I hope it don't stay black long," said Steve.

"I got to be going," said Max. But he waited. "What you want to transact with Keela? You come a long way to see him." He stared at Steve with his eyes wide open now, and interested.

"Well, I was goin' to give him some money or somethin', I guess, if I ever found him, only now I ain't got any," said Steve defiantly.

"O.K.," said Max. "Here's some change for you, boy. Just take it. Go on back in the house. Go on."

Little Lee Roy took the money speechlessly, and then fell upon his yellow crutches and hopped with miraculous rapidity away through the door. Max stared after him for a moment.

"As for you"—he brushed himself off, turned to Steve and then said, "When did you eat last?"

"Well, I'll tell you," said Steve.

"Not here," said Max. "I didn't go to ask you a question. Just follow me. We serve eats at Max's Place, and I want to play the juke box. You eat, and I'll listen to the juke box."

"Well . . ." said Steve. "But when it cools off I got to catch a ride some place."

"Today while all you all was gone, and not a soul in de house," said Little Lee Roy at the supper table that night, "two white mens come heah to de house. Wouldn't come in. But talks to me about de ole times when I use to be wid de circus—"

"Hush up, Pappy," said the children.

Critical Questions

NOTE THAT in "The Gioconda Smile" Huxley uses an omniscient point of view; that is, he does not limit himself to what it would be possible for a spectator to observe. He gets at the thoughts of his characters, especially the thoughts of the chief character, Mr. Hutton; and he is aware of and comments on the meaning of actions and emotions. Generally speaking the comments seem to be Mr. Hutton's; but some are obviously Huxley's, in his own person. What does Huxley gain by this shifting point of view? Is the device justified by the gain?

In "Keela, the Outcast Indian Maiden," on the other hand, Eudora Welty limits herself to recording what an observer might see. In the stage directions accompanying the dialogue, she seldom gives more than a gesture or a description of a voice tone. The reader has to reconstruct the emotions and motivations of the characters. How does this opacity affect the tone of the story? Note that Eudora Welty sets the characters of Max and Steve quite explicitly in the passage beginning, " 'Look,' said Steve finally, his voice trembling. 'I guess I was supposed to feel bad like this, and you wasn't' " (page 341).

Note the first two speeches of Max. Explain the repeated " 'Bud?' " That is, what emotion is implied by the question?

Note Max's speech (page 337): "'Yea, what man?' said Max in a hopeless voice." Why is he hopeless?

What is the effect of the final conversation between Little Lee Roy and his children?

Noon Wine

KATHERINE ANNE PORTER (1894–)

Time: 1896–1905
Place: Small South Texas Farm

THE TWO grubby small boys with tow-colored hair who were digging among the ragweed in the front yard sat back on their heels and said, "Hello," when the tall bony man with straw-colored hair turned in at their gate. He did not pause at the gate; it had swung back, conveniently half open, long ago, and was now sunk so firmly on its broken hinges no one thought of trying to close it. He did not even glance at the small boys, much less give them good-day. He just clumped down his big square dusty shoes one after the other steadily, like a man following a plow, as if he knew the place well and knew where he was going and what he would find there. Rounding the right-hand corner of the house under the row of chinaberry trees, he walked up to the side porch where Mr. Thompson was pushing a big swing churn back and forth.

Mr. Thompson was a tough weather-beaten man with stiff black hair and a week's growth of black whiskers. He was a noisy proud man who held his neck so straight his whole face stood level with his Adam's apple, and the whiskers continued down his neck and disappeared into a black thatch under his open collar. The churn rumbled and swished like the belly of a trotting horse, and Mr. Thompson seemed somehow to be driving a horse with one hand, reining it in and urging it forward; and every now and then he turned halfway around and squirted a tremendous spit of tobacco juice out over the steps. The door stones were brown and gleaming with fresh tobacco juice. Mr. Thompson had been churning quite a while and he was tired of it. He was just fetching a mouthful of juice to squirt again when the stranger came around the corner and stopped. Mr. Thompson saw a narrow-chested man with blue eyes so pale they were almost white, looking and not looking at him from a long gaunt face, under white eyebrows. Mr. Thompson judged him to be another of these Irishmen, by his long upper lip.

"Howdy do, sir," said Mr. Thompson politely, swinging his churn.

"I need work," said the man, clearly enough but with some kind of foreign accent Mr. Thompson couldn't place. It wasn't Cajun and it wasn't Nigger and it wasn't Dutch, so it had him stumped. "You need a man here?"

Mr. Thompson gave the churn a great shove and it swung back and forth several times on its own momentum. He sat on the steps, shot his quid into the grass, and said, "Set down. Maybe we can make a deal. I been kinda lookin' round for somebody. I had two niggers but they got into a cutting scrape up the creek last week, one of 'em dead now and the other in the hoosegow at Cold Springs. Neither one of 'em worth killing, come right down to it. So it looks like I'd better get somebody. Where'd you work last?"

"North Dakota," said the man, folding himself down on the other end of the steps, but not as if he were tired. He folded up and settled down as if it would be a long time before he got up again. He never had looked at Mr. Thompson, but there wasn't anything sneaking in his eye, either. He didn't seem to be looking anywhere else. His eyes sat in his head and let things pass by them. They didn't seem to be expecting to see anything worth looking at. Mr. Thompson waited a long time for the man to say something more, but he had gone into a brown study.

"North Dakota," said Mr. Thompson, trying to remember where that was. "That's a right smart distance off, seems to me."

"I can do everything on farm," said the man; "cheap. I need work."

Mr. Thompson settled himself to get down to business. "My name's Thompson, Mr. Royal Earle Thompson," he said.

"I'm Mr. Helton," said the man, "Mr. Olaf Helton." He did not move.

"Well, now," said Mr. Thompson in his most carrying voice, "I guess we'd better talk turkey."

When Mr. Thompson expected to drive a bargain he always grew very hearty and jovial. There was nothing wrong with him except that he hated like the devil to pay wages. He said so himself. "You furnish grub and a shack," he said, "and then you got to pay 'em besides. It ain't right. Besides the wear and tear on your implements," he said, "they just let everything go to rack and ruin." So he began to laugh and shout his way through the deal.

"Now, what I want to know is, how much you fixing to gouge outa me?" he brayed, slapping his knee. After he had kept it up as long as he could, he quieted down, feeling a little sheepish, and cut himself a chew. Mr. Helton was staring out somewhere between the barn and the orchard, and seemed to be sleeping with his eyes open.

"I'm good worker," said Mr. Helton as from the tomb. "I get dollar a day."

Mr. Thompson was so shocked he forgot to start laughing again at the top of his voice until it was nearly too late to do any good. "Haw, haw," he bawled. "Why, for a dollar a day I'd hire out myself. What kinda work is it where they pay you a dollar a day?"

"Wheatfields, North Dakota," said Mr. Helton, not even smiling.

Mr. Thompson stopped laughing. "Well, this ain't any wheat-field by a long shot. This is more of a dairy farm," he said, feeling apologetic. "My wife, she was set on a dairy, she seemed to like working around with cows and calves, so I humored her. But it was a mistake," he said. "I got nearly everything to do, anyhow. My wife ain't very strong. She's sick today, that's a fact. She's been porely for the last few days. We plant a little feed, and a corn patch, and there's the orchard, and a few pigs and chickens, but our main hold is the cows. Now just speakin' as one man to another, there ain't any money in it. Now I can't give you no dollar a day because ackshally I don't make that much out of it. No, sir, we get along on a lot less than a dollar a day, I'd say, if we figger up everything in the long run. Now, I paid seven dollars a month to the two niggers, three-fifty each, and grub, but what I say is, one middlin'-good white man ekals a whole passel of niggers any day in the week, so I'll give you seven dollars and you eat at the table with us, and you'll be treated like a white man, as the feller says—"

"That's all right," said Mr. Helton. "I take it."

"Well, now I guess we'll call it a deal, hey?" Mr. Thompson jumped up as if he had remembered important business. "Now, you just take hold of that churn and give it a few swings, will you, while I ride to town on a coupla little errands. I ain't been able to leave the place all week. I guess you know what to do with butter after you get it, don't you?"

"I know," said Mr. Helton without turning his head. "I know butter business." He had a strange drawling voice, and even when he spoke only two words his voice waved slowly up and down and the emphasis was in the wrong place. Mr. Thompson wondered what kind of foreigner Mr. Helton could be.

"Now just where did you say you worked last?" he asked, as if he expected Mr. Helton to contradict himself.

"North Dakota," said Mr. Helton.

"Well, one place is good as another once you get used to it," said Mr. Thompson, amply. "You're a forriner, ain't you?"

"I'm a Swede," said Mr. Helton, beginning to swing the churn.

Mr. Thompson let forth a booming laugh, as if this was the best joke on somebody he'd ever heard. "Well, I'll be damned," he said at the top of his voice. "A Swede: well, now, I'm afraid you'll get pretty lonesome around here. I never seen any Swedes in this neck of the woods."

"That's all right," said Mr. Helton. He went on swinging the churn as if he had been working on the place for years.

"In fact, I might as well tell you, you're practically the first Swede I ever laid eyes on."

"That's all right," said Mr. Helton.

Mr. Thompson went into the front room where Mrs. Thompson was lying down, with the green shades drawn. She had a bowl of water by her on the table and a wet cloth over her eyes. She took the cloth off at the sound of Mr. Thompson's boots and said, "What's all the noise out there? Who is it?"

"Got a feller out there says he's a Swede, Ellie," said Mr. Thompson; "says he knows how to make butter."

"I hope it turns out to be the truth," said Mrs. Thompson. "Looks like my head never will get any better."

"Don't you worry," said Mr. Thompson. "You fret too much. Now I'm gointa ride into town and get a little order of groceries."

"Don't you linger, now, Mr. Thompson," said Mrs. Thompson. "Don't go to the hotel." She meant the saloon; the proprietor also had rooms for rent upstairs.

"Just a coupla little toddies," said Mr. Thompson, laughing loudly, "never hurt anybody."

"I never took a dram in my life," said Mrs. Thompson, "and what's more I never will."

"I wasn't talking about the womenfolks," said Mr. Thompson.

The sound of the swinging churn rocked Mrs. Thompson first into a gentle doze, then a deep drowse from which she waked suddenly knowing that the swinging had stopped a good while ago. She sat up shading her weak eyes from the flat strips of late summer sunlight between the sill and the lowered shades. There she was, thank God, still alive, with supper to cook but no churning on hand, and her head still bewildered, but easy. Slowly she realized she had been hearing a new sound even in her sleep. Somebody was playing a tune on the harmonica, not merely shrilling up and down making a sickening noise, but really playing a pretty tune, merry and sad.

She went out through the kitchen, stepped off the porch, and stood facing the east, shading her eyes. When her vision cleared and settled, she saw a long, pale-haired man in blue jeans sitting in the doorway of the hired man's shack, tilted back in a kitchen chair, blowing away at the harmonica with his eyes shut. Mrs. Thompson's heart fluttered and sank. Heavens, he looked lazy and worthless, he did, now. First a lot of no-count fiddling darkies and then a no-count white man. It was just like Mr. Thompson to take on that kind. She did wish he would be more considerate, and take a little trouble with his business. She wanted to believe in her husband, and there were too many times when she couldn't. She wanted to believe that tomorrow, or at least the day after, life, such a battle at best, was going to be better.

She walked past the shack without glancing aside, stepping carefully, bent at the waist because of the nagging pain in her side, and went to the springhouse, trying to harden her mind to speak very plainly to that new hired man if he had not done his work.

The milk house was only another shack of weather-beaten boards nailed together hastily years before because they needed a milk house; it was meant to be temporary, and it was; already shapeless, leaning this way and that over a perpetual cool trickle of water that fell from a little grot, almost choked with pallid ferns. No one else in the whole countryside had such a spring on his land. Mr. and Mrs. Thompson felt they had a fortune in that spring, if ever they got around to doing anything with it.

Rickety wooden shelves clung at hazard in the square around the small pool where the larger pails of milk and butter stood, fresh and sweet in the cold water. One hand supporting her flat, pained side, the other shading her eyes, Mrs. Thompson leaned over and peered into the pails. The cream had been skimmed and set aside, there was a rich roll of butter, the wooden molds and shallow pans had been scrubbed and scalded for the first time in who knows when, the barrel was full of buttermilk ready for the pigs and the weanling calves, the hard packed-dirt floor had been swept smooth. Mrs. Thompson straightened up again, smiling tenderly. She had been ready to scold him, a poor man who needed a job, who had just come there and who might not have been expected to do things properly at first. There was nothing she could do to make up for the injustice she had done him in her thoughts but to tell him how she appreciated his good clean work, finished already, in no time at all. She ventured near the door of the shack with her careful steps; Mr. Helton opened his eyes, stopped playing, and brought his chair down straight, but did not look at her, or get up. She was a little frail woman with long thick brown hair in a braid, a suffering patient mouth and diseased eyes which cried easily. She wove her fingers into an eyeshade, thumbs on temples, and winking her tearful lids, said with a polite little manner, "Howdy do, sir. I'm Miz Thompson, and I wanted to tell you I think you did real well in the milk house. It's always been a hard place to keep."

He said, "That's all right," in a slow voice, without moving.

Mrs. Thompson waited a moment. "That's a pretty tune you're playing. Most folks don't seem to get much music out of a harmonica."

Mr. Helton sat humped over, long legs sprawling, his spine in a bow, running his thumb over the square mouth-stops; except for his moving hand he might have been asleep. The harmonica was a big shiny new one, and Mrs. Thompson, her gaze wandering about, counted five others, all good and expensive, standing in a row on the shelf beside his cot. "He must carry them around in his jumper pocket," she thought, and noted there was not a sign of any other possession lying about. "I see you're mighty fond of music," she said. "We used to have an old accordion, and Mr. Thompson could play it right smart, but the little boys broke it up."

Mr. Helton stood up rather suddenly, the chair clattered under him, his knees straightened though his shoulders did not, and he looked at the floor as if he were listening carefully. "You know how little boys are," said Mrs. Thompson. "You'd better set them harmonicas on a high shelf or they'll be after them. They're great hands for getting into things. I try to learn 'em, but it don't do much good."

Mr. Helton, in one wide gesture of his long arms, swept his harmonicas up against his chest, and from there transferred them in a row to the ledge where the roof joined to the wall. He pushed them back almost out of sight.

"That'll do, maybe," said Mrs. Thompson. "Now I wonder," she said, turning and closing her eyes helplessly against the stronger western light, "I wonder what became of them little tads. I can't keep up with them." She had a way of speaking about her children as if they were rather troublesome nephews on a prolonged visit.

"Down by the creek," said Mr. Helton, in his hollow voice. Mrs. Thompson, pausing confusedly, decided he had answered her question. He stood in silent patience, not exactly waiting for her to go, perhaps, but pretty plainly not waiting for anything else. Mrs. Thompson was perfectly accustomed to all kinds of men full of all kinds of cranky ways. The point was, to find out just how Mr. Helton's crankiness was different from any other man's, and then get used to it, and let him feel at home. Her father had been cranky, her brothers and uncles had all been set in their ways and none of them alike; and every hired man she'd ever seen had quirks and crotchets of his own. Now here was Mr. Helton, who was a Swede, who wouldn't talk, and who played the harmonica besides.

"They'll be needing something to eat," said Mrs. Thompson in a vague friendly way, "pretty soon. Now I wonder what I ought to be thinking about for supper? Now what do you like to eat, Mr. Helton? We always have plenty of good butter and milk and cream, that's a blessing. Mr. Thompson says we ought to sell all of it, but I say my family comes first." Her little face went all out of shape in a pained blind smile.

"I eat anything," said Mr. Helton, his words wandering up and down.

He *can't* talk, for one thing, thought Mrs. Thompson; it's a shame to keep at him when he don't know the language good. She took a slow step away from the shack, looking back over her shoulder. "We usually have cornbread except on Sundays," she told him. "I suppose in your part of the country you don't get much good cornbread."

Not a word from Mr. Helton. She saw from her eye-corner that he had sat down again, looking at his harmonica, chair tilted. She hoped he would remember it was getting near milking time. As she moved away, he started playing again, the same tune.

Milking time came and went. Mrs. Thompson saw Mr. Helton going back and forth between the cow barn and the milk house. He swung along in an easy lope, shoulders bent, head hanging, the big buckets balancing like a pair of scales at the ends of his bony arms. Mr. Thompson rode in from town sitting straighter than usual, chin in, a towsack full of supplies swung behind the saddle. After a trip to the barn, he came into the kitchen full of good will, and gave Mrs. Thompson a hearty smack on the cheek after dusting her face off with his tough whiskers. He had been to the hotel, that was plain. "Took a look around the premises, Ellie," he shouted. "That Swede sure is grinding out the labor. But he is the closest mouthed feller I ever met up with in all my days. Looks like he's scared he'll crack his jaw if he opens his front teeth."

Mrs. Thompson was stirring up a big bowl of buttermilk cornbread. "You smell like a toper, Mr. Thompson," she said with perfect dignity. "I wish you'd get one of the little boys to bring me in an extra load of firewood. I'm thinking about baking a batch of cookies tomorrow."

Mr. Thompson, all at once smelling the liquor on his own breath, sneaked out, justly rebuked, and brought in the firewood himself. Arthur and Herbert, grubby from thatched head to toes, from skin to shirt, came stamping in yelling for supper. "Go wash your faces and comb your hair," said Mrs. Thompson, automatically. They retired to the porch. Each one put his hand under the pump and wet his forelock, combed it down with his fingers, and returned at once to the kitchen, where all the fair prospects of life were centered. Mrs. Thompson set an extra plate and commanded Arthur, the eldest, eight years old, to call Mr. Helton for supper.

Arthur, without moving from the spot, bawled like a bull calf, "Saaaaaay, Hellllllton, suuuuuupper's ready!" and added in a lower voice, "You big Swede!"

"Listen to me," said Mrs. Thompson, "that's no way to act. Now you go out there and ask him decent, or I'll get your daddy to give you a good licking."

Mr. Helton loomed, long and gloomy, in the doorway. "Sit right there," boomed Mr. Thompson, waving his arm. Mr. Helton swung his square shoes across the kitchen in two steps, slumped onto the bench and sat. Mr. Thompson occupied his chair at the head of the table, the two boys scrambled into place opposite Mr. Helton, and Mrs. Thompson sat at the end nearest the stove. Mrs. Thompson clasped her hands, bowed her head and said aloud hastily, "Lord, for all these and Thy other blessings we thank Thee in Jesus' name, amen," trying to finish before Herbert's rusty little paw reached the nearest dish. Otherwise she would be duty-bound to send him away from the table, and growing children need their meals. Mr. Thompson and Arthur always waited, but Herbert, aged six, was too young to take training yet.

Mr. and Mrs. Thompson tried to engage Mr. Helton in conversation, but it was a failure. They tried first the weather, and then the crops, and then the cows, but Mr. Helton simply did not reply.

Mr. Thompson then told something funny he had seen in town. It was about some of the other old grangers at the hotel, friends of his, giving beer to a goat, and the goat's subsequent behavior. Mr. Helton did not seem to hear. Mrs. Thompson laughed dutifully, but she didn't think it was very funny. She had heard it often before, though Mr. Thompson, each time he told it, pretended it had happened that self-same day. It must have happened years ago if it ever happened at all, and it had never been a story that Mrs. Thompson thought suitable for mixed company. The whole thing came of Mr. Thompson's weakness for a dram too much now and then, though he voted for local option at every election. She passed the food to Mr. Helton, who took a helping of everything, but not much, not enough to keep him up to his full powers if he expected to go on working the way he had started.

At last, he took a fair-sized piece of cornbread, wiped his plate up as clean as if it had been licked by a hound dog, stuffed his mouth full, and, still chewing, slid off the bench and started for the door.

"Good night, Mr. Helton," said Mrs. Thompson, and the other Thompsons took it up in a scattered chorus. "Good night, Mr. Helton!"

"Good night," said Mr. Helton's wavering voice grudgingly from the darkness.

"Gude not," said Arthur, imitating Mr. Helton.

"Gude not," said Herbert, the copy-cat.

"You don't do it right," said Arthur. "Now listen to me. Guuuuuude naht," and he ran a hollow scale in a luxury of successful impersonation. Herbert almost went into a fit with joy.

"Now you *stop* that," said Mrs. Thompson. "He can't help the way he talks. You ought to be ashamed of yourselves, both of you, making fun of a poor stranger like that. How'd you like to be a stranger in a strange land?"

"I'd like it," said Arthur. "I think it would be fun."

"They're both regular heathens, Ellie," said Mr. Thompson. "Just plain ignoramuses." He turned the face of awful fatherhood upon his young. "You're both going to get sent to school next year, and that'll knock some sense into you."

"I'm going to git sent to the 'formatory when I'm old enough," piped up Herbert. "That's where I'm goin'."

"Oh, you are, are you?" asked Mr. Thompson. "Who says so?"

"The Sunday School Supintendant," said Herbert, a bright boy showing off.

"You see?" said Mr. Thompson, staring at his wife. "What did I tell you?" He became a hurricane of wrath. "Get to bed, you two," he roared until his Adam's apple shuddered. "Get now before I take the hide off you!" They got, and shortly from their attic bedroom the sounds of scuffling and snorting and giggling and growling filled the house and shook the kitchen ceiling.

Mrs. Thompson held her head and said in a small uncertain voice, "It's no use picking on them when they're so young and tender. I can't stand it."

"My goodness, Ellie," said Mr. Thompson, "we've got to raise 'em. We can't just let 'em grow up hog wild."

She went on in another tone. "That Mr. Helton seems all right, even if he can't be made to talk. Wonder how he comes to be so far from home."

"Like I said, he isn't no whamper-jaw," said Mr. Thompson, "but he sure knows how to lay out the work. I guess that's the main thing around here. Country's full of fellers trampin' round looking for work."

Mrs. Thompson was gathering up the dishes. She now gathered up Mr. Thompson's plate from under his chin. "To tell you the honest truth," she remarked, "I think it's a mighty good change to have a man round the place who knows how to work and keep his mouth shut. Means he'll keep out of our business. Not that we've got anything to hide, but it's convenient."

"That's a fact," said Mr. Thompson. "Haw, haw," he shouted suddenly. "Means you can do all the talking, huh?"

"The only thing," went on Mrs. Thompson, "is this: he don't eat hearty enough to suit me. I like to see a man set down and relish a good meal. My granma used to say it was no use putting dependence on a man who won't set down and make out his dinner. I hope it won't be that way this time."

"Tell *you* the truth, Ellie," said Mr. Thompson, picking his teeth with a fork and leaning back in the best of good humors, "I always thought your granma was a ter'ble ole fool. She'd just say the first thing that popped into her head and call it God's wisdom."

"My granma wasn't anybody's fool. Nine times out of ten she knew what she was talking about. I always say, the first thing you think is the best thing you can say."

"Well," said Mr. Thompson, going into another shout, "you're so *ree*fined about that goat story, you just try speaking out in mixed comp'ny sometime! You just try it. S'pose you happened to be thinking about a hen and a rooster, hey? I reckon you'd shock the Babtist preacher!" He gave her a good pinch on her thin little rump. "No more meat on you than a rabbit," he said, fondly. "Now I like 'em cornfed."

Mrs. Thompson looked at him open-eyed and blushed. She could see better by lamplight. "Why, Mr. Thompson, sometimes I think you're the evilest-minded man that ever lived." She took a handful of hair on the crown of his head and gave it a good, slow pull. "That's to show you how it feels, pinching so hard when you're supposed to be playing," she said, gently.

In spite of his situation in life, Mr. Thompson had never been able to outgrow his deep conviction that running a dairy and chasing after chickens was woman's work. He was fond of saying that he could plow a furrow, cut sorghum, shuck corn, handle a team, build a corn crib, as well as any man. Buying and selling, too, were man's work. Twice a week he drove the spring wagon to market with the fresh butter, a few eggs, fruits in their proper season, sold them, pocketed the change, and spent it as seemed best, being careful not to dig into Mrs. Thompson's pin money.

But from the first the cows worried him, coming up regularly twice a day to be milked, standing there reproaching him with their smug female faces. Calves worried him, fighting the rope and strangling themselves until their eyes bulged, trying to get at the teat. Wrestling with a calf unmanned him, like having to change a baby's diaper. Milk worried him, coming bitter sometimes, drying up, turning sour. Hens worried him, cackling, clucking, hatching out when you least expected it and leading their broods into the barnyard where the horses could step on them; dying of roup and wryneck and getting plagues of chicken lice; laying eggs all over God's creation so that half of them were spoiled before a man could find them, in spite of a rack of nests Mrs. Thompson had set out for them in the feed room. Hens were a blasted nuisance.

Slopping hogs was hired man's work, in Mr. Thompson's opinion. Killing hogs was a job for the boss, but scraping them and cutting them up was for the hired man again; and again woman's proper work was dressing meat, smoking, pickling, and making lard and sausage. All his carefully limited fields of activity were related somehow to Mr. Thompson's feeling for the appearance of things, his own appearance in the sight of God and man. "It don't *look* right," was his final reason for not doing anything he did not wish to do.

It was his dignity and his reputation that he cared about, and there were only a few kinds of work manly enough for Mr. Thompson to undertake with his own hands. Mrs. Thompson, to whom so many forms of work would have been becoming, had simply gone down on him early. He saw, after a while, how short-sighted it had been of him to expect much from Mrs. Thompson; he had fallen in love with her delicate waist and lace-trimmed petticoats and big blue eyes, and, though all those charms had disappeared, she had in the meantime become Ellie to him, not at all the same person as Miss Ellen Bridges, popular Sunday School teacher in the Mountain City First Baptist Church, but his dear wife, Ellie, who was not strong. Deprived as he was, however, of the main support in life which a man might expect in marriage, he had almost without knowing it resigned himself to failure. Head erect, a prompt payer of taxes, yearly subscriber to the preacher's salary, land owner and father of a family, employer, a hearty good fellow among men, Mr. Thompson knew, without putting it into words, that he had been going steadily down hill. God amighty, it did look like somebody around the place might take a rake in hand now and then and clear up the clutter around the barn and the kitchen steps. The wagon shed was so full of broken-down machinery and ragged harness and old wagon wheels and battered milk pails and rotting lumber you could hardly drive in there any more. Not a soul on the place would raise a hand to it, and as for him, he had all he could do with his regular work. He would sometimes in the slack season sit for hours worrying about it, squirting tobacco on the ragweeds growing in a thicket against the wood pile, wondering what a fellow could do, handicapped as he was. He looked forward to the boys growing up soon; he was going to put them through the mill just as his own father had done with him when he was a boy; they were going to learn how to take hold and run the place right. He wasn't going to overdo it, but those two boys were going to earn their salt, or he'd know why. Great big lubbers sitting around whittling! Mr. Thompson sometimes grew quite enraged with them, when imagining their possible future, big lubbers sitting around whittling or thinking about fishing trips. Well, he'd put a stop to that, mighty damn quick.

As the seasons passed, and Mr. Helton took hold more and more, Mr. Thompson began to relax in his mind a little. There seemed to be nothing the fellow couldn't do, all in the day's work and as a matter of course. He got up at five o'clock in the morning, boiled his own coffee and fried his own bacon and was out in the cow lot before Mr. Thompson had even begun to yawn, stretch, groan, roar and thump around looking for his jeans. He milked the cows, kept the milk house, and churned the butter; rounded the hens up and somehow persuaded them to lay in the nests, not under the house and behind the haystacks; he fed them regularly and they hatched out until you couldn't set a foot down for them. Little by little the piles of trash around the barns and house disappeared. He carried buttermilk and corn to the hogs, and curried cockleburs out of the horses' manes. He was gentle with the calves, if a little grim with the cows and hens; judging by his conduct, Mr. Helton had never heard of the difference between man's and woman's work on a farm.

In the second year, he showed Mr. Thompson the picture of a cheese press in a mail order catalogue, and said, "This is a good thing. You buy this, I make cheese." The press was bought and Mr. Helton did make cheese, and it was sold, along with the increased butter and the crates of eggs. Sometimes Mr. Thompson felt a little contemptuous of Mr. Helton's ways. It did seem kind of picayune for a man to go around picking up half a dozen ears of corn that had fallen off the wagon on the way from the field, gathering up fallen fruit to feed to the pigs, storing up old nails and stray parts of machinery, spending good time stamping a fancy pattern on the butter before it went to market. Mr. Thompson, sitting up high on the spring-wagon seat, with the decorated butter in a five-gallon lard can wrapped in wet towsack, driving to town, chirruping to the horses and snapping the reins over their backs, sometimes thought that Mr. Helton was a pretty meeching sort of fellow; but he never gave way to these feelings, he knew a good thing when he had it. It was a fact the hogs were in better shape and sold for more money. It was a fact that Mr. Thompson stopped buying feed, Mr. Helton managed the crops so well. When beef- and hog-slaughtering time came, Mr. Helton knew how to save the scraps that Mr. Thompson had thrown away, and wasn't above scraping guts and filling them with sausages that he made by his own methods. In all, Mr. Thompson had no grounds for complaint. In the third year, he raised Mr. Helton's wages, though Mr. Helton had not asked for a raise. The fourth year, when Mr. Thompson was not only out of debt but had a little cash in the bank, he raised Mr. Helton's wages again, two dollars and a half a month each time.

"The man's worth it, Ellie," said Mr. Thompson, in a glow

of self-justification for his extravagance. "He's made this place pay, and I want him to know I appreciate it."

Mr. Helton's silence, the pallor of his eyebrows and hair, his long, glum jaw and eyes that refused to see anything, even the work under his hands, had grown perfectly familiar to the Thompsons. At first, Mrs. Thompson complained a little. "It's like sitting down at the table with a disembodied spirit," she said. "You'd think he'd find something to say, sooner or later."

"Let him alone," said Mr. Thompson. "When he gets ready to talk, he'll talk."

The years passed, and Mr. Helton never got ready to talk. After his work was finished for the day, he would come up from the barn or the milk house or the chicken house, swinging his lantern, his big shoes clumping like pony hoofs on the hard path. They, sitting in the kitchen in the winter, or on the back porch in summer, would hear him drag out his wooden chair, hear the creak of it tilted back, and then for a little while he would play his single tune on one or another of his harmonicas. The harmonicas were in different keys, some lower and sweeter than the others, but the same changeless tune went on, a strange tune, with sudden turns in it, night after night, and sometimes even in the afternoons when Mr. Helton sat down to catch his breath. At first the Thompsons liked it very much, and always stopped to listen. Later there came a time when they were fairly sick of it, and began to wish to each other that he would learn a new one. At last they did not hear it any more, it was as natural as the sound of the wind rising in the evenings, or the cows lowing, or their own voices.

Mrs. Thompson pondered now and then over Mr. Helton's soul. He didn't seem to be a church-goer, and worked straight through Sunday as if it were any common day of the week. "I think we ought to invite him to go to hear Dr. Martin," she told Mr. Thompson. "It isn't very Christian of us not to ask him. He's not a forward kind of man. He'd wait to be asked."

"Let him alone," said Mr. Thompson. "The way I look at

it, his religion is every man's own business. Besides, he ain't got any Sunday clothes. He wouldn't want to go to church in them jeans and jumpers of his. I don't know what he does with his money. He certainly don't spend it foolishly."

Still, once the notion got into her head, Mrs. Thompson could not rest until she invited Mr. Helton to go to church with the family next Sunday. He was pitching hay into neat little piles in the field back of the orchard. Mrs. Thompson put on smoked glasses and a sunbonnet and walked all the way down there to speak to him. He stopped and leaned on his pitchfork, listening, and for a moment Mrs. Thompson was almost frightened at his face. The pale eyes seemed to glare past her, the eyebrows frowned, the long jaw hardened. "I got work," he said bluntly, and lifting his pitchfork he turned from her and began to toss the hay. Mrs. Thompson, her feelings hurt, walked back thinking that by now she should be used to Mr. Helton's ways, but it did seem like a man, even a foreigner, could be just a little polite when you gave him a Christian invitation. "He's not polite, that's the only thing I've got against him," she said to Mr. Thompson. "He just can't seem to behave like other people. You'd think he had a grudge against the world," she said. "I sometimes don't know what to make of it."

In the second year something had happened that made Mrs. Thompson uneasy, the kind of thing she could not put into words, hardly into thoughts, and if she had tried to explain to Mr. Thompson it would have sounded worse than it was, or not bad enough. It was that kind of queer thing that seems to be giving a warning, and yet, nearly always nothing comes of it. It was on a hot, still spring day, and Mrs. Thompson had been down to the garden patch to pull some new carrots and green onions and string beans for dinner. As she worked, sunbonnet low over her eyes, putting each kind of vegetable in a pile by itself in her basket, she noticed how neatly Mr. Helton weeded, and how rich the soil was. He had spread it all over with manure from the barns, and worked it in, in the fall, and the vegetables were coming up fine and full. She walked back under the nubbly little fig trees where the unpruned branches leaned almost to the ground, and the thick leaves made a cool screen. Mrs. Thompson was always looking for shade to save her eyes. So she, looking idly about, saw through the screen a sight that struck her as very strange. If it had been a noisy spectacle, it would have been quite natural. It was the silence that struck her. Mr. Helton was shaking Arthur by the shoulders, ferociously, his face most terribly fixed and pale. Arthur's head snapped back and forth and he had not stiffened in resistance, as he did when Mrs. Thompson tried to shake him. His eyes were rather frightened, but surprised, too, probably more surprised than anything else. Herbert stood by meekly, watching. Mr. Helton dropped Arthur, and seized Herbert, and shook him with the same methodical ferocity, the same face of hatred. Herbert's mouth crumpled as if he would cry, but he made no sound. Mr. Helton let him go, turned and strode into the shack, and the little boys ran, as if for their lives, without a word. They disappeared around the corner to the front of the house.

Mrs. Thompson took time to set her basket on the kitchen table, to push her sunbonnet back on her head and draw it forward again, to look in the stove and make certain the fire was going, before she followed the boys. They were sitting huddled together under a clump of chinaberry trees in plain sight of her bedroom window, as if it were a safe place they had discovered.

"What are you doing?" asked Mrs. Thompson.

They looked hang-dog from under their foreheads and Arthur mumbled, "Nothin'."

"Nothing *now*, you mean," said Mrs. Thompson, severely. "Well, I have plenty for you to do. Come right in here this minute and help me fix vegetables. This minute."

They scrambled up very eagerly and followed her close. Mrs. Thompson tried to imagine what they had been up to; she did not like the notion of Mr. Helton taking it on himself to correct her little boys, but she was afraid to ask them for reasons. They might tell her a lie, and she would have to overtake them in it, and whip them. Or she would have to pretend to believe them, and they would get in the habit of lying. Or they might tell her the truth, and it would be something she would have to whip them for. The very thought of it gave her a headache. She supposed she might ask Mr. Helton, but it was not her place to ask. She would wait and tell Mr. Thompson, and let him get at the bottom of it. While her mind ran on, she kept the little boys hopping. "Cut those carrot tops closer, Herbert, you're just being careless. Arthur, stop breaking up the beans so little. They're little enough already. Herbert, you go get an armload of wood. Arthur, you take these onions and wash them under the pump. Herbert, as soon as you're done here, you get a broom and sweep out this kitchen. Arthur, you get a shovel and take up the ashes. Stop picking your nose, Herbert. How often must I tell you? Arthur, you go look in the top drawer of my bureau, left-hand side, and bring me the vaseline for Herbert's nose. Herbert, come here to me. . . ."

They galloped through their chores, their animal spirits rose with activity, and shortly they were out in the front yard again, engaged in a wrestling match. They sprawled and fought, scrambled, clutched, rose and fell shouting, as aimlessly, noisily, monotonously as two puppies. They imitated various animals, not a human sound from them, and their dirty faces were streaked with sweat. Mrs. Thompson, sitting at her window, watched them with baffled pride and tenderness, they were so sturdy and healthy and growing so fast; but uneasily, too, with her pained little smile and the tears rolling from her eyelids that clinched themselves against the sunlight. They were so idle and careless, as if they had no future in this world, and no immortal souls to save, and oh, what had they been up to that Mr. Helton had shaken them, with his face positively dangerous?

In the evening before supper, without a word to Mr. Thompson of the curious fear the sight had caused her, she told him that Mr. Helton had shaken the little boys for some reason. He stepped out to the shack and spoke to Mr. Helton. In five minutes he was back, glaring at his young. "He says them brats been fooling with his harmonicas, Ellie, blowing in them and getting them all dirty and full of spit and they don't play good."

"Did he say all that?" asked Mrs. Thompson. "It doesn't seem possible."

"Well, that's what he meant, anyhow," said Mr. Thompson. "He didn't say it just that way. But he acted pretty worked up about it."

"That's a shame," said Mrs. Thompson, "a perfect shame. Now we've got to do something so they'll remember they mustn't go into Mr. Helton's things."

"I'll tan their hides for them," said Mr. Thompson. "I'll take a calf rope to them if they don't look out."

"Maybe you'd better leave the whipping to me," said Mrs. Thompson. "You haven't got a light enough hand for children."

"That's just what's the matter with them now," shouted Mr. Thompson, "rotten spoiled and they'll wind up in the penitentiary. You don't half whip 'em. Just little love taps. My pa used to knock me down with a stick of stove wood or anything else that came handy."

"Well, that's not saying it's right," said Mrs. Thompson. "I don't hold with that way of raising children. It makes them run away from home. I've seen too much of it."

"I'll break every bone in 'em," said Mr. Thompson, simmering down, "if they don't mind you better and stop being so bullheaded."

"Leave the table and wash your face and hands," Mrs. Thompson commanded the boys, suddenly. They slunk out and dabbled at the pump and slunk in again, trying to make themselves small. They had learned long ago that their mother always made them wash when there was trouble ahead. They looked at their plates. Mr. Thompson opened up on them.

"Well, now, what you got to say for yourselves about going into Mr. Helton's shack and ruining his harmonicas?"

The two little boys wilted, their faces drooped into the grieved hopeless lines of children's faces when they are brought to the terrible bar of blind adult justice; their eyes telegraphed each other in panic, "Now we're really going to catch a licking"; in despair, they dropped their buttered cornbread on their plates, their hands lagged on the edge of the table.

"I ought to break your ribs," said Mr. Thompson, "and I'm a good mind to do it."

"Yes, sir," whispered Arthur, faintly.

"Yes, sir," said Herbert, his lip trembling.

"Now, papa," said Mrs. Thompson in a warning tone. The children did not glance at her. They had no faith in her good will. She had betrayed them in the first place. There was no trusting her. Now she might save them and she might not. No use depending on her.

"Well, you ought to get a good thrashing. You deserve it, don't you, Arthur?"

Arthur hung his head. "Yes, sir."

"And the next time I catch either of you hanging around Mr. Helton's shack, I'm going to take the hide off *both* of you, you hear me, Herbert?"

Herbert mumbled and choked, scattering his cornbread. "Yes, sir."

"Well, now sit up and eat your supper and not another word out of you," said Mr. Thompson, beginning on his own food. The little boys perked up somewhat and started chewing, but every time they looked around they met their parents' eyes, regarding them steadily. There was no telling when they would think of something new. The boys ate warily, trying not to be seen or heard, the cornbread sticking, the buttermilk gurgling, as it went down their gullets.

"And something else, Mr. Thompson," said Mrs. Thompson after a pause. "Tell Mr. Helton he's to come straight to us when they bother him, and not to trouble shaking them himself. Tell him we'll look after that."

"They're so mean," answered Mr. Thompson, staring at them. "It's a wonder he don't just kill 'em off and be done with it." But there was something in the tone that told Arthur and Herbert that nothing more worth worrying about was going to happen this time. Heaving deep sighs, they sat up, reaching for the food nearest them.

"Listen," said Mrs. Thompson, suddenly. The little boys stopped eating. "Mr. Helton hasn't come for his supper. Arthur, go and tell Mr. Helton he's late for supper. Tell him nice, now."

Arthur, miserably depressed, slid out of his place and made for the door, without a word.

There were no miracles of fortune to be brought to pass on a small dairy farm. The Thompsons did not grow rich, but they kept out of the poor house, as Mr. Thompson was fond of saying, meaning he had got a little foothold in spite of Ellie's poor health, and unexpected weather, and strange declines in market prices, and his own mysterious handicaps which weighed him down. Mr. Helton was the hope and the prop of the family, and all the Thompsons became fond of him, or at any rate they ceased to regard him as in any way peculiar, and looked upon him, from a distance they did not know how to bridge, as a good man and a good friend. Mr. Helton went his way, worked, played his tune. Nine years passed. The boys grew up and learned to work. They could not remember the time when Ole Helton hadn't been there: a grouchy cuss, Brother Bones; Mr. Helton, the dairymaid; that Big Swede. If he had heard them, he might have been annoyed at some of the names they called him. But he did not hear them, and besides they meant no harm—or at least such harm as existed was all there, in the names; the boys referred to their father as the Old Man, or the Old Geezer, but not to his face. They lived through by main strength all the grimy, secret, oblique phases of growing up and got past the crisis safely if anyone does. Their parents could see they were good solid boys with hearts of gold in spite of their rough ways. Mr. Thompson was relieved to find that, without knowing how he had done it, he had succeeded in raising a set of boys who were not trifling whittlers. They were such good boys Mr. Thompson began to believe they were born that way, and that he had never spoken a harsh word to them in their lives, much less thrashed them. Herbert and Arthur never disputed his word.

Mr. Helton, his hair wet with sweat, plastered to his dripping forehead, his jumper streaked dark and light blue and clinging to his ribs, was chopping a little firewood. He chopped slowly, struck the ax into the end of the chopping log, and piled the wood up neatly. He then disappeared round the house into his shack, which shared with the wood pile a good shade from a row of mulberry trees. Mr. Thompson was lolling in a swing chair on the front porch, a place he had never liked. The chair was new, and Mrs. Thompson had wanted it on the front porch, though the side porch was the place for it, being cooler; and Mr. Thompson wanted to sit in the chair, so there he was. As soon as the new wore off of it, and Ellie's pride in it was exhausted, he would move it round to the side porch. Meantime the August heat was almost unbearable, the air so thick you could poke a hole in it. The dust was inches thick on everything, though Mr. Helton sprinkled the whole yard regularly every night. He even shot the hose upward and washed the tree tops and the roof of the house. They had laid waterpipes to the kitchen and an outside faucet. Mr. Thompson must have dozed, for he opened his eyes and shut his mouth just in time to save his face before a stranger who had driven up to the front gate. Mr. Thompson stood up, put on his hat, pulled up his jeans, and watched while the stranger tied his team, attached to a light spring wagon, to the hitching post. Mr. Thompson recognized the team and wagon. They were from a livery stable in Buda. While the stranger was opening the gate, a strong gate that Mr. Helton had built and set firmly on its hinges several years back, Mr. Thompson strolled down the path to greet him and find out what in God's world a man's business might be that would bring him out at this time of day, in all this dust and welter.

He wasn't exactly a fat man. He was more like a man who had been fat recently. His skin was baggy and his clothes were too big for him, and he somehow looked like a man who should be fat, ordinarily, but who might have just got over a spell of sickness. Mr. Thompson didn't take to his looks at all, he couldn't say why.

The stranger took off his hat. He said in a loud hearty voice, "Is this Mr. Thompson, Mr. Royal Earle Thompson?"

"That's my name," said Mr. Thompson, almost quietly, he was so taken aback by the free manner of the stranger.

"My name is Hatch," said the stranger, "Mr. Homer T. Hatch, and I've come to see you about buying a horse."

"I reckon you've been misdirected," said Mr. Thompson. "I haven't got a horse for sale. Usually if I've got anything like that to sell," he said, "I tell the neighbors and tack up a little sign on the gate."

The fat man opened his mouth and roared with joy, showing rabbit teeth brown as shoeleather. Mr. Thompson saw nothing to laugh at, for once. The stranger shouted, "That's just an old joke of mine." He caught one of his hands in the other and shook hands with himself heartily. "I always say something like that when I'm calling on a stranger, because I've noticed that when a feller says he's come to buy something nobody takes him for a suspicious character. You see? Haw, haw, haw."

His joviality made Mr. Thompson nervous, because the expression in the man's eyes didn't match the sounds he was making. "Haw, haw," laughed Mr. Thompson obligingly, still not seeing the joke. "Well, that's all wasted on me because I never take any man for a suspicious character 'til he shows hisself to be one. Says or does something," he explained. "Until that happens, one man's as good as another, so far's *I'm* concerned."

"Well," said the stranger, suddenly very sober and sensible, "I ain't come neither to buy nor sell. Fact is, I want to see you about something that's of interest to us both. Yes, sir, I'd like to have a little talk with you, and it won't cost you a cent."

"I guess that's fair enough," said Mr. Thompson, reluctantly. "Come on around the house where there's a little shade."

They went round and seated themselves on two stumps under a chinaberry tree.

"Yes, sir, Homer T. Hatch is my name and America is my nation," said the stranger. "I reckon you must know the name? I used to have a cousin named Jameson Hatch lived up the country a ways."

"Don't think I know the name," said Mr. Thompson. "There's some Hatchers settled somewhere around Mountain City."

"Don't know the old Hatch family," cried the man in deep concern. He seemed to be pitying Mr. Thompson's ignorance. "Why, we came over from Georgia fifty years ago. Been here long yourself?"

"Just all my whole life," said Mr. Thompson, beginning to feel peevish. "And my pa and my grampap before me. Yes, sir, we've been right here all along. Anybody wants to find a Thompson knows where to look for him. My grampap immigrated in 1836."

"From Ireland, I reckon?" said the stranger.

"From Pennsylvania," said Mr. Thompson. "Now what makes you think we came from Ireland?"

The stranger opened his mouth and began to shout with merriment, and he shook hands with himself as if he hadn't met himself for a long time. "Well, what I always says is, a feller's got to come from *somewhere*, ain't he?"

While they were talking, Mr. Thompson kept glancing at the face near him. He certainly did remind Mr. Thompson of somebody, or maybe he really had seen the man himself somewhere. He couldn't just place the features. Mr. Thompson finally decided it was just that all rabbit-teethed men looked alike.

"That's right," acknowledged Mr. Thompson, rather sourly, "but what I always say is, Thompsons have been settled here for so long it don't make much difference any more *where* they come from. Now a course, this is the slack season, and we're all just laying round a little, but nevertheless we've all got our chores to do, and I don't want to hurry you, and so if you've come to see me on business maybe we'd better get down to it."

"As I said, it's not in a way, and again in a way it is," said the fat man. "Now I'm looking for a man named Helton, Mr. Olaf Eric Helton, from North Dakota, and I was told up around the country a ways that I might find him here, and I wouldn't mind having a little talk with him. No, siree, I sure wouldn't mind, if it's all the same to you."

"I never knew his middle name," said Mr. Thompson, "but Mr. Helton is right here, and been here now for going on nine years. He's a mighty steady man, and you can tell anybody I said so."

"I'm glad to hear that," said Mr. Homer T. Hatch. "I like to hear of a feller mending his ways and settling down. Now when I knew Mr. Helton he was pretty wild, yes, sir, wild is what he was, he didn't know his own mind atall. Well, now, it's going to be a great pleasure to me to meet up with an old friend and find him all settled down and doing well by hisself."

"We've all got to be young once," said Mr. Thompson. "It's like the measles, it breaks out all over you, and you're a nuisance to yourself and everybody else, but it don't last, and it usually don't leave no ill effects." He was so pleased with this notion he forgot and broke into a guffaw. The stranger folded his arms over his stomach and went into a kind of fit, roaring until he had tears in his eyes. Mr. Thompson stopped shouting and eyed the stranger uneasily. Now he liked a good laugh as well as any man, but there ought to be a little moderation. Now this feller laughed like a perfect lunatic, that was a fact. And he wasn't laughing because he really thought things were funny, either. He was laughing for reasons of his own. Mr. Thompson fell into a moody silence, and waited until Mr. Hatch settled down a little.

Mr. Hatch got out a very dirty blue cotton bandanna and wiped his eyes. "That joke just about caught me where I live," he said, almost apologetically. "Now I wish I could think up things as funny as that to say. It's a gift. It's . . ."

"If you want to speak to Mr. Helton, I'll go and round him up," said Mr. Thompson, making motions as if he might get up. "He may be in the milk house and he may be setting in his shack this time of day." It was drawing towards five o'clock. "It's right around the corner," he said.

"Oh, well, there ain't no special hurry," said Mr. Hatch. "I've been wanting to speak to him for a good long spell now and I guess a few minutes more won't make no difference. I just more wanted to locate him, like. That's all."

Mr. Thompson stopped beginning to stand up, and unbuttoned one more button of his shirt, and said, "Well, he's here, and he's this kind of man, that if he had any business with you he'd like to get it over. He don't dawdle, that's one thing you can say for him."

Mr. Hatch appeared to sulk a little at these words. He wiped his face with the bandanna and opened his mouth to speak, when round the house there came the music of Mr. Helton's harmonica. Mr. Thompson raised a finger. "There he is," said Mr. Thompson. "Now's your time."

Mr. Hatch cocked an ear towards the east side of the house and listened for a few seconds, a very strange expression on his face.

"I know that tune like I know the palm of my own hand," said Mr. Thompson, "but I never heard Mr. Helton say what it was."

"That's a kind of Scandahoovian song," said Mr. Hatch. "Where I come from they sing it a lot. In North Dakota, they sing it. It says something about starting out in the morning feeling so good you can't hardly stand it, so you drink up all your likker before noon. All the likker, y' understand, that you was saving for the noon lay-off. The words ain't much, but it's a pretty tune. It's a kind of drinking song." He sat there drooping a little, and Mr. Thompson didn't like his expression. It was a satisfied expression, but it was more like the cat that et the canary.

"So far as I know," said Mr. Thompson, "he ain't touched a

drop since he's been on the place, and that's nine years this coming September. Yes, sir, nine years, so far as I know, he ain't wetted his whistle once. And that's more than I can say for myself," he said, meekly proud.

"Yes, that's a drinking song," said Mr. Hatch. "I used to play 'Little Brown Jug' on the fiddle when I was younger than I am now," he went on, "but this Helton, he just keeps it up. He just sits and plays it by himself."

"He's been playing it off and on for nine years right here on the place," said Mr. Thompson, feeling a little proprietary.

"And he was certainly singing it as well, fifteen years before that, in North Dakota," said Mr. Hatch. "He used to sit up in a straitjacket, practically, when he was in the asylum—"

"What's that you say?" said Mr. Thompson. "What's that?"

"Shucks, I didn't mean to tell you," said Mr. Hatch, a faint leer of regret in his drooping eyelids. "Shucks, that just slipped out. Funny, now I'd made up my mind I wouldn' say a word, because it would just make a lot of excitement, and what I say is, if a man has lived harmless and quiet for nine years it don't matter if he *is* loony, does it? So long's he keeps quiet and don't do nobody harm."

"You mean they had him in a straitjacket?" asked Mr. Thompson, uneasily. "In a lunatic asylum?"

"They sure did," said Mr. Hatch. "That's right where they had him, from time to time."

"They put my Aunt Ida in one of them things in the State asylum," said Mr. Thompson. "She got vi'lent, and they put her in one of these jackets with long sleeves and tied her to an iron ring in the wall, and Aunt Ida got so wild she broke a blood vessel and when they went to look after her she was dead. I'd think one of them things was dangerous."

"Mr. Helton used to sing his drinking song when he was in a straitjacket," said Mr. Hatch. "Nothing ever bothered him, except if you tried to make him talk. That bothered him, and he'd get vi'lent, like your Aunt Ida. He'd get vi'lent and then they'd put him in the jacket and go off and leave him, and he'd lay there perfickly contented, so far's you could see, singing his song. Then one night he just disappeared. Left, you might say, just went, and nobody ever saw hide or hair of him again. And then I come along and find him here," said Mr. Hatch, "all settled down and playing the same song."

"He never acted crazy to me," said Mr. Thompson. "He always acted like a sensible man, to me. He never got married, for one thing, and he works like a horse, and I bet he's got the first cent I paid him when he landed here, and he don't drink, and he never says a word, much less swear, and he don't waste time runnin' around Saturday nights, and if he's crazy," said Mr. Thompson, "why, I think I'll go crazy myself for a change."

"Haw, ha," said Mr. Hatch, "heh, he, that's good! Ha, ha, ha, I hadn't thought of it jes like that. Yeah, that's right. Let's all go crazy and get rid of our wives and save our money, hey?" He smiled unpleasantly, showing his little rabbit teeth.

Mr. Thompson felt he was being misunderstood. He turned around and motioned toward the open window back of the honeysuckle trellis. "Let's move off down here a little," he said. "I oughta thought of that before." His visitor bothered Mr. Thompson. He had a way of taking the words out of Mr. Thompson's mouth, turning them around and mixing them up until Mr. Thompson didn't know himself what he had said. "My wife's not very strong," said Mr. Thompson. "She's been kind of invalid now goin' on fourteen years. It's mighty tough on a poor man, havin' sickness in the family. She had four operations," he said proudly, "one right after the other, but they didn't do any good. For five years handrunnin', I just turned every nickel I made over to the doctors. Upshot is, she's a mighty delicate woman."

"My old woman," said Mr. Homer T. Hatch, "had a back like a mule, yes, sir. That woman could have moved the barn with her bare hands if she'd ever took the notion. I used to say, it was a good thing she didn't know her own stren'th. She's dead now, though. That kind wear out quicker than the puny ones. I never had much use for a woman always complainin'. I'd get rid of her mighty quick, yes, sir, mighty quick. It's just as you say: a dead loss, keepin' one of 'em up."

This was not at all what Mr. Thompson had heard himself say; he had been trying to explain that a wife as expensive as his was a credit to a man. "She's a mighty reasonable woman," said Mr. Thompson, feeling baffled, "but I wouldn't answer for what she'd say or do if she found out we'd had a lunatic on the place all this time." They had moved away from the window; Mr. Thompson took Mr. Hatch the front way, because if he went the back way they would have to pass Mr. Helton's shack. For some reason he didn't want the stranger to see or talk to Mr. Helton. It was strange, but that was the way Mr. Thompson felt.

Mr. Thompson sat down again, on the chopping log, offering his guest another tree stump. "Now, I mighta got upset myself at such a thing, once," said Mr. Thompson, "but now I *deefy* anything to get me lathered up." He cut himself an enormous plug of tobacco with his horn-handled pocketknife, and offered it to Mr. Hatch, who then produced his own plug and, opening a huge bowie knife with a long blade sharply whetted, cut off a large wad and put it in his mouth. They then compared plugs and both of them were astonished to see how different men's ideas of good chewing tobacco were.

"Now, for instance," said Mr. Hatch, "mine is lighter colored. That's because, for one thing, there ain't any sweetenin' in this plug. I like it dry, natural leaf, medium strong."

"A little sweetenin' don't do no harm so far as I'm concerned," said Mr. Thompson, "but it's got to be mighty little. But with me, now, I want a strong leaf, I want it heavy-cured, as the feller says. There's a man near here, named Williams, Mr. John Morgan Williams, who chews a plug—well, sir, it's black as your hat and soft as melted tar. It fairly drips with molasses, jus' plain molasses, and it chews like licorice. Now, I don't call that a good chew."

"One man's meat," said Mr. Hatch, "is another man's poison.

Now, such a chew would simply gag me. I couldn't begin to put it in my mouth."

"Well," said Mr. Thompson, a tinge of apology in his voice, "I jus' barely tasted it myself, you might say. Just took a little piece in my mouth and spit it out again."

"I'm dead sure I couldn't even get that far," said Mr. Hatch. "I like a dry natural chew without any artificial flavorin' of any kind."

Mr. Thompson began to feel that Mr. Hatch was trying to make out he had the best judgment in tobacco, and was going to keep up the argument until he proved it. He began to feel seriously annoyed with the fat man. After all, who was he and where did he come from? Who was he to go around telling other people what kind of tobacco to chew?

"Artificial flavorin'," Mr. Hatch went on, doggedly, "is jes put in to cover up a cheap leaf and make a man think he's gettin' somethin' more than he *is* gettin'. Even a little sweetenin' is a sign of a cheap leaf, you can mark my words."

"I've always paid a fair price for my plug," said Mr. Thompson, stiffly. "I'm not a rich man and I don't go round settin' myself up for one, but I'll say this, when it comes to such things as tobacco, I buy the best on the market."

"Sweetenin', even a little," began Mr. Hatch, shifting his plug and squirting tobacco juice at a dry-looking little rose bush that was having a hard enough time as it was, standing all day in the blazing sun, its roots clenched in the baked earth, "is the sign of—"

"About this Mr. Helton, now," said Mr. Thompson, determinedly, "I don't see no reason to hold it against a man because he went loony once or twice in his lifetime and so I don't expect to take no steps about it. Not a step. I've got nothin' against the man, he's always treated me fair. They's things and people," he went on, " 'nough to drive any man loony. The wonder to me is, more men don't wind up in straitjackets, the way things are going these days and times."

"That's right," said Mr. Hatch, promptly, entirely too promptly, as if he were turning Mr. Thompson's meaning back on him. "You took the words right out of my mouth. There ain't every man in a straitjacket that ought to be there. Ha, ha, you're right all right. You got the idea."

Mr. Thompson sat silent and chewed steadily and stared at a spot on the ground about six feet away and felt a slow muffled resentment climbing from somewhere deep down in him, climbing and spreading all through him. What was this fellow driving at? What was he trying to say? It wasn't so much his words, but his looks and his way of talking: that droopy look in the eye, that tone of voice, as if he was trying to mortify Mr. Thompson about something. Mr. Thompson didn't like it, but he couldn't get hold of it either. He wanted to turn around and shove the fellow off the stump, but it wouldn't look reasonable. Suppose something happened to the fellow when he fell off the stump, just for instance, if he fell on the ax and cut himself, and then someone should ask Mr. Thompson why he shoved him, and what could a man say? It would look mighty funny, it would sound mighty strange to say, Well, him and me fell out over a plug of tobacco. He might just shove him anyhow and then tell people he was a fat man not used to the heat and while he was talking he got dizzy and fell off by himself, or something like that, and it wouldn't be the truth either, because it wasn't the heat and it wasn't the tobacco. Mr. Thompson made up his mind to get the fellow off the place pretty quick, without seeming to be anxious, and watch him sharp till he was out of sight. It doesn't pay to be friendly with strangers from another part of the country. They're always up to something, or they'd stay at home where they belong.

"And they's some people," said Mr. Hatch, "would jus' as soon have a loonatic around their house as not, they can't see no difference between them and anybody else. I always say, if that's the way a man feels, don't care who he associates with, why, why, that's his business, not mine. I don't wanta have a thing to do with it. Now back home in North Dakota, we don't feel that way. I'd like to a seen anybody hiring a loonatic there, aspecially after what he done."

"I didn't understand your home was North Dakota," said Mr. Thompson. "I thought you said Georgia."

"I've got a married sister in North Dakota," said Mr. Hatch, "married a Swede, but a white man if ever I saw one. So I say *we* because we got into a little business together out that way. And it seems like home, kind of."

"What did he do?" asked Mr. Thompson, feeling very uneasy again.

"Oh, nothin' to speak of," said Mr. Hatch, jovially, "jus' went loony one day in the hayfield and shoved a pitchfork right square through his brother, when they was makin' hay. They was goin' to execute him, but they found out he had went crazy with the heat, as the feller says, and so they put him in the asylum. That's all he done. Nothin' to get lathered up about, ha, ha, ha!" he said, and taking out his sharp knife he began to slice off a chew as carefully as if he were cutting cake.

"Well," said Mr. Thompson, "I don't deny that's news. Yes, sir, news. But I still say somethin' must have drove him to it. Some men make you feel like giving 'em a good killing just by lookin' at you. His brother may a been a mean ornery cuss."

"Brother was going to get married," said Mr. Hatch; "used to go courtin' his girl nights. Borrowed Mr. Helton's harmonica to give her a serenade one evenin', and lost it. Brand new harmonica."

"He thinks a heap of his harmonicas," said Mr. Thompson. "Only money he ever spends, now and then he buys hisself a new one. Must have a dozen in that shack, all kinds and sizes."

"Brother wouldn't buy him a new one," said Mr. Hatch, "so Mr. Helton just ups, as I says, and runs his pitchfork through his brother. Now you know he musta been crazy to get all worked up over a little thing like that."

"Sounds like it," said Mr. Thompson, reluctant to agree in anything with this intrusive and disagreeable fellow. He kept thinking he couldn't remember when he had taken such a dislike to a man on first sight.

"Seems to me you'd get pretty sick of hearin' the same tune year in, year out," said Mr. Hatch.

"Well, sometimes I think it wouldn't do no harm if he learned a new one," said Mr. Thompson, "but he don't, so there's nothin' to be done about it. It's a pretty good tune, though."

"One of the Scandahoovians told me what it meant, that's how I come to know," said Mr. Hatch. "Especially that part about getting so gay you jus' go ahead and drink up all the likker you got on hand before noon. It seems like up in them Swede countries a man carries a bottle of wine around with him as a matter of course, at least that's the way I understood it. Those fellers will tell you anything, though—" He broke off and spat.

The idea of drinking any kind of liquor in this heat made Mr. Thompson dizzy. The idea of anybody feeling good on a day like this, for instance, made him tired. He felt he was really suffering from the heat. The fat man looked as if he had grown to the stump; he slumped there in his damp, dark clothes too big for him, his belly slack in his pants, his wide black felt hat pushed off his narrow forehead red with prickly heat. A bottle of good cold beer, now, would be a help, thought Mr. Thompson, remembering the four bottles sitting deep in the pool at the spring-house, and his dry tongue squirmed in his mouth. He wasn't going to offer this man anything, though, not even a drop of water. He wasn't even going to chew any more tobacco with him. He shot out his quid suddenly, and wiped his mouth on the back of his hand, and studied the head near him attentively. The man was no good, and he was there for no good, but what was he up to? Mr. Thompson made up his mind he'd give him a little more time to get his business, whatever it was, with Mr. Helton over, and then if he didn't get off the place he'd kick him off.

Mr. Hatch, as if he suspected Mr. Thompson's thoughts, turned his eyes, wicked and pig-like, on Mr. Thompson. "Fact is," he said, as if he had made up his mind about something, "I might need your help in the little matter I've got on hand, but it won't cost you any trouble. Now, this Mr. Helton here, like I tell you, he's a dangerous escaped loonatic, you might say. Now fact is, in the last twelve years or so I musta rounded up twenty-odd escaped loonatics, besides a couple of escaped convicts that I just run into by accident, like. I don't make a business of it, but if there's a reward, and there usually is a reward, of course, I get it. It amounts to a tidy little sum in the long run, but that ain't the main question. Fact is, I'm for law and order, I don't like to see lawbreakers and loonatics at large. It ain't the place for them. Now I reckon you're bound to agree with me on that, aren't you?"

Mr. Thompson said, "Well, circumstances alters cases, as the feller says. Now, what I know of Mr. Helton, he ain't dangerous, as I told you." Something serious was going to happen, Mr. Thompson could see that. He stopped thinking about it. He'd just let this fellow shoot off his head and then see what could be done about it. Without thinking he got out his knife and plug and started to cut a chew, then remembered himself and put them back in his pocket.

"The law," said Mr. Hatch, "is solidly behind me. Now this Mr. Helton, he's been one of my toughest cases. He's kept my record from being practically one hundred per cent. I knew him before he went loony, and I know the fam'ly, so I undertook to help out rounding him up. Well, sir, he was gone slick as a whistle, for all we knew the man was as good as dead long while ago. Now we never might have caught up with him, but do you know what he did? Well, sir, about two weeks ago his old mother gets a letter from him, and in that letter, what do you reckon she found? Well, it was a check on that little bank in town for eight hundred and fifty dollars, just like that; the letter wasn't nothing much, just said he was sending her a few little savings, she might need something, but there it was, name, postmark, date, everything. The old woman practically lost her mind with joy. She's gettin' childish, and it looked like she kinda forgot that her only living son killed his brother and went loony. Mr.

Helton said he was getting along all right, and for her not to tell nobody. Well, natchally, she couldn't keep it to herself, with that check to cash and everything. So that's how I come to know." His feelings got the better of him. "You coulda knocked me down with a feather." He shook hands with himself and rocked, wagging his head, going "Heh, heh," in his throat. Mr. Thompson felt the corners of his mouth turning down. Why, the dirty low-down hound, sneaking around spying into other people's business like that. Collecting blood money, that's what it was! Let him talk!

"Yea, well, that musta been a surprise all right," he said, trying to hold his voice even. "I'd say a surprise."

"Well, siree," said Mr. Hatch, "the more I got to thinking about it, the more I just come to the conclusion that I'd better look into the matter a little, and so I talked to the old woman. She's pretty decrepit, now, half blind and all, but she was all for taking the first train out and going to see her son. I put it up to her square—how she was too feeble for the trip, and all. So, just as a favor to her, I told her for my expenses I'd come down and see Mr. Helton and bring her back all the news about him. She gave me a new shirt she made herself by hand, and a big Swedish kind of cake to bring to him, but I musta mislaid them along the road somewhere. It don't reely matter, though, he prob'ly ain't in any state of mind to appreciate 'em."

Mr. Thompson sat up and turning round on the log looked at Mr. Hatch and asked as quietly as he could, "And now what are you aiming to do? That's the question."

Mr. Hatch slouched up to his feet and shook himself. "Well, I come all prepared for a little scuffle," he said. "I got the handcuffs," he said, "but I don't want no violence if I can help it. I didn't want to say nothing around the countryside, making an uproar. I figured the two of us could overpower him." He reached into his big inside pocket and pulled them out. Handcuffs, for God's sake, thought Mr. Thompson. Coming round on a peaceable afternoon worrying a man, and making trouble, and fishing handcuffs out of his pocket on a decent family homestead, as if it was all in the day's work.

Mr. Thompson, his head buzzing, got up too. "Well," he said, roundly, "I want to tell you I think you've got a mighty sorry job on hand, you sure must be hard up for something to do, and now I want to give you a good piece of advice. You just drop the idea that you're going to come here and make trouble for Mr. Helton, and the quicker you drive that hired rig away from my front gate the better I'll be satisfied."

Mr. Hatch put one handcuff in his outside pocket, the other dangling down. He pulled his hat down over his eyes, and reminded Mr. Thompson of a sheriff, somehow. He didn't seem in the least nervous, and didn't take up Mr. Thompson's words. He said, "Now listen just a minute, it ain't reasonable to suppose that a man like yourself is going to stand in the way of getting an escaped loonatic back to the asylum where he belongs. Now I know it's enough to throw you off, coming sudden like this, but fact is I counted on your being a respectable man and helping me out to see that justice is done. Now a course, if you won't help, I'll have to look around for help somewheres else. It won't look very good to your neighbors that you was harbring an escaped loonatic who killed his own brother, and then you refused to give him up. It will look mighty funny."

Mr. Thompson knew almost before he heard the words that it would look funny. It would put him in a mighty awkward position. He said, "But I've been trying to tell you all along that the man ain't loony now. He's been perfectly harmless for nine years. He's—he's—"

Mr. Thompson couldn't think how to describe how it was with Mr. Helton. "Why, he's been like one of the family," he said, "the best standby a man ever had." Mr. Thompson tried to see his way out. It was a fact Mr. Helton might go loony again any minute, and now this fellow talking around the country would put Mr. Thompson in a fix. It was a terrible position. He couldn't think of any way out. "You're crazy," Mr. Thompson roared suddenly, "you're the crazy one around here, you're crazier than he ever was! You get off this place or I'll handcuff you and turn you over to the law. You're trespassing," shouted Mr. Thompson. "Get out of here before I knock you down!"

He took a step towards the fat man, who backed off, shrinking, "Try it, try it, go ahead!" and then something happened that Mr. Thompson tried hard afterwards to piece together in his mind, and in fact it never did come straight. He saw the fat man with his long bowie knife in his hand, he saw Mr. Helton come round the corner on the run, his long jaw dropped, his arms swinging, his eyes wild. Mr. Helton came in between them, fists doubled up, then stopped short, glaring at the fat man, his big frame seemed to collapse, he trembled like a shied horse; and then the fat man drove at him, knife in one hand, handcuffs in the other. Mr. Thompson saw it coming, he saw the blade going into Mr. Helton's stomach, he knew he had the ax out of the log in his own hands, felt his arms go up over his head and bring the ax down on Mr. Hatch's head as if he were stunning a beef.

Mrs. Thompson had been listening uneasily for some time to the voices going on, one of them strange to her, but she was too tired at first to get up and come out to see what was going on. The confused shouting that rose so suddenly brought her up to her feet and out across the front porch without her slippers, hair half-braided. Shading her eyes, she saw first Mr. Helton, running all stooped over through the orchard, running like a man with dogs after him; and Mr. Thompson supporting himself on the ax handle was leaning over shaking by the shoulder a man Mrs. Thompson had never seen, who lay doubled up with the top of his head smashed and the blood running away in a greasy-looking puddle. Mr. Thompson without taking his hand from the man's shoulder, said in a thick voice, "He killed Mr. Helton, he killed him, I saw him do it. I had to knock him out," he called loudly, "but he won't come to."

Mrs. Thompson said in a faint scream, "Why, yonder goes Mr. Helton," and she pointed. Mr. Thompson pulled himself up and looked where she pointed. Mrs. Thompson sat down slowly against the side of the house and began to slide forward on her face; she felt as if she were drowning, she couldn't rise to the top somehow, and her only thought was she was glad the boys were not there, they were out, fishing at Halifax, oh, God, she was glad the boys were not there.

Mr. and Mrs. Thompson drove up to their barn about sunset. Mr. Thompson handed the reins to his wife, got out to open the big door, and Mrs. Thompson guided old Jim in under the roof. The buggy was gray with dust and age, Mrs. Thompson's face was gray with dust and weariness, and Mr. Thompson's face, as he stood at the horse's head and began unhitching, was gray except for the dark blue of his freshly shaven jaws and chin, gray and blue and caved in, but patient, like a dead man's face.

Mrs. Thompson stepped down to the hard packed manure of the barn floor, and shook out her light flower-sprigged dress. She wore her smoked glasses, and her wide shady leghorn hat with the wreath of exhausted pink and blue forget-me-nots hid her forehead, fixed in a knot of distress.

The horse hung his head, raised a huge sigh and flexed his stiffened legs. Mr. Thompson's words came up muffled and hollow. "Poor ole Jim," he said, clearing his throat, "he looks pretty sunk in the ribs. I guess he's had a hard week." He lifted the harness up in one piece, slid it off and Jim walked out of the shafts halting a little. "Well, this is the last time," Mr. Thompson said, still talking to Jim. "Now you can get a good rest."

Mrs. Thompson closed her eyes behind her smoked glasses. The last time, and high time, and they should never have gone at all. She did not need her glasses any more, now the good darkness was coming down again, but her eyes ran full of tears steadily, though she was not crying, and she felt better with the glasses, safer, hidden away behind them. She took out her handkerchief with her hands shaking as they had been shaking ever since *that day*, and blew her nose. She said, "I see the boys have lighted the lamps. I hope they've started the stove going."

She stepped along the rough path holding her thin dress and starched petticoats around her, feeling her way between the sharp small stones, leaving the barn because she could hardly bear to be near Mr. Thompson, advancing slowly towards the house because she dreaded going there. Life was all one dread, the faces of her neighbors, of her boys, of her husband, the face of the whole world, the shape of her own house in the darkness, the very smell of the grass and the trees were horrible to her. There was no place to go, only one thing to do, bear it somehow—but how? She asked herself that question often. How was she going to keep on living now? Why had she lived at all? She wished now she had died one of those times when she had been so sick, instead of living on for this.

The boys were in the kitchen; Herbert was looking at the funny pictures from last Sunday's newspapers, the Katzenjammer Kids and Happy Hooligan. His chin was in his hands and his elbows on the table, and he was really reading and looking at the pictures, but his face was unhappy. Arthur was building the fire, adding kindling a stick at a time, watching it catch and blaze. His face was heavier and darker than Herbert's, but he was a little sullen by nature; Mrs. Thompson thought, he takes things harder, too. Arthur said, "Hello, Momma," and went on with his work. Herbert swept the papers together and moved over on the bench. They were big boys—fifteen and seventeen, and Arthur as tall as his father. Mrs. Thompson sat down beside Herbert, taking off her hat. She said, "I guess you're hungry. We were late today. We went the Log Hollow road, it's rougher than ever." Her pale mouth drooped with a sad fold on either side.

"I guess you saw the Mannings, then," said Herbert.

"Yes, and the Fergusons, and the Allbrights, and that new family McClellan."

"Anybody say anything?" asked Herbert.

"Nothing much, you know how it's been all along, some of them keeps saying, yes, they know it was a clear case and a fair trial and they say how glad they are your papa came out so well, and all that, some of 'em do, anyhow, but it looks like they don't really take sides with him. I'm about wore out," she said, the tears rolling again from under her dark glasses. "I don't know what good it does, but your papa can't seem to rest unless he's telling how it happened. I don't know."

"I don't think it does any good, not a speck," said Arthur, moving away from the stove. "It just keeps the whole question stirred up in people's minds. Everybody will go round telling what he heard, and the whole thing is going to get worse mixed up than ever. It just makes matters worse. I wish you could get Papa to stop driving round the country talking like that."

"Your papa knows best," said Mrs. Thompson. "You oughtn't to criticize him. He's got enough to put up with without that."

Arthur said nothing, his jaw stubborn. Mr. Thompson came in, his eyes hollowed out and dead-looking, his thick hands gray white and seamed from washing them clean every day before he started out to see the neighbors to tell them his side of the story. He was wearing his Sunday clothes, a thick pepper-and-salt-colored suit with a black string tie.

Mrs. Thompson stood up, her head swimming. "Now you-all get out of the kitchen, it's too hot in here and I need room. I'll get us a little bite of supper, if you'll just get out and give me some room."

They went as if they were glad to go, the boys outside, Mr. Thompson into his bedroom. She heard him groaning to himself as he took off his shoes, and heard the bed creak as he lay down. Mrs. Thompson opened the icebox and felt the sweet coldness flow out of it; she had never expected to have an icebox, much less did she hope to afford to keep it filled with ice. It still seemed like a miracle, after two or three years. There was the food, cold and clean, all ready to be warmed over. She would never have had that icebox if Mr. Helton hadn't happened along one day, just by the strangest luck; so saving, and so managing, so good, thought Mrs. Thompson, her heart swelling until she feared she would faint again, standing there with the door open and leaning her head upon it. She simply could not bear to remember Mr. Helton, with his long sad face and silent ways, who had always been so quiet and harmless, who had worked so hard and helped Mr. Thompson so much, running through the hot fields and woods, being hunted like a mad dog, everybody turning out with ropes and guns and sticks to catch and tie him. Oh, God, said Mrs. Thompson in a long dry moan, kneeling before the icebox and fumbling inside for the dishes, even if they did pile mattresses all over the jail floor and against the walls, and five men there to hold him to keep him from hurting himself any more, he was already hurt too badly, he couldn't have lived anyway. Mr. Barbee, the sheriff, told her about it. He said, well, they didn't aim to harm him but they had to catch him, he was crazy as a loon; he picked up rocks and tried to brain every man that got near him. He had two harmonicas in his jumper pocket, said the sheriff, but they fell out in the scuffle, and Mr. Helton tried to pick 'em up again, and that's when they finally got him. "They *had* to be rough, Miz Thompson, he fought like a wildcat." Yes, thought Mrs. Thompson again with the same bitterness, of course, they had to be rough. They always have to be rough. Mr. Thompson can't argue with a man and get him off the place peaceably; no, she thought, standing up and shutting the icebox, he has to kill somebody, he has to be a murderer and ruin his boys' lives and cause Mr. Helton to be killed like a mad dog.

Her thoughts stopped with a little soundless explosion, cleared and began again. The rest of Mr. Helton's harmonicas were still in the shack, his tune ran in Mrs. Thompson's head at certain times of the day. She missed it in the evenings. It seemed so strange she had never known the name of that song, nor what it meant, until after Mr. Helton was gone. Mrs. Thompson, trembling in the knees, took a drink of water at the sink and poured the red beans into the baking dish, and began to roll the pieces of chicken in flour to fry them. There was a time, she said to herself, when I thought I had neighbors and friends, there was a time when we could hold up our heads, there was a time when my husband hadn't killed a man and I could tell the truth to anybody about anything.

Mr. Thompson, turning on his bed, figured that he had done all he could, he'd just try to let the matter rest from now on. His lawyer, Mr. Burleigh, had told him right at the beginning, "Now you keep calm and collected. You've got a fine case, even if you haven't got witnesses. Your wife must sit in court, she'll be a powerful argument with the jury. You just plead not guilty and I'll do the rest. The trial is going to be a mere formality, you haven't got a thing to worry about. You'll be clean out of this before you know it." And to make talk Mr. Burleigh had got to telling about all the men he knew around the country who for one reason or another had been forced to kill somebody, always in self-defense, and there just wasn't anything to it at all. He even told about how his own father in the old days had shot and killed a man just for setting foot inside his gate when he told him not to. "Sure, I shot the scoundrel," said Mr. Burleigh's father, "in self-defense; I *told* him I'd shoot him if he set his foot in my yard, and he did, and I did." There had been bad blood between them for years, Mr. Burleigh said, and his father had waited a long time to catch the other fellow in the wrong, and when he did he certainly made the most of his opportunity.

"But Mr. Hatch, as I told you," Mr. Thompson had said, "made a pass at Mr. Helton with his bowie knife. That's why I took a hand."

"All the better," said Mr. Burleigh. "That stranger hadn't any right coming to your house on such an errand. Why, hell," said Mr. Burleigh, "that wasn't even manslaughter you committed. So now you just hold your horses and keep your shirt on. And don't say one word without I tell you."

Wasn't even manslaughter. Mr. Thompson had to cover Mr.

Hatch with a piece of wagon canvas and ride to town to tell the sheriff. It had been hard on Ellie. When they got back, the sheriff and the coroner and two deputies, they found her sitting beside the road, on a low bridge over a gulley, about half a mile from the place. He had taken her up behind his saddle and got her back to the house. He had already told the sheriff that his wife had witnessed the whole business, and now he had time, getting her to her room and in bed, to tell her what to say if they asked anything. He had left out the part about Mr. Helton being crazy all along, but it came out at the trial. By Mr. Burleigh's advice Mr. Thompson had pretended to be perfectly ignorant; Mr. Hatch hadn't said a word about that. Mr. Thompson pretended to believe that Mr. Hatch had just come looking for Mr. Helton to settle old scores, and the two members of Mr. Hatch's family who had come down to try to get Mr. Thompson convicted didn't get anywhere at all. It hadn't been much of a trial, Mr. Burleigh saw to that. He had charged a reasonable fee, and Mr. Thompson had paid him and felt grateful, but after it was over Mr. Burleigh didn't seem pleased to see him when he got to dropping into the office to talk it over, telling him things that had slipped his mind at first: trying to explain what an ornery low hound Mr. Hatch had been, anyhow. Mr. Burleigh seemed to have lost his interest; he looked sour and upset when he saw Mr. Thompson at the door. Mr. Thompson kept saying to himself that he'd got off, all right, just as Mr. Burleigh had predicted, but, but—and it was right there that Mr. Thompson's mind stuck, squirming like an angleworm on a fishhook: he had killed Mr. Hatch, and he was a murderer. That was the truth about himself that Mr. Thompson couldn't grasp, even when he said the word to himself. Why, he had not even once *thought* of killing anybody, much less Mr. Hatch, and if Mr. Helton hadn't come out so unexpectedly, hearing the row, why, then—but then, Mr. Helton had come on the run that way to help him. What he couldn't understand was what happened next. He had seen Mr. Hatch go after Mr. Helton with the knife, he had seen the point, blade up, go into Mr. Helton's stomach and slice up like you slice a hog, but when they finally caught Mr. Helton there wasn't a knife scratch on him. Mr. Thompson knew he had the ax in his own hands and felt himself lifting it, but he couldn't remember hitting Mr. Hatch. He couldn't remember it. He couldn't. He remembered only that he had been determined to stop Mr. Hatch from cutting Mr. Helton. If he was given a chance he could explain the whole matter. At the trial they hadn't let him talk. They just asked questions and he answered yes or no, and they never did get to the core of the matter. Since the trial, now, every day for a week he had washed and shaved and put on his best clothes and had taken Ellie with him to tell every neighbor he had that he never killed Mr. Hatch on purpose, and what good did it do? Nobody believed him. Even when he turned to Ellie and said, "You was there, you saw it, didn't you?" and Ellie spoke up, saying, "Yes, that's the truth. Mr. Thompson was trying to save Mr. Helton's life," and he added, "If you don't believe me, you can believe my wife. She won't lie," Mr. Thompson saw something in all their faces that disheartened him, made him feel empty and tired out. They didn't believe he was not a murderer.

Even Ellie never said anything to comfort him. He hoped she would say finally, "I remember now, Mr. Thompson, I really did come round the corner in time to see everything. It's not a lie, Mr. Thompson. Don't you worry." But as they drove together in silence, with the days still hot and dry, shortening for fall, day after day, the buggy jolting in the ruts, she said nothing; they grew to dread the sight of another house, and the people in it: all houses looked alike now, and the people—old neighbors or new—had the same expression when Mr. Thompson told them why he had come and began his story. Their eyes looked as if someone had pinched the eyeball at the back; they shriveled and the light went out of them. Some of them sat with fixed tight smiles trying to be friendly. "Yes, Mr. Thompson, we know how you must feel. It must be terrible for you, Mrs. Thompson. Yes, you know, I've about come to the point where I believe in such a thing as killing in self-defense. Why, certainly, we believe you, Mr. Thompson, why shouldn't we believe you? Didn't you have a perfectly fair and above-board trial? Well, now, natchally, Mr. Thompson, we think you done right."

Mr. Thompson was satisfied they didn't think so. Sometimes the air around him was so thick with their blame he fought and pushed with his fists, and the sweat broke out all over him, he shouted his story in a dust-choked voice, he would fairly bellow at last: "My wife, here, you know her, she was there, she saw and heard it all, if you don't believe me, ask her, she won't lie!" and Mrs. Thompson, with her hands knotted together, aching, her chin trembling, would never fail to say: "Yes, that's right, that's the truth—"

The last straw had been laid on today, Mr. Thompson decided. Tom Allbright, an old beau of Ellie's, why, he had squired Ellie around a whole summer, had come out to meet them when they drove up, and standing there bareheaded had stopped them from getting out. He had looked past them with an embarrassed frown on his face, telling them his wife's sister was there with a raft of young ones, and the house was pretty full and everything upset, or he'd ask them to come in. "We've been thinking of trying to get up to your place one of these days," said Mr. Allbright, moving away trying to look busy, "we've been mighty occupied up here of late." So they had to say, "Well, we just happened to be driving this way," and go on. "The Allbrights," said Mrs. Thompson, "always was fair-weather friends." "They look out for number one, that's a fact," said Mr. Thompson. But it was cold comfort to them both.

Finally Mrs. Thompson had given up. "Let's go home," she said. "Old Jim's tired and thirsty, and we've gone far enough."

Mr. Thompson said, "Well, while we're out this way, we might as well stop at the McClellans'." They drove in, and asked a little cotton-haired boy if his mamma and papa were at home. Mr. Thompson wanted to see them. The little boy stood gazing with his mouth open, then galloped into the house shouting, "Mommer, Popper, come out hyah. That man that kilt Mr. Hatch has come ter see yer!"

The man came out in his sock feet, with one gallus up, the other broken and dangling, and said, "Light down, Mr. Thompson, and come in. The ole woman's washing, but she'll git here." Mrs. Thompson, feeling her way, stepped down and sat in a broken rocking-chair on the porch that sagged under her feet. The woman of the house, barefooted, in a calico wrapper, sat on the edge of the porch, her fat sallow face full of curiosity. Mr. Thompson began, "Well, as I reckon you happen to know, I've had some strange troubles lately, and, as the feller says, it's not the kind of trouble that happens to a man every day in the year, and there's some things I don't want no misunderstanding about in the neighbors' minds, so—" He halted and stumbled forward, and the two listening faces took on a mean look, a greedy, despising look, a look that said plain as day, "My, you must be a purty sorry feller to come round worrying about what *we* think, *we* know you wouldn't be here if you had anybody else to turn to—my, I wouldn't lower myself that much, myself." Mr. Thompson was ashamed of himself, he was suddenly in a rage, he'd like to knock their dirty skunk heads together, the low-down white trash—but he held himself down and went on to the end. "My wife will tell you," he said, and this was the hardest place, because Ellie always without moving a muscle seemed to stiffen as if somebody had threatened to hit her; "ask my wife, she won't lie."

"It's true, I saw it—"

"Well, now," said the man, drily, scratching his ribs inside his shirt, "that sholy is too bad. Well, now, I kaint see what we've got to do with all this here, however. I kaint see no good reason for us to git mixed up in these murder matters, I shore kaint. Whichever way you look at it, it ain't none of my business. However, it's mighty nice of you-all to come around and give us the straight of it, fur we've heerd some mighty queer yarns about it, mighty queer, I golly you couldn't hardly make head ner tail of it."

"Evvybody goin' round shootin' they heads off," said the woman. "Now we don't hold with killin'; the Bible says—"

"Shet yer trap," said the man, "and keep it shet 'r I'll shet it fer yer. Now it shore looks like to me—"

"We mustn't linger," said Mrs. Thompson, unclasping her hands. "We've lingered too long now. It's getting late, and we've far to go." Mr. Thompson took the hint and followed her. The man and the woman lolled against their rickety porch poles and watched them go.

Now lying on his bed, Mr. Thompson knew the end had come. Now, this minute, lying in the bed where he had slept with Ellie for eighteen years; under this roof where he had laid the shingles when he was waiting to get married; there as he was with his whiskers already sprouting since his shave that morning; with his fingers feeling his bony chin, Mr. Thompson felt he was a dead man. He was dead to his other life, he had got to the end of something without knowing why, and he had to make a fresh start, he did not know how. Something different was going to begin, he didn't know what. It was in some way not his business. He didn't feel he was going to have much to do with it. He got up, aching, hollow, and went out to the kitchen where Mrs. Thompson was just taking up the supper.

"Call the boys," said Mrs. Thompson. They had been down to the barn, and Arthur put out the lantern before hanging it on a nail near the door. Mr. Thompson didn't like their silence. They had hardly said a word about anything to him since that day. They seemed to avoid him, they ran the place together as if he wasn't there, and attended to everything without asking him for any advice. "What you boys been up to?" he asked, trying to be hearty. "Finishing your chores?"

"No, sir," said Arthur, "there ain't much to do. Just greasing some axles." Herbert said nothing. Mrs. Thompson bowed her head: "For these and all Thy blessings. . . . Amen," she whispered weakly, and the Thompsons sat there with their eyes down and their faces sorrowful, as if they were at a funeral.

Every time he shut his eyes, trying to sleep, Mr. Thompson's mind started up and began to run like a rabbit. It jumped from one thing to another, trying to pick up a trail here or there that would straighten out what had happened that day he killed Mr. Hatch. Try as he might, Mr. Thompson's mind would not go anywhere that it had not already been, he could not see anything but what he had seen once, and he knew that was not right. If he had not seen straight that first time, then everything about his killing Mr. Hatch was wrong from start to finish, and there was nothing more to be done about it, he might just as well give up. It still seemed to him that he had done, maybe not the right thing, but the only thing he could do, that day, but had he? *Did he have to kill Mr. Hatch?* He had never seen a man he hated more, the minute he laid eyes on him. He knew in his bones the fellow was there for trouble. What seemed so funny now was this: Why hadn't he just told Mr. Hatch to get out before he ever even got in?

Mrs. Thompson, her arms crossed on her breast, was lying beside him, perfectly still, but she seemed awake, somehow. "Asleep, Ellie?"

After all, he might have got rid of him peaceably, or maybe he might have had to overpower him and put those handcuffs on him and turn him over to the sheriff for disturbing the peace. The most they could have done was to lock Mr. Hatch up while he cooled off for a few days, or fine him a little something. He would try to think of things he might have said to Mr. Hatch. Why, let's see, I could just have said, Now look here, Mr. Hatch, I want to talk to you as man to man. But his brain would go empty. What could he have said or done? But if he *could* have done anything else almost except kill Mr. Hatch, then nothing would have happened to Mr. Helton. Mr. Thompson hardly ever thought of Mr. Helton. His mind just skipped over him and went on. If he stopped to think about Mr. Helton he'd never in God's world get anywhere. He tried to imagine how it might all have been, this very night even, if Mr. Helton were still safe and sound out in his shack playing his tune about feeling so good in the morning, drinking up all the wine so you'd feel even better; and Mr. Hatch safe in jail somewhere, mad as hops, maybe, but out of harm's way and ready to listen to reason and to repent of his meanness, the dirty, yellow-livered hound coming around persecuting an innocent man and ruining a whole family that never harmed him! Mr. Thompson felt the veins of his forehead start up, his fists clutched as if they seized an ax handle, the sweat broke out on him, he bounded up from the bed with a yell smothered in his throat, and Ellie started up after him, crying out, "Oh, oh, don't! Don't! Don't!" as if she were having a nightmare. He stood shaking until his bones rattled in him, crying hoarsely, "Light the lamp, light the lamp, Ellie."

Instead, Mrs. Thompson gave a shrill weak scream, almost the same scream he had heard on that day she came around the house when he was standing there with the ax in his hand. He could not see her in the dark, but she was on the bed, rolling violently. He felt for her in horror, and his groping hands found her arms, up, and her own hands pulling her hair straight out from her head, her neck strained back, and the tight screams strangling her. He shouted out for Arthur, for Herbert. "Your mother!" he bawled, his voice cracking. As he held Mrs. Thompson's arms, the boys came tumbling in, Arthur with the lamp above his head. By this light Mr. Thompson saw Mrs. Thompson's eyes, wide open, staring dreadfully at him, the tears pouring. She sat up at sight of the boys, and held out one arm towards them, the hand wagging in a crazy circle, then dropped on her back again, and suddenly went limp. Arthur set the lamp on the table and turned on Mr. Thompson. "She's scared," he said, "she's scared to death." His face was in a knot of rage, his fists were doubled up, he faced his father as if he meant to strike him. Mr. Thompson's jaw fell, he was so surprised he stepped back from the bed. Herbert went to the other side. They stood on each side of Mrs. Thompson and watched Mr. Thompson as if he were a dangerous wild beast. "What did you do to her?" shouted Arthur, in a grown man's voice. "You touch her again and I'll blow your heart out!" Herbert was pale and his cheek twitched, but he was on Arthur's side; he would do what he could to help Arthur.

Mr. Thompson had no fight left in him. His knees bent as he stood, his chest collapsed. "Why, Arthur," he said, his words crumbling and his breath coming short. "She's fainted again. Get the ammonia." Arthur did not move. Herbert brought the bottle, and handed it, shrinking, to his father.

Mr. Thompson held it under Mrs. Thompson's nose. He poured a little in the palm of his hand and rubbed it on her forehead. She gasped and opened her eyes and turned her head away from him. Herbert began a doleful hopeless sniffling. "Mamma," he kept saying, "Mamma, don't die."

"I'm all right," Mrs. Thompson said. "Now don't you worry around. Now Herbert, you mustn't do that. I'm all right." She closed her eyes. Mr. Thompson began pulling on his best pants; he put on his socks and shoes. The boys sat on each side of the bed, watching Mrs. Thompson's face. Mr. Thompson put on his shirt and coat. He said, "I reckon I'll ride over and get the doctor. Don't look like all this fainting is a good sign. Now you just keep watch until I get back." They listened, but said nothing. He said, "Don't you get any notions in your head. I never did your mother any harm in my life, on purpose." He went out, and, looking back, saw Herbert staring at him from under his brows, like a stranger. "You'll know how to look after her," said Mr. Thompson.

Mr. Thompson went through the kitchen. There he lighted the lantern, took a thin pad of scratch paper and a stub pencil from the shelf where the boys kept their schoolbooks. He swung the lantern on his arm and reached into the cupboard where he kept the guns. The shotgun was there to his hand, primed and ready, a man never knows when he may need a shotgun. He went out of the house without looking around, or looking back when he had left it, passed his barn without seeing it, and struck out to the farthest end of his fields, which ran for half a mile to the east. So many blows had been struck at Mr. Thompson and from so many directions he couldn't stop any more to find out where he was hit. He walked on, over plowed ground and over meadow, going through barbed wire fences cautiously, putting his gun through first; he could almost see in the dark, now his eyes were used to it. Finally he came to the last fence; here he sat down, back against a post, lantern at his side, and, with the pad on his knee, moistened the stub pencil and began to write:

"Before Almighty God, the great judge of all before who I am about to appear, I do hereby solemnly swear that I did not take the life of Mr. Homer T. Hatch on purpose. It was done in defense of Mr. Helton. I did not aim to hit him with the ax but only to keep him off Mr. Helton. He aimed a blow at Mr. Helton who was not looking for it. It was my belief at the time that Mr. Hatch would of taken the life of Mr. Helton if I did not interfere. I have told all this to the judge and the jury and they let me off but nobody believes it. This is the only way I can prove I am not a cold blooded murderer like everybody seems to think. If I had been in Mr. Helton's place he would of done the same for me. I still think I done the only thing there was to do. My wife—"

Mr. Thompson stopped here to think a while. He wet the pencil point with the tip of his tongue and marked out the last two words. He sat a while blacking out the words until he had made a neat oblong patch where they had been, and started again:

"It was Mr. Homer T. Hatch who came to do wrong to a harmless man. He caused all this trouble and he deserved to die but I am sorry it was me who had to kill him."

He licked the point of his pencil again, and signed his full name carefully, folded the paper and put it in his outside pocket. Taking off his right shoe and sock, he set the butt of the shotgun along the ground with the twin barrels pointed towards his head. It was very awkward. He thought about this a little, leaning his head against the gun mouth. He was trembling and his head was drumming until he was deaf and blind, but he lay down flat on the earth on his side, drew the barrel under his chin and fumbled for the trigger with his great toe. That way he could work it.

The Rocking-Horse Winner

D. H. LAWRENCE (1885–1930)

THERE WAS a woman who was beautiful, who started with all the advantages, yet she had no luck. She married for love, and the love turned to dust. She had bonny children, yet she felt they had been thrust upon her, and she could not love them. They looked at her coldly, as if they were finding fault with her. And hurriedly she felt she must cover up some fault in herself. Yet what it was that she must cover up she never knew. Nevertheless, when her children were present, she always felt the centre of her heart go hard. This troubled her, and in her manner she was all the more gentle and anxious for her children, as if she loved them very much. Only she herself knew that at the centre of her heart was a hard little place that could not feel love, no, not for anybody. Everybody else said of her: "She is such a good mother. She adores her children." Only she herself, and her children themselves, knew it was not so. They read it in each other's eyes.

There were a boy and two little girls. They lived in a pleasant house, with a garden, and they had discreet servants, and felt themselves superior to anyone in the neighbourhood.

Although they lived in style, they felt always an anxiety in the house. There was never enough money. The mother had a small income, and the father had a small income, but not nearly enough for the social position which they had to keep up. The father went into town to some office. But though he had good prospects, these prospects never materialized. There was always the grinding sense of the shortage of money, though the style was always kept up.

At last the mother said: "I will see if I can't make something." But she did not know where to begin. She racked her brains, and tried this thing and the other, but could not find anything successful. The failure made deep lines come into her face. Her children were growing up, they would have to go to school. There must be more money, there must be more money. The father, who was always very handsome and expensive in his tastes, seemed as if he never would be able to do anything worth doing. And the mother, who had a great belief in herself, did not succeed any better, and her tastes were just as expensive.

And so the house came to be haunted by the unspoken phrase: There must be more money! There must be more money! The children could hear it all the time, though nobody said it aloud. They heard it at Christmas, when the expensive and splendid toys filled the nursery. Behind the shining modern rocking-horse, behind the smart doll's-house, a voice would start whispering: "There must be more money! There must be more money!" And the children would stop playing, to listen for a moment. They would look into each other's eyes, to see if they had all heard. And each one saw in the eyes of the other two that they too had heard. "There must be more money! There must be more money!"

It came whispering from the springs of the still-swaying rocking-horse, and even the horse, bending his wooden, champing head, heard it. The big doll, sitting so pink and smirking in her new pram, could hear it quite plainly, and seemed to be smirking all the more self-consciously because of it. The foolish puppy, too, that took the place of the teddy-bear, he was looking so extraordinarily foolish for no other reason but that he heard the secret whisper all over the house: "There must be more money!"

Yet nobody ever said it aloud. The whisper was everywhere, and therefore no one spoke it. Just as no one ever says: "We are breathing!" in spite of the fact that breath is coming and going all the time.

"Mother," said the boy Paul one day, "why don't we keep a car of our own? Why do we always use uncle's, or else a taxi?"

"Because we're the poor members of the family," said the mother.

"But why are we, mother?"

"Well—I suppose," she said slowly and bitterly, "it's because your father has no luck."

The boy was silent for some time.

"Is luck money, mother?" he asked, rather timidly.

"No, Paul. Not quite. It's what causes you to have money."

"Oh!" said Paul vaguely. "I thought when Uncle Oscar said filthy lucker, it meant money."

"Filthy lucre does mean money," said the mother. "But it's lucre, not luck."

"Oh!" said the boy. "Then what is luck, mother?"

"It's what causes you to have money. If you're lucky you have money. That's why it's better to be born lucky than rich. If you're rich, you may lose your money. But if you're lucky, you will always get more money."

"Oh! Will you? And is father not lucky?"

"Very unlucky, I should say," she said bitterly.

The boy watched her with unsure eyes.

"Why?" he asked.

"I don't know. Nobody ever knows why one person is lucky and another unlucky."

"Don't they? Nobody at all? Does nobody know?"

"Perhaps God. But He never tells."

"He ought to, then. And aren't you lucky either, mother?"

"I can't be, if I married an unlucky husband."

"But by yourself, aren't you?"

"I used to think I was, before I married. Now I think I am very unlucky indeed."

"Why?"

"Well—never mind! Perhaps I'm not really," she said.

The child looked at her, to see if she meant it. But he saw, by the lines of her mouth, that she was only trying to hide something from him.

"Well, anyhow," he said stoutly, "I'm a lucky person."

"Why?" said his mother, with a sudden laugh.

He stared at her. He didn't even know why he had said it.

"God told me," he asserted, brazening it out.

"I hope He did, dear!" she said, again with a laugh, but rather bitter.

"He did, mother!"

"Excellent!" said the mother, using one of her husband's exclamations.

The boy saw she did not believe him; or, rather, that she paid no attention to his assertion. This angered him somewhat, and made him want to compel her attention.

He went off by himself, vaguely, in a childish way, seeking for the clue to "luck." Absorbed, taking no heed of other people, he went about with a sort of stealth, seeking inwardly for luck. He wanted luck, he wanted it, he wanted it. When the two girls were playing dolls in the nursery, he would sit on his big rocking-horse, charging madly into space, with a frenzy that made the little girls peer at him uneasily. Wildly the horse careered, the waving dark hair of the boy tossed, his eyes had a strange glare in them. The little girls dared not speak to him.

When he had ridden to the end of his mad little journey, he climbed down and stood in front of his rocking-horse, staring fixedly into its lowered face. Its red mouth was slightly open, its big eye was wide and glassy-bright.

"Now!" he would silently command the snorting steed. "Now, take me to where there is luck! Now take me!"

And he would slash the horse on the neck with the little whip he had asked Uncle Oscar for. He knew the horse could take him to where there was luck, if only he forced it. So he would mount again, and start on his furious ride, hoping at last to get there. He knew he could get there.

"You'll break your horse, Paul!" said the nurse.

"He's always riding like that! I wish he'd leave off!" said his elder sister Joan.

But he only glared down on them in silence. Nurse gave him up. She could make nothing of him. Anyhow he was growing beyond her.

One day his mother and his Uncle Oscar came in when he was on one of his furious rides. He did not speak to them.

"Hallo, you young jockey! Riding a winner?" said his uncle.

"Aren't you growing too big for a rocking-horse? You're not a very little boy any longer, you know," said his mother.

But Paul only gave a blue glare from his big, rather close-set eyes. He would speak to nobody when he was in full tilt. His mother watched him with an anxious expression on her face.

At last he suddenly stopped forcing his horse into the mechanical gallop, and slid down.

"Well, I got there!" he announced fiercely, his blue eyes still flaring, and his sturdy long legs straddling apart.

"Where did you get to?" asked his mother.

"Where I wanted to go," he flared back at her.

"That's right, son!" said Uncle Oscar. "Don't you stop till you get there. What's the horse's name?"

"He doesn't have a name," said the boy.

"Gets on without all right?" asked the uncle.

"Well, he has different names. He was called Sansovino last week."

"Sansovino, eh? Won the Ascot. How did you know his name?"

"He always talks about horse-races with Bassett," said Joan.

The uncle was delighted to find that his small nephew was

posted with all the racing news. Bassett, the young gardener, who had been wounded in the left foot in the war and had got his present job through Oscar Cresswell, whose batman he had been, was a perfect blade of the "turf." He lived in the racing events, and the small boy lived with him.

Oscar Cresswell got it all from Bassett.

"Master Paul comes and asks me, so I can't do more than tell him, sir," said Bassett, his face terribly serious, as if he were speaking of religious matters.

"And does he ever put anything on a horse he fancies?"

"Well—I don't want to give him away—he's a young sport, a fine sport, sir. Would you mind asking him yourself? He sort of takes a pleasure in it, and perhaps he'd feel I was giving him away, sir, if you don't mind."

Bassett was serious as a church.

The uncle went back to his nephew, and took him off for a ride in the car.

"Say, Paul, old man, do you ever put anything on a horse?" the uncle asked.

The boy watched the handsome man closely.

"Why, do you think I oughtn't to?" he parried.

"Not a bit of it! I thought perhaps you might give me a tip for the Lincoln."

The car sped on into the country, going down to Uncle Oscar's place in Hampshire.

"Honour bright?" said the nephew.

"Honour bright, son!" said the uncle.

"Well, then, Daffodil."

"Daffodil! I doubt it, sonny. What about Mirza?"

"I only know the winner," said the boy. "That's Daffodil."

"Daffodil, eh?"

There was a pause. Daffodil was an obscure horse comparatively.

"Uncle!"

"Yes, son?"

"You won't let it go any further, will you? I promised Bassett."

"Bassett be damned, old man! What's he got to do with it?"

"We're partners. We've been partners from the first. Uncle, he lent me my first five shillings, which I lost. I promised him, honour bright, it was only between me and him; only you gave me that ten-shilling note I started winning with, so I thought you were lucky. You won't let it go any further, will you?"

The boy gazed at his uncle from those big, hot, blue eyes, set rather close together. The uncle stirred and laughed uneasily.

"Right you are, son! I'll keep your tip private. Daffodil, eh? How much are you putting on him?"

"All except twenty pounds," said the boy. "I keep that in reserve."

The uncle thought it a good joke.

"You keep twenty pounds in reserve, do you, you young romancer? What are you betting, then?"

"I'm betting three hundred," said the boy gravely. "But it's between you and me, Uncle Oscar! Honour bright?"

The uncle burst into a roar of laughter.

"It's between you and me all right, you young Nat Gould," he said, laughing. "But where's your three hundred?"

"Bassett keeps it for me. We're partners."

"You are, are you! And what is Bassett putting on Daffodil?"

"He won't go quite as high as I do, I expect. Perhaps he'll go a hundred and fifty."

"What, pennies?" laughed the uncle.

"Pounds," said the child, with a surprised look at his uncle. "Bassett keeps a bigger reserve than I do."

Between wonder and amusement Uncle Oscar was silent. He pursued the matter no further, but he determined to take his nephew with him to the Lincoln races.

"Now, son," he said, "I'm putting twenty on Mirza, and I'll put five for you on any horse you fancy. What's your pick?"

"Daffodil, uncle."

"No, not the fiver on Daffodil!"

"I should if it was my own fiver," said the child.

"Good! Good! Right you are! A fiver for me and a fiver for you on Daffodil."

The child had never been to a race-meeting before, and his eyes were blue fire. He pursed his mouth tight, and watched. A Frenchman just in front had put his money on Lancelot. Wild with excitement, he flayed his arms up and down, yelling "Lancelot! Lancelot!" in his French accent.

Daffodil came in first, Lancelot second, Mirza third. The child, flushed and with eyes blazing, was curiously serene. His uncle brought him four five-pound notes, four to one.

"What am I to do with these?" he cried, waving them before the boy's eyes.

"I suppose we'll talk to Bassett," said the boy. "I expect I have fifteen hundred now; and twenty in reserve; and this twenty."

His uncle studied him for some moments.

"Look here, son!" he said. "You're not serious about Bassett and that fifteen hundred, are you?"

"Yes, I am. But it's between you and me, uncle. Honour bright!"

"Honour bright all right, son! But I must talk to Bassett."

"If you'd like to be a partner, uncle, with Bassett and me, we could all be partners. Only, you'd have to promise, honour bright, uncle, not to let it go beyond us three. Bassett and I are lucky, and you must be lucky, because it was your ten shillings I started winning with. . . ."

Uncle Oscar took both Bassett and Paul into Richmond Park for an afternoon, and there they talked.

"It's like this, you see, sir," Bassett said. "Master Paul would get me talking about racing events, spinning yarns, you know, sir. And he was always keen on knowing if I'd made or if I'd lost. It's about a year since, now, that I put five shillings on Blush of Dawn for him—and we lost. Then the luck turned, with that ten shillings he had from you, that we put on Singhalese. And since that time, it's been pretty steady, all things considering. What do you say, Master Paul?"

"We're all right when we're sure," said Paul. "It's when we're not quite sure that we go down."

"Oh, but we're careful then," said Bassett.

"But when are you sure?" smiled Uncle Oscar.

"It's Master Paul, sir," said Bassett, in a secret, religious voice. "It's as if he had it from heaven. Like Daffodil, now, for the Lincoln. That was as sure as eggs."

"Did you put anything on Daffodil?" asked Oscar Cresswell.

"Yes, sir. I made my bit."

"And my nephew?"

Bassett was obstinately silent, looking at Paul.

"I made twelve hundred, didn't I, Bassett? I told uncle I was putting three hundred on Daffodil."

"That's right," said Bassett, nodding.

"But where's the money?" asked the uncle.

"I keep it safe locked up, sir. Master Paul he can have it any minute he likes to ask for it."

"What, fifteen hundred pounds?"

"And twenty! And forty, that is, with the twenty he made on the course."

"It's amazing!" said the uncle.

"If Master Paul offers you to be partners, sir, I would, if I were you; if you'll excuse me," said Bassett.

Oscar Cresswell thought about it.

"I'll see the money," he said.

They drove home again, and sure enough, Bassett came round to the garden-house with fifteen hundred pounds in notes. The twenty pounds reserve was left with Joe Glee, in the Turf Commission deposit.

"You see, it's all right, uncle, when I'm sure! Then we go strong, for all we're worth. Don't we, Bassett?"

"We do that, Master Paul."

"And when are you sure?" said the uncle, laughing.

"Oh, well, sometimes I'm absolutely sure, like about Daffodil," said the boy; "and sometimes I have an idea; and sometimes I haven't even an idea, have I, Bassett? Then we're careful, because we mostly go down."

"You do, do you! And when you're sure, like about Daffodil, what makes you sure, sonny?"

"Oh, well, I don't know," said the boy uneasily. "I'm sure, you know, uncle; that's all."

"It's as if he had it from heaven, sir," Bassett reiterated.

"I should say so!" said the uncle.

But he became a partner. And when the Leger was coming on, Paul was "sure" about Lively Spark, which was a quite inconsiderable horse. The boy insisted on putting a thousand on the horse, Bassett went for five hundred, and Oscar Cresswell two hundred. Lively Spark came in first, and the betting had been ten to one against him. Paul had made ten thousand.

"You see," he said, "I was absolutely sure of him."

Even Oscar Cresswell had cleared two thousand.

"Look here, son," he said, "this sort of thing makes me nervous."

"It needn't, uncle! Perhaps I shan't be sure again for a long time."

"But what are you going to do with your money?" asked the uncle.

"Of course," said the boy, "I started it for mother. She said she had no luck, because father is unlucky, so I thought if I was lucky, it might stop whispering."

"What might stop whispering?"

"Our house. I hate our house for whispering."

"What does it whisper?"

"Why—why"—the boy fidgeted—"why, I don't know. But it's always short of money, you know, uncle."

"I know it, son, I know it."

"You know people send mother writs, don't you, uncle?"

"I'm afraid I do," said the uncle.

"And then the house whispers, like people laughing at you behind your back. It's awful, that is! I thought if I was lucky . . ."

"You might stop it," added the uncle.

The boy watched him with big blue eyes that had an uncanny cold fire in them, and he said never a word.

"Well, then!" said the uncle. "What are we doing?"

"I shouldn't like mother to know I was lucky," said the boy.

"Why not, son?"

"She'd stop me."

"I don't think she would."

"Oh!"—and the boy writhed in an odd way—"I don't want her to know, uncle."

"All right, son! We'll manage it without her knowing."

They managed it very easily. Paul, at the other's suggestion, handed over five thousand pounds to his uncle, who deposited it with the family lawyer, who was then to inform Paul's mother that a relative had put five thousand pounds into his hands, which sum was to be paid out a thousand pounds at a time, on the mother's birthday, for the next five years.

"So she'll have a birthday present of a thousand pounds for five successive years," said Uncle Oscar. "I hope it won't make it all the harder for her later."

Paul's mother had her birthday in November. The house had been "whispering" worse than ever lately, and, even in spite of his luck, Paul could not bear up against it. He was very anxious to see the effect of the birthday letter, telling his mother about the thousand pounds.

When there were no visitors, Paul now took his meals with his parents, as he was beyond the nursery control. His mother went into town nearly every day. She had discovered that she had an odd knack of sketching furs and dress materials, so she worked secretly in the studio of a friend who was the chief "artist" for the leading drapers. She drew the figures of ladies in furs and ladies in silk and sequins for the newspaper advertisements. This young woman artist earned several thousand pounds a year, but Paul's mother only made several hundreds, and she was again dissatisfied. She so wanted to be first in something, and she did not succeed, even in making sketches for drapery advertisements.

She was down to breakfast on the morning of her birthday. Paul watched her face as she read her letters. He knew the lawyer's letter. As his mother read it, her face hardened and became more expressionless. Then a cold, determined look came on her mouth. She hid the letter under the pile of others, and said not a word about it.

"Didn't you have anything nice in the post for your birthday, mother?" said Paul.

"Quite moderately nice," she said, her voice cold and absent.

She went away to town without saying more.

But in the afternoon Uncle Oscar appeared. He said Paul's mother had had a long interview with the lawyer, asking if the whole five thousand could be advanced at once, as she was in debt.

"What do you think, uncle?" said the boy.

"I leave it to you, son."

"Oh, let her have it, then! We can get some more with the other," said the boy.

"A bird in the hand is worth two in the bush, laddie!" said Uncle Oscar.

"But I'm sure to know for the Grand National; or the Lincolnshire; or else the Derby. I'm sure to know for one of them," said Paul.

So Uncle Oscar signed the agreement, and Paul's mother touched the whole five thousand. Then something very curious happened. The voices in the house suddenly went mad, like a chorus of frogs on a spring evening. There were certain new furnishings, and Paul had a tutor. He was really going to Eton, his father's school, in the following autumn. There were flowers in the winter, and a blossoming of the luxury Paul's mother had been used to. And yet the voices in the house, behind the sprays of mimosa and almond blossom, and from under the piles of iridescent cushions, simply trilled and screamed in a sort of ecstasy: "There must be more money! Oh-h-h, there must be more money. Oh, now, now-w! Now-w-w—there must be more money!—more than ever! More than ever!"

It frightened Paul terribly. He studied away at his Latin and Greek with his tutors. But his intense hours were spent with Bassett. The Grand National had gone by: he had not "known," and had lost a hundred pounds. Summer was at hand. He was in agony for the Lincoln. But even for the Lincoln he didn't "know" and he lost fifty pounds. He became wild-eyed and strange, as if something were going to explode in him.

"Let it alone, son! Don't you bother about it!" urged Uncle Oscar. But it was as if the boy couldn't really hear what his uncle was saying.

"I've got to know for the Derby! I've got to know for the Derby!" the child reiterated, his big blue eyes blazing with a sort of madness.

His mother noticed how overwrought he was.

"You'd better go to the seaside. Wouldn't you like to go now to the seaside, instead of waiting? I think you'd better," she said, looking down at him anxiously, her heart curiously heavy because of him.

But the child lifted his uncanny blue eyes.

"I couldn't possibly go before the Derby, mother!" he said. "I couldn't possibly!"

"Why not?" she said, her voice becoming heavy when she was opposed. "Why not? You can still go from the seaside to see the Derby with your Uncle Oscar, if that's what you wish. No need for you to wait here. Besides, I think you care too much about these races. It's a bad sign. My family has been a gambling family, and you won't know till you grow up how much damage it has done. But it has done damage. I shall have to send Bassett away, and ask Uncle Oscar not to talk racing to you, unless you promise to be reasonable about it; go away to the seaside and forget it. You're all nerves!"

"I'll do what you like, mother, so long as you don't send me away till after the Derby," the boy said.

"Send you away from where? Just from this house?"

"Yes," he said, gazing at her.

"Why, you curious child, what makes you care about this house so much, suddenly? I never knew you loved it."

He gazed at her without speaking. He had a secret within a secret, something he had not divulged, even to Bassett or to his Uncle Oscar.

But his mother, after standing undecided and a little bit sullen for some moments, said:

"Very well, then! Don't go to the seaside till after the Derby, if you don't wish it. But promise me you won't let your nerves go to pieces. Promise you won't think so much about horse-racing and events, as you call them!"

"Oh, no," said the boy casually. "I won't think much about them, mother. You needn't worry. I wouldn't worry, mother, if I were you."

"If you were me and I were you," said his mother, "I wonder what we should do!"

"But you know you needn't worry, mother, don't you?" the boy repeated.

"I should be awfully glad to know it," she said wearily.

"Oh, well, you can, you know. I mean, you ought to know you needn't worry," he insisted.

"Ought I? Then I'll see about it," she said.

Paul's secret of secrets was his wooden horse, that which had no name. Since he was emancipated from a nurse and a nursery-governess, he had had his rocking-horse removed to his own bedroom at the top of the house.

"Surely, you're too big for a rocking-horse!" his mother had remonstrated.

"Well, you see, mother, till I can have a real horse, I like to have some sort of animal about," had been his quaint answer.

"Do you feel he keeps you company?" she laughed.

"Oh, yes! He's very good, he always keeps me company, when I'm there," said Paul.

So the horse, rather shabby, stood in an arrested prance in the boy's bedroom.

The Derby was drawing near, and the boy grew more and more tense. He hardly heard what was spoken to him, he was very frail, and his eyes were really uncanny. His mother had sudden seizures of uneasiness about him. Sometimes, for half-an-hour, she would feel a sudden anxiety about him that was almost anguish. She wanted to rush to him at once, and know he was safe.

Two nights before the Derby, she was at a big party in town, when one of her rushes of anxiety about her boy, her first-born, gripped her heart till she could hardly speak. She fought with the feeling, might and main, for she believed in common sense. But it was too strong. She had to leave the dance and go downstairs to telephone to the country. The children's nursery-governess was terribly surprised and startled at being rung up in the night.

"Are the children all right, Miss Wilmot?"

"Oh, yes, they are quite all right."

"Master Paul? Is he all right?"

"He went to bed as right as a trivet. Shall I run up and look at him?"

"No," said Paul's mother reluctantly. "No! Don't trouble. It's all right. Don't sit up. We shall be home fairly soon." She did not want her son's privacy intruded upon.

"Very good," said the governess.

It was about one o'clock when Paul's mother and father drove up to their house. All was still. Paul's mother went to her room and slipped off her white fur coat. She had told her maid not to wait up for her. She heard her husband downstairs, mixing a whisky-and-soda.

And then, because of the strange anxiety at her heart, she stole upstairs to her son's room. Noiselessly she went along the upper corridor. Was there a faint noise? What was it?

She stood, with arrested muscles, outside his door, listening. There was a strange, heavy, and yet not loud noise. Her heart stood still. It was a soundless noise, yet rushing and powerful.

Something huge, in violent, hushed motion. What was it? What in God's name was it? She ought to know. She felt that she knew the noise. She knew what it was.

Yet she could not place it. She couldn't say what it was. And on and on it went, like a madness.

Softly, frozen with anxiety and fear, she turned the door-handle.

The room was dark. Yet in the space near the window, she heard and saw something plunging to and fro. She gazed in fear and amazement.

Then suddenly she switched on the light, and saw her son, in his green pyjamas, madly surging on the rocking-horse. The blaze of light suddenly lit him up, as he urged the wooden horse, and lit her up, as she stood, blonde, in her dress of pale green and crystal, in the doorway.

"Paul!" she cried. "Whatever are you doing?"

"It's Malabar!" he screamed, in a powerful, strange voice. "It's Malabar."

His eyes blazed at her for one strange and senseless second, as he ceased urging his wooden horse. Then he fell with a crash to the ground, and she, all her tormented motherhood flooding upon her, rushed to gather him up.

But he was unconscious, and unconscious he remained, with some brain-fever. He talked and tossed, and his mother sat stonily by his side.

"Malabar! It's Malabar! Bassett, Bassett, I know! It's Malabar!"

So the child cried, trying to get up and urge the rocking-horse that gave him his inspiration.

"What does he mean by Malabar?" asked the heart-frozen mother.

"I don't know," said the father stonily.

"What does he mean by Malabar?" she asked her brother Oscar.

"It's one of the horses running for the Derby," was the answer.

And, in spite of himself, Oscar Cresswell spoke to Bassett, and himself put a thousand on Malabar: at fourteen to one.

The third day of the illness was critical: they were waiting for a change. The boy, with his rather long, curly hair, was tossing ceaselessly on the pillow. He neither slept nor regained consciousness, and his eyes were like blue stones. His mother sat, feeling her heart had gone, turned actually into a stone.

In the evening, Oscar Cresswell did not come, but Bassett sent a message, saying could he come up for one moment, just one moment? Paul's mother was very angry at the intrusion, but on second thought she agreed. The boy was the same. Perhaps Bassett might bring him to consciousness.

The gardener, a shortish fellow with a little brown moustache, and sharp little brown eyes, tiptoed into the room, touched his imaginary cap to Paul's mother, and stole to the bedside, staring with glittering, smallish eyes, at the tossing, dying child.

"Master Paul!" he whispered. "Master Paul! Malabar come in first all right, a clean win. I did as you told me. You've made over seventy thousand pounds, you have; you've got over eighty thousand. Malabar came in all right, Master Paul."

"Malabar! Malabar! Did I say Malabar, mother? Did I say Malabar? Do you think I'm lucky, mother? I knew Malabar, didn't I? Over eighty thousand pounds! I call that lucky, don't you, mother? Over eighty thousand pounds! I knew, didn't I know I knew? Malabar came in all right. If I ride my horse till I'm sure, then I tell you, Bassett, you can go as high as you like. Did you go for all you were worth, Bassett?"

"I went a thousand on it, Master Paul."

"I never told you, mother, that if I can ride my horse, and get there, then I'm absolutely sure—oh, absolutely! Mother, did I ever tell you? I am lucky."

"No, you never did," said the mother.

But the boy died in the night.

And even as he lay dead, his mother heard her brother's voice saying to her: "My God, Hester, you're eighty-odd thousand to the good and a poor devil of a son to the bad. But, poor devil, poor devil, he's best gone out of a life where he rides his rocking-horse to find a winner."

Critical Analysis

This story could be described, on one level, as a tale of a boy who gave his life in a futile attempt to provide his insatiable mother with enough money. Approached differently, it might be seen as a kind of ghost story in which the main interest lies in the mystery of the unexplained power which enabled the boy to pick the winner in a horse race. Incomplete or distorted analyses of the story might pursue either of these directions and neglect the other. A close examination of Lawrence's methods, however, will show how the two elements fit together and how the story at once arouses and satisfies the reader's interest in a melodramatic suspense, in "psychology," and in a theme.

The story begins very simply: "There was a woman who was beautiful, who started with all the advantages, yet she had no luck." It is almost the style of a fairy tale, and the fresh, naive style is important in putting the reader in the frame of mind necessary for the story which is to follow. We must, in fact, believe something which has no obvious natural explanation, so we are urged subtly to adopt for a moment that kind of wonder and suspension of disbelief which we used to feel when we read Grimm or Hans Christian Andersen. As the story progresses, however, this style changes and becomes more intense. It is directly related to the mounting excitement of the story, with the psychological element in it.

How much is psychological and how much is moral? In the first place, the reader must recognize that the attitude toward horse racing and betting on the horses is thoroughly British; there is no hint in the story of disapproval of betting *as such*. The moral concern is rather over the quality in some people which always makes them want more money. This moral concern is developed psychologically: the need for more money in the family is presented, not as something that anybody says, not as an external fact established in the story by a glance at the family bank book or the mention of a pile of bills on the first of the month, but as something *felt.*

> And so the house came to be haunted by the unspoken phrase: There must be more money! There must be more money!

This is the kind of haunted house which even the most skeptical reader will be prepared to accept, and Lawrence reinforces the effect by relating the whisper to the children's expensive toys:

> The children could hear it all the time, though nobody said it aloud. They heard it at Christmas, when the expensive and splendid toys filled the nursery. Behind the shining modern rocking-horse, behind the smart doll's house, a voice would start whispering. . . .

It is a short step from this point to attributing the feeling to the toys themselves: ". . . even the horse, bending his wooden, champing head, heard it." By this innocent and subtle method the reader is prepared for the tremendous role of the rocking horse in the climax of the story. But even more important, the *antagonist* in the story has been created. Here is the force against which the hero is to throw himself and perish.

If such a disembodied force is to be a character in the story, there must be careful handling of the characters who are people, so that the composition does not become confused. Notice how vague are the outlines of Paul's mother and father. The father is described as going into town to "some office," and when the mother tries to earn money, she is said to try "this thing and the other." The mother is not even named—she is always Paul's mother—until the very end of the story, when she is no longer Paul's mother and the author allows Oscar to call her by her name, Hester.

The central role of Paul in the story demands careful attention. Frequently Lawrence takes us close to the point of view of Paul, and some readers might say that the vagueness about his father's business or his mother's attempts to make money merely indicates the normal child's vagueness about such matters. But the story cannot really be told from Paul's point of view, for several reasons. The suspense of the story would be ruined if the reader knew immediately all that went on in Paul's mind. The "secret within a secret" could not be held back from the reader. Moreover, the emotional quality of the ending would be changed; if we had followed the story exclusively through Paul's eyes and feelings, the ending would be pathetic and maudlin. As it is, there is enough distance so that a tragic feeling is possible.

As mediators between the reader's natural skepticism and the fantasy element in the plot stand Uncle Oscar and Bassett. They are both men of practical common sense, Bassett with his repeated "It's as if he had it from heaven" and his respectful suggestion to his social superior that when you have a good thing you shouldn't refuse it just because you don't understand it—"If Master Paul offers you to be partners, sir, I would, if I were you; if you'll excuse me"—and Uncle Oscar with his sense of humor and his cautious indulgence of his nephew. Oscar is developed very fully. He is introduced first unobtrusively, as the owner of the car which Paul's family borrows, as the source of the phrase "filthy lucre" which confused Paul, as the donor of the whip, the unconscious planter of the idea of "riding a winner" and the donor of the ten shillings which started Paul on his winning streak. When Oscar emerges into the foreground as an important character, he serves the purpose of expressing the reader's doubts. "Oscar Cresswell thought about it. 'I'll see the money,' he said." But the joke is on Uncle Oscar, as it will be on the reader if he is too skeptical. When the Leger is run, Oscar bets only two hundred pounds, while the humble and conservative Bassett bets five hundred and the boy a thousand. When their horse wins at the odds of ten to one, Paul is not a bit surprised: " 'You see,' he said, 'I was absolutely sure of him.' Even Oscar Cresswell had cleared two thousand. 'Look here, son,' he said, 'this sort of thing makes me nervous.' " Lawrence exploits the comic irony of Cresswell's situation, but not to the extent of forfeiting our sympathy with him. So his final bet, on Malabar in the Derby, is made "in spite of himself." And Uncle Oscar is saved to be the speaker of the epitaph for Paul.

Despite the skill and subtlety with which the characters are presented, this is not primarily a story of character. Certain symbols in the story have much more vitality than any of the people in it, and as we have already pointed out, one of the chief characters is not a person but a feeling, a fear, expressed in the unspoken whispers which are as real as breathing. From the very first sentence of the story, "luck" is used as a symbol. In the story as a whole, it seems to be the opposite of, or a substitute for, love. Paul's pursuit of "luck" might be translated as a pursuit of love, if he had been able to understand rightly what he wanted. Then why, if this is what Lawrence means, does he not say so? The answer must be that love is not a concept, to be understood rationally, any more than "luck" is. It must be felt. And he very carefully shows that the absence of love on the part of Paul's mother is not mere failure in kindness, gentleness, or consideration: she is a good mother in these respects, and everybody says so. It is "a hard little place" at the center of her heart; she knows it is there and her children know it is there. "They read it in each other's eyes."

The dialogue between Paul and his mother on the subject of luck is very interesting. Superficially, it is merely a step in the education of the boy; he is learning about an adult idea. But notice how much more Lawrence conveys in this dialogue than is actually expressed in the speeches of the characters; the mother's answers are given "slowly and bitterly," "bitterly," "again with a laugh, but rather bitter." Paul, on the other hand, shows more from his silences than he does from his words. "The boy was silent for some time." "The boy watched her with unsure eyes." "The child looked at her, to see if she meant it." It is in this dialogue that the boy's hunger for love is betrayed, distorted into the pursuit of luck. But Lawrence is writing a story in which suspense is important, and the revelations here are carefully controlled. Very unobtrusively he prepares for the bitter irony of the end:

> "Well, anyhow," he said stoutly, "I'm a lucky person."
> "Why?" said his mother, with a sudden laugh.

Paul's last words, as he lies dying, return to this:

> "Mother, did I ever tell you? I am lucky."
> "No, you never did," said the mother.
> But the boy died in the night.

The condemnation of the mother could hardly be more violent, but the irony does not stop here. It continues, to underline Oscar's last words and to force upon us the feeling that Paul was luckier than he knew.

The last three-fourths of the story is devoted to the discovery of Paul's secret; this is done gradually, with some humor, as the character of Uncle Oscar emerges. But at the same time the desperation of the mother increases, the whispering increases so that after the birthday and the mother's receipt of five thousand pounds the voices are screaming. What we have is a building up of Paul's confidence and strength as Uncle Oscar and Bassett seem mere attendants on him, but at the same time the antagonist is growing in strength too, and the way is prepared for the great tragic climax. Lawrence does full justice to the theatrical quality of the scene; the mother's uneasiness at the party, the vague, mysterious noise, the dark bedroom and the sudden blaze of light bringing out the two figures, the boy in his green pyjamas "madly surging" and the mother "as she stood, blonde, in her dress of pale green and crystal, in the doorway." The difference between them is immediately shown in their lines,

"Paul!" she cried. "Whatever are you doing?"
"It's Malabar!" he screamed, in a powerful, strange voice.

Even in all this theatricality the values of the symbols are not lost. Paul's fever and the mother's coldness (now become a coldness of the heart somewhat different from her first state) show us the equivalents in feeling of love and luck.

The Rocking-Horse Winner is not a cheap story with the obvious sentimental moral that life without love is worse than death; it is not a psychological thriller about a boy with extrasensory perception who dies in the act of trying to predict the outcome of the Derby; it is not merely a satire on people who never have enough money, no matter how much they have. Each of these descriptions is wrong because it is incomplete, because it does violence to the particular and individual character of the story. A satisfactory analysis must be one which responds to the way in which Lawrence has woven together character and symbol, theme and plot tension. These elements do not exist separately, they must be seen in relationship to each other. The only reason for taking them apart is to put them back together again and appreciate them more fully.

The Celestial Omnibus

E. M. FORSTER (1879–)

THE BOY who resided at Agathox Lodge, 28, Buckingham Park Road, Surbiton, had often been puzzled by the old sign-post that stood almost opposite. He asked his mother about it, and she replied that it was a joke, and not a very nice one, which had been

THE CELESTIAL OMNIBUS is reprinted from *The Celestial Omnibus* by E. M. Forster, by permission of Alfred A. Knopf, Inc.

made many years back by some naughty young men, and that the police ought to remove it. For there were two strange things about this sign-post: firstly, it pointed up a blank alley, and, secondly, it had painted on it, in faded characters, the words, "To Heaven."

"What kind of young men were they?" he asked.

"I think your father told me that one of them wrote verses, and was expelled from the University and came to grief in other ways. Still, it was a long time ago. You must ask your father about it. He will say the same as I do, that it was put up as a joke."

"So it doesn't mean anything at all?"

She sent him upstairs to put on his best things, for the Bonses were coming to tea, and he was to hand the cakestand.

It struck him, as he wrenched on his tightening trousers, that he might do worse than ask Mr. Bons about the sign-post. His father, though very kind, always laughed at him—shrieked with laughter whenever he or any other child asked a question or spoke. But Mr. Bons was serious as well as kind. He had a beautiful house and lent one books, he was a churchwarden, and a candidate for the County Council; he had donated to the Free Library enormously, he presided over the Literary Society, and had Members of Parliament to stop with him—in short, he was probably the wisest person alive.

Yet even Mr. Bons could only say that the sign-post was a joke—the joke of a person named Shelley.

"Of course!" cried the mother; "I told you so, dear. That was the name."

"Had you ever heard of Shelley?" asked Mr. Bons.

"No," said the boy, and hung his head.

"But is there no Shelley in the house?"

"Why, yes!" exclaimed the lady, in much agitation. "Dear Mr. Bons, we aren't such Philistines as that. Two at the least. One a wedding present, and the other, smaller print, in one of the spare rooms."

"I believe we have seven Shelleys," said Mr. Bons, with a slow smile. Then he brushed the cake crumbs off his stomach, and, together with his daughter, rose to go.

The boy, obeying a wink from his mother, saw them all the way to the garden gate, and when they had gone he did not at once return to the house, but gazed for a little up and down Buckingham Park Road.

His parents lived at the right end of it. After No. 39 the quality of the houses dropped very suddenly, and 64 had not even a separate servants' entrance. But at the present moment the whole road looked rather pretty, for the sun had just set in splendour, and the inequalities of rent were drowned in a saffron afterglow. Small birds twittered, and the breadwinners' train shrieked musically down through the cutting—that wonderful cutting which has drawn to itself the whole beauty out of Surbiton, and clad itself, like any Alpine valley, with the glory of the fir and the silver birch and the primrose. It was this cutting that had first stirred desires within the boy—desires for something just a little different, he knew not what, desires that would return whenever things were sunlit, as they were this evening, running up and down inside him, up and down, up and down, till he would feel quite unusual all over, and as likely as not would want to cry. This evening he was even sillier, for he slipped across the road towards the sign-post and began to run up the blank alley.

The alley runs between high walls—the walls of the gardens of "Ivanhoe" and "Bella Vista," respectively. It smells a little all the way, and is scarcely twenty yards long, including the turn at the end. So not unnaturally the boy soon came to a standstill. "I'd like to kick that Shelley," he exclaimed, and glanced idly at a piece of paper which was pasted on the wall. Rather an odd piece of paper, and he read it carefully before he turned back. This is what he read:

S. AND C.R.C.C.

ALTERATION IN SERVICE

Owing to lack of patronage the Company are regretfully compelled to suspend the hourly service, and to retain only the

Sunrise and Sunset Omnibuses,

which will run as usual. It is to be hoped that the public will patronize an arrangement which is intended for their convenience. As an extra inducement, the Company will, for the first time, now issue

Return Tickets!

(available one day only), which may be obtained of the driver. Passengers are again reminded that *no tickets are issued at the other end*, and that no complaints in this connection will receive consideration from the Company. Nor will the Company be responsible for any negligence or stupidity on the part of Passengers, nor for Hailstorms, Lightning, Loss of Tickets, nor for any Act of God.

For the Direction.

Now he had never seen this notice before, nor could he imagine where the omnibus went to. S. of course was for Surbiton, and R.C.C. meant Road Car Company. But what was the meaning of the other C.? Coombe and Malden, perhaps, or possibly "City." Yet it could not hope to compete with the South-Western. The whole thing, the boy reflected, was run on hopelessly unbusiness-like lines. Why no tickets from the other end? And what an hour to start! Then he realized that unless the notice was a hoax, an omnibus must have been starting just as he was wishing the Bonses good-bye. He peered at the ground through the gathering dusk, and there he saw what might or might not be the marks of wheels. Yet nothing had come out of the alley. And he had never seen an omnibus at any time in the Buckingham Park Road. No:

it must be a hoax, like the sign-post, like the fairy tales, like the dreams upon which he would wake suddenly in the night. And with a sigh he stepped from the alley—right into the arms of his father.

Oh, how his father laughed! "Poor, poor Popsey!" he cried. "Diddums! Diddums! Diddums think he'd walky-palky up to Evink!" And his mother, also convulsed with laughter, appeared on the steps of Agathox Lodge.

"Don't, Bob!" she gasped. "Don't be so naughty! Oh, you'll kill me! Oh, leave the boy alone!"

But all that evening the joke was kept up. The father implored to be taken too. Was it a very tiring walk? Need one wipe one's shoes on the door-mat? And the boy went to bed feeling faint and sore, and thankful for only one thing—that he had not said a word about the omnibus. It was a hoax, yet through his dreams it grew more and more real, and the streets of Surbiton, through which he saw it driving, seemed instead to become hoaxes and shadows. And very early in the morning he woke with a cry, for he had had a glimpse of its destination.

He struck a match, and its light fell not only on his watch but also on his calendar, so that he knew it to be half-an-hour to sunrise. It was pitch dark, for the fog had come down from London in the night, and all Surbiton was wrapped in its embraces. Yet he sprang out and dressed himself, for he was determined to settle once for all which was real: the omnibus or the streets. "I shall be a fool one way or the other," he thought, "until I know." Soon he was shivering in the road under the gas lamp that guarded the entrance to the alley.

To enter the alley itself required some courage. Not only was it horribly dark, but he now realized that it was an impossible terminus for an omnibus. If it had not been for a policeman, whom he heard approaching through the fog, he would never have made the attempt. The next moment he had made the attempt and failed. Nothing. Nothing but a blank alley and a very silly boy gaping at its dirty floor. It *was* a hoax. "I'll tell papa and mamma," he decided. "I deserve it. I deserve that they should know. I am too silly to be alive." And he went back to the gate of Agathox Lodge.

There he remembered that his watch was fast. The sun was not risen; it would not rise for two minutes. "Give the bus every chance," he thought cynically, and returned into the alley.

But the omnibus was there.

II

It had two horses, whose sides were still smoking from their journey, and its two great lamps shone through the fog against the alley's walls, changing their cobwebs and moss into tissues of fairyland. The driver was huddled up in a cape. He faced the blank wall, and how he had managed to drive in so neatly and so silently was one of the many things that the boy never discovered. Nor could he imagine how ever he would drive out.

"Please," his voice quavered through the foul brown air, "please, is that an omnibus?"

"Omnibus est," said the driver, without turning round. There was a moment's silence. The policeman passed, coughing, by the entrance of the alley. The boy crouched in the shadow, for he did not want to be found out. He was pretty sure, too, that it was a Pirate; nothing else, he reasoned, would go from such odd places and at such odd hours.

"About when do you start?" He tried to sound nonchalant.

"At sunrise."

"How far do you go?"

"The whole way."

"And can I have a return ticket which will bring me all the way back?"

"You can."

"Do you know, I half think I'll come." The driver made no answer. The sun must have risen, for he unhitched the brake. And scarcely had the boy jumped in before the omnibus was off.

How? Did it turn? There was no room. Did it go forward?

There was a blank wall. Yet it was moving—moving at a stately pace through the fog, which had turned from brown to yellow. The thought of warm bed and warmer breakfast made the boy feel faint. He wished he had not come. His parents would not have approved. He would have gone back to them if the weather had not made it impossible. The solitude was terrible; he was the only passenger. And the omnibus, though well-built, was cold and somewhat musty. He drew his coat round him, and in so doing chanced to feel his pocket. It was empty. He had forgotten his purse.

"Stop!" he shouted. "Stop!" And then, being of a polite disposition, he glanced up at the painted notice-board so that he might call the driver by name. "Mr. Browne! stop; oh, do please stop!"

Mr. Browne did not stop, but he opened a little window and looked in at the boy. His face was a surprise, so kind it was and modest.

"Mr. Browne, I've left my purse behind. I've not got a penny. I can't pay for the ticket. Will you take my watch, please? I am in the most awful hole."

"Tickets on this line," said the driver, "whether single or return, can be purchased by coinage from no terrene mint. And a chronometer, though it had solaced the vigils of Charlemagne, or measured the slumbers of Laura, can acquire by no mutation the double-cake that charms the fangless Cerberus of Heaven!" So saying, he handed in the necessary ticket, and, while the boy said "Thank you," continued, "Titular pretensions, I know it well, are vanity. Yet they merit no censure when uttered on a laughing lip, and in an homonymous world are in some sort useful, since they do serve to distinguish one Jack from his fellow. Remember me, therefore, as Sir Thomas Browne."

"Are you a Sir? Oh, sorry!" He had heard of these gentlemen drivers. "It *is* good of you about the ticket. But if you go on at this rate, however does your bus pay?"

"It does not pay. It was not intended to pay. Many are the

faults of my equipage; it is compounded too curiously of foreign woods; its cushions tickle erudition rather than promote repose; and my horses are nourished not on the evergreen pastures of the moment, but on the dried bents and clovers of Latinity. But that it pays!—that error at all events was never intended and never attained."

"Sorry again," said the boy rather hopelessly. Sir Thomas looked sad, fearing that, even for a moment, he had been the cause of sadness. He invited the boy to come up and sit beside him on the box, and together they journeyed on through the fog, which was now changing from yellow to white. There were no houses by the road; so it must be either Putney Heath or Wimbledon Common.

"Have you been a driver always?"

"I was a physician once."

"But why did you stop? Weren't you good?"

"As a healer of bodies I had scant success, and several score of my patients preceded me. But as a healer of the spirit I have succeeded beyond my hopes and my deserts. For though my draughts were not better nor subtler than those of other men, yet, by reason of the cunning goblets wherein I offered them, the queasy soul was ofttimes tempted to sip and be refreshed."

"The queasy soul," the boy murmured; "if the sun sets with trees in front of it, and you suddenly come strange all over, is that a queasy soul?"

"Have you felt that?"

"Why, yes."

After a pause he told the boy a little, a very little, about the journey's end. But they did not chatter much, for the boy, when he liked a person, would as soon sit silent in his company as speak, and this, he discovered, was also the mind of Sir Thomas Browne and of many others with whom he was to be acquainted. He heard, however, about the young man Shelley, who was now quite a famous person, with a carriage of his own, and about some of the other drivers who are in the service of the Company.

Meanwhile the light grew stronger, though the fog did not disperse. It was now more like mist than fog, and at times would travel quickly across them, as if it was part of a cloud. They had been ascending, too, in a most puzzling way; for over two hours the horses had been pulling against the collar, and even if it were Richmond Hill they ought to have been at the top long ago. Perhaps it was Epsom, or even the North Downs; yet the air seemed keener than that which blows on either. And as to the name of their destination, Sir Thomas Browne was silent.

Crash!

"Thunder, by Jove!" said the boy, "and not so far off either. Listen to the echoes! It's more like mountains."

He thought, not very vividly, of his father and mother. He saw them sitting down to sausages and listening to the storm. He saw his own empty place. Then there would be questions, alarms, theories, jokes, consolations. They would expect him back at lunch. To lunch he would not come, nor to tea, but he would be in for dinner, and so his day's truancy would be over. If he had had his purse he would have bought them presents—not that he should have known what to get them.

Crash!

The peal and the lightning came together. The cloud quivered as if it were alive, and torn streamers of mist rushed past. "Are you afraid?" asked Sir Thomas Browne.

"What is there to be afraid of? Is it much farther?"

The horses of the omnibus stopped just as a ball of fire burst up and exploded with a ringing noise that was deafening but clear, like the noise of a blacksmith's forge. All the cloud was shattered.

"Oh, listen, Sir Thomas Browne! No, I mean look; we shall get a view at last. No, I mean listen; that sounds like a rainbow!"

The noise had died into the faintest murmur, beneath which another murmur grew, spreading stealthily, steadily, in a curve that widened but did not vary. And in widening curves a rainbow was spreading from the horses' feet into the dissolving mists.

"But how beautiful! What colours! Where will it stop? It is more like the rainbows you can tread on. More like dreams."

The colour and the sound grew together. The rainbow spanned an enormous gulf. Clouds rushed under it and were pierced by it, and still it grew, reaching forward, conquering the darkness, until it touched something that seemed more solid than a cloud.

The boy stood up. "What is that out there?" he called. "What does it rest on, out at that other end?"

In the morning sunshine a precipice shone forth beyond the gulf. A precipice—or was it a castle? The horses moved. They set their feet upon the rainbow.

"Oh, look!" the boy shouted. "Oh, listen! Those caves—or are they gateways? Oh, look between those cliffs at those ledges. I see people! I see trees!"

"Look also below," whispered Sir Thomas. "Neglect not the diviner Acheron."

The boy looked below, past the flames of the rainbow that licked against their wheels. The gulf also had cleared, and in its depths there flowed an everlasting river. One sunbeam entered and struck a green pool, and as they passed over he saw three maidens rise to the surface of the pool, singing, and playing with something that glistened like a ring.

"You down in the water—" he called.

They answered, "You up on the bridge—" There was a burst of music. "You up on the bridge, good luck to you. Truth in the depth, truth on the height."

"You down in the water, what are you doing?"

Sir Thomas Browne replied: "They sport in the mancipiary possession of their gold"; and the omnibus arrived.

III

The boy was in disgrace. He sat locked up in the nursery of Agathox Lodge, learning poetry for a punishment. His father had said, "My boy! I can pardon anything but untruthfulness," and had caned him, saying at each stroke, "There is *no* omnibus, *no* driver, *no* bridge, *no* mountain; you are a *truant*, a *gutter snipe*, a *liar*." His father could be very stern at times. His mother had begged him to say he was sorry. But he could not say that. It was the greatest day of his life, in spite of the caning and the poetry at the end of it.

He had returned punctually at sunset—driven not by Sir Thomas Browne, but by a maiden lady who was full of quiet fun. They had talked of omnibuses and also of barouche landaus. How far away her gentle voice seemed now! Yet it was scarcely three hours since he had left her up the alley.

His mother called through the door. "Dear, you are to come down and to bring your poetry with you."

He came down, and found that Mr. Bons was in the smoking-room with his father. It had been a dinner party.

"Here is the great traveller!" said his father grimly. "Here is the young gentleman who drives in an omnibus over rainbows, while young ladies sing to him." Pleased with his wit, he laughed.

"After all," said Mr. Bons, smiling, "there is something a little like it in Wagner. It is odd how, in quite illiterate minds, you will find glimmers of Artistic Truth. The case interests me. Let me plead for the culprit. We have all romanced in our time, haven't we?"

"Hear how kind Mr. Bons is," said his mother, while his father said, "Very well. Let him say his Poem, and that will do. He is going away to my sister on Tuesday, and *she* will cure him of this alley-slopering." (Laughter.) "Say your Poem."

The boy began. "'Standing aloof in giant ignorance.'"

His father laughed again—roared. "One for you, my son! 'Standing aloof in giant ignorance!' I never knew these poets talked sense. Just describes you. Here, Bons, you go in for poetry. Put him through it, will you, while I fetch up the whisky?"

"Yes, give me the Keats," said Mr. Bons. "Let him say his Keats to me."

So for a few moments the wise man and the ignorant boy were left alone in the smoking-room.

"'Standing aloof in giant ignorance, of thee I dream and of the Cyclades, as one who sits ashore and longs perchance to visit—'"[1]

"Quite right. To visit what?"

"'To visit dolphin coral in deep seas,'" said the boy, and burst into tears.

"Come, come! why do you cry?"

"Because—because all these words that only rhymed before, now that I've come back they're me."

Mr. Bons laid the Keats down. The case was more interesting than he had expected. "*You?*" he exclaimed. "This sonnet, *you?*"

"Yes—and look further on: 'Aye, on the shores of darkness there is light, and precipices show untrodden green.' It *is* so, sir. All these things are true."

"I never doubted it," said Mr. Bons, with closed eyes.

"You—then you believe me? You believe in the omnibus and the driver and the storm and that return ticket I got for nothing and—"

"Tut, tut! No more of your yarns, my boy. I meant that I never doubted the essential truth of Poetry. Some day, when you have read more, you will understand what I mean."

"But, Mr. Bons, it *is* so. There *is* light upon the shores of darkness. I have seen it coming. Light and a wind."

"Nonsense," said Mr. Bons.

"If I had stopped! They tempted me. They told me to give up my ticket—for you cannot come back if you lose your ticket. They called from the river for it, and indeed I was tempted, for I have never been so happy as among those precipices. But I thought of my mother and father, and that I must fetch them. Yet they will not come, though the road starts opposite our house. It has all happened as the people up there warned me, and Mr.

[1] *Editors' note:* The boy is reciting Keats's sonnet *To Homer,* given in full in the first part of this book.

Bons has disbelieved me like everyone else. I have been caned. I shall never see that mountain again."

"What's that about me?" said Mr. Bons, sitting up in his chair very suddenly.

"I told them about you, and how clever you were, and how many books you had, and they said, 'Mr. Bons will certainly disbelieve you.' "

"Stuff and nonsense, my young friend. You grow impertinent. I—well—I will settle the matter. Not a word to your father. I will cure you. Tomorrow evening I will myself call here to take you for a walk, and at sunset we will go up this alley opposite and hunt for your omnibus, you silly little boy."

His face grew serious, for the boy was not disconcerted, but leapt about the room singing, "Joy! joy! I told them you would believe me. We will drive together over the rainbow. I told them that you would come." After all, could there be anything in the story? Wagner? Keats? Shelley? Sir Thomas Browne? Certainly the case was interesting.

And on the morrow evening, though it was pouring with rain, Mr. Bons did not omit to call at Agathox Lodge.

The boy was ready, bubbling with excitement, and skipping about in a way that rather vexed the President of the Literary Society. They took a turn down Buckingham Park Road, and then—having seen that no one was watching them—slipped up the alley. Naturally enough (for the sun was setting) they ran straight against the omnibus.

"Good heavens!" exclaimed Mr. Bons. "Good gracious heavens!"

It was not the omnibus in which the boy had driven first, nor yet that in which he had returned. There were three horses—black, gray, and white, the gray being the finest. The driver, who turned round at the mention of goodness and of heaven, was a sallow man with terrifying jaws and sunken eyes. Mr. Bons, on seeing him, gave a cry as if of recognition, and began to tremble violently.

The boy jumped in.

"Is it possible?" cried Mr. Bons. "Is the impossible possible?"

"Sir; come in, sir. It is such a fine omnibus. Oh, here is his name —Dan someone."

Mr. Bons sprang in too. A blast of wind immediately slammed the omnibus door, and the shock jerked down all the omnibus blinds, which were very weak on their springs.

"Dan . . . Show me. Good gracious heavens! We're moving."

"Hooray!" said the boy.

Mr. Bons became flustered. He had not intended to be kidnapped. He could not find the door-handle nor push up the blinds. The omnibus was quite dark, and by the time he had struck a match, night had come on outside also. They were moving rapidly.

"A strange, a memorable adventure," he said, surveying the interior of the omnibus, which was large, roomy, and constructed with extreme regularity, every part exactly answering to every other part. Over the door (the handle of which was outside) was written, "Lasciate ogni baldanza voi che entrate"—at least, that was what was written, but Mr. Bons said that it was Lashy arty something, and that baldanza was a mistake for speranza. His voice sounded as if he was in church. Meanwhile, the boy called to the cadaverous driver for two return tickets. They were handed in without a word. Mr. Bons covered his face with his hand and again trembled. "Do you know who that is!" he whispered, when the little window had shut upon them. "It is the impossible."

"Well, I don't like him as much as Sir Thomas Browne, though I shouldn't be surprised if he had even more in him."

"More in him?" He stamped irritably. "By accident you have made the greatest discovery of the century, and all you can say is that there is more in this man. Do you remember those vellum books in my library, stamped with red lilies? This—sit still, I bring you stupendous news!—*this is the man who wrote them.*"

The boy sat quite still. "I wonder if we shall see Mrs. Gamp?" he asked, after a civil pause.

"Mrs.—?"

"Mrs. Gamp and Mrs. Harris. I like Mrs. Harris. I came upon them quite suddenly. Mrs. Gamp's bandboxes have moved over the rainbow so badly. All the bottoms have fallen out, and two of the pippins off her bedstead tumbled into the stream."

"Out there sits the man who wrote my vellum books!" thundered Mr. Bons, "and you talk to me of Dickens and of Mrs. Gamp?"

"I know Mrs. Gamp so well," he apologized. "I could not help being glad to see her. I recognized her voice. She was telling Mrs. Harris about Mrs. Prig."

"Did you spend the whole day in her elevating company?"

"Oh, no. I raced. I met a man who took me out beyond to a race-course. You run, and there are dolphins out at sea."

"Indeed. Do you remember the man's name?"

"Achilles. No; he was later. Tom Jones."

Mr. Bons sighed heavily. "Well, my lad, you have made a miserable mess of it. Think of a cultured person with your opportunities! A cultured person would have known all these characters and known what to have said to each. He would not have wasted his time with a Mrs. Gamp or a Tom Jones. The creations of Homer, of Shakespeare, and of Him who drives us now, would alone have contented him. He would not have raced. He would have asked intelligent questions."

"But, Mr. Bons," said the boy humbly, "you will be a cultured person. I told them so."

"True, true, and I beg you not to disgrace me when we arrive. No gossiping. No running. Keep close to my side, and never speak to these Immortals unless they speak to you. Yes, and give me the return tickets. You will be losing them."

The boy surrendered the tickets, but felt a little sore. After all, he had found the way to this place. It was hard first to be disbelieved and then to be lectured. Meanwhile, the rain had stopped, and moonlight crept into the omnibus through the cracks in the blinds.

"But how is there to be a rainbow?" cried the boy.

"You distract me," snapped Mr. Bons. "I wish to meditate on beauty. I wish to goodness I was with a reverent and sympathetic person."

The lad bit his lip. He made good resolutions. He would imitate Mr. Bons all the visit. He would not laugh, or run, or sing, or do any of the vulgar things that must have disgusted his new friends last time. He would be very careful to pronounce their names properly, and to remember who knew whom. Achilles did not know Tom Jones—at least, so Mr. Bons said. The Duchess of Malfi was older than Mrs. Gamp—at least, so Mr. Bons said. He would be self-conscious, reticent, and prim. He would never say he liked anyone. Yet, when the blind flew up at a chance touch of his head, all these good resolutions went to the winds, for the omnibus had reached the summit of a moonlit hill, and there was the chasm, and there, across it, stood the old precipices, dreaming, with their feet in the everlasting river. He exclaimed, "The mountain! Listen to the new tune in the water! Look at the camp fires in the ravines," and Mr. Bons, after a hasty glance, retorted, "Water? Camp fires? Ridiculous rubbish. Hold your tongue. There is nothing at all."

Yet, under his eyes, a rainbow formed, compounded not of sunlight and storm, but of moonlight and the spray of the river. The three horses put their feet upon it. He thought it the finest rainbow he had seen, but did not dare to say so, since Mr. Bons said that nothing was there. He leant out—the window had opened—and sang the tune that rose from the sleeping waters.

"The prelude of Rhinegold?" said Mr. Bons suddenly. "Who taught you these *leit motifs?*" He, too, looked out of the window. Then he behaved very oddly. He gave a choking cry and fell back onto the omnibus floor. He writhed and kicked. His face was green.

"Does the bridge make you dizzy?" the boy asked.

"Dizzy!" gasped Mr. Bons. "I want to go back. Tell the driver."

But the driver shook his head.

"We are nearly there," said the boy. "They are asleep. Shall I call? They will be so pleased to see you, for I have prepared them."

Mr. Bons moaned. They moved over the lunar rainbow, which ever and ever broke away behind their wheels. How still the night was! Who would be sentry at the Gate?

"I am coming," he shouted, again forgetting the hundred resolutions. "I am returning—I, the boy."

"The boy is returning," cried a voice to other voices, who repeated, "The boy is returning."

"I am bringing Mr. Bons with me."

Silence.

"I should have said Mr. Bons is bringing me with him."

Profound silence.

"Who stands sentry?"

"Achilles."

And on the rocky causeway, close to the springing of the rainbow bridge, he saw a young man who carried a wonderful shield.

"Mr. Bons, it is Achilles, armed."

"I want to go back," said Mr. Bons.

The last fragment of the rainbow melted, the wheels sang upon the living rock, the door of the omnibus burst open. Out leapt the boy—he could not resist—and sprang to meet the warrior, who, stooping suddenly, caught him on his shield.

"Achilles!" he cried, "let me get down, for I am ignorant and vulgar, and I must wait for that Mr. Bons of whom I told you yesterday."

But Achilles raised him aloft. He crouched on the wonderful shield, on heroes and burning cities, on vineyards graven in gold, on every dear passion, every joy, on the entire image of the Mountain that he had discovered, encircled, like it, with an everlasting stream. "No, no," he protested, "I am not worthy. It is Mr. Bons who must be up here."

But Mr. Bons was whimpering, and Achilles trumpeted and cried, "Stand upright upon my shield!"

"Sir, I did not mean to stand! something made me stand. Sir, why do you delay? Here is only the great Achilles, whom you knew."

Mr. Bons screamed, "I see no one. I see nothing. I want to go back." Then he cried to the driver, "Save me! Let me stop in your chariot. I have honoured you. I have quoted you. I have bound you in vellum. Take me back to my world."

The driver replied, "I am the means and not the end. I am the food and not the life. Stand by yourself, as that boy has stood. I cannot save you. For poetry is a spirit; and they that would worship it must worship in spirit and in truth."

Mr. Bons—he could not resist—crawled out of the beautiful omnibus. His face appeared, gaping horribly. His hands followed, one gripping the step, the other beating the air. Now his shoulders emerged, his chest, his stomach. With a shriek of "I see London," he fell—fell against the hard, moonlit rock, fell into it as if it were water, fell through it, vanished, and was seen by the boy no more.

"Where have you fallen to, Mr. Bons? Here is a procession arriving to honour you with music and torches. Here come the men and women whose names you know. The mountain is awake, the river is awake, over the race-course the sea is awaking those dolphins, and it is all for you. They want you—"

There was the touch of fresh leaves on his forehead. Someone had crowned him.

ΤΕΛΟΣ

✦

From the *Kingston Gazette*, *Surbiton Times*, and *Raynes Park Observer*.

The body of Mr. Septimus Bons has been found in a shockingly mutilated condition in the vicinity of the Bermondsey gasworks. The deceased's pockets contained a sovereign-purse, a silver cigar-case, a bijou pronouncing dictionary, and a couple of omnibus tickets. The unfortunate gentleman had apparently been hurled from a considerable height. Foul play is suspected, and a thorough investigation is pending by the authorities.

The Dead

JAMES JOYCE (1882–1941)

LILY, the caretaker's daughter, was literally run off her feet. Hardly had she brought one gentleman into the little pantry behind the office on the ground floor and helped him off with his overcoat than the wheezy hall-door bell clanged again and she had to scamper along the bare hallway to let in another guest. It was well for her she had not to attend to the ladies also. But Miss Kate and Miss Julia had thought of that and had converted the bathroom upstairs into a ladies' dressing-room. Miss Kate and Miss Julia were there, gossiping and laughing and fussing, walking after each other to the head of the stairs, peering down over the banisters and calling down to Lily to ask her who had come.

It was always a great affair, the Misses Morkan's annual dance. Everybody who knew them came to it, members of the family, old friends of the family, the members of Julia's choir, any of Kate's pupils that were grown up enough, and even some of Mary Jane's pupils too. Never once had it fallen flat. For years and years it had gone off in splendid style, as long as anyone could remember; ever since Kate and Julia, after the death of their brother

Pat, had left the house in Stoney Batter and taken Mary Jane, their only niece, to live with them in the dark, gaunt house on Usher's Island, the upper part of which they had rented from Mr. Fulham, the corn-factor on the ground floor. That was a good thirty years ago if it was a day. Mary Jane, who was then a little girl in short clothes, was now the main prop of the household, for she had the organ in Haddington Road. She had been through the Academy and gave a pupils' concert every year in the upper room of the Antient Concert Rooms. Many of her pupils belonged to the better-class families on the Kingstown and Dalkey line. Old as they were, her aunts also did their share. Julia, though she was quite grey, was still the leading soprano in Adam and Eve's, and Kate, being too feeble to go about much, gave music lessons to beginners on the old square piano in the back room. Lily, the caretaker's daughter, did housemaid's work for them. Though their life was modest, they believed in eating well; the best of everything: diamond-bone sirloins, three-shilling tea and the best bottled stout. But Lily seldom made a mistake in the orders, so that she got on well with her three mistresses. They were fussy, that was all. But the only thing they would not stand was back answers.

Of course, they had good reason to be fussy on such a night. And then it was long after ten o'clock and yet there was no sign of Gabriel and his wife. Besides they were dreadfully afraid that Freddy Malins might turn up screwed. They would not wish for worlds that any of Mary Jane's pupils should see him under the influence; and when he was like that it was sometimes very hard to manage him. Freddy Malins always came late, but they wondered what could be keeping Gabriel: and that was what brought them every two minutes to the banisters to ask Lily had Gabriel or Freddy come.

"O, Mr. Conroy," said Lily to Gabriel when she opened the door for him, "Miss Kate and Miss Julia thought you were never coming. Good-night, Mrs. Conroy."

"I'll engage they did," said Gabriel, "but they forget that my wife here takes three mortal hours to dress herself."

He stood on the mat, scraping the snow from his goloshes, while Lily led his wife to the foot of the stairs and called out:

"Miss Kate, here's Mrs. Conroy."

Kate and Julia came toddling down the dark stairs at once. Both of them kissed Gabriel's wife, said she must be perished alive, and asked was Gabriel with her.

"Here I am as right as the mail, Aunt Kate! Go on up. I'll follow," called out Gabriel from the dark.

He continued scraping his feet vigorously while the three women went upstairs, laughing, to the ladies' dressing-room. A light fringe of snow lay like a cape on the shoulders of his overcoat and like toecaps on the toes of his goloshes; and, as the buttons of his overcoat slipped with a squeaking noise through the snow-stiffened frieze, a cold, fragrant air from out-of-doors escaped from crevices and folds.

"Is it snowing again, Mr. Conroy?" asked Lily.

She had preceded him into the pantry to help him off with his overcoat. Gabriel smiled at the three syllables she had given his surname and glanced at her. She was a slim, growing girl, pale in complexion and with hay-coloured hair. The gas in the pantry made her look still paler. Gabriel had known her when she was a child and used to sit on the lowest step nursing a rag doll.

"Yes, Lily," he answered, "and I think we're in for a night of it."

He looked up at the pantry ceiling, which was shaking with the stamping and shuffling of feet on the floor above, listened for a moment to the piano and then glanced at the girl, who was folding his overcoat carefully at the end of a shelf.

"Tell me, Lily," he said in a friendly tone, "do you still go to school?"

"O no, sir," she answered. "I'm done schooling this year and more."

"O, then," said Gabriel gaily, "I suppose we'll be going to your wedding one of these fine days with your young man, eh?"

The girl glanced back at him over her shoulder and said with great bitterness:

"The men that is now is only all palaver and what they can get out of you."

Gabriel coloured, as if he felt he had made a mistake and, without looking at her, kicked off his goloshes and flicked actively with his muffler at his patent-leather shoes.

He was a stout, tallish young man. The high colour of his cheeks pushed upwards even to his forehead, where it scattered itself in a few formless patches of pale red; and on his hairless face there scintillated restlessly the polished lenses and the bright gilt rims of the glasses which screened his delicate and restless eyes. His glossy black hair was parted in the middle and brushed in a long curve behind his ears where it curled slightly beneath the groove left by his hat.

When he had flicked lustre into his shoes he stood up and pulled his waistcoat down more tightly on his plump body. Then he took a coin rapidly from his pocket.

"O Lily," he said, thrusting it into her hands, "it's Christmas-time, isn't it? Just . . . here's a little . . ."

He walked rapidly towards the door.

"O no, sir!" cried the girl, following him. "Really, sir, I wouldn't take it."

"Christmas-time! Christmas-time!" said Gabriel, almost trotting to the stairs and waving his hand to her in deprecation.

The girl, seeing that he had gained the stairs, called out after him:

"Well, thank you, sir."

He waited outside the drawing-room door until the waltz should finish, listening to the skirts that swept against it and to the shuffling of feet. He was still discomposed by the girl's bitter and sudden retort. It had cast a gloom over him which he tried to dispel by arranging his cuffs and the bows of his tie. He then took from his waistcoat pocket a little paper and glanced at the headings he had made for his speech. He was undecided about the lines from Robert Browning, for he feared they would be above the heads of his hearers. Some quotation that they would recognise from Shakespeare or from the Melodies would be better. The indelicate clacking of the men's heels and the shuffling of their soles reminded him that their grade of culture differed from his. He would only make himself ridiculous by quoting poetry to them which they could not understand. They would think that he was airing his superior education. He would fail with them just as he had failed with the girl in the pantry. He had taken up a wrong tone. His whole speech was a mistake from first to last, an utter failure.

Just then his aunts and his wife came out of the ladies' dressing-room. His aunts were two small, plainly dressed old women. Aunt Julia was an inch or so the taller. Her hair, drawn low over the tops of her ears, was grey; and grey also, with darker shadows, was her large flaccid face. Though she was stout in build and stood erect, her slow eyes and parted lips gave her the appearance of a woman who did not know where she was or where she was going. Aunt Kate was more vivacious. Her face, healthier than her sister's, was all puckers and creases, like a shrivelled red apple, and her hair, braided in the same old-fashioned way, had not lost its ripe nut colour.

They both kissed Gabriel frankly. He was their favourite nephew, the son of their dead elder sister, Ellen, who had married T. J. Conroy of the Port and Docks.

"Gretta tells me you're not going to take a cab back to Monkstown tonight, Gabriel," said Aunt Kate.

"No," said Gabriel, turning to his wife, "we had quite enough of that last year, hadn't we? Don't you remember, Aunt Kate, what a cold Gretta got out of it? Cab windows rattling all the way, and the east wind blowing in after we passed Merrion. Very jolly it was. Gretta caught a dreadful cold."

Aunt Kate frowned severely and nodded her head at every word.

"Quite right, Gabriel, quite right," she said. "You can't be too careful."

"But as for Gretta there," said Gabriel, "she'd walk home in the snow if she were let."

Mrs. Conroy laughed.

"Don't mind him, Aunt Kate," she said. "He's really an awful bother, what with green shades for Tom's eyes at night and making him do the dumb-bells, and forcing Eva to eat the stirabout. The poor child! And she simply hates the sight of it! . . . O, but you'll never guess what he makes me wear now!"

She broke out into a peal of laughter and glanced at her husband, whose admiring and happy eyes had been wandering from her dress to her face and hair. The two aunts laughed heartily, too, for Gabriel's solicitude was a standing joke with them.

"Goloshes!" said Mrs. Conroy. "That's the latest. Whenever it's wet underfoot I must put on my goloshes. Tonight even, he wanted me to put them on, but I wouldn't. The next thing he'll buy me will be a diving suit."

Gabriel laughed nervously and patted his tie reassuringly, while Aunt Kate nearly doubled herself, so heartily did she enjoy the joke. The smile soon faded from Aunt Julia's face and her mirthless eyes were directed towards her nephew's face. After a pause she asked:

"And what are goloshes, Gabriel?"

"Goloshes, Julia!" exclaimed her sister. "Goodness me, don't you know what goloshes are? You wear them over your . . . over your boots, Gretta, isn't it?"

"Yes," said Mrs. Conroy. "Guttapercha things. We both have a pair now. Gabriel says everyone wears them on the Continent."

"O, on the Continent," murmured Aunt Julia, nodding her head slowly.

Gabriel knitted his brows and said, as if he were slightly angered:

"It's nothing very wonderful, but Gretta thinks it very funny because she says the word reminds her of Christy Minstrels."

"But tell me, Gabriel," said Aunt Kate, with brisk tact. "Of course, you've seen about the room. Gretta was saying . . ."

"O, the room is all right," replied Gabriel. "I've taken one in the Gresham."

"To be sure," said Aunt Kate, "by far the best thing to do. And the children, Gretta, you're not anxious about them?"

"O, for one night," said Mrs. Conroy. "Besides, Bessie will look after them."

"To be sure," said Aunt Kate again. "What a comfort it is to have a girl like that, one you can depend on! There's that Lily, I'm sure I don't know what has come over her lately. She's not the girl she was at all."

Gabriel was about to ask his aunt some questions on this point, but she broke off suddenly to gaze after her sister, who had wandered down the stairs and was craning her neck over the banisters.

"Now, I ask you," she said almost testily, "where is Julia going? Julia! Julia! Where are you going?"

Julia, who had gone half way down one flight, came back and announced blandly: "Here's Freddy."

At the same moment a clapping of hands and a final flourish of the pianist told that the waltz had ended. The drawing-room door was opened from within and some couples came out. Aunt Kate drew Gabriel aside hurriedly and whispered into his ear:

"Slip down, Gabriel, like a good fellow and see if he's all right, and don't let him up if he's screwed. I'm sure he's screwed. I'm sure he is."

Gabriel went to the stairs and listened over the banisters. He could hear two persons talking in the pantry. Then he recognised Freddy Malins' laugh. He went down the stairs noisily.

"It's such a relief," said Aunt Kate to Mrs. Conroy, "that Gabriel is here. I always feel easier in my mind when he's here. . . . Julia, there's Miss Daly and Miss Power will take some refreshment. Thanks for your beautiful waltz, Miss Daly. It made lovely time."

A tall wizen-faced man, with a stiff grizzled moustache and swarthy skin, who was passing out with his partner, said:

"And may we have some refreshment, too, Miss Morkan?"

"Julia," said Aunt Kate summarily, "and here's Mr. Browne and Miss Furlong. Take them in, Julia, with Miss Daly and Miss Power."

"I'm the man for the ladies," said Mr. Browne, pursing his lips until his moustache bristled and smiling in all his wrinkles. "You know, Miss Morkan, the reason they are so fond of me is—"

He did not finish his sentence, but, seeing that Aunt Kate was out of earshot, at once led the three young ladies into the back room. The middle of the room was occupied by two square tables placed end to end, and on these Aunt Julia and the caretaker were straightening and smoothing a large cloth. On the sideboard were arrayed dishes and plates, and glasses and bundles of knives and forks and spoons. The top of the closed square piano served also as a sideboard for viands and sweets. At a smaller sideboard in one corner two young men were standing, drinking hop-bitters.

Mr. Browne led his charges thither and invited them all, in jest, to some ladies' punch, hot, strong and sweet. As they said they never took anything strong, he opened three bottles of lemonade for them. Then he asked one of the young men to move aside, and, taking hold of the decanter, filled out for himself a goodly measure of whisky. The young men eyed him respectfully while he took a trial sip.

"God help me," he said, smiling, "it's the doctor's orders."

His wizened face broke into a broader smile, and the three young ladies laughed in musical echo to his pleasantry, swaying their bodies to and fro, with nervous jerks of their shoulders. The boldest said:

"O, now, Mr. Browne, I'm sure the doctor never ordered anything of the kind."

Mr. Browne took another sip of his whisky and said, with sidling mimicry:

"Well, you see, I'm like the famous Mrs. Cassidy, who is reported to have said: 'Now, Mary Grimes, if I don't take it, make me take it, for I feel I want it.' "

His hot face had leaned forward a little too confidentially and he had assumed a very low Dublin accent so that the young ladies, with one instinct, received his speech in silence. Miss Furlong, who was one of Mary Jane's pupils, asked Miss Daly what was the name of the pretty waltz she had played; and Mr. Browne, seeing that he was ignored, turned promptly to the two young men who were more appreciative.

A red-faced young woman, dressed in pansy, came into the room, excitedly clapping her hands and crying:

"Quadrilles! Quadrilles!"

Close on her heels came Aunt Kate, crying:

"Two gentlemen and three ladies, Mary Jane!"

"O, here's Mr. Bergin and Mr. Kerrigan," said Mary Jane. "Mr. Kerrigan, will you take Miss Power? Miss Furlong, may I get you a partner, Mr. Bergin. O, that'll just do now."

"Three ladies, Mary Jane," said Aunt Kate.

The two young gentlemen asked the ladies if they might have the pleasure, and Mary Jane turned to Miss Daly.

"O, Miss Daly, you're really awfully good, after playing for the last two dances, but really we're so short of ladies tonight."

"I don't mind in the least, Miss Morkan."

"But I've a nice partner for you, Mr. Bartell D'Arcy, the tenor. I'll get him to sing later on. All Dublin is raving about him."

"Lovely voice, lovely voice!" said Aunt Kate.

As the piano had twice begun the prelude to the first figure Mary Jane led her recruits quickly from the room. They had hardly gone when Aunt Julia wandered slowly into the room, looking behind her at something.

"What is the matter, Julia?" asked Aunt Kate anxiously. "Who is it?"

Julia, who was carrying in a column of table-napkins, turned to her sister and said, simply, as if the question had surprised her:

"It's only Freddy, Kate, and Gabriel with him."

In fact right behind her Gabriel could be seen piloting Freddy Malins across the landing. The latter, a young man of about forty, was of Gabriel's size and build, with very round shoulders. His face was fleshy and pallid, touched with colour only at the thick hanging lobes of his ears and at the wide wings of his nose. He had coarse features, a blunt nose, a convex and receding brow, tumid and protruded lips. His heavy-lidded eyes and the disorder of his scanty hair made him look sleepy. He was laughing heartily in a high key at a story which he had been telling Gabriel on the stairs and at the same time rubbing the knuckles of his left fist backwards and forwards into his left eye.

"Good evening, Freddy," said Aunt Julia.

Freddy Malins bade the Misses Morkan good-evening in what seemed an offhand fashion by reason of the habitual catch in his voice and then, seeing that Mr. Browne was grinning at him from the sideboard, crossed the room on rather shaky legs and began to repeat in an undertone the story he had just told to Gabriel.

"He's not so bad, is he?" said Aunt Kate to Gabriel.

Gabriel's brows were dark but he raised them quickly and answered:

"O, no, hardly noticeable."

"Now, isn't he a terrible fellow!" she said. "And his poor mother made him take the pledge on New Year's Eve. But come on, Gabriel, into the drawing-room."

Before leaving the room with Gabriel she signalled to Mr. Browne by frowning and shaking her forefinger in warning to and fro. Mr. Browne nodded in answer and, when she had gone, said to Freddy Malins:

"Now, then, Teddy, I'm going to fill you out a good glass of lemonade just to buck you up."

Freddy Malins, who was nearing the climax of his story, waved the offer aside impatiently but Mr. Browne, having first called Freddy Malins' attention to a disarray in his dress, filled out and handed him a full glass of lemonade. Freddy Malins' left hand accepted the glass mechanically, his right hand being engaged in the mechanical readjustment of his dress. Mr. Browne, whose face was once more wrinkling with mirth, poured out for himself a glass of whisky while Freddy Malins exploded, before he had well reached the climax of his story, in a kink of high-pitched bronchitic laughter and, setting down his untasted and overflowing glass, began to rub the knuckles of his left fist backwards and forwards into his left eye, repeating words of his last phrase as well as his fit of laughter would allow him.

. . . .

Gabriel could not listen while Mary Jane was playing her Academy piece, full of runs and difficult passages, to the hushed drawing-room. He liked music but the piece she was playing had no melody for him and he doubted whether it had any melody for the other listeners, though they had begged Mary Jane to play something. Four young men, who had come from the refreshment-room to stand in the doorway at the sound of the piano, had gone away quietly in couples after a few minutes. The only persons who seemed to follow the music were Mary Jane herself, her hands racing along the key-board or lifted from it at the pauses like those of a priestess in momentary imprecation, and Aunt Kate standing at her elbow to turn the page.

Gabriel's eyes, irritated by the floor, which glittered with beeswax under the heavy chandelier, wandered to the wall above the piano. A picture of the balcony scene in *Romeo and Juliet* hung there and beside it was a picture of the two murdered princes in the Tower which Aunt Julia had worked in red, blue and brown wools when she was a girl. Probably in the school they had gone to as girls that kind of work had been taught for one year. His mother had worked for him as a birthday present a waistcoat of purple tabinet, with little foxes' heads upon it, lined with brown satin and having round mulberry buttons. It was strange that his mother had had no musical talent though Aunt Kate used to call her the brains carrier of the Morkan family. Both she and Julia had always seemed a little proud of their serious and matronly sister. Her photograph stood before the pierglass. She held an open book on her knees and was pointing out something in it to Constantine who, dressed in a man-o'-war suit, lay at her feet. It was she who had chosen the names of her sons for she was very sensible of the dignity of family life. Thanks to her, Constantine was now senior curate in Balbriggan and, thanks to her, Gabriel himself had taken his degree in the Royal University. A shadow passed over his face as he remembered her sullen opposition to his marriage. Some slighting phrases she had used still rankled in his memory; she had once spoken of Gretta as being country cute and that was not true of Gretta at all. It was Gretta who had nursed her during all her last long illness in their house at Monkstown.

He knew that Mary Jane must be near the end of her piece for she was playing again the opening melody with runs of scales after every bar and while he waited for the end the resentment died down in his heart. The piece ended with a trill of octaves in the treble and a final deep octave in the bass. Great applause greeted Mary Jane as, blushing and rolling up her music nervously, she escaped from the room. The most vigorous clapping came from the four young men in the doorway who had gone away to the refreshment-room at the beginning of the piece but had come back when the piano had stopped.

Lancers were arranged. Gabriel found himself partnered with Miss Ivors. She was a frank-mannered talkative young lady, with a freckled face and prominent brown eyes. She did not wear a low-cut bodice and the large brooch which was fixed in the front of her collar bore on it an Irish device and motto.

When they had taken their places she said abruptly:

"I have a crow to pluck with you."

"With me?" said Gabriel.

She nodded her head gravely.

"What is it?" asked Gabriel, smiling at her solemn manner.

"Who is G. C.?" answered Miss Ivors, turning her eyes upon him.

Gabriel coloured and was about to knit his brows, as if he did not understand, when she said bluntly:

"O, innocent Amy! I have found out that you write for *The Daily Express*. Now, aren't you ashamed of yourself?"

"Why should I be ashamed of myself?" asked Gabriel, blinking his eyes and trying to smile.

"Well, I'm ashamed of you," said Miss Ivors frankly. "To say you'd write for a paper like that. I didn't think you were a West Briton."

A look of perplexity appeared on Gabriel's face. It was true that he wrote a literary column every Wednesday in *The Daily Express*, for which he was paid fifteen shillings. But that did not make him a West Briton surely. The books he received for review were almost more welcome than the paltry cheque. He loved to feel the covers and turn over the pages of newly printed books. Nearly every day when his teaching in the college was ended he used to wander down the quays to the second-hand booksellers, to Hickey's on Bachelor's Walk, to Webb's or Massey's on Aston's Quay, or to O'Clohissey's in the by-street. He did not know how to meet her charge. He wanted to say that literature was above politics. But they were friends of many years' standing and their careers had been parallel, first at the University and then as teachers: he could not risk a grandiose phrase with her. He continued blinking his eyes and trying to smile and murmured lamely that he saw nothing political in writing reviews of books.

When their turn to cross had come he was still perplexed and inattentive. Miss Ivors promptly took his hand in a warm grasp and said in a soft friendly tone:

"Of course, I was only joking. Come, we cross now."

When they were together again she spoke of the University question and Gabriel felt more at ease. A friend of hers had shown her his review of Browning's poems. That was how she had found out the secret: but she liked the review immensely. Then she said suddenly:

"O, Mr. Conroy, will you come for an excursion to the Aran

Isles this summer? We're going to stay there a whole month. It will be splendid out in the Atlantic. You ought to come. Mr. Clancy is coming, and Mr. Kilkelly and Kathleen Kearney. It would be splendid for Gretta too if she'd come. She's from Connacht, isn't she?"

"Her people are," said Gabriel shortly.

"But you will come, won't you?" said Miss Ivors, laying her warm hand eagerly on his arm.

"The fact is," said Gabriel, "I have just arranged to go—"

"Go where?" asked Miss Ivors.

"Well, you know, every year I go for a cycling tour with some fellows and so—"

"But where?" asked Miss Ivors.

"Well, we usually go to France or Belgium or perhaps Germany," said Gabriel awkwardly.

"And why do you go to France and Belgium," said Miss Ivors, "instead of visiting your own land?"

"Well," said Gabriel, "it's partly to keep in touch with the languages and partly for a change."

"And haven't you your own language to keep in touch with—Irish?" asked Miss Ivors.

"Well," said Gabriel, "if it comes to that, you know, Irish is not my language."

Their neighbours had turned to listen to the cross-examination. Gabriel glanced right and left nervously and tried to keep his good humour under the ordeal which was making a blush invade his forehead.

"And haven't you your own land to visit," continued Miss Ivors, "that you know nothing of, your own people, and your own country?"

"O, to tell you the truth," retorted Gabriel suddenly, "I'm sick of my own country, sick of it!"

"Why?" asked Miss Ivors.

Gabriel did not answer for his retort had heated him.

"Why?" repeated Miss Ivors.

They had to go visiting together and, as he had not answered her, Miss Ivors said warmly:

"Of course, you've no answer."

Gabriel tried to cover his agitation by taking part in the dance with great energy. He avoided her eyes for he had seen a sour expression on her face. But when they met in the long chain he was surprised to feel his hand firmly pressed. She looked at him from under her brows for a moment quizzically until he smiled. Then, just as the chain was about to start again, she stood on tiptoe and whispered into his ear:

"West Briton!"

When the lancers were over Gabriel went away to a remote corner of the room where Freddy Malins' mother was sitting. She was a stout feeble old woman with white hair. Her voice had a catch in it like her son's and she stuttered slightly. She had been told that Freddy had come and that he was nearly all right. Gabriel asked her whether she had had a good crossing. She lived with her married daughter in Glasgow and came to Dublin on a visit once a year. She answered placidly that she had had a beautiful crossing and that the captain had been most attentive to her. She spoke also of the beautiful house her daughter kept in Glasgow, and of all the friends they had there. While her tongue rambled on Gabriel tried to banish from his mind all memory of the unpleasant incident with Miss Ivors. Of course the girl or woman, or whatever she was, was an enthusiast but there was a time for all things. Perhaps he ought not to have answered her like that. But she had no right to call him a West Briton before people, even in joke. She had tried to make him ridiculous before people, heckling him and staring at him with her rabbit's eyes.

He saw his wife making her way towards him through the waltzing couples. When she reached him she said into his ear:

"Gabriel, Aunt Kate wants to know won't you carve the goose as usual. Miss Daly will carve the ham and I'll do the pudding."

"All right," said Gabriel.

"She's sending in the younger ones first as soon as this waltz is over so that we'll have the table to ourselves."

"Were you dancing?" asked Gabriel.

"Of course I was. Didn't you see me? What row had you with Molly Ivors?"

"No row. Why? Did she say so?"

"Something like that. I'm trying to get that Mr. D'Arcy to sing. He's full of conceit, I think."

"There was no row," said Gabriel moodily, "only she wanted me to go for a trip to the west of Ireland and I said I wouldn't."

His wife clasped her hands excitedly and gave a little jump.

"O, do go, Gabriel," she cried. "I'd love to see Galway again."

"You can go if you like," said Gabriel coldly.

She looked at him for a moment, then turned to Mrs. Malins and said:

"There's a nice husband for you, Mrs. Malins."

While she was threading her way back across the room Mrs. Malins, without adverting to the interruption, went on to tell Gabriel what beautiful places there were in Scotland and beautiful scenery. Her son-in-law brought them every year to the lakes and they used to go fishing. Her son-in-law was a splendid fisher. One day he caught a beautiful big fish and the man in the hotel cooked it for their dinner.

Gabriel hardly heard what she said. Now that supper was coming near he began to think again about his speech and about the quotation. When he saw Freddy Malins coming across the room to visit his mother Gabriel left the chair free for him and retired into the embrasure of the window. The room had already cleared and from the back room came the clatter of plates and knives. Those who still remained in the drawing-room seemed tired of dancing and were conversing quietly in little groups. Gabriel's warm trembling fingers tapped the cold pane of the window. How cool it must be outside! How pleasant it would be to walk out alone, first along by the river and then through the park! The snow would be lying on the branches of the trees and forming a bright cap on the top of the Wellington Monument. How much more pleasant it would be there than at the supper-table!

He ran over the headings of his speech: Irish hospitality, sad memories, the Three Graces, Paris, the quotation from Browning. He repeated to himself a phrase he had written in his review: "One feels that one is listening to a thought-tormented music." Miss Ivors had praised the review. Was she sincere? Had she really any life of her own behind all her propagandism? There had never been any ill-feeling between them until that night. It unnerved him to think that she would be at the supper-table, looking up at him while he spoke with her critical quizzing eyes. Perhaps she would not be sorry to see him fail in his speech. An idea came into his mind and gave him courage. He would say, alluding to Aunt Kate and Aunt Julia: "Ladies and Gentlemen, the generation which is now on the wane among us may have had its faults but for my part I think it had certain qualities of hospitality, of humour, of humanity, which the new and very serious and hyper-educated generation that is growing up around us seems to me to lack." Very good: that was one for Miss Ivors. What did he care that his aunts were only two ignorant old women?

A murmur in the room attracted his attention. Mr. Browne was advancing from the door, gallantly escorting Aunt Julia, who leaned upon his arm, smiling and hanging her head. An irregular musketry of applause escorted her also as far as the piano and then, as Mary Jane seated herself on the stool, and Aunt Julia, no longer smiling, half turned so as to pitch her voice fairly into the room, gradually ceased. Gabriel recognised the prelude. It was that of an old song of Aunt Julia's—*Arrayed for the Bridal*. Her voice, strong and clear in tone, attacked with great spirit the runs which embellish the air and though she sang very rapidly she did not miss even the smallest of the grace notes. To follow the voice, without looking at the singer's face, was to feel and share the excitement of swift and secure flight. Gabriel applauded loudly with all the others at the close of the song and loud applause was borne in from the invisible supper-table. It sounded so genuine that a little colour struggled into Aunt Julia's face as she bent to replace in the music-stand the old leather-bound song-book that had her initials on the cover. Freddy Malins, who had listened with his head perched sideways to hear her better, was still applauding when everyone else had ceased and talking animatedly to his mother who nodded her head gravely and slowly in acquiescence. At last, when he could clap no more, he stood up suddenly and hurried across the room to Aunt Julia whose hand he seized and held in both his hands, shaking it when words failed him or the catch in his voice proved too much for him.

"I was just telling my mother," he said, "I never heard you sing so well, never. No, I never heard your voice so good as it is tonight. Now! Would you believe that now? That's the truth. Upon my word and honour that's the truth. I never heard your voice sound so fresh and so . . . so clear and fresh, never."

Aunt Julia smiled broadly and murmured something about compliments as she released her hand from his grasp. Mr. Browne extended his open hand towards her and said to those who were near him in the manner of a showman introducing a prodigy to an audience:

"Miss Julia Morkan, my latest discovery!"

He was laughing very heartily at this himself when Freddy Malins turned to him and said:

"Well, Browne, if you're serious you might make a worse discovery. All I can say is I never heard her sing half so well as long as I am coming here. And that's the honest truth."

"Neither did I," said Mr. Browne. "I think her voice has greatly improved."

Aunt Julia shrugged her shoulders and said with meek pride:

"Thirty years ago I hadn't a bad voice as voices go."

"I often told Julia," said Aunt Kate emphatically, "that she was simply thrown away in that choir. But she never would be said by me."

She turned as if to appeal to the good sense of the others

against a refractory child while Aunt Julia gazed in front of her, a vague smile of reminiscence playing on her face.

"No," continued Aunt Kate, "she wouldn't be said or led by anyone, slaving there in that choir night and day, night and day. Six o'clock on Christmas morning! And all for what?"

"Well, isn't it for the honour of God, Aunt Kate?" asked Mary Jane, twisting round on the piano-stool and smiling.

Aunt Kate turned fiercely on her niece and said:

"I know all about the honour of God, Mary Jane, but I think it's not at all honourable for the pope to turn out the women out of the choirs that have slaved there all their lives and put little whipper-snappers of boys over their heads. I suppose it is for the good of the Church if the pope does it. But it's not just, Mary Jane, and it's not right."

She had worked herself into a passion and would have continued in defence of her sister for it was a sore subject with her but Mary Jane, seeing that all the dancers had come back, intervened pacifically:

"Now, Aunt Kate, you're giving scandal to Mr. Browne who is of the other persuasion."

Aunt Kate turned to Mr. Browne, who was grinning at this allusion to his religion, and said hastily:

"O, I don't question the pope's being right. I'm only a stupid old woman and I wouldn't presume to do such a thing. But there's such a thing as common everyday politeness and gratitude. And if I were in Julia's place I'd tell that Father Healey straight up to his face . . ."

"And besides, Aunt Kate," said Mary Jane, "we really are all hungry and when we are hungry we are all very quarrelsome."

"And when we are thirsty we are also quarrelsome," added Mr. Browne.

"So that we had better go to supper," said Mary Jane, "and finish the discussion afterwards."

On the landing outside the drawing-room Gabriel found his wife and Mary Jane trying to persuade Miss Ivors to stay for supper. But Miss Ivors, who had put on her hat and was buttoning her cloak, would not stay. She did not feel in the least hungry and she had already overstayed her time.

"But only for ten minutes, Molly," said Mrs. Conroy. "That won't delay you."

"To take a pick itself," said Mary Jane, "after all your dancing."

"I really couldn't," said Miss Ivors.

"I am afraid you didn't enjoy yourself at all," said Mary Jane hopelessly.

"Ever so much, I assure you," said Miss Ivors, "but you really must let me run off now."

"But how can you get home?" asked Mrs. Conroy.

"O, it's only two steps up the quay."

Gabriel hesitated a moment and said:

"If you will allow me, Miss Ivors, I'll see you home if you are really obliged to go."

But Miss Ivors broke away from them.

"I won't hear of it," she cried. "For goodness' sake go in to your suppers and don't mind me. I'm quite well able to take care of myself."

"Well, you're the comical girl, Molly," said Mrs. Conroy frankly.

"*Beannacht libh*," cried Miss Ivors, with a laugh, as she ran down the staircase.

Mary Jane gazed after her, a moody puzzled expression on her face, while Mrs. Conroy leaned over the banisters to listen for the hall-door. Gabriel asked himself was he the cause of her abrupt departure. But she did not seem to be in ill humour: she had gone away laughing. He stared blankly down the staircase.

At the moment Aunt Kate came toddling out of the supper-room, almost wringing her hands in despair.

"Where is Gabriel?" she cried. "Where on earth is Gabriel? There's everyone waiting in there, stage to let, and nobody to carve the goose!"

"Here I am, Aunt Kate!" cried Gabriel, with sudden animation, "ready to carve a flock of geese, if necessary."

A fat brown goose lay at one end of the table and at the other end, on a bed of creased paper strewn with sprigs of parsley, lay a great ham, stripped of its outer skin and peppered over with crust crumbs, a neat paper frill round its shin and beside this was a round of spiced beef. Between these rival ends ran parallel lines of side-dishes: two little minsters of jelly, red and yellow; a shallow dish full of blocks of blancmange and red jam, a large green leaf-shaped dish with a stalk-shaped handle, on which lay bunches of purple raisins and peeled almonds, a companion dish on which lay a solid rectangle of Smyrna figs, a dish of custard topped with grated nutmeg, a small bowl full of chocolates and sweets wrapped in gold and silver papers and a glass vase in which stood some tall celery stalks. In the centre of the table there stood, as sentries to a fruit-stand which upheld a pyramid of oranges and American apples, two squat old-fashioned decanters of cut glass, one containing port and the other dark sherry. On the closed square piano a pudding in a huge yellow dish lay in waiting and behind it were three squads of bottles of stout and ale and minerals, drawn up according to the colours of their uniforms, the first two black, with brown and red labels, the third and smallest squad white, with transverse green sashes.

Gabriel took his seat boldly at the head of the table and, having looked to the edge of the carver, plunged his fork firmly into the goose. He felt quite at ease now for he was an expert carver and liked nothing better than to find himself at the head of a well-laden table.

"Miss Furlong, what shall I send you?" he asked. "A wing or a slice of the breast?"

"Just a small slice of the breast."

"Miss Higgins, what for you?"

"O, anything at all, Mr. Conroy."

While Gabriel and Miss Daly exchanged plates of goose and plates of ham and spiced beef Lily went from guest to guest with a dish of hot floury potatoes wrapped in a white napkin. This was Mary Jane's idea and she had also suggested apple sauce for the goose but Aunt Kate had said that plain roast goose without any apple sauce had always been good enough for her and she hoped she might never eat worse. Mary Jane waited on her pupils and saw that they got the best slices and Aunt Kate and Aunt Julia opened and carried across from the piano bottles of stout and ale for the gentlemen and bottles of minerals for the ladies. There was a great deal of confusion and laughter and noise, the noise of orders and counter-orders, of knives and forks, of corks and glass-stoppers. Gabriel began to carve second helpings as soon as he had finished the first round without serving himself. Everyone protested loudly so that he compromised by taking a long draught of stout for he had found the carving hot work. Mary Jane settled down quietly to her supper but Aunt Kate and Aunt Julia were still toddling round the table, walking on each other's heels, getting in each other's way and giving each other unheeded orders. Mr. Browne begged of them to sit down and eat their suppers and so did Gabriel but they said there was time enough, so that, at last, Freddy Malins stood up and, capturing Aunt Kate, plumped her down on her chair amid general laughter.

When everyone had been well served Gabriel said, smiling:

"Now, if anyone wants a little more of what vulgar people call stuffing let him or her speak."

A chorus of voices invited him to begin his own supper and Lily came forward with three potatoes which she had reserved for him.

"Very well," said Gabriel amiably, as he took another preparatory draught, "kindly forget my existence, ladies and gentlemen, for a few minutes."

He set to his supper and took no part in the conversation with which the table covered Lily's removal of the plates. The subject of talk was the opera company which was then at the Theatre Royal. Mr. Bartell D'Arcy, the tenor, a dark-complexioned young man with a smart moustache, praised very highly the leading contralto of the company but Miss Furlong thought she had a rather vulgar style of production. Freddy Malins said there was a Negro chieftain singing in the second part of the Gaiety pantomime who had one of the finest tenor voices he had ever heard.

"Have you heard him?" he asked Mr. Bartell D'Arcy across the table.

"No," answered Mr. Bartell D'Arcy carelessly.

"Because," Freddy Malins explained, "now I'd be curious to hear your opinion of him. I think he has a grand voice."

"It takes Teddy to find out the really good things," said Mr. Browne familiarly to the table.

"And why couldn't he have a voice too?" asked Freddy Malins sharply. "Is it because he's only a black?"

Nobody answered this question and Mary Jane led the table back to the legitimate opera. One of her pupils had given her a pass for *Mignon.* Of course it was very fine, she said, but it made her think of poor Georgina Burns. Mr. Browne could go back farther still, to the old Italian companies that used to come to Dublin—Tietjens, Ilma de Murzka, Campanini, the great Trebelli, Giuglini, Ravelli, Aramburo. Those were the days, he said, when there was something like singing to be heard in Dublin. He told too of how the top gallery of the old Royal used to be packed night after night, of how one night an Italian tenor had sung five encores to *Let me like a Soldier fall*, introducing a high C every time, and of how the gallery boys would sometimes in their enthusiasm unyoke the horses from the carriage of some great *prima donna* and pull her themselves through the streets to her hotel. Why did they never play the grand old operas now, he asked, *Dinorah, Lucrezia Borgia?* Because they could not get the voices to sing them: that was why.

"O, well," said Mr. Bartell D'Arcy, "I presume there are as good singers today as there were then."

"Where are they?" asked Mr. Browne defiantly.

"In London, Paris, Milan," said Mr. Bartell D'Arcy warmly. "I suppose Caruso, for example, is quite as good, if not better than any of the men you have mentioned."

"Maybe so," said Mr. Browne. "But I may tell you I doubt it strongly."

"O, I'd give anything to hear Caruso sing," said Mary Jane.

"For me," said Aunt Kate, who had been picking a bone, "there was only one tenor. To please me, I mean. But I suppose none of you ever heard of him."

"Who was he, Miss Morkan?" asked Mr. Bartell D'Arcy politely.

"His name," said Aunt Kate, "was Parkinson. I heard him when he was in his prime and I think he had then the purest tenor voice that was ever put into a man's throat."

"Strange," said Mr. Bartell D'Arcy. "I never even heard of him."

"Yes, yes, Miss Morkan is right," said Mr. Browne. "I remember hearing of old Parkinson but he's too far back for me."

"A beautiful, pure, sweet, mellow English tenor," said Aunt Kate with enthusiasm.

Gabriel having finished, the huge pudding was transferred to the table. The clatter of forks and spoons began again. Gabriel's wife served out spoonfuls of the pudding and passed the plates down the table. Midway down they were held up by Mary Jane, who replenished them with raspberry or orange jelly or with blancmange and jam. The pudding was of Aunt Julia's making and she received praises for it from all quarters. She herself said that it was not quite brown enough.

"Well, I hope, Miss Morkan," said Mr. Browne, "that I'm brown enough for you because, you know, I'm all brown."

All the gentlemen, except Gabriel, ate some of the pudding out of compliment to Aunt Julia. As Gabriel never ate sweets the celery had been left for him. Freddy Malins also took a stalk of celery and ate it with his pudding. He had been told that celery was a capital thing for the blood and he was just then under doctor's care. Mrs. Malins, who had been silent all through the supper, said that her son was going down to Mount Melleray in a week or so. The table then spoke of Mount Melleray, how bracing the air was down there, how hospitable the monks were and how they never asked for a penny-piece from their guests.

"And do you mean to say," asked Mr. Browne incredulously, "that a chap can go down there and put up there as if it were a hotel and live on the fat of the land and then come away without paying anything?"

"O, most people give some donation to the monastery when they leave," said Mary Jane.

"I wish we had an institution like that in our Church," said Mr. Browne candidly.

He was astonished to hear that the monks never spoke, got up at two in the morning and slept in their coffins. He asked what they did it for.

"That's the rule of the order," said Aunt Kate firmly.

"Yes, but why?" asked Mr. Browne.

Aunt Kate repeated that it was the rule, that was all. Mr. Browne still seemed not to understand. Freddy Malins explained to him, as best he could, that the monks were trying to make up for the sins committed by all the sinners in the outside world. The explanation was not very clear for Mr. Browne grinned and said:

"I like that idea very much but wouldn't a comfortable spring bed do them as well as a coffin?"

"The coffin," said Mary Jane, "is to remind them of their last end."

As the subject had grown lugubrious it was buried in a silence of the table during which Mrs. Malins could be heard saying to her neighbour in an indistinct undertone:

"They are very good men, the monks, very pious men."

The raisins and almonds and figs and apples and oranges and chocolates and sweets were now passed about the table and Aunt Julia invited all the guests to have either port or sherry. At first Mr. Bartell D'Arcy refused to take either but one of his neighbours nudged him and whispered something to him upon which he allowed his glass to be filled. Gradually as the last glasses were being filled the conversation ceased. A pause followed, broken only by the noise of the wine and by unsettlings of chairs. The Misses Morkan, all three, looked down at the tablecloth. Someone coughed once or twice and then a few gentlemen patted the table gently as a signal for silence. The silence came and Gabriel pushed back his chair and stood up.

The patting at once grew louder in encouragement and then ceased altogether. Gabriel leaned his ten trembling fingers on the tablecloth and smiled nervously at the company. Meeting a row of upturned faces he raised his eyes to the chandelier. The piano was playing a waltz tune and he could hear the skirts sweeping against the drawing-room door. People, perhaps, were standing in the snow on the quay outside, gazing up at the lighted windows and listening to the waltz music. The air was pure there. In the distance lay the park where the trees were weighted with snow. The Wellington Monument wore a gleaming cap of snow that flashed westward over the white field of Fifteen Acres.

He began:

"Ladies and Gentlemen,

"It has fallen to my lot this evening, as in years past, to perform a very pleasing task but a task for which I am afraid my poor powers as a speaker are all too inadequate."

"No, no!" said Mr. Browne.

"But, however that may be, I can only ask you tonight to take the will for the deed and to lend me your attention for a few moments while I endeavour to express to you in words what my feelings are on this occasion.

"Ladies and Gentlemen, it is not the first time that we have gathered together under this hospitable roof, around this hospitable board. It is not the first time that we have been the recipients—or perhaps, I had better say, the victims—of the hospitality of certain good ladies."

He made a circle in the air with his arm and paused. Everyone laughed or smiled at Aunt Kate and Aunt Julia and Mary Jane who all turned crimson with pleasure. Gabriel went on more boldly:

"I feel more strongly with every recurring year that our country has no tradition which does it so much honour and which it should guard so jealously as that of its hospitality. It is a tradition that is unique as far as my experience goes (and I have visited not a few places abroad) among the modern nations. Some would say, perhaps, that with us it is rather a failing than anything to be boasted of. But granted even that, it is, to my mind, a princely failing, and one that I trust will long be cultivated among us. Of one thing, at least, I am sure. As long as this one roof shelters the good ladies aforesaid—and I wish from my heart it may do so for many and many a long year to come—the tradition of genuine warm-hearted courteous Irish hospitality, which our forefathers have handed down to us and which we in turn must hand down to our descendants, is still alive among us."

A hearty murmur of assent ran round the table. It shot through Gabriel's mind that Miss Ivors was not there and that she had gone away discourteously: and he said with confidence in himself:

"Ladies and Gentlemen,

"A new generation is growing up in our midst, a generation actuated by new ideas and new principles. It is serious and enthusiastic for these new ideas and its enthusiasm, even when it is misdirected, is, I believe, in the main sincere. But we are living in a sceptical and, if I may use the phrase, a thought-tormented age: and sometimes I fear that this new generation, educated or hypereducated as it is, will lack those qualities of humanity, of hospitality, of kindly humour which belonged to an older day. Listening tonight to the names of all those great singers of the past it seemed to me, I must confess, that we were living in a less spacious age. Those days might, without exaggeration, be called spacious days: and if they are gone beyond recall let us hope, at least, that in gatherings such as this we shall still speak of them with pride and affection, still cherish in our hearts the memory of those dead and gone great ones whose fame the world will not willingly let die."

"Hear, hear!" said Mr. Browne loudly.

"But yet," continued Gabriel, his voice falling into a softer inflection, "there are always in gatherings such as this sadder thoughts that will recur to our minds: thoughts of the past, of youth, of changes, of absent faces that we miss here tonight. Our path through life is strewn with many such sad memories: and were we to brood upon them always we could not find the heart to go on bravely with our work among the living. We have all of us living duties and living affections which claim, and rightly claim, our strenuous endeavours.

"Therefore, I will not linger on the past. I will not let any gloomy moralising intrude upon us here tonight. Here we are gathered together for a brief moment from the bustle and rush of our everyday routine. We are met here as a friends, in the spirit of good-fellowship, as colleagues, also to a certain extent, in the true spirit of *camaraderie*, and as the guests of—what shall I call them?—the Three Graces of the Dublin musical world."

The table burst into applause and laughter at this allusion. Aunt Julia vainly asked each of her neighbours in turn to tell her what Gabriel had said.

"He says we are the Three Graces, Aunt Julia," said Mary Jane.

Aunt Julia did not understand but she looked up, smiling, at Gabriel, who continued in the same vein:

"Ladies and Gentlemen,

"I will not attempt to play tonight the part that Paris played on another occasion. I will not attempt to choose between them. The task would be an invidious one and one beyond my poor powers. For when I view them in turn, whether it be our chief hostess herself, whose good heart, whose too good heart, has become a byword with all who know her, or her sister, who seems to be gifted with perennial youth and whose singing must have been a surprise and a revelation to us all tonight, or, last but not least, when I consider our youngest hostess, talented, cheerful, hard-working and the best of nieces, I confess, Ladies and Gentlemen, that I do not know to which of them I should award the prize."

Gabriel glanced down at his aunts and, seeing the large smile on Aunt Julia's face and the tears which had risen to Aunt Kate's eyes, hastened to his close. He raised his glass of port gallantly, while every member of the company fingered a glass expectantly, and said loudly:

"Let us toast them all three together. Let us drink to their health, wealth, long life, happiness and prosperity and may they long continue to hold the proud and self-won position which they hold in their profession and the position of honour and affection which they hold in our hearts."

All the guests stood up, glass in hand, and turning towards the three seated ladies, sang in unison, with Mr. Browne as leader:

For they are jolly gay fellows,
For they are jolly gay fellows,
For they are jolly gay fellows,
Which nobody can deny.

Aunt Kate was making frank use of her handkerchief and even Aunt Julia seemed moved. Freddy Malins beat time with his pudding-fork and the singers turned towards one another, as if in melodious conference, while they sang with emphasis:

Unless he tells a lie,
Unless he tells a lie,

Then, turning once more towards their hostesses, they sang:

For they are jolly gay fellows,
For they are jolly gay fellows,
For they are jolly gay fellows,
Which nobody can deny.

The acclamation which followed was taken up beyond the door of the supper-room by many of the other guests and renewed time after time, Freddy Malins acting as officer with his fork on high.

. . . .

The piercing morning air came into the hall where they were standing so that Aunt Kate said:

"Close the door, somebody. Mrs. Malins will get her death of cold."

"Browne is out there, Aunt Kate," said Mary Jane.

"Browne is everywhere," said Aunt Kate, lowering her voice.

Mary Jane laughed at her tone.

"Really," she said archly, "he is very attentive."

"He has been laid on here like the gas," said Aunt Kate in the same tone, "all during the Christmas."

She laughed herself this time good-humouredly and then added quickly:

"But tell him to come in, Mary Jane, and close the door. I hope to goodness he didn't hear me."

At that moment the hall-door was opened and Mr. Browne came in from the doorstep, laughing as if his heart would break. He was dressed in a long green overcoat with mock astrakhan cuffs and collar and wore on his head an oval fur cap. He pointed down the snow-covered quay from where the sound of shrill prolonged whistling was borne in.

"Teddy will have all the cabs in Dublin out," he said.

Gabriel advanced from the little pantry behind the office, struggling into his overcoat and, looking round the hall, said:

"Gretta not down yet?"

"She's getting on her things, Gabriel," said Aunt Kate.

"Who's playing up there?" asked Gabriel.

"Nobody. They're all gone."

"O no, Aunt Kate," said Mary Jane. "Bartell D'Arcy and Miss O'Callaghan aren't gone yet."

"Someone is fooling at the piano anyhow," said Gabriel.

Mary Jane glanced at Gabriel and Mr. Browne and said with a shiver:

"It makes me feel cold to look at you two gentlemen muffled up like that. I wouldn't like to face your journey home at this hour."

"I'd like nothing better this minute," said Mr. Browne stoutly, "than a rattling fine walk in the country or a fast drive with a good spanking goer between the shafts."

"We used to have a very good horse and trap at home," said Aunt Julia sadly.

"The never-to-be-forgotten Johnny," said Mary Jane, laughing.

Aunt Kate and Gabriel laughed too.

"Why, what was wonderful about Johnny?" asked Mr. Browne.

"The late lamented Patrick Morkan, our grandfather, that is," explained Gabriel, "commonly known in his later years as the old gentleman, was a glue-boiler."

"O, now, Gabriel," said Aunt Kate, laughing, "he had a starch mill."

"Well, glue or starch," said Gabriel, "the old gentleman had a horse by the name of Johnny. And Johnny used to work in the old gentleman's mill, walking round and round in order to drive the mill. That was all very well; but now comes the tragic part about Johnny. One fine day the old gentleman thought he'd like to drive out with the quality to a military review in the park."

"The Lord have mercy on his soul," said Aunt Kate compassionately.

"Amen," said Gabriel. "So the old gentleman, as I said, harnessed Johnny and put on his very best tall hat and his very best stock collar and drove out in grand style from his ancestral mansion somewhere near Back Lane, I think."

Everyone laughed, even Mrs. Malins, at Gabriel's manner and Aunt Kate said:

"O, now, Gabriel, he didn't live in Back Lane, really. Only the mill was there."

"Out from the mansion of his forefathers," continued Gabriel, "he drove with Johnny. And everything went on beautifully until Johnny came in sight of King Billy's statue: and whether he fell in love with the horse King Billy sits on or whether he thought he was back again in the mill, anyhow he began to walk round the statue."

Gabriel paced in a circle round the hall in his goloshes amid the laughter of the others.

"Round and round he went," said Gabriel, "and the old gentleman, who was a very pompous old gentleman, was highly indignant. 'Go on, sir! What do you mean, sir? Johnny! Johnny! Most extraordinary conduct! Can't understand the horse!' "

The peal of laughter which followed Gabriel's imitation of the incident was interrupted by a resounding knock at the hall door. Mary Jane ran to open it and let in Freddy Malins. Freddy Malins, with his hat well back on his head and his shoulders humped with cold, was puffing and steaming after his exertions.

"I could only get one cab," he said.

"O, we'll find another along the quay," said Gabriel.

"Yes," said Aunt Kate. "Better not keep Mrs. Malins standing in the draught."

Mrs. Malins was helped down the front steps by her son and Mr. Browne and, after many manœuvres, hoisted into the cab. Freddy Malins clambered in after her and spent a long time settling her on the seat, Mr. Browne helping him with advice. At last she was settled comfortably and Freddy Malins invited Mr. Browne into the cab. There was a good deal of confused talk, and then Mr. Browne got into the cab. The cabman settled his rug over his knees, and bent down for the address. The confusion grew greater and the cabman was directed differently by Freddy Malins and Mr. Browne, each of whom had his head out through a window of the cab. The difficulty was to know where to drop Mr. Browne along the route, and Aunt Kate, Aunt Julia and Mary Jane helped the discussion from the doorstep with cross-directions and contradictions and abundance of laughter. As for Freddy Malins he was speechless with laughter. He popped his head in and out of the window every moment to the great danger of his hat, and told his mother how the discussion was progressing, till at last Mr. Browne shouted to the bewildered cabman above the din of everybody's laughter:

"Do you know Trinity College?"

"Yes, sir," said the cabman.

"Well, drive bang up against Trinity College gates," said Mr. Browne, "and then we'll tell you where to go. You understand now?"

"Yes, sir," said the cabman.

"Make like a bird for Trinity College."

"Right, sir," said the cabman.

The horse was whipped up and the cab rattled off along the quay amid a chorus of laughter and adieus.

Gabriel had not gone to the door with the others. He was in a dark part of the hall gazing up the staircase. A woman was standing near the top of the first flight, in the shadow also. He could not see her face but he could see the terra-cotta and salmon-pink panels of her skirt which the shadow made appear black and white. It was his wife. She was leaning on the banisters, listening to something. Gabriel was surprised at her stillness and strained his ear to listen also. But he could hear little save the noise of laughter and dispute on the front steps, a few chords struck on the piano and a few notes of a man's voice singing.

He stood still in the gloom of the hall, trying to catch the air that the voice was singing and gazing up at his wife. There was grace and mystery in her attitude as if she were a symbol of something. He asked himself what is a woman standing on the stairs in the shadow, listening to distant music, a symbol of. If he were a painter he would paint her in that attitude. Her blue felt hat would show off the bronze of her hair against the darkness and the dark panels of her skirt would show off the light ones. *Distant Music* he would call the picture if he were a painter.

The hall-door was closed; and Aunt Kate, Aunt Julia and Mary Jane came down the hall, still laughing.

"Well, isn't Freddy terrible?" said Mary Jane. "He's really terrible."

Gabriel said nothing but pointed up the stairs towards where his wife was standing. Now that the hall-door was closed the voice and the piano could be heard more clearly. Gabriel held up his hand for them to be silent. The song seemed to be in the old Irish tonality and the singer seemed uncertain both of his words and of his voice. The voice, made plaintive by distance and by the singer's hoarseness, faintly illuminated the cadence of the air with words expressing grief:

O, the rain falls on my heavy locks
And the dew wets my skin,
My babe lies cold . . .

"O," exclaimed Mary Jane. "It's Bartell D'Arcy singing and he wouldn't sing all the night. O, I'll get him to sing a song before he goes."

"O, do, Mary Jane," said Aunt Kate.

Mary Jane brushed past the others and ran to the staircase, but before she reached it the singing stopped and the piano was closed abruptly.

"O, what a pity!" she cried. "Is he coming down, Gretta?"

Gabriel heard his wife answer yes and saw her come down towards them. A few steps behind her were Mr. Bartell D'Arcy and Miss O'Callaghan.

"O, Mr. D'Arcy," cried Mary Jane, "it's downright mean of you to break off like that when we were all in raptures listening to you."

"I have been at him all the evening," said Miss O'Callaghan, "and Mrs. Conroy, too, and he told us he had a dreadful cold and couldn't sing."

"O, Mr. D'Arcy," said Aunt Kate, "now that was a great fib to tell."

"Can't you see that I'm as hoarse as a crow?" said Mr. D'Arcy roughly.

He went into the pantry hastily and put on his overcoat. The others, taken aback by his rude speech, could find nothing to say. Aunt Kate wrinkled her brows and made signs to the others to drop the subject. Mr. D'Arcy stood swathing his neck carefully and frowning.

"It's the weather," said Aunt Julia, after a pause.

"Yes, everybody has colds," said Aunt Kate readily, "everybody."

"They say," said Mary Jane, "we haven't had snow like it for thirty years; and I read this morning in the newspapers that the snow is general all over Ireland."

"I love the look of snow," said Aunt Julia sadly.

"So do I," said Miss O'Callaghan. "I think Christmas is never really Christmas unless we have the snow on the ground."

"But poor Mr. D'Arcy doesn't like the snow," said Aunt Kate, smiling.

Mr. D'Arcy came from the pantry, fully swathed and buttoned, and in a repentant tone told them the history of his cold. Everyone gave him advice and said it was a great pity and urged him to be very careful of his throat in the night air. Gabriel watched his wife, who did not join in the conversation. She was standing right under the dusty fanlight and the flame of the gas lit up the rich bronze of her hair, which he had seen her drying at the fire a few days before. She was in the same attitude and seemed unaware of the talk about her. At last she turned towards them and Gabriel saw that there was colour on her cheeks and that her eyes were shining. A sudden tide of joy went leaping out of his heart.

"Mr. D'Arcy," she said, "what is the name of that song you were singing?"

"It's called *The Lass of Aughrim*," said Mr. D'Arcy, "but

I couldn't remember it properly. Why? Do you know it?"

"*The Lass of Aughrim,*" she repeated. "I couldn't think of the name."

"It's a very nice air," said Mary Jane. "I'm sorry you were not in voice tonight."

"Now, Mary Jane," said Aunt Kate, "don't annoy Mr. D'Arcy. I won't have him annoyed."

Seeing that all were ready to start she shepherded them to the door, where good-night was said:

"Well, good-night, Aunt Kate, and thanks for the pleasant evening."

"Good-night, Gabriel. Good-night, Gretta!"

"Good-night, Aunt Kate, and thanks ever so much. Good-night, Aunt Julia."

"O, good-night, Gretta, I didn't see you."

"Good-night, Mr. D'Arcy. Good-night, Miss O'Callaghan."

"Good-night, Miss Morkan."

"Good-night, again."

"Good-night, all. Safe home."

"Good-night. Good night."

The morning was still dark. A dull, yellow light brooded over the houses and the river; and the sky seemed to be descending. It was slushy underfoot; and only streaks and patches of snow lay on the roofs, on the parapets of the quay and on the area railings. The lamps were still burning redly in the murky air and, across the river, the palace of the Four Courts stood out menacingly against the heavy sky.

She was walking on before him with Mr. Bartell D'Arcy, her shoes in a brown parcel tucked under one arm and her hands holding her skirt up from the slush. She had no longer any grace of attitude, but Gabriel's eyes were still bright with happiness. The blood went bounding along his veins; and the thoughts went rioting through his brain, proud, joyful, tender, valorous.

She was walking on before him so lightly and so erect that he longed to run after her noiselessly, catch her by the shoulders and say something foolish and affectionate into her ear. She seemed to him so frail that he longed to defend her against something and then to be alone with her. Moments of their secret life together burst like stars upon his memory. A heliotrope envelope was lying beside his breakfast-cup and he was caressing it with his hand. Birds were twittering in the ivy and the sunny web of the curtain was shimmering along the floor: he could not eat for happiness. They were standing on the crowded platform and he was placing a ticket inside the warm palm of her glove. He was standing with her in the cold, looking in through a grated window at a man making bottles in a roaring furnace. It was very cold. Her face, fragrant in the cold air, was quite close to his; and suddenly he called out to the man at the furnace:

"Is the fire hot, sir?"

But the man could not hear with the noise of the furnace. It was just as well. He might have answered rudely.

A wave of yet more tender joy escaped from his heart and went coursing in warm flood along his arteries. Like the tender fire of stars moments of their life together, that no one knew of or would ever know of, broke upon and illumined his memory. He longed to recall to her those moments, to make her forget the years of their dull existence together and remember only their moments of ecstasy. For the years, he felt, had not quenched his soul or hers. Their children, his writing, her household cares had not quenched all their souls' tender fire. In one letter that he had written to her then he had said: "Why is it that words like these seem to me so dull and cold? Is it because there is no word tender enough to be your name?"

Like distant music these words that he had written years before were borne towards him from the past. He longed to be alone with her. When the others had gone away, when he and she were in the room in the hotel, then they would be alone together. He would call her softly:

"Gretta!"

Perhaps she would not hear at once: she would be undressing.

Then something in his voice would strike her. She would turn and look at him. . . .

At the corner of Winetavern Street they met a cab. He was glad of its rattling noise as it saved him from conversation. She was looking out of the window and seemed tired. The others spoke only a few words, pointing out some building or street. The horse galloped along wearily under the murky morning sky, dragging his old rattling box after his heels, and Gabriel was again in a cab with her, galloping to catch the boat, galloping to their honeymoon.

As the cab drove across O'Connell Bridge Miss O'Callaghan said:

"They say you never cross O'Connell Bridge without seeing a white horse."

"I see a white man this time," said Gabriel.

"Where?" asked Mr. Bartell D'Arcy.

Gabriel pointed to the statue, on which lay patches of snow. Then he nodded familiarly to it and waved his hand.

"Good-night, Dan," he said gaily.

When the cab drew up before the hotel, Gabriel jumped out and, in spite of Mr. Bartell D'Arcy's protest, paid the driver. He gave the man a shilling over his fare. The man saluted and said:

"A prosperous New Year to you, sir."

"The same to you," said Gabriel cordially.

She leaned for a moment on his arm in getting out of the cab and while standing at the curbstone, bidding the others good-night. She leaned lightly on his arm, as lightly as when she had danced with him a few hours before. He had felt proud and happy then, happy that she was his, proud of her grace and wifely carriage. But now, after the kindling again of so many memories, the first touch of her body, musical and strange and perfumed, sent through him a keen pang of lust. Under cover of her silence he pressed her arm closely to his side; and, as they stood at the hotel door, he felt that they had escaped from their lives and duties, escaped from home and friends and run away together with wild and radiant hearts to a new adventure.

An old man was dozing in a great hooded chair in the hall. He lit a candle in the office and went before them to the stairs. They followed him in silence, their feet falling in soft thuds on the thickly carpeted stairs. She mounted the stairs behind the porter, her head bowed in the ascent, her frail shoulders curved as with a burden, her skirt girt tightly about her. He could have flung his arms about her hips and held her still, for his arms were trembling with desire to seize her and only the stress of his nails against the palms of his hands held the wild impulse of his body in check. The porter halted on the stairs to settle his guttering candle. They halted, too, on the steps below him. In the silence Gabriel could hear the falling of the molten wax into the tray and the thumping of his own heart against his ribs.

The porter led them along a corridor and opened a door. Then he set his unstable candle down on a toilet-table and asked at what hour they were to be called in the morning.

"Eight," said Gabriel.

The porter pointed to the tap of the electric-light and began a muttered apology, but Gabriel cut him short.

"We don't want any light. We have light enough from the street. And I say," he added, pointing to the candle, "you might remove that handsome article, like a good man."

The porter took up his candle again, but slowly, for he was surprised by such a novel idea. Then he mumbled good-night and went out. Gabriel shot the lock to.

A ghastly light from the street lamp lay in a long shaft from one window to the door. Gabriel threw his overcoat and hat on a couch and crossed the room towards the window. He looked down into the street in order that his emotion might calm a little. Then he turned and leaned against a chest of drawers with his back to the light. She had taken off her hat and cloak and was standing before a large swinging mirror, unhooking her waist. Gabriel paused for a few moments, watching her, and then said:

"Gretta!"

She turned away from the mirror slowly and walked along the shaft of light towards him. Her face looked so serious and weary that the words would not pass Gabriel's lips. No, it was not the moment yet.

"You looked tired," he said.

"I am a little," she answered.

"You don't feel ill or weak?"

"No, tired: that's all."

She went on to the window and stood there, looking out. Gabriel waited again and then, fearing that diffidence was about to conquer him, he said abruptly:

"By the way, Gretta!"

"What is it?"

"You know that poor fellow Malins?" he said quickly.

"Yes. What about him?"

"Well, poor fellow, he's a decent sort of chap, after all," continued Gabriel in a false voice. "He gave me back that sovereign I lent him, and I didn't expect it, really. It's a pity he wouldn't keep away from that Browne, because he's not a bad fellow, really."

He was trembling now with annoyance. Why did she seem so abstracted? He did not know how he could begin. Was she annoyed, too, about something? If she would only turn to him or come to him of her own accord! To take her as she was would be brutal. No, he must see some ardour in her eyes first. He longed to be master of her strange mood.

"When did you lend him the pound?" she asked, after a pause.

Gabriel strove to restrain himself from breaking out into brutal language about the sottish Malins and his pound. He longed to cry to her from his soul, to crush her body against his, to overmaster her. But he said:

"O, at Christmas, when he opened that little Christmas-card shop in Henry Street."

He was in such a fever of rage and desire that he did not

hear her come from the window. She stood before him for an instant, looking at him strangely. Then, suddenly raising herself on tiptoe and resting her hands lightly on his shoulders, she kissed him.

"You are a very generous person, Gabriel," she said.

Gabriel, trembling with delight at her sudden kiss and at the quaintness of her phrase, put his hands on her hair and began smoothing it back, scarcely touching it with his fingers. The washing had made it fine and brilliant. His heart was brimming over with happiness. Just when he was wishing for it she had come to him of her own accord. Perhaps her thoughts had been running with his. Perhaps she had felt the impetuous desire that was in him, and then the yielding mood had come upon her. Now that she had fallen to him so easily, he wondered why he had been so diffident.

He stood, holding her head between his hands. Then, slipping one arm swiftly about her body and drawing her towards him, he said softly:

"Gretta, dear, what are you thinking about?"

She did not answer nor yield wholly to his arm. He said again, softly:

"Tell me what it is, Gretta. I think I know what is the matter. Do I know?"

She did not answer at once. Then she said in an outburst of tears:

"O, I am thinking about that song, *The Lass of Aughrim*."

She broke loose from him and ran to the bed and, throwing her arms across the bed-rail, hid her face. Gabriel stood stock-still for a moment in astonishment and then followed her. As he passed in the way of the cheval-glass he caught sight of himself in full length, his broad, well-filled shirt-front, the face whose expression always puzzled him when he saw it in a mirror, and his glimmering gilt-rimmed eyeglasses. He halted a few paces from her and said:

"What about the song? Why does that make you cry?"

She raised her head from her arms and dried her eyes with the back of her hand like a child. A kinder note than he had intended went into his voice.

"Why, Gretta?" he asked.

"I am thinking about a person long ago who used to sing that song."

"And who was the person long ago?" asked Gabriel, smiling.

"It was a person I used to know in Galway when I was living with my grandmother," she said.

The smile passed away from Gabriel's face. A dull anger began to gather again at the back of his mind and the dull fires of his lust began to glow angrily in his veins.

"Someone you were in love with?" he asked ironically.

"It was a young boy I used to know," she answered, "named Michael Furey. He used to sing that song, *The Lass of Aughrim*. He was very delicate."

Gabriel was silent. He did not wish her to think that he was interested in this delicate boy.

"I can see him so plainly," she said, after a moment. "Such eyes as he had: big, dark eyes! And such an expression in them—an expression!"

"O, then, you are in love with him?" said Gabriel.

"I used to go out walking with him," she said, "when I was in Galway."

A thought flew across Gabriel's mind.

"Perhaps that was why you wanted to go to Galway with that Ivors girl?" he said coldly.

She looked at him and asked in surprise:

"What for?"

Her eyes made Gabriel feel awkward. He shrugged his shoulders and said:

"How do I know? To see him, perhaps."

She looked away from him along the shaft of light towards the window in silence.

"He is dead," she said at length. "He died when he was only seventeen. Isn't it a terrible thing to die so young as that?"

"What was he?" asked Gabriel, still ironically.

"He was in the gasworks," she said.

Gabriel felt humiliated by the failure of his irony and by the evocation of this figure from the dead, a boy in the gasworks. While he had been full of memories of their secret life together, full of tenderness and joy and desire, she had been comparing him in her mind with another. A shameful consciousness of his own person assailed him. He saw himself as a ludicrous figure, acting as a pennyboy for his aunts, a nervous, well-meaning sentimentalist, orating to vulgarians and idealising his own clownish lusts, the pitiable fatuous fellow he had caught a glimpse of in the mirror. Instinctively he turned his back more to the light lest she might see the shame that burned upon his forehead.

He tried to keep up his tone of cold interrogation, but his voice when he spoke was humble and indifferent.

"I suppose you were in love with this Michael Furey, Gretta," he said.

"I was great with him at that time," she said.

Her voice was veiled and sad. Gabriel, feeling now how vain it would be to try to lead her whither he had purposed, caressed one of her hands and said, also sadly:

"And what did he die of so young, Gretta? Consumption, was it?"

"I think he died for me," she answered.

A vague terror seized Gabriel at this answer, as if, at that hour when he had hoped to triumph, some impalpable and vindictive being was coming against him, gathering forces against him in its vague world. But he shook himself free of it with an effort of reason and continued to caress her hand. He did not question her again, for he felt that she would tell him of herself. Her hand was warm and moist: it did not respond to his touch, but he continued to caress it just as he had caressed her first letter to him that spring morning.

"It was in the winter," she said, "about the beginning of the winter when I was going to leave my grandmother's and come up here to the convent. And he was ill at the time in his lodgings in Galway and wouldn't be let out, and his people in Oughterard were written to. He was in decline, they said, or something like that. I never knew rightly."

She paused for a moment and sighed.

"Poor fellow," she said. "He was very fond of me and he was such a gentle boy. We used to go out together, walking, you know, Gabriel, like the way they do in the country. He was going to study singing only for his health. He had a very good voice, poor Michael Furey."

"Well; and then?" asked Gabriel.

"And then when it came to the time for me to leave Galway and come up to the convent he was much worse and I wouldn't be let see him so I wrote him a letter saying I was going up to Dublin and would be back in the summer, and hoping he would be better then."

She paused for a moment to get her voice under control, and then went on:

"Then the night before I left, I was in my grandmother's house in Nuns' Island, packing up, and I heard gravel thrown up against the window. The window was so wet I couldn't see, so I ran downstairs as I was and slipped out the back into the garden and there was the poor fellow at the end of the garden, shivering."

"And did you not tell him to go back?" asked Gabriel.

"I implored of him to go home at once and told him he would get his death in the rain. But he said he did not want to live. I can see his eyes as well as well! He was standing at the end of the wall where there was a tree."

"And did he go home?" asked Gabriel.

"Yes, he went home. And when I was only a week in the convent he died and he was buried in Oughterard, where his people came from. O, the day I heard that, that he was dead!"

She stopped, choking with sobs, and, overcome by emotion, flung herself face downward on the bed, sobbing in the quilt. Gabriel held her hand for a moment longer, irresolutely, and then, shy of intruding on her grief, let it fall gently and walked quietly to the window.

She was fast asleep.

Gabriel, leaning on his elbow, looked for a few moments unresentfully on her tangled hair and half-open mouth, listening to her deep-drawn breath. So she had had that romance in her life: a man had died for her sake. It hardly pained him now to think how poor a part he, her husband, had played in her life. He watched her while she slept, as though he and she had never lived together as man and wife. His curious eyes rested long upon her face and on her hair: and, as he thought of what she must have been then, in that time of her first girlish beauty, a strange, friendly pity for her entered his soul. He did not like to say even to himself that her face was no longer beautiful, but he knew that it was no longer the face for which Michael Furey had braved death.

Perhaps she had not told him all the story. His eyes moved to the chair over which she had thrown some of her clothes. A petticoat string dangled to the floor. One boot stood upright, its limp upper fallen down: the fellow of it lay upon its side. He wondered at his riot of emotions of an hour before. From what had it proceeded? From his aunt's supper, from his own foolish speech, from the wine and dancing, the merry-making when saying good-night in the hall, the pleasure of the walk along the river in the snow. Poor Aunt Julia! She, too, would soon be a shade with the shade of Patrick Morkan and his horse. He had caught that haggard look upon her face for a moment when she was singing *Arrayed for the Bridal.* Soon, perhaps, he would be sitting in that same drawing-room, dressed in black, his silk hat on his knees. The blinds would be drawn down and Aunt Kate would be sitting beside him, crying and blowing her nose and telling him how Julia had died. He would cast about in his mind for some words that might console her, and would find only lame and useless ones. Yes, yes: that would happen very soon.

The air of the room chilled his shoulders. He stretched himself cautiously along under the sheets and lay down beside his wife. One by one, they were all becoming shades. Better pass boldly into that other world, in the full glory of some passion, than fade and wither dismally with age. He thought of how she who lay beside him had locked in her heart for so many years that image of her lover's eyes when he had told her that he did not wish to live.

Generous tears filled Gabriel's eyes. He had never felt like that himself towards any woman, but he knew that such a feeling must be love. The tears gathered more thickly in his eyes and in the partial darkness he imagined he saw the form of a young man standing under a dripping tree. Other forms were near. His soul had approached that region where dwell the vast hosts of the dead. He was conscious of, but could not apprehend, their wayward and flickering existence. His own identity was fading out into a grey impalpable world: the solid world itself, which these dead had one time reared and lived in, was dissolving and dwindling.

A few light taps upon the pane made him turn to the window. It had begun to snow again. He watched sleepily the flakes, silver and dark, falling obliquely against the lamplight. The time had come for him to set out on his journey westward. Yes, the newspapers were right: snow was general all over Ireland. It was falling on every part of the dark central plain, on the treeless hills, falling softly upon the Bog of Allen and, farther westward, softly falling into the dark mutinous Shannon waves. It was falling, too, upon every part of the lonely churchyard on the hill where Michael Furey lay buried. It lay thickly drifted on the crooked crosses and headstones, on the spears of the little gate, on the barren thorns. His soul swooned slowly as he heard the snow falling faintly through the universe and faintly falling, like the descent of their last end, upon all the living and the dead.

Critical Questions

WHAT ARE the moments when emotion is most poignantly felt in the story? What is the stimulus for the emotion in each instance? Could the expression be called sentimental? (Distinguish between sentimental treatment and sentimental subject.)

At what points in the story does Gabriel Conroy reveal himself most clearly? Is Joyce's treatment of Gabriel sympathetic, neutral or satirical?

Do the characters strike you as free or frustrated? Consider Lily, Aunt Kate and Aunt Julia, Miss Ivors, Bartell D'Arcy, Gretta, Gabriel. What do Freddy Malins and Mr. Browne contribute to the story?

Discuss the possible symbolic value in the story of Johnny (Grandfather's horse), the snow, Michael Furey.

How do you account for the length and the proportions of the story, its narrative method, and the considerable attention to apparently insignificant details?

What effect is created by the last three paragraphs? Consider in some detail the style of the last paragraph.

Joyce said that in *The Dubliners,* of which "The Dead" (1907) is the last story, his intention was to write "a chapter of the moral history of my country and I chose Dublin for the scene because that city seemed to me to be the centre of paralysis." What are the most important surface features of the life of the city seen in "The Dead"? The most important profound traits?

Although "The Dead" can be read with enjoyment without reference to its autobiographical elements or its relation to all the stories in *The Dubliners,* a student of the story should know that *The Dubliners,* like Joyce's *Ulysses,* has analogues in Homer's *Odyssey*. The understanding of Joyce's creative method in the story will be increased by a knowledge of the parts of the original tale that Joyce retells. (For an interesting article on the analogues see Richard Levin and Charles Shattuck's "A New Reading of Joyce's *Dubliners*," reprinted from *Accent*, Winter, 1944, in Seon Givens, ed.; *James Joyce: Two Decades of Criticism* [1948], pp. 87–92.)

The Essays

The essays in *The Critical Reader* have been chosen with two purposes in mind: to provide for discussion some interesting ideas that will not be too far removed from the background and concerns of the average student; and to give a sampling of modern prose style—or at least of the styles of a number of consciously artistic prose writers.

Many of the essays bear directly on common prejudices and superstitions of our time. Boas, for example, has something to say to anyone who is about to become a member of the educated classes and is, therefore, in danger of succumbing to old theories of an intellectual aristocracy. Lawrence's modern primitivism may somewhat startle anyone reared in the mythology of an industrial civilization. Liebling adds a footnote to contemporary editorials on the freedom of the press, and to discussions of democratic freedoms—popular subjects for the present and the immediate future. Mencken's essay is likely to raise the question of stock responses to death, and especially to the death of a famous man; moreover, it is a serious comment on middle-class suspicion of culture and knowledge, and on the intolerance encouraged by this suspicion. In addition the critical reader should want to consider the justice of Mencken's attack on Bryan. Sharp's essay offers an interesting comment on Lawrence's, and of course raises the whole issue of social planning, and that in a field where the effect of individual operations can be easily visualized; what college is not close to a slum? Gertrude Stein and Dunham may arouse some skepticism of two very popular nostrums for social ills. And what Commager has to say, it is obvious, will be of critical importance to all citizens during the next few years.

It was once conventional to divide essays into the formal and the informal. The formal essay included all those which explained or analyzed or criticized; and the informal all those which made small comments on life, generally with a smile or a chuckle. Informal essays are still written; [1] for example, in a current magazine there is a column in which brief comments are made on men who are always in a hurry, on ours as an age of the facsimile (canned soup, canned music, canned conversation), on the curious relationship between the psychoanalyst and his patient, and so on. *The New Yorker* "Talk of the Town" is today, perhaps, the best example of the informal essay, though typically the pieces in "Talk of the Town" are more sharply pointed and have a more incisive tone than the informal essay of the nineteenth century.

At any rate the division of essays into formal and informal is not very meaningful. Presumably the adjectives apply to the predominant tone of the two types. Consider the way one textbook describes the process of writing a formal essay: "It is a fine thing to be serious, to draw one's self up to a formal task of explaining a machine or analyzing an idea or criticizing a novel. . . ." But obviously many factual, analytical, or critical papers are not formal in tone. A better classification might be worked out in terms of the actual writing problems involved in various kinds of exposition. These problems depend on the personality of the author, on the subject of the piece, on its probable audience, and on its intent—whether the writer wants to explain something, to convince someone, or to move someone toward accepting some attitude. One might also note that some pieces of exposition are the product of reflection or of research, whereas others are based on immediate observation.

Many of the essays in this volume are obviously examples of criticism; their individual forms, however, vary because of differ-

[1] In *The Critical Reader* "I Hate Thursday," "Progress and Change," and "Preface to a Life" might be called informal essays.

ences in the author, the audience, or the intention. Compare Boas' essay with Dunham's, or Dobrée's with Hemingway's. "Jean le Nègre" and "Your United States" are examples of autobiographical narrative; but the latter verges on straight reportage. What determines this difference in effect? Similar questions could be asked about the other essays in this volume. The point is that any rigid classification of expository writing is quite unsatisfactory. What one has to do is to consider the nature of each individual piece before one can find out what makes it take the form it does.

The editors assume that critical papers are a necessary part of the approach they have suggested in the Introduction, and further that such papers, if submitted in a college course, will be subjected to high standards in content and form. They hope that the essays, especially those that deal with literature, will be in some way suggestive to students, if only to the extent of convincing a few that they need not write stiffly and impersonally just because their audience happens to be an English teacher. Above everything else, the essays are intended to demonstrate that a man writing can still be a man speaking to people; with his style sometimes only tidied up, at other times artfully contrived, but nowadays never very far from the rhythms and patterns of the spoken language.

The analyses of the essays, therefore, are designed to provide a vocabulary to use in discussing the qualities of a prose style and a method by which some of the qualities can be discovered. This intention is, of course, subordinate to the purpose stated in the Introduction, but for two reasons it should not be slighted or considered an improper activity. In the first place, the editors believe that a student of writing will often become more careful of his own writing when he can see how careful others have been of theirs. This simple proposition is often overlooked in the tedious search for new and stimulating ideas; and it is hardly probable that a decent English style can be provoked merely by discussing provocative ideas. In the second place, the editors assume with

Coleridge that the parts of a work of literature can be abstracted, analyzed, and evaluated as things in themselves, apart from their relations in the work as a whole, always provided that this activity be recognized for what it is, a preliminary step in criticism.

Preface to a Life

JAMES THURBER (1894–)

BENVENUTO CELLINI said that a man should be at least forty years old before he undertakes so fine an enterprise as that of setting down the story of his life. He said also that an autobiographer should have accomplished something of excellence. Nowadays nobody who has a typewriter pays any attention to the old master's quaint rules. I myself have accomplished nothing of excellence except a remarkable and, to some of my friends, unaccountable expertness in hitting empty ginger ale bottles with small rocks at a distance of thirty paces. Moreover, I am not yet forty years old. But the grim date moves toward me apace; my legs are beginning to go, things blur before my eyes, and the faces of the rose-lipped maids I knew in my twenties are misty as dreams.

At forty my faculties may have closed up like flowers at evening, leaving me unable to write my memoirs with a fitting and discreet inaccuracy or, having written them, unable to carry them to the publisher's. A writer verging into the middle years lives in dread of losing his way to the publishing house and wandering down to the Bowery or the Battery, there to disappear like Ambrose Bierce. He has sometimes also the kindred dread of turning a sudden corner and meeting himself sauntering along in the opposite direction. I have known writers at this dangerous and

PREFACE TO A LIFE is reprinted by permission. From *My Life and Hard Times*, tricky age to phone their homes from their offices, or their offices from their homes, ask for themselves in a low tone, and then, having fortunately discovered that they were "out," to collapse in hard-breathing relief. This is particularly true of writers of light pieces running from a thousand to two thousand words.

The notion that such persons are gay of heart and carefree is curiously untrue. They lead, as a matter of fact, an existence of jumpiness and apprehension. They sit on the edge of the chair of Literature. In the house of Life they have the feeling that they have never taken off their overcoats. Afraid of losing themselves in the larger flight of the two-volume novel, or even the one-volume novel, they stick to short accounts of their misadventures because they never get so deep into them but that they feel they can get out. This type of writing is not a joyous form of self-expression but the manifestation of a twitchiness at once cosmic and mundane. Authors of such pieces have, nobody knows why, a genius for getting into minor difficulties: they walk into the wrong apartments, they drink furniture polish for stomach bitters, they drive their cars into the prize tulip beds of haughty neighbors, they playfully slap gangsters, mistaking them for old school friends. To call such persons "humorists," a loose-fitting and ugly word, is to miss the nature of their dilemma and the dilemma of their nature. The little wheels of their invention are set in motion by the damp hand of melancholy.

Such a writer moves about restlessly wherever he goes, ready to get the hell out at the drop of a pie-pan or the lift of a skirt. His gestures are the ludicrous reflexes of the maladjusted; his repose is the momentary inertia of the nonplussed. He pulls the blinds against the morning and creeps into smoky corners at night. He talks largely about small matters and smally about great affairs. His ears are shut to the ominous rumblings of the dynasties of the world moving toward a cloudier chaos than ever before, but he hears with an acute perception the startling sounds that rabbits make twisting in the bushes along a country road at night and a cold chill comes upon him when the comic supplement of a Sunday newspaper blows unexpectedly out of an areaway and envelopes his knees. He can sleep while the commonwealth crumbles but a strange sound in the pantry at three in the morning will strike terror into his stomach. He is not afraid, or much aware, of the menaces of empire but he keeps looking behind him as he walks along darkening streets out of the fear that he is being softly followed by little men padding along in single file, about a foot and a half high, large-eyed, and whiskered.

It is difficult for such a person to conform to what Ford Madox Ford in his book of recollections has called the sole reason for writing one's memoirs: namely, to paint a picture of one's time. Your short-piece writer's time is not Walter Lippmann's time, or Stuart Chase's time, or Professor Einstein's time. It is his own personal time, circumscribed by the short boundaries of his pain and his embarrassment, in which what happens to his digestion, the rear axle of his car, and the confused flow of his relationships with six or eight persons and two or three buildings is of greater importance than what goes on in the nation or in the universe. He knows vaguely that the nation is not much good any more; he has read that the crust of the earth is shrinking alarmingly and that the universe is growing steadily colder, but he does not believe that any of the three is in half as bad shape as he is.

Enormous strides are made in star-measurement, theoretical economics, and the manufacture of bombing planes, but he usually doesn't find out about them until he picks up an old copy of "Time" on a picnic grounds or in the summer house of a friend. He is aware that billions of dollars are stolen every year by bankers and politicians, and that thousands of people are out of work, but these conditions do not worry him a tenth as much as the conviction that he has wasted three months on a stupid psychoanalyst or the suspicion that a piece he has been working on for two long days was done much better and probably more quickly by Robert Benchley in 1924.

The "time" of such a writer, then, is hardly worth reading about if the reader wishes to find out what was going on in the world while the writer in question was alive and at what might be laughingly called "his best." All that the reader is going to find out is what happened to the writer. The compensation, I suppose, must lie in the comforting feeling that one has had, after all, a pretty sensible and peaceful life, by comparison. It is unfortunate, however, that even a well-ordered life can not lead anybody safely around the inevitable doom that waits in the skies. As F. Hopkinson Smith long ago pointed out, the claw of the sea-puss gets us all in the end.

Suggestions for Study

THIS ESSAY is a fine example of the flexibility of modern prose. It bristles with alliteration and literary allusions; some of its figures are characteristic of the most elaborate and purple prose in the language—for example, "the nature of their dilemma and the dilemma of their nature" and "talks largely about small matters and smally about great affairs," which seem to be examples of a kind of chiasmus. Yet the final effect of the piece is one of lightness, indeed of a rather plain style. The deception is accomplished, I suppose, because the sentences are so unobtrusive. (On this point compare the essay by Mencken, which is so much more emphatic in its rhythms.) Another cause is undoubtedly the number of homely or colloquial allusions ("get the hell out at the drop of a pie-pan or the lift of a skirt," but note the play on the colloquial expression "drop of a hat" and the psychological truism suggested by "lift of a skirt"), each of which seems deliberately placed to counter some serious statement or obviously artistic figure. Perhaps the most conspicuous ornament in the essay is its imagery, which here, as in a good deal of modern prose, replaces the classic figures of sound and sense: compare the sentence "He is not afraid, or much aware, of the menaces of empire but keeps looking behind him as he walks along darkening streets out of the fear that he is being softly followed by little men padding along in single file, about a foot and a half high, large-eyed, and whiskered."

The organization of the essay is very simple. It begins, deceptively enough, with a conventional and straight-faced introduction, complete even to the elaborate literary allusion. This, however, lasts only until the mention of his "unaccountable expertness in hitting empty ginger ale bottles with small rocks at a distance of thirty paces." After that the parody of backward glances takes over and continues to the end of the second paragraph. The remainder of the essay is divided into three sections, in which Thurber talks about the mind, the experience, and the significance of the comic writer.

Much of the effect of the essay is created by the unexpected and suggestive combinations of details drawn from widely separated areas of experience.

> His ears are shut to the ominous rumblings of the dynasties of the world moving toward a cloudier chaos than ever before, but he hears with an acute perception the startling sounds that rabbits make twisting in the bushes along a country road at night and a cold chill comes upon him when the comic supplement of a Sunday newspaper blows unexpectedly out of an areaway and envelops his knees.

> The little wheels of their invention are set in motion by the damp hand of melancholy.

> A writer verging into the middle years lives in dread of losing his way to the publishing house and wandering down to the Bowery or the Battery, there to disappear like Ambrose Bierce.

At first reading, these sentences—the whole essay, for that matter—may seem to be only rather sophisticated examples of the humorist's trick of assembling incongruous elements for their shock effect. But properly read, they can be seen as parts of a fundamental design, which prepares the reader for the last two sentences.

Considering these two sentences and others of like nature, what is the underlying idea of the essay? What is its exact tone?

I Hate Thursday

THOMAS HORNSBY FERRIL (1896–   )

I HATE Thursday. On Thursday I get mean. All my bestial traits hold carnival. My household might include six other days, but on Thursday I'm even mean to me. I don't want to have myself around. I'm uncivil to my sugar company associates at the office. I sulk through lunch. I ask impossible questions nobody knows any answer to. I come home at night without the horse meat.

"Did you bring the horse meat for Loper, dear?"

"No I didn't bring the damned horse meat . . . and I don't intend to . . . and he's your dog anyhow . . . and leave me alone . . . and if the telephone rings we're not going to waltz night . . . and we're not going to the Budapest quartet . . . and we don't even live here . . . and where the hell is that clipping on Dumbarton Oaks I left under the shirts to go to the Chinaman?"

I go to the library and feel sorry for myself. I put a piece of paper into the typewriter.

"Did you read the mail, darling?"

"ME, ME, ME! It's always me that has to read the mail in this family! Throw the damned stuff out!" But I add meekly, "Who were the letters from? Anything interesting?"

Nothing happens to the paper in my typewriter. I go to the window and stare at the tranquil city. Thoughtful people are tucked into bed reading detective stories and learning about tomorrow from Drew Pearson. Out there somewhere in the blackness one of my friends is in his basement making Heppelwhite chairs. Why can't I make Heppelwhite chairs? Why have I no artistic hobbies? Out there somewhere Thursday's domestics are

I HATE THURSDAY is reprinted from *I Hate Thursday* by Thomas Hornsby Ferril.

at the movies and their masters and mistresses are drinking beer in pleasant cheeseburger stands, discussing nylons and Attlee. Why can't I? I return to the typewriter, I oil it, I wind the ribbon back and forth. My fingers wander idly over the ivory keys. How many billion years would it take a monkey, hitting the keys at random, to turn out "The Lost Chord"? Ho hum! It goads me into hitting the keys myself. In the upper left-hand corner I put

RMH

1-col 10 pt.

That means *Rocky Mountain Herald* and tells the printer how to set it up. Then my first sentence begins to take form. I have picked up three new expressions in the past ten days and they all want to get in on the first sentence—"foreseeable future," "central fact" and "telegony." I rule out telegony because it can't possibly do me or anybody else any good. It means "hypothetical influence of a sire on subsequent offspring by a different sire." But the other two are all right, so here goes:

"In the foreseeable future of India one central fact is clear . . ."

Very very clear!

The foreseeable future? The day before the San Francisco earthquake? The day before the crash of '29? The day of Pearl Harbor when all the brass hats were at Griffith stadium cheering the Washington Redskins to foreseeable touchdowns?

And what is this central fact that's so clear about India? The one central fact I'm sure of is that when we were diagramming sentences in Room 27 in the eighth grade at Whittier School I didn't do too well with "In India it is a sin to kill a spider." I angrily jerk the paper from the typewriter and throw it to the wolves.

This Thursday business gets me down because we have a one-horse weekly newspaper in the family that I think I ought to write for, and I don't have to at all. It goes to press on Friday, the *Rocky Mountain Herald*, a sort of step-dog heirloom established in Denver eighty-six years ago. The *Herald* has eight pages of which up to seven are filled with legal notices and a front page we call "the pearls"—pearls of wisdom, pearls of great price, pearls before swine. My father ran the paper for ages and, as his eyesight failed, my wife Helen would go down to read proof on legals, make out bills and paste up affidavits that looked like valentines. In 1939, on his death, she took over and has become, alas, expert in the legal business. The *Herald* rides her like an incubus, no vacations, no fun, no nothing. We call it the Rocky Mountain Albatross.

Nothing makes you madder than feeling incompetent to undertake something you don't have to do at all. That's me. I don't have to write for the *Herald*. Nobody has to write for weekly papers because nobody does anything else. A weekly is the most written-for thing in the world, thanks to what we call boiler-plate, the syndicated material you buy by the yard, all set up ready to go. Boiler-plate is like the wreck in *Swiss Family Robinson*, everything you could dream of is there for the asking. "Do you, Ernest, swim out to the wreck and fetch me what Walter Lippmann is muttering about Bretton Woods." Presto! It's done.

Boiler-plate is the digest of digests, the tomb and resurrection of the printed word. Boiler-plate tells you about baby opossums and how to take out inkstains, it gives you Washington-merry-go-rounds galore, Walter Winchells a dime a dozen, Baukages, Dorothy Thompsons; it flashes spot news about normal precipitation in Patagonia and what Harry Emerson Fosdick thinks about the atomic bomb. It's the battle royal of semantics with Darwinian victories. Think of a quotation from Homer proving its fitness to survive against a 1945 smear of pectin, just the right amount of pectin, milady, to keep your jelly from collapsing. And intersmeared with Homer and pectin will be a doleful reminder that a crumb of bread, thrown in jest, made Prescott, the historian, blind for life. You'll never throw another crumb of bread as long as you live! Whatever the world forgets, the boiler-plate remembers; it is the corruption and regeneration of all truth; it points with pride, it views with alarm, it relieves the stresses of life with comical jokes and assuages life's transitoriness with poetry that tugs at the heartstrings.

Why anyone should try to compete with boiler-plate I do not know, myself of all people, for it trails clouds of glory far above my poor powers to add or detract. When I try to figure out why I feel I have to write for the *Herald*, it comes down to admitting that I like to run off at the mouth and am gloomy when I'm not trying to. But before you heave the first stone, may I suggest that you also ought to have a weekly paper in your family—a one-horse one-wife paper, an anchor, a millstone, an albatross to impose discipline and humility, but, more than that, a temptation to put into print what you most approve in your own conversation and furtive dreams. Know what it's like to feel your own inadequacy in a world of words, of half-truths, of propaganda, of plausibility. They say you don't know a thing unless you can write it down. Your weekly is a garden with no forbidden fruit and a gallows to hang your stupidity on.

There are, I hasten to add, Thursday compensations, but they irk me worse than the boiler-plate. For some strange reason a weekly paper is a lodestone to people who can't help writing any more than I can. Take the pitiful case of H. L. Davis of Oregon who, in my opinion, stands head and shoulders above other western writing men. Davis won the Harper seventy-five hundred dollar prize and the Pulitzer prize for his novel *Honey in the Horn.* Why does he write year in, year out, anonymously for the *Rocky Mountain Herald?* I look at those big welcome Manila envelopes he sends in and cuss him from hell to breakfast for knowing enough to say what I can't say at all and doing it all for nothing. And there's Richard Peete, peerless yarn spinner of the western bar. Dick has written nearly four hundred consecutive anecdotes about lawyers. Davis and Peete remind me of Irvin Cobb's story about the girl who gave away thousands of dollars worth of a reasonably valuable commodity before she found she could sell it. The *Herald* could run a year on its stock pile of free contributions from kind friends who don't know any better.

Clearly, Thursday shouldn't throw me into a dither, but I think I know why it does. Every waking hour of every day affects me more or less the same way. I am constantly reminded of how little I know about the world I live in. Putting paper into a typewriter simply emphasizes the predicament. What ought to be a statement of truth turns into verbal manipulation of ignorance. Not that I'm against verbal manipulation. I love puns, limericks, double-crostics. Life would be poor without word games. But the trouble is that we are living in a world of word games, most of them so seriously contrived that we don't take them for games at all. We can't tell a White paper from a charade. We read something about India or Russia without realizing that the man who wrote it didn't know what he was talking about. He was just a monkey with the typewriter keys falling his way. He keeps up with the fashions in words, inexorable as fashions in lipsticks—the central fact, the foreseeable future.

But when I finally pin myself down to why I loathe and abhor my Thursday complexes, I'm happy to confess and proud to boast that I am a perfectionist. Being such, I've worked up a condoning martyrdom. I tolerate all the wretched stuff I write as the Son of Heaven has to tolerate the imperial privy, or must have before Douglas Mikado demoted him to mortality. Only the perfectionist can be careless, like Robert Frost saying "I ain't" or "it don't." I have no difficulty in bringing myself around to saying: "At least I understand what I'm up to and thoroughly disapprove of it, but I'm big, I'm under pressure, I embrace multitudes, I forgive myself. My friends will understand, the rest don't matter." Let every writer, I continue, be judged by his best moments, and let his careless moments be patently careless, for no literary sin is more abominable than to polish a bad fact or a no-fact-at-all into beautiful plausible prose. They told me in school that Walter Pater would write prose on paper ruled in groups of three lines and that he'd go through an essay first on the top line, then the second, then to ultimate perfection on the third. If so, how wicked! All stylists are embezzlers.

Two kinds of writing, since I am a perfectionist, seem eminently eloquent to me and, the older I grow, the more I become viciously intolerant of anything else. I refer to the best writing of knowledge and the best writing of feeling, in a word, pure science and pure poetry. I find science and poetry antipodal and complementary, never competitive. Competition occurs only in the scrambled middle ground between the two poles where we feel much and know little about very complex subjects and finally achieve neither good fact, good fiction, good history, good nonsense or good poetry. Mass word production, the impact of literacy on deadlines, has a good deal to do with it, but I don't blame the newspapers and radio alone. I blame the general frenzy to be timely which destroys all sense of time. This new book on China or sixty million jobs must be done while the subject is hot.

Forget China or sixty million jobs and apply my principles of perfection to something that is never spot news or controversial, say, a falcon. Let the falcon test the writing of fact and feeling. On the first score, fact, I envy and salute the writer who can tell what kind of falcon it is, describe its habits, its habitat, its life behavior, its biological composition. If the lights and liver of the bird lead him into atomic biochemistry, the mystery of life itself, let him end as we all must end in some final faith in manifestation, but let him stop where he has to stop: "I know this much this far and I can't go further." However stumbling the syntax, that kind of writing is, to me, downright magnificent. Would that we might write with the same integrity about India or the sterling bloc! The other kind of magnificent writing begins with immediate faith in manifestation, the writing of perfect feeling, poetry. Our falcon is now flying over the prairie. Knowledge doesn't help though it may qualify the experience, for the wonder in the heart of an ornithologist may differ from the wonder in the heart of a child. But deep feeling is common to both. You summon words. What's the falcon like, no, not like, what *is* it? How can you realize this experience, more than realize it, make it *realler* than it is? You want to hold it, keep it forever, communicate it to someone else. Wonder, desire, memory, innumerable impacts, as unmistakable as they are undefinable, grope for the concrete ecstatic statement and, if achieved, it is poetry of the purest character.

There are other ways to write about the falcon and you can have them. Planned Falconhood! Marxist Falcons! Baptist Falcons! The Falcon Looks at Democracy! Go to it! It's a free country! Write about the falcon just as you do about India or the sterling bloc. But it's not for me. I'll curl up in my chair and read the geodetic survey or "The Battle Hymn of the Republic," which I don't have to put through any filters of how much fact, how much feeling? I'll take my emotion straight, Ring Lardner or Shakespeare's sixty-sixth sonnet and let the wisdom trickle through without resistance or effort on my part.

Don't be a perfectionist! That's what they tell you. It's impractical. After all, life is just a bowl of Munichs. Give-and-take must solve our problems. Our old colored washerwoman Josephine used to say, "You don't have to throw razors and chairs, there's always a nice way." Maybe so, but we spend too much time looking for it. Being forever driven to compromise, we woo and glorify it. We let adoration of compromise front for the stupidities that make compromise necessary. So behaving, we bow and scrape to stupidity itself. We say "Let's make the best of it" but we mean the easiest. The best is perfection. Perfectionists created the atomic bomb and a perfectionist created the "Ode to a Grecian Urn." If we must put up with less, let it growl and hiss in our acid gizzards as something we hate very much every day in the week. I give you my horrible Thursdays. May they make you wretched too! Many happy returns!

Suggestions for Study

THE PARAGRAPH that begins "Boiler-plate is the digest of digests" is a fair sample of Ferril's style. In a little more than one hundred and fifty words, there are thirteen main and five subordinate predications. Of the thirteen independent clauses, eleven begin with the subject immediately followed by the verb. How do these qualities affect the sound of the prose?

How many sentences in the essay follow the pattern of the sentence beginning "Boiler-plate tells you about baby opossums"? How many sentences in the essay contain imperatives? What is the average length in words and syllables of Ferril's sentences? (Count the words and syllables in twenty-five or thirty sentences selected from different sections of the essay, say five or so consecutive sentences from several pages. The syllabic length is probably more important than the length in words.)

The diction in this essay is worth attention. What is the source of such expressions as "throw it to the wolves" and "head and shoulders above"? In "The *Herald* rides her like an incubus," comment on the choice of the verb. Comment on the verb in "But before you heave the first stone." What is the meaning of "battle royal of semantics with Darwinian victories"? From what level of the vocabulary does a word like *milady* come?

In each of the following sentences Ferril wants to make a serious point.

Whatever the world forgets, the boiler-plate remembers; it is the corruption and regeneration of all truth; it points with pride, it views with alarm, it relieves the stresses of life with comical jokes and assuages life's transitoriness with poetry that tugs at the heartstrings.

Wonder, desire, memory, innumerable impacts, as unmistakable as they are undefinable, grope for the concrete ecstatic statement and, if achieved, it is poetry of the purest character.

Compare the first sentence with the last two sentences of Thurber's "Preface to a Life." What is the most obvious difference in the diction? Bonamy Dobrée quotes William Puttenham, who wrote in the sixteenth century: "Style is a constant and continual phrase or tenour of speaking and writing, extending to the whole tale or process of the poem or history, and not properly to any piece or member of the tale; but is of words, speeches, and sentences together, a certain contrived form and quality . . . such as he . . . will not, peradventure cannot, easily alter into any other." Mr. Dobrée goes on to suggest that when we read we are "aware of a voice." What kind of voice (or mind, one might say) does Ferril seem to have?

Compare the second of the sentences quoted above (p. 502) with the three quoted in the comment that follows Thurber's "Preface." Who tells you more about his subject, Ferril or Thurber?

In "I Hate Thursday" allusions seem to be the chief device for stylistic ornamentation. There are allusions to history, contemporary events, and personalities, to literature of all kinds (a popular song as well as Whitman, *The Swiss Family Robinson* as well as Walter Pater), to folklore (the monkey at the typewriter), to common experience (parsing sentences like "In India it is a sin to kill a spider"). Identify and classify as many allusions as you can. Which seem to be the most effective?

Progress and Change

E. B. WHITE (1899–)

My friends in the city tell me that the Sixth Avenue El is coming down, but that's a hard thing for anyone to believe who once lived in its fleeting and audible shadow. The El was the most distinguished and outstanding vein on the town's neck, a varicosity tempting to the modern surgeon. One wonders whether New York can survive this sort of beauty operation, performed in the name of civic splendor and rapid transit.

A resident of the city grew accustomed to the heavenly railroad which swung implausibly in air, cutting off his sun by day, wandering in and out of his bedchamber by night. The presence of the structure and the passing of the trains were by all odds the most pervasive of New York's influences. Here was a sound which, if it ever got in the conch of your ear, was ineradicable—forever singing, like the sea. It punctuated the morning with brisk tidings of repetitious adventure, and it accompanied the night with sad but reassuring sounds of life-going-on—the sort of threnody which cricket and katydid render for suburban people sitting on screened porches, the sort of lullaby which the whippoorwill sends up to the Kentucky farm wife on a summer evening.

I spent a lot of time, once, doing nothing in the vicinity of Sixth Avenue. Naturally I know something of the El's fitful charm. It was, among other things, the sort of railroad you would occasionally ride just for the hell of it, a higher existence into which you would escape unconsciously and without destination. Let's say you had just emerged from the Childs' on the west side of Sixth Avenue between 14th and 15th Streets, where you had

had a bowl of vegetable soup and a stack of wheat cakes. The syrup still was a cloying taste on your tongue. You intended to go back to the apartment and iron a paragraph, or wash a sock. But miraculously, at the corner of 14th, there rose suddenly in front of you a flight of marble stairs all wrapt in celestial light, with treads of shining steel, and risers richly carved with the names of the great, and a canopy overhead where danced the dust in the shafts of golden sunshine. As in a trance, you mounted steadily to the pavilion above, where there was an iron stove and a man's hand visible through a mousehole. And the first thing you knew you were in South Ferry, with another of life's inestimable journeys behind you—and before you the dull, throbbing necessity of getting uptown again.

For a number of years I went to work every morning on the uptown trains of the Sixth Avenue El. I had it soft, because my journey wasn't at the rush hour and I often had the platform of the car to myself. It was a good way to get where you wanted to go, looking down on life at just the right speed, and peeking in people's windows, where the sketchy pantomime of potted plant and half-buttoned undershirt and dusty loft provided a curtain raiser to the day. The railroad was tolerant and allowed its passengers to loll outdoors if they wished; and on mornings when the air was heady that was the place to be—with the sudden whiff of the candy factory telling you that your ride was half over, and the quick eastward glance through 24th Street to check your time with the clock in the Metropolitan Tower, visible for the tenth part of a second.

The El always seemed to me to possess exactly the right degree of substantiality: it seemed reasonably strong and able to carry its load, and competent with that easy slovenly competence of an old drudge; yet it was perceptibly a creature of the clouds, the whole structure vibrating ever so slightly following the final grasping success of the applied brake. The El had giddy spells, too—days when a local train would shake off its patient, plodding manner and soar away in a flight of sheer whimsy, skipping stations in a drunken fashion and scaring the pants off everybody. To go roaring past a scheduled stop, hell bent for 53rd Street and the plunge into space, was an experience which befell every El rider more than once. On this line a man didn't have to be a locomotophobe to suffer from visions of a motorman's lifeless form slumped over an open throttle. And if the suspense got too great and you walked nervously to the front of the train the little window in the booth gave only the most tantalizing view of the driver—three inert fingers of a gloved hand, or a *Daily News* wedged in some vital cranny.

One thing I always admired about the El was the way it tormented its inexperienced customers. Veterans like myself, approaching a station stop, knew to a fraction of an inch how close it was advisable to stand to the little iron gates on the open type cars. But visitors to town had no such information. When the train halted and the guard, pulling his two levers, allowed the gates to swing in and take the unwary full in the stomach, there was always a dim pleasure in it for the rest of us. Life has little enough in the way of reward; these small moments of superiority are not to be despised.

The El turned the Avenue into an arcade. That, in a way, was its chief contribution. It made Sixth Avenue as distinct from Fifth as Fifth is from Jones Street. Its pillars, straddling the car tracks in the long channel of the night, provided the late cruising taxicab with the supreme challenge, and afforded the homing pedestrian, his wine too much with him, forest sanctuary and the friendly accommodation of a tree.

Of course I have read about the great days of the El, when it was the railroad of the élite and when financial giants rode elegantly home from Wall Street in its nicely appointed coaches. But I'm just as glad I didn't meet the El until after it had lost its money. Its lazy crescendos, breaking into one's dreams, will always stick in the mind—and the soiled hands of the guards on the bellcords, and the brusque, husky-throated bells that had long ago lost their voices, cuing each other along the whole length of the train. Yes, at this distance it's hard to realize that the Sixth Avenue El is just a problem in demolition. I can't for the life of me imagine what New York will have to offer in its place. It will have to be something a good deal racier, a good deal more open and aboveboard, than a new subway line.

Suggestions for Study

THIS SELECTION ought to be compared with Ferril's "I Hate Thursday," not only for its rhythm, sound, and diction, but also for the quality of mind which it reveals.

In the first three paragraphs of "Progress and Change," most of the sentences begin with the subject, which is followed more or less closely by the verb. Occasionally adverbial modifiers—"Here was a sound . . ." "Naturally I know . . ." "As in a trance . . ."—and a couple of initial conjunctions take some of the weight from the subject-verb nexus. What other characteristics of the sentence structure have this effect? In addition to sentence length in words and syllables, number of predications, number of subordinate clauses, consider here the effect of such rhythm-groups as "civic splendor and rapid transit," "forever singing, like the sea," "suburban people sitting on screened porches," "sends up to the Kentucky farm wife on a summer evening." Note in the third and fourth sentences of the second paragraph that the dashes replace neutral or colorless predications like "it was" or "which was," the effect of which would be to break the back of the rhythm. But then, what about the position of "once" in the first sentence of the third paragraph? Is it possible to justify the heavy emphasis which this word receives?

Note the many examples of alliteration and also the subtle handling of literary allusions.

The most conspicuous characteristic of the passage is its delicate play with fact and fancy. "It was, among other things, the sort of railroad you would occasionally ride just for the hell of it, a higher existence into which you would escape unconsciously and without destination. Let's say you had just emerged from the Childs' on the west side of Sixth Avenue between 14th and 15th Streets, where you had had a bowl of vegetable soup and a stack of wheat cakes. The syrup still was a cloying taste on your tongue. You intended to go back to the apartment and iron a paragraph, or wash a sock." Analyze the diction of the passage, paying especial attention to the background of the details.

Describe the attitude toward modern life expressed in this passage. Consider also the sentence "As in a trance, you mounted steadily to the pavilion above, where there was an iron stove and a man's hand visible through a mousehole."

Your United States

GERTRUDE STEIN (1874–1946)

I USED to say that I would not go to America until I was a real lion a real celebrity at that time of course I did not really think I was going to be one. But now we were coming and I was going to be one. In America everybody is but some are more than others. I was more than others. New York was coming nearer and we were nervous but not really nervous enough. You never are when a thing is really happening.

So the statue of liberty began and Staten Island. And just then we saw the boat coming. Everybody who has ever done anything has seen reporters. After all there always are newspapers and one has always read them. They are not interesting like books or detective stories but one does read them. Well anyway there we all

YOUR UNITED STATES by Gertrude Stein is reprinted from *The Atlantic Monthly*, October 1937, by permission of Carl Van Vechten.

were and it was very lively and I liked it, I always like talking and I like asking questions and I like to know who everybody is and where they come from.

Strangeness always goes off very quickly, that is one of the troubles with travelling but then the pleasure of looking if you like to look is always a pleasure. Alice Toklas began to complain she said why do they call Paris la ville lumière, she always prefers that anything should be American, I said because when they did there were more lights there than anywhere, you cannot blame them that they still think so although there are more lights here than anywhere. And there were. And more beautifully strung as lights than anywhere except in Spain, and we were walking along and talking and all of a sudden I noticed that Alice Toklas was looking queer and I said what is it and she said my knees are shaking and I said what is it and she said I just happened to see it, the side of the building. She just had happened to see it, and if you do just happen to see one of those buildings well her knees had not shaken not since the first bomb in 1915 had fallen in Paris so the sky scrapers are something.

So then we went on and people said how do you do nicely and we said how do you do to them and we thought how pleasantly New York was like Bilignin where in the country everybody says how do you do in passing the way they do in any country place in the country and then we saw a fruit store and we went in. How do you do Miss Stein said the man, how do you do, I said, and how do you like it, he said, very much, I said, he said it must be pleasant coming back after thirty years, and I said it certainly was. He was so natural about knowing my name that it was not surprising and yet we had not expected anything like that to happen. If anything is natural enough it is not surprising and then we went out again on an Avenue and the elevated railroad looked just like it had ever so long ago and then we saw an electric sign moving around a building and it said Gertrude Stein has come and that was upsetting. Anybody saying how do you do to you and knowing your name may be upsetting but on the whole it is natural enough but to suddenly see your name is always upsetting. Of course it has happened to me pretty often and I like it to happen just as often but always it does give me a little shock of recognition and non-recognition. It is one of the things most worrying in the subject of identity.

Well anyway we went home to the hotel as the English say the Americans say and so we did always come to say and we went to bed and so after the thirty years we went to sleep in beds in a hotel in America.

The next day was a different thing everything was happening and nothing was as strange as it had been, we could see it and we were looking but it would never be again what yesterday had been.

Lecturing was to begin. Carl Van Vechten had arranged that I was to give one a little privately so as to get used to everything. Thank him.

And then Potter of the university extension of Columbia came to see me and he was a nice man. He had been the first person to ask me to lecture, and this was the university extension of Columbia. We had had a pleasant correspondence and there were to be four lectures and he had described the audience as being a few hundred and after the private lecture this was to be my first one.

He said he was pleased that everybody now that everybody had been so excited at my coming everybody was coming to hear me lecture and that there would be many over a thousand in the audience. I lost everything, I was excited and I said but in that case I would not come. What do you mean, he said, well, I said, I have written these lectures they are hard lectures to read and it will be hard to listen to them, anybody not used to lecturing cannot hold the attention of more than a roomful of that I was certain and I certainly was not going to read a difficult lecture to more than a thousand of them, you said that there would be no more than five hundred and if there are more than that I will not come. But what can I do, said Potter. I do not know anything about that, I said, but if there are more than five hundred there I will not come. Does she mean it, said he perplexedly to Alice Toklas, If she says so, said Alice Toklas, she probably will not come. What can I do, said Potter, I do not know, I said, but I am definitely not going to read a difficult lecture to more than five hundred people, it cannot be done, I said. Well, he said and he was a nice man and he left. Of course I was awfully upset I was to speak the next evening before two hundred and that was bad enough. Carl Van Vechten had arranged all that but here was all this trouble and then I was not accustomed to heated apartments, we heat very sparingly in Paris and beside Paris is moist, the food is dry and the air is moist and in New York the food was moist and the air was dry, so gradually I was certain that there was something the matter with my throat and I would not be able to speak anywhere. Anyway before we went to bed Potter telegraphed, everything arranged I have done the impossible sleep peacefully. And that was over. Nothing is immediately over with me but that was over.

Carl Van Vechten said that they had asked him to introduce me for the first lecture and he did not think I would care to be introduced and I said I would not. And I could refuse him because that would be alright and if I refused him then I could never of course accept any one. Beside it was silly everybody knew who I was if not why did they come and why should I sit and get nervous while somebody else was talking. So it was decided from then on that there would be no introduction nobody on the platform a table for me to lean on and five hundred to listen.

But my throat was not any better and so we telephoned to the nice doctor we had met on the Champlain and he came and he said there was nothing the matter, of course there was nothing the matter but it was a pleasure when he said there was nothing the matter and he gave me something and it was a comfort and I was almost ready to begin lecturing. Many people say you go on being afraid when you are alone on the platform but after the first one I never was again. Not at all.

The wooden houses of America excited me as nothing else in America excited me, the sky-scrapers and the streets of course and everybody knowing you of course but not like the wooden houses everywhere. I never stopped being excited by the wooden houses everywhere. I liked them all. Almost best I liked those near the railway stations old ones not very old ones but still old ones with long flat wooden surfaces, painted sometimes not and many near automobile dumps. I liked them all. I do like a flat surface that is the reason I like pictures and do not like sculpture and I like paint even if it is not painted and wood painted or not painted has the color of paint and it takes paint so much better than plaster. In France and in Spain I like barracks because they have so much flat surface but almost I liked best American wooden houses and there are so many of them an endless number of them and endless varieties in them. It is what in America is very different, each one has something and well taken care of or neglect helps them, helps them to be themselves each one of them. Nobody could get tired of them and then the windows they put in. That is one thing any American can do he can put windows in a building and wherever they are they are interesting. Windows in a building are the most interesting thing in America. It is hard to remember them because they are so interesting. Every wooden house has windows and the windows are put in in a way that is interesting. Of course the sky scrapers it is a wrong name because in America there is no sky there is air but no sky of course that has a lot to do with why there really is no painting in America no real painting but it is not necessary when there are houses and windows and air. Less and less there are curtains and shutters on the windows bye and bye there are not shutters and no curtains at all and that worried me and I asked everybody about that. But the reason is easy enough. Everybody in America is nice and everybody is honest except those who want to break in. If they want to break in shutters will not stop them so why have them and other people looking in, well as everybody is a public something and anybody can know anything about any one and can know any one then why shut the shutters and the curtains and keep any one from seeing, they all know what they are going to see so why look. I gradually began to realise all this.

We went to Cambridge over night and I spoke in Radcliffe and at the Signet Club at Harvard. It was funny about Cambridge it was the one place where there was nothing that I recognised nothing. Considering that I had spent four years there it was sufficiently astonishing that nothing was there that I remembered nothing at all. New York Washington East Oakland Baltimore San Francisco were just about as they were they were changed of course but I could find my way there anywhere but Cambridge not at all. I did not go back again perhaps I might have begun again but that day Cambridge was so different that it was as if I had never been there there was nothing there that had any relation to any place that had been there. I lost Cambridge then and there. That is funny.

In between everything I wandered around the streets of New York. The ten cent stores did disappoint me but the nut stores not. In the ten cent stores there was nothing that I wanted and what there was there was not for ten cents. Alice Toklas says they were not a disappointment but nothing in America was a disappointment to her but they were really they were. But the nut stores I had first known of their existence accidentally from Carl Van Vechten when he happened to say that he one day met Henry McBride as Henry was coming out and Carl was going into a nut store. What is that we had asked excitedly what is a nut store. Then later when he was back in New York he did not forget to send us an ad. of a nut store and now here we were and there they were. I was always looking into them.

I also lectured in Brooklyn and that was interesting it was a nice audience but it was not because of that but because I met Marianne Moore and because an attentive young man accidentally closed the door on my thumb and we had to go into a drug store to have it fixed. It was dirty the drug store, one of the few things really dirty in America are the drug stores but the people in them sitting up and eating and drinking milk and coffee that part of the drug store was clean that fascinated me. After that I was always going in to buy a detective novel just to watch the people sitting on the stools. It was like a piece of provincial life in a real city. The people sitting on the stools and eating in the drug store all looked and acted as if they lived in a small country town. You could not imagine them ever being out in the streets of New York, nor the drug store itself being in New York. I never had enough of going into them.

Then we began to have trouble with Chicago, not with the city but with the arrangements for lecturing. There is always war and peace anywhere and we always have a good deal of both of these things and we proceeded to have them. You have to have peace after war and you have to have war after peace and then there is the tug of war when both sides pull and any side starts then the other side goes, there was a good deal of Chicago I like Chicago. I liked Texas and Chicago. Chicago because we had a good deal of trouble with it and Texas because we had none.

We had said that I would lecture in a university any university for one hundred dollars and mostly well really gradually I liked that best and in Chicago nobody in the university had asked me but still I had been asked. It turned out that some students were arranging it and they were to charge a dollar apiece for anybody and of course I did not want that. If I had wanted that everything would have been different and I did not want that. So the trouble began. Everywhere else it had all been easy but here the trouble began. For the first time they were making arrangements that did not please me and I was beginning to say so, and the long distance telephoning that we had heard that everybody did began. So we went on struggling. I said I would not go unless they arranged it the way we wanted it and there we were.

I had not seen the opera [1] played naturally not because we were not here and now they were to give a ten days of it in Chicago. They telephoned to us would we go but then how could we go. We wanted to go but how could we go it would take too long. We always think that everything takes long. Well it does.

They telephoned there is plenty of time if you come by airplane. Of course we could not do that we telephoned back, why not, they said, because we never have we said, we will pay you your trip the two of you forward and back they said, we want to see the opera we said but we are afraid. Carl Van Vechten was there while all this was going on, what is it, we explained, oh nonsense he said of course you will fly, we telephoned back if Carl Van Vechten can go with us we will fly, alright they telephoned back we will pay for the three of you. Alright we said and we had to do it. Everybody is afraid but some are more afraid than others. Everything can scare me but most of the things that are frightening are things that I can do without and really mostly unless they happen to come unexpectedly do not frighten me. I was much more easily frightened before the war. Since the war nothing is so frightening not the dark nor alone in a room or anything on a road or a dog or a moon but two things yes, indigestion and high places they are frightening. One well one always hopes that that will not happen but high places well there is nothing to do about them. I was not really surprised that being high was not frightening.

It was then in a kind of way that I really began to know what the ground looked like. Quarter sections make a picture and going over America like that made any one know why the post cubist painting was what it was. The wandering line of Masson was there the mixed line of Picasso coming and coming again and following itself into a beginning was there, the simple solution of Braque was there and I suppose Leger might be there but I did

[1] *Four Saints in Three Acts.*

not see it not over there. Particularly the track of a waggon making a perfect circle and then going back to the corner from where they had come and later in the South as finally we went everywhere by air and always wanted the front seat so I could look down and what is the use, the earth does look like that and even if none of them had seen it and they had not very likely had not but since every one was going to see it they had to see it like that.

So we landed in Chicago and there were many there to meet us, and naturally I had to tell them all about it, somebody always took me away and there were always lots of them there, and I always have something to say and I like to say anything I say.

So we went and rested and then we went to hear the opera. I was less excited about that than I had expected to be. It was my opera but it was so far away.

So we flew back again to New York, Carl was not then with us but it was alright, flying was now a natural thing for us to be doing.

In New York that time Alfred Harcourt asked us to come and week end with them and to go and see the Yale Dartmouth football game.

Two things are always the same the dance and war. One might say anything is the same but the dance and war are particularly the same because one can see them.

That is the way it is. Well anyway we liked going with Harcourt to see the football game. First we drove all through New England not all through later on we drove through a great deal more of it but it was our first driving through it in a motor-car.

I was fascinated with the way everybody did what they should. When I first began driving a car myself in Chicago and in California I was surprised at the slowness of the driving, in France you drive much faster, you are supposed not to have accidents but you drive as fast as you like and in America you drive very slowly forty-five miles an hour is slow, and when lights tell you to stop they all stop and they never pass each other going up a hill or around a curve and yet so many get hurt. It was a puzzle to me.

During the war Clemenceau remarked that one of the things that was most striking was the way the nations were not at all as they were supposed to be, the Englishman was noted for his calm and the English soldiers tended more to be hysterical than any other one, the Americans were supposed to be so quick and they were so slow, the French were supposed to be so gay and they were so solemn. A young French soldier who was one of those who taught the American soldiers how to use the French mitrailleuse told me that to his surprise the Americans understood very quickly the mechanics of the gun but their physical reaction in action was very slow very much slower than the French one, consequently it took more Americans to do anything than it did Frenchmen and so of course it was done less quickly. He also told a story of when he posted the Americans as sentry, he told them that when they heard a sound like quack quack it was not a duck it was a german and he said he told them this and they always understood and then when it was the German they did not disappear quickly enough and the German got them.

Well anyway when we were there at the ball-ground everything was orderly and we went in. The players were longer and thinner than I remembered them, both sides were, they did not seem to have such bulky clothing on them, they seem to move more. But there are two things about football that anybody can like. They live by numbers, numbers are everything to them and their preparation is like any savage dancing, they do what red Indians do when they are dancing and their movement is angular like the red Indians move. When they lean over and when they are on their hands and feet and when they are squatting they are like an Indian dance.

As I say it was not a very exciting game and those around us came to know that I was there, a very little boy came from somewhere and he asked me to write my name, I did. And then from everywhere came programs and would I write my name and then there was a man he was very drunk and his wife was coaxing him along I suppose it was his wife and anyway she was coaxing him along and he said he had to see me he just had to see me and I just had to see him, I did see him and he did see me, and then his wife kept coaxing him and slowly he went away.

And then we took a plane again to Chicago. By that time it was winter.

We saw it was winter from the windows of the Drake Hotel. I had not seen winter for many years and Alice Toklas had never seen it. We liked it.

So we went on spending our two weeks in Chicago, the Hutchins asking us to dinner, Bobsy and Barney Goodspeed were to be there and Thornton Wilder.

We went to dinner it was a good dinner. We were at dinner but Hutchins the president of Chicago University was not there later he came in with Mortimer Adler.

Hutchins was tired and we all sat down again together and then he began talking about what he had been doing. He and Adler were having special classes and in them they were talking over all the ideas that had been important in the world's history. Every week they took a new idea and the man who had written it and the class read it and then they had a conversation about it.

What are the ideas that are important I asked him. Here said he is the list of them I took the list and looked it over. Ah I said I noticed that none of the books read at any time by them were originally written in English, was that intentional I asked him. No he said but in English there have really been no ideas expressed. Then I gather that to you there are no ideas which are not sociological or governmental ideas. Well are there he said, well yes I said. Government is the least interesting thing in human life, creation and the expression of that creation is a damn sight more interesting, yes I know and I began to get excited yes I know, naturally you are teachers and teaching is your occupation and naturally what you call ideas are easy to teach and so you are convinced that they are the only ideas but the real ideas are not the relation of human beings as groups but a human being to himself inside him and that is an idea that is more interesting than humanity in groups, after all the minute that there are a lot of them they do not do it for themselves but somebody does it for them and that is a darn sight less interesting. Then Adler began and I have forgotten what the detail of it was but we were saying violent things to each other and I was telling him that anybody could tell by looking that he was a man who would be singularly unsusceptible to ideas that are created within oneself that he would take to either inside or outside regulation but not to creation, and Hutchins was saying well if you can improve upon what we are doing I challenge you to do it take our class next week and I said of course I will and then Adler said something and I was standing next to him and violently telling him and everybody was excited and the maid came and said Madame the police. Adler went a little white and we all stopped and then burst out laughing. Fanny Butcher had arranged that Alice Toklas and I should go off that evening in the homicidal squad car and they had come and there they were waiting. Well we all said good-night and we went off with the policemen.

We drove around, we had just missed one homicide it was the only one that happened that evening and it had not been interesting it had been a family affair and everybody could understand everything. The sergeant said he was afraid not much would happen, it was raining and when it rained nobody moved around and if nobody moved around there could not be any homicide unless it was a family affair as this one had been and that was not interesting some day he said when it was a really nice night I will let you know and then you will see something but we did like that night when nothing was happening and we did not stay long enough in Chicago to have a nice night.

So we stayed our two weeks in Chicago and Mrs. Goodspeed took us to the opera and to concerts, one of them was Lohengrin and the other was Salome.

And then the Hutchins asked us to come and nobody was to

know anything not even Thornton or Mrs. Goodspeed and we went to dinner and then I went to take over their class with them.

So we all sat around a long table and Hutchins and Adler and I presiding, at least we were not to be but there we were as if we were, well anyway I began talking.

I began to talk and they not Hutchins and Adler but the others began to talk and pretty soon we were all talking about epic poetry and what it was it was exciting we found out a good deal some of it I used in one of the four lectures I wrote for the course I came back to give them but it was all that after all in epic poetry you can have an epic because the death of the man meant the end of everything and now nothing is ending by the death of any one because something is already happening. Well we all came out and they liked it and I liked it and Hutchins said to me as he and I were walking, you did make them all talk more than we can make them and a number of them talked who never talked before and it was very nice of him to say it and he added and if you will come back I will be glad to have you do some teaching and I said I would and he said he would let me know and then I said you see why they talk to me is that I am like them I do not know the answer, you you say you do not know but you do know if you did not know the answer you could not spend your life in teaching but I I really do not know, I really do not, I do not even know whether there is a question let alone having an answer for a question. To me when a thing is really interesting it is when there is no question and no answer, if there is then already the subject is not interesting and it is so, that is the reason that anything for which there is a solution is not interesting, that is the trouble with governments and Utopias and teaching, the things not that can be learnt but that can be taught are not interesting. Well anyway we went away.

It was winter and it went on being winter and we went away to places where we had never been, we went to Wisconsin and Ohio and Indiana and Minnesota and Michigan. We went to Minneapolis. It was still winter but not as winter as it had been in Wisconsin.

It was at this time that my real interest in reporters began. Reporters are mostly young college men who are interested in writing and naturally I was interested in talking with them. Once it may have been in Cleveland or Indianapolis I was talking there were two or three of them and a photographer with them and I said you know it is funny but the photographer is the one of the lot of you who looks as if he were intelligent and was listening now why is that, you do I said to the photographer you do understand what I am talking about dont you. Of course I do he said you see I can listen to what you say because I dont have to remember what you are saying, they cant listen because they have got to remember.

I liked the photographers, there is one who came in and said he was sent to do a lay out of me. A lay out, I said yes he said what is that I said oh he said it is four or five pictures of you doing anything. Alright I said what do you want me to do. Why he said there is your airplane bag suppose you unpack it, Oh I said Miss Toklas always does that oh no I could not do that, well he said there is the telephone suppose you telephone well I said yes but I never do Miss Toklas always does that, well he said what can you do, well I said I can take my hat on and take my hat off and I can put my coat on and I can take it off and I like water I can drink a glass of water alright he said do that so I did that and he photographed while I did that and the next morning there was the lay out and I had done it.

So we went on lecturing at colleges and even in schools in New England. I lectured in mens colleges and in womens colleges, the mens I liked best was Wesleyan, and after the lecture I liked talking to the Wesleyan men. We talked about and that has always been a puzzle to me why American men think that success is everything when they know that eighty per cent of them are not going to succeed more than to just keep going and why if they are not why they do not keep on being interested in the things that interested them when they were college men and why American men different from English American men do not get more interesting as they get older. We talked about that a lot at Wesleyan. Then I liked Mount Holyoke, I liked that the best of the womens colleges in New England, we talked there mostly about the theatre and as they were really interested it was interesting. Afterwards it seemed rather strange to me that the two colleges which were really made to make missionaries were more interesting than those that had been made to make culture and the other professions. It made me wonder a lot about what it is to be American.

I went to the Choate school and they were charming to me. The boys from twelve to sixteen listened really listened to everything I had to say and I talked to them about whether one's contemporaries were really contemporary. And then later the next morning we had a talk about that. I had been much struck by the Choate school literary magazine which did have extraordinary good writing in it, and now the Utica High School has sent me a Gertrude Stein number and again it is striking how well they are writing. It is a bother.

Once long ago René Crevel and I talked about education. I said that french boys believed in the teaching of their teachers. American boys did not. Later on I talked with François d'Aiguy about this. He said french boys who went to the lycées which are controlled by the government did believe in what the teachers believed, and therefore they never did revolt, but boys who went to what in France they call a boîte, a box that is to the religious schools, the catholic schools, they did not have to believe what the teachers believe, they could and did believe in Catholicism but they did not have to believe what the teacher believed and so they did have some intellectual freedom. I said to the Choate teachers I wonder if the boys can ever come to be themselves because you are all so reasonable and so sweet to them that inevitably they are convinced too soon. Is not that the trouble with American education that if they are to be convinced at all they are convinced too soon is it not the trouble with any republican education. Other than republican education does not convince them so most of them do not have any conviction and the few who have are not convinced too soon.

When I first heard about Oklahoma I always thought it was in the northwest, until I really saw it and saw it so close to Texas did I really believe that it is where it does exist. Oklahoma City with its towers that is its sky scrapers coming right up out of the flat oil country was as exciting as when going to Alsace just after the armistice we first saw the Strasbourg cathedral. They do come up wonderfully out of that flat country and it was exciting and seeing the oil wells and the funny shapes they made the round things as well as the Eiffel tower ones gave me a feeling like I have in going to Marseilles and seeing the chimneys come out of the earth and there are no houses or anything near them, it always is a strange looking country that produces that kind of thing, of course Alice Toklas' father had once almost had an oil well they dug and dug but naturally the oil did not gush, naturally not these things never do happen to any one one knows, if it could happen to them you would not be very likely to know them most naturally not. We did later see in California some small oil fields and the slow movement of the oil wells make it perfectly alright that in America the prehistoric beasts moved slowly. America is funny that way everything is quick but really everybody does move slowly, and the movement of the oil well that slow movement very well that slow movement is the country and it makes it prehistoric and large shapes and moving slowly very very slowly so slowly that they do almost stand still. I do think Americans are slow minded, it seems quick but they are slow minded yes they are.

We were to go to dinner at Beverly Hills which is the same as Hollywood this I have said we were to meet Dashiell Hammett and Charlie Chaplin and Anita Loos and her husband and Mamoulian who was directing everything and we did. Of course I liked Charlie Chaplin he is a gentle person like any Spanish gypsy bullfighter he is very like my favorite one Gallo who could not kill a bull but he could make him move better than any one ever could and he himself not having any grace in person could move one as no one else ever did, and Charlie Chaplin was like Gallo. Gypsies are intelligent I do not think Charlie Chaplin is one perhaps not but he might have been, anyway we naturally talked about the cinema, and he explained something. He said naturally it was disappointing, he had known the silent films and in that they could do something that the theatre had not done they could change the rhythm but if you had a voice accompanying naturally after that you could never change the rhythm you were always held by the rhythm that the voice gave them. We talked a little about the Four Saints and what my idea had been, I said that what was most exciting was when nothing was happening, I said that saints should naturally do nothing if you were a saint that was enough and a saint existing was everything, if you made them do anything then there was nothing to it they were just like any one so I wanted to write a drama where no one did anything where there was no action and I had and it was the Four Saints and it was exciting, he said yes he could understand that, I said the films would become like the newspapers just a daily habit and not at all exciting or interesting, after all the business of an artist is to be really exciting and he is only exciting when nothing is happening, if anything happens then it is like any other one, after all Hamlet Shakespeare's most interesting play has really nothing happening except that they live and die but it is not that that is interesting and I said I was sure that it is true that an interesting thing is when there is nothing happening, I said that the moon excited dogs because it did nothing, lights coming and going do not excite them and now that they have seen so many of them the poor things can no longer see the moon and so no lights can excite them, well we did not say all this but that is what we meant, he wanted the sentiment of movement invented by himself and I wanted the sentiment of doing nothing invented by myself, anyway we both liked talking but each one had to stop to be polite and let the other say something. After dinner they all gathered around me and asked me what I thought of the cinema, I told them what I had been telling Charlie Chaplin, it seemed to worry them and at last I found out what was bothering them they wanted to know how I had succeeded in getting so much publicity, I said by having a small audience, I said if you have a big audience you have no publicity, this seemed to worry them and naturally it would worry them they wanted the publicity and the big audience, and really to have the biggest publicity you have to have a small one, yes alright the biggest publicity comes from the reallest poetry and the reallest poetry has a small audience not a big one, but it is really exciting and therefore it has the biggest publicity, alright that is it. Well after a little while we left, it had been an amusing evening.

We went to Berkeley and they had invited me I think it was the Phi Beta Kappa to lunch, and during the lunch there were a lot of them there everybody asked a question not everybody but a good many, they thought I answered them very well the only thing I remember is their asking why I do not write as I talk and I said to them if they had invited Keats for lunch and they asked him an ordinary question would they expect him to answer with the Ode To The Nightingale. It is funny everybody knows but of course everybody knows that writing poetry that writing anything is a private matter and of course if you do it in private then it is not what you do in public. We used to say when we were children if you do it in private you will do it in public and we did not then say if you do it in public you will do it in private. Well anyway when you say what you do say you say it in public but when you write what you do write you write it in private if not you do not write it, that is what writing is, and in private you are you and in public you are in public and everybody knows that, just read Webster's Mr. and Mrs. everybody knows that but when they ask questions well then they are neither public nor private they are just fat-headed yes yes. That is what Virgil Thomson says yes yes. What is the use of asking questions, either you know your answer or you do not, mostly you do know your answer and certainly any question has no answer so why question the answer or answer the question.

And so we took the airplane to go back to Chicago we stopped at Omaha and really we did not stop in Chicago only for the night and then we went on back to New York. The Rockefeller Center building was finished it all was a pleasure and that was a pleasure and they all seemed as pleased to see me as they had been, Alice Toklas said they now said there goes Miss Stein before they had said there goes Gertrude Stein well anyway having them say it was still a pleasure and then everything was all over and we got on the Champlain to go back to Paris again.

Before we went on the Champlain I asked Bennett Cerf about my writing, I always want what I have written to be printed and it has not always happened no not mostly happened and now I timidly said something to him, he said it is very simple whatever you decide each year you want printed you tell me and I will publish that thing, just like that I said, just like that, he said, you do the deciding, and so we happily very happily went on to the Champlain.

Suggestions for Study

THIS SELECTION is more "normal" than a good deal of Gertrude Stein's prose. The words are chosen for their meanings (not for their rhythm and sound, as they were when she was chiefly interested, she said, in arousing feelings), and there is none of that elaborate play of rhythmic repetition of phrase which exasperated readers who were looking for effects that they had been used to in conventional literature, and who were reluctant to allow to Gertrude Stein the syntactical freedom that they readily granted to Shakespeare. In punctuation and sentence structure, however, the passage is unconventional. The sentences are, presumably, intended to suggest the movement of the mind as it "closes in" on thought. (The expression is Mr. Wilder's, in a short and sensible article in the October issue of '47.) The punctuation can best be explained in Gertrude Stein's own words: "A long complicated sentence should force itself upon you, make you know yourself knowing it and the comma, well at most a comma is a poor period that lets you stop and take a breath but if you want to take a breath you ought to know yourself that you want to take a breath." [1]

Mr. Wilder says that Gertrude Stein once replied to the objections of a friend, "But what's the difficulty? Just read the words on the paper. They're in English. Just read them. Be simple and you'll understand these things." This may explain how to read such paragraphs as those on Miss Toklas' reaction to skyscrapers and on the airplane ride to Chicago. But a reader should remember that in our time it is difficult to write simply about the simple (compare what Mrs. Woolf has to say about Chaucer's poetry in "The Pastons and Chaucer"), and that even the simplest response of an original mind like Gertrude Stein's is likely to be unconventional and therefore hard to describe and equally hard to understand, because the writer cannot fall back on the stock phrases that evoke stock responses.

Gertrude Stein had a considerable influence on many modern writers. Can you find evidence of this influence in other selections in the book? (Since Gertrude Stein's style was a powerful one, you may feel its influence. Before you try to imitate it, be sure you know what she was trying to do, and be sure that what you want to do needs a style like hers.)

What was Gertrude Stein saying about America in the paragraphs on the wooden houses, on the drugstores, on the flight to Chicago, and on the movies?

Analyze Gertrude Stein's criticism of American education.

[1] Quoted in *Current Expressions of Fact and Opinion*, edited by Harrison G. Platt, Jr., and Porter G. Perrin (Chicago, 1941), p. 427.

Cagliari

D. H. LAWRENCE (1885–1930)

There is a very little crowd waiting on the quay: mostly men with their hands in their pockets. But, thank Heaven, they have a certain aloofness and reserve. They are not like the tourist-parasites of these post-war days, who move to the attack with a terrifying cold vindictiveness the moment one emerges from any vehicle. And some of these men look really poor. There are no poor Italians any more: at least, loafers.

Strange the feeling round the harbour: as if everybody had gone away. Yet there are people about. It is "festa" however, Epiphany. But it is so different from Sicily: none of the suave Greek-Italian charms, none of the airs and graces, none of the glamour. Rather bare, rather stark, rather cold and yellow—somehow like Malta, without Malta's foreign liveliness. Thank Goodness no one wants to carry my knapsack. Thank Goodness no one has a fit at the sight of it. Thank Heaven no one takes any notice. They stand cold and aloof, and don't move.

We make our way through the Customs: then through the Dazio, the City Customs-house. Then we are free. We set off up a steep, new, broad road, with little trees on either side. But stone, arid, new, wide stone, yellowish under the cold sky—and abandoned-seeming. Though, of course, there are people about. The north wind blows bitingly.

We climb a broad flight of steps, always upwards, up the wide, precipitous, dreary boulevard with sprouts of trees. Looking for the Hotel, and dying with hunger.

At last we find it, the Scala di Ferro: through a courtyard with green plants. And at last a little man with lank, black hair, like an esquimo, comes smiling. He is one brand of Sardinian—esquimo looking. There is no room with two beds: only single rooms. And thus we are led off, if you please, to the "bagnio": the bathing-establishment wing, on the dank ground floor. Cubicles on either side a stone passage, and in every cubicle a dark stone bath, and a little bed. We can have each a little bath cubicle. If there's nothing else for it, there isn't: but it seems dank and cold and horrid, underground. And one thinks of all the unsavory "assignations" at these old bagnio places. True, at the end of the passage are seated two carabinieri. But whether to ensure respectability or not, Heaven knows. We are in the baths, that's all.

The esquimo returns after five minutes, however. There *is* a bedroom in the house. He is pleased, because he didn't like putting us into the bagnio. Where he found the bedroom I don't know. But there it was, large, sombre, cold, and over the kitchen fumes of a small inner court like a well. But perfectly clean and all right. And the people seemed warm and good-natured, like human beings. One has got so used to the non-human ancient-souled Sicilians, who are suave and so completely callous.

After a really good meal we went out to see the town. It was after three o'clock and everywhere was shut up like an English Sunday. Cold, stony Cagliari: in summer you must be sizzling hot, Cagliari, like a kiln. The men stood about in groups, but without the intimate Italian watchfulness that never leaves a passer-by alone.

Strange, stony Cagliari. We climbed up a street like a corkscrew stairway. And we saw announcements of a children's fancy-dress ball. Cagliari is very steep. Half-way up there is a strange place called the bastions, a large, level space like a drill-ground with trees, curiously suspended over the town, and sending off a long shoot like a wide viaduct, across above the corkscrew street that comes climbing up. Above this bastion place the town still rises steeply to the Cathedral and the fort. What is so curious is that this terrace or bastion is so large, like some big recreation ground, that it is almost dreary, and one cannot understand its being suspended in mid-air. Down below is the little circle of the harbour. To the left a low, malarial-looking sea plain, with tufts of palm trees and Arab-looking houses. From this runs out the long spit of land towards that black-and-white watch-fort, the white road trailing forth. On the right, most curiously, a long strange spit of sand runs in a causeway far across the shallows of the bay, with the open sea on one hand, and vast, end-of-the-world lagoons on the other. There are peaky, dark mountains beyond this—just as across the vast bay are gloomy hills. It is a strange, strange landscape: as if here the world left off. The bay is vast in itself; and all these curious things happening at its head: this curious, craggy-studded town, like a great stud of house-covered rock jutting up out of the bay flats: around it on one side the weary, Arab-looking palm-desolated malarial plain, and on the other side great salt lagoons, dead beyond the sand-bar: these backed again by serried, clustered mountains, suddenly, while away beyond the plain, hills rise to sea again. Land and sea both seem to give out, exhausted, at the bay head: the world's end. And into this world's end starts up Cagliari, and on either side, sudden, serpent-crest hills.

But it still reminds me of Malta: lost between Europe and Africa and belonging to nowhere. Belonging to nowhere, never having belonged to anywhere. To Spain and the Arabs and the Phœnicians most. But as if it had never really had a fate. No fate. Left outside of time and history.

The spirit of the place is a strange thing. Our mechanical age tries to override it. But it does not succeed. In the end the strange, sinister spirit of the place, so diverse and adverse in differing places, will smash our mechanical oneness into smithereens, and all that we think the real thing will go off with a pop, and we shall be left staring.

On the great parapet above the Municipal Hall and above the corkscrew high-street a thick fringe of people is hanging, looking down. We go to look too: and behold, below there is the entrance to the ball. Yes, there is a china shepherdess in pale blue and powdered hair, crook, ribbons, Marie Antoinette satin daintiness and all, slowly and haughtily walking up the road, and gazing superbly round. She is not more than twelve years old, moreover. Two servants accompany her. She gazes supremely from right to left as she goes, mincingly, and I would give her the prize for haughtiness. She is perfect—a little too haughty for Watteau, but "marquise" to a T. The people watch in silence. There is no yelling and screaming and running. They watch in a suitable silence.

Comes a carriage with two fat bay horses slithering, almost swimming up the corkscrew high-street. That in itself is a "tour-de-force": for Cagliari doesn't have carriages. Imagine a street like a corkscrew stair, paved with slippery stone. And imagine two bay horses rowing their way up it: they did not walk a single stride. But they arrived. And there fluttered out three strangely exquisite children, two frail, white satin Pierrots and a white satin Pierrette. They were like fragile winter butterflies with black spots. They had a curious, indefinable remote elegance, something conventional and "fin-de-siècle." But not our century. The wonderful artificial delicacy of the eighteenth. The boys had big, perfect ruffs round their necks: and behind were slung old, cream-colored Spanish shawls, for warmth. They were frail as tobacco flowers, and with remote, cold elegance they fluttered by the carriage, from which emerged a large black-satin Mama. Fluttering their queer little butterfly feet on the pavement, hovering round the large Mama like three frail-tissued ghosts, they found their way past the solid, seated Carabinieri into the hall.

Arrived a primrose-brocade beau, with ruffles, and his hat under his arm: about twelve years old. Walking statelily, without a qualm up the steep twist of the street. Or perhaps so perfect in his self-consciousness that it became an elegant "aplomb" in him. He was a genuine eighteenth-century exquisite, rather stiffer than the French, maybe, but completely in the spirit. Curious, curious children! They had a certain stand-offish superbness, and not a single trace of misgiving. For them, their "noblesse" was indisputable. For the first time in my life I recognized the true cold superbness of the old "noblesse." They had not a single qualm about their own perfect representing of the higher order of being.

Followed another white satin "marquise," with a maid-servant. They are strong on the eighteenth century in Cagliari. Perhaps it is the last bright reality to them. The nineteenth hardly counts.

Curious the children in Cagliari. The poor seem thoroughly poor-bare-footed urchins, gay and wild in the narrow dark streets. But the more well-to-do children are so fine: so extraordinarily elegantly dressed. It quite strikes one of a heap. Not so much the grown-ups. The children. All the "chic," all the fashion, all the originality is expended on the children. And with a great deal of success. Better than Kensington Gardens very often. And they promenade with Papa and Mama with such alert assurance, having quite brought it off, their fashionable get-up. Who would have expected it?

Oh narrow, dark, and humid streets going up to the Cathedral, like crevices. I narrowly miss a huge pail of slop-water which comes crashing down from heaven. A small boy who was playing in the street, and whose miss is not quite a clean miss, looks up with that naïve, impersonal wonder with which children stare at a star or a lamp-lighter.

The Cathedral must have been a fine old pagan stone fortress once. Now it has come, as it were, through the mincing machine of the ages, and oozed out baroque and sausagey, a bit like the horrible baldachins in St. Peter's at Rome. None the less it is homely and hole-and-cornery, with a rather ragged high mass trailing across the pavement towards the high altar, since it is almost sunset, and Epiphany. It feels as if one might squat in a corner and play marbles and eat bread and cheese and be at home: a comfortable old-time churchey feel.

There is some striking filet lace on the various altar-cloths. And St. Joseph must be a prime saint. He has an altar and a verse of invocation praying for the dying.

"Oh, St. Joseph, true potential father of Our Lord." What can it profit a man, I wonder, to be the potential father of anybody! For the rest I am not Baedeker.

The top of Cagliari is the fortress: the old gate, the old ramparts, of honey-combed, fine yellowish sandstone. Up in a great sweep goes the rampart wall, Spanish and splendid, dizzy. And the road creeping down again at the foot, down the back of the hill. There lies the country: that dead plain with its bunch of palms and a fainting sea, and inland again, hills. Cagliari must be on a single, loose, lost bluff of rock.

From the terrace just below the fortress, above the town, not behind it, we stand and look at the sunset. It is all terrible, taking place beyond the knotted, serpent-crested hills that lie, bluey and velvety, beyond the waste lagoons. Dark, sultry, heavy crimson the west is, hanging sinisterly, with those gloomy blue cloud-bars and cloud-banks drawn across. All behind the blue-gloomy peaks stretches the curtain of sinister, smouldering red, and away to the sea. Deep below lie the sea-meres. They seem miles and miles, and utterly waste. But the sand-bar crosses like a bridge, and has a road. All the air is dark, a sombre bluish tone. The great west burns inwardly, sullenly, and gives no glow, yet a deep red. It is cold.

We go down the steep streets, smelly, dark, dank, and very cold. No wheeled vehicle can scramble up them, presumably. People live in one room. Men are combing their hair or fastening their collars in the doorways. Evening is here, and it is a feast day.

At the bottom of the street we come to a little bunch of masked youths, one in a long yellow frock and a frilled bonnet, another like an old woman, another in red twill. They are arm in arm and are accosting the passers-by. The q-b [1] gives a cry, and looks for escape. She has a terror of maskers, a terror that comes from childhood. To say the truth, so have I. We hasten invisibly down the far side of the street, and come out under the bastions. Then we go down our own familiar wide, short, cold boulevard to the sea.

At the bottom, again, is a carriage with more maskers. Carnival is beginning. A man dressed as a peasant woman in native costume is clambering with his great wide skirts and wide strides on to the box, and, flourishing his ribboned whip, is addressing a little crowd of listeners. He opens his mouth wide and goes on with a long yelling harangue of taking a drive with his mother—another man in old-woman's gaudy finery and wig who sits already bobbing on the box. The would-be daughter flourishes, yells, and prances up there on the box of the carriage. The crowd listens attentively and mildly smiles. It all seems real to them. The q-b hovers in the distance, half-fascinated, and watches. With a great flourish of whip and legs—showing his frilled drawers—the masker pulls round to drive along the boulevard by the sea—the only place where one can drive.

The big street by the sea is the Via Roma. It has the cafés on one side and across the road the thick tufts of trees intervening between the sea and us. Among these thick tufts of sea-front trees the little steam tram, like a little train, bumps to rest, after having wound round the back of the town.

The Via Roma is all social Cagliari. Including the cafés with their outdoor tables on the one side of the road, and the avenue

[1] *Editors' note:* q-b: The queen-bee, Lawrence's wife.

strand on the other, it is very wide, and at evening it contains the whole town. Here, and here alone carriages can spank along, very slowly, officers can ride, and the people can promenade "en masse."

We were amazed at the sudden crowd we found ourselves amongst—like a short, dense river of people streaming slowly in a mass. There is practically no vehicular traffic—only the steady dense streams of human beings of all sorts, all on a human footing. It must have been something like this in the streets of imperial Rome, where no chariots might drive and humanity was all on foot.

Little bunches of maskers, and single maskers danced and strutted along in the thick flow under the trees. If you are a mask you don't walk like a human being: you dance and prance along extraordinaryily like the life-size marionettes, conducted by wires from above. That is how you go: with that odd jauntiness as if lifted and propelled by wires from the shoulders. In front of me went a charming coloured harlequin, all in diamond-shaped colours, and beautiful as a piece of china. He tripped with the light, fantastic trip, quite alone in the thick crowd, and quite blithe. Came two little children hand in hand in brilliant scarlet and white costumes sauntering calmly. They did not do the mask trip. After a while a sky-blue girl with a high hat and full skirts, very short, that went flip-flip-flip, as a ballet dancer's, whilst she strutted; after her a Spanish grandee capering like a monkey. They threaded among the slow stream of the crowd. Appeared Dante and Beatrice, in Paradise apparently, all in white sheet-robes, and with silver wreaths on their heads, arm in arm, and prancing very slowly and majestically, yet with the long lilt as if hitched along by wires from above. They were very good: all the well-known vision come to life, Dante incorporate, and white as a shroud, with his tow-haired, silver-crowned, immortal Beatrice on his arm, strutting the dark avenues. He had the nose and cheek-bones and banded cheek, and the stupid wooden look, and offered a modern criticism on the Inferno.

It had become quite dark, the lamps were lighted. We crossed the road to the Café Roma, and found a table on the pavement among the crowd. In a moment we had our tea. The evening was cold, with ice in the wind. But the crowd surged on, back and forth, back and forth, slowly. At the tables were seated mostly men, taking coffee or vermouth or aqua vitae, all familiar and easy, without the modern self-consciousness. There was a certain pleasant, natural robustness of spirit, and something of a feudal free-and-easiness. Then arrived a family, with children, and nurse in her native costume. They all sat at table together, perfectly easy with one another, though the marvellous nurse seemed to be seated below the salt. She was bright as a poppy, in a rose-scarlet dress of fine cloth, with a curious little waistcoat of emerald green and purple, and a bodice of soft, homespun linen with great full sleeves. On her head she had a rose-scarlet and white head-dress, and she wore great studs of gold filigree, and similar ear-rings. The feudal-bourgeois family drank its syrup-drinks and watched the crowd. Most remarkable is the complete absence of self-consciousness. They all have a perfect natural "sang-froid," the nurse in her marvellous native costume is as thoroughly at her ease as if she were in her own village street. She moves and speaks and calls to a passer-by without the slightest constraint, and much more, without the slightest presumption. She is below the invisible salt, the invisible but insuperable salt. And it strikes me the salt-barrier is a fine thing for both parties: they both remain natural and human on either side of it, instead of becoming devilish, scrambling and pushing at the barricade.

The crowd is across the road, under the trees near the sea. On this side stroll occasional pedestrians. And I see my first peasant in costume. He is an elderly, upright, handsome man, beautiful in the black-and-white costume. He wears the full-sleeved white shirt and the close black bodice of thick, native frieze, cut low. From this sticks out a short kilt or frill, of the same black frieze, a band of which goes between the legs, between the full loose drawers of coarse linen. The drawers are banded below the knee into tight black frieze gaiters. On his head he has the long black stocking cap, hanging down behind. How handsome he is, and so beautifully male! He walks with his hands loose behind his back, slowly, upright, and aloof. The lovely unapproachableness, indomitable. And the flash of the black and white, the slow stride of the full white drawers, the black gaiters and black cuirass with the bolero, then the great white sleeves and white breast again, and once more the black cap—what marvellous massing of the contrast, marvellous, and superb, as on a magpie.—How beautiful maleness is, if it finds its right expression.—And how perfectly ridiculous it is made in modern clothes.

There is another peasant too, a young one with a swift eye and hard cheek and hard, dangerous thighs. He has folded his stocking cap, so that it comes forward to his brow like a phrygian cap. He wears close knee breeches and close sleeved waistcoat of thick brownish stuff that looks like leather. Over the waistcoat a sort of cuirass of black, rusty sheepskin, the curly wool outside. So he strides, talking to a comrade. How fascinating it is, after the soft Italians, to see these limbs in their close knee-breeches, so definite, so manly, with the old fierceness in them still. One realises, with horror, that the race of men is almost extinct in Europe. Only Christ-like heroes and woman-worshipping Don Juans, and rabid equality-mongrels. The old, hardy, indomitable male is gone. His fierce singleness is quenched. The last sparks are dying out in Sardinia and Spain. Nothing left but the herd-proletariat and the herd-equality mongrelism, and the wistful poisonous self-sacrificial cultured soul. How detestable.

But that curious, flashing, black-and-white costume! I seem to have known it before: to have worn it even: to have dreamed it. To have dreamed it: to have had actual contact with it. It belongs in some way to something in me—to my past, perhaps. I don't know. But the uneasy sense of blood-familiarity haunts me. I *know* I have known it before. It is something of the same uneasiness I feel before Mount Eryx: but without the awe this time.

In the morning the sun was shining from a blue, blue sky, but the shadows were deadly cold, and the wind like a flat blade of ice. We went out running to the sun. The hotel could not give us coffee and milk: only a little black coffee. So we descended to the sea-front again, to the Via Roma, and to our café. It was Friday: people seemed to be bustling in from the country with huge baskets.

The Café Roma had coffee and milk, but no butter. We sat and watched the movement outside. Tiny Sardinian donkeys, the tiniest things ever seen, trotted their infinitesimal little paws along the road, drawing little wagons like handcarts. Their proportion is so small, that they make a boy walking at their side look like a tall man, while a natural man looks like a Cyclops stalking hugely and cruelly. It is ridiculous for a grown man to have one of these little creatures, hardly bigger than a fly, hauling his load for him. One is pulling a chest of drawers on a cart, and it seems to have a whole house behind it. Nevertheless it plods bravely, away beneath the load, a wee thing.

They tell me there used to be flocks of these donkeys, feeding half wild on the wild, moor-like hills of Sardinia. But the war—and also the imbecile wantonness of the war-masters—consumed these flocks too, so that few are left. The same with the cattle. Sardinia, home of cattle, hilly little Argentine of the Mediterranean, is now almost deserted. It is war, say the Italiana.—And also the wanton, imbecile, foul lavishness of the war-masters. It was not alone the war which exhausted the world. It was the deliberate evil wastefulness of the war-makers in their own countries. Italy ruined Italy.

Two peasants in black-and-white are strolling in the sun, flashing. And my dream of last evening was not a dream. And my nostalgia for something I know not what was not an illusion. I feel it again, at once, at the sight of the men in frieze and linen, a heart yearning for something I have known, and which I want back again.

It is market day. We turn up the Largo Carlo-Felice, the second wide gap of a street, a vast but very short boulevard, like the end of something. Cagliari is like that: all bits and bobs. And by the side of the pavement are many stalls, stalls selling combs and collar-studs, cheap mirrors, handkerchiefs, shoddy Manchester goods, bed-ticking, boot-paste, poor crockery, and so on. But we see also Madame of Cagliari going marketing, with a servant accompanying her, carrying a huge grass-woven basket: or returning from marketing, followed by a small boy supporting one of these huge grass-woven baskets—like huge dishes—on his head, piled with bread, eggs, vegetables, a chicken, and so forth. Therefore we follow Madame going marketing, and find ourselves in the vast market house, and it fairly glows with eggs: eggs in these great round dish-baskets of golden grass: but eggs in piles, in mounds, in heaps, a Sierra Nevada of eggs, glowing warm white. How they glow! I have never noticed it before. But they give off a warm, pearly effulgence into the air, almost a warmth. A pearly-gold heat seems to come out of them. Myriads of eggs, glowing avenues of eggs.

And they are marked—60 centimes, 65 centimes. Ah, cries the q-b, I must live in Cagliari—For in Sicily the eggs cost 1.50 each.

This is the meat and poultry and bread market. There are stalls of new, various-shaped bread, brown and bright: there are tiny stalls of marvellous native cakes, which I want to taste, there is a great deal of meat and kid: and there are stalls of cheese, all cheeses, all shapes, all whitenesses, all the cream-colours, on into daffodil yellow. Goat cheese, sheeps cheese, Swiss cheese, Parmegiano, stracchino, caciocavallo, torolone, how many cheeses I don't know the names of! But they cost about the same as in Sicily, eighteen francs, twenty francs, twenty-five francs the kilo. And there is lovely ham—thirty and thirty-five francs the kilo. There is a little fresh butter too—thirty or thirty-two francs the kilo. Most of the butter, however, is tinned in Milan. It costs the same as the fresh. There are splendid piles of salted black olives, and huge bowls of green salted olives. There are chickens and ducks and wild-fowl: at eleven and twelve and fourteen francs a kilo. There is mortadella, the enormous Bologna sausage, thick as a church pillar: 16 francs: and there are various sorts of smaller sausage, salami, to be eaten in slices. A wonderful abundance of food, glowing and shining. We are rather late for fish, especially on Friday. But a barefooted man offers us two weird objects from the Mediterranean, which teems with marine monsters.

The peasant women sit behind their wares, their home-woven linen skirts, hugely full, and of various colours, ballooning round them. The yellow baskets give off a glow of light. There is a sense of profusion once more. But alas no sense of cheapness: save the eggs. Every month, up goes the price of everything.

"I must come and live in Cagliari, to do my shopping here," says the q-b. "I must have one of those big grass baskets."

We went down to the little street—but saw more baskets emerging from a broad flight of stone stairs, enclosed. So up we went—and found ourselves in the vegetable market. Here the q-b was happier still. Peasant women, sometimes barefoot, sat in their tight little bodices and voluminous, coloured skirts behind the piles of vegetables, and never have I seen a lovelier show. The intense deep green of spinach seemed to predominate, and out of that came the monuments of curd-white and black-purple cauliflowers: but marvellous cauliflowers, like a flower-show, the purple ones intense as great bunches of violets. From this green, white, and purple massing struck out the vivid rose-scarlet and blue crimson of radishes, large radishes like little turnips, in piles. Then the long, slim, grey-purple buds of artichokes, and dangling clusters of dates, and piles of sugar-dusty white figs and sombre-looking black figs, and bright burnt figs: basketfuls and basketfuls of figs. A few baskets of almonds, and many huge walnuts. Basket-pans of native raisins. Scarlet peppers like trumpets: magnificent fennels, so white and big and succulent: baskets of new potatoes: scaly kohlrabi: wild asparagus in bunches, yellow-budding sparacelli: big, clean-fleshed carrots: feathery salads with white hearts: long, brown-purple onions and then, of course pyramids of big oranges, pyramids of pale apples, and baskets of brilliant shiny mandarini, the little tangerine oranges with their green-black leaves. The green and vivid-coloured world of fruit-gleams I have never seen in such splendour as under the market roof at Cagliari: so raw and gorgeous. And all quite cheap, the one remaining cheapness, except potatoes. Potatoes of any sort are 1.40 or 1.50 the kilo.

"Oh!" cried the q-b, "If I don't live at Cagliari and come and do my shopping here, I shall die with one of my wishes unfulfilled."

But out of the sun it was cold, nevertheless. We went into the streets to try and get warm. The sun was powerful. But alas, as in southern towns generally, the streets are sunless as wells.

So the q-b and I creep slowly along the sunny bits, and then perforce are swallowed by shadow. We look at the shops. But there is not much to see. Little, frowsy provincial shops, on the whole.

But a fair number of peasants in the streets, and peasant women in rather ordinary costume: tight-bodiced, volume-skirted dresses of hand-woven linen or thickish cotton. The prettiest is of dark-blue-and-red, stripes-and-lines, intermingled, so made that the dark-blue gathers round the waist into one colour, the myriad pleats hiding all the rosy red. But when she walks, the full-petticoated peasant woman, then the red goes flash-flash-flash, like a bird showing its colours. Pretty that looks in the sombre street. She has a plain, light bodice with a peak: sometimes a little vest, and great full white sleeves, and usually a handkerchief or shawl loose knotted. It is charming the way they walk, with quick, short steps. When all is said and done, the most attractive costume for women in my eye, is the tight little bodice and the many-pleated skirt, full and vibrating with movement. It has a charm which modern elegance lacks completely—a bird-like play in movement.

They are amusing, these peasant girls and women: so brisk and defiant. They have straight backs, like little walls, and decided, well-drawn brows. And they are amusingly on the alert. There is no eastern creeping. Like sharp, brisk birds they dart along the streets, and you feel they would fetch you a bang over the head as leave as look at you. Tenderness, thank heaven, does not seem to be a Sardinian quality. Italy is so tender—like cooked macaroni—yards and yards of soft tenderness ravelled round everything. Here men don't idealise women, by the looks of things. Here they don't make these great leering eyes, the inevitable yours-to-command look of Italian males. When the men from the country look at these women, then it is Mind-yourself, my lady. I should think the grovelling Madonna-worship is not much of a Sardinian feature. These women have to look out for themselves, keep their own back-bone stiff and their knuckles hard. Man is going to be male Lord if he can. And woman isn't going to give him too much of his own way, either. So there you have it, the fine old martial split between the sexes. It is tonic and splendid, really, after so much sticky intermingling and backboneless Madonna-worship. The Sardinian isn't looking for the "noble woman nobly planned." No, thank you. He wants that young madam over there, a young stiff-necked generation that she is. Far better sport than with the nobly-planned sort: hollow frauds that they are. Better sport too than with a Carmen, who gives herself away too much. In these women there is something shy and defiant and un-get-atable. The defiant, splendid split between the sexes, each absolutely determined to defend his side, her side, from assault. So the meeting has a certain wild, salty savour, each the deadly unknown to the other. And at the same time, each his own, her own native pride and courage, taking the dangerous leap and scrambling back.

Give me the old, salty way of love. How I am nauseated with sentiment and nobility, the macaroni slithery-slobbery mess of modern adorations.

One sees a few fascinating faces in Cagliari: those great dark unlighted eyes. There are fascinating dark eyes in Sicily, bright, big, with an impudent point of light, and a curious roll, and long lashes: the eyes of old Greece, surely. But here one sees eyes of soft, blank darkness, all velvet, with no imp looking out of them. And they strike a stranger, older note: before the soul became self-conscious: before the mentality of Greece appeared in the world. Remote, always remote, as if the intelligence lay deep within the cave, and never came forward. One searches into the gloom for one second, while the glance lasts. But without being able to penetrate to the reality. It recedes, like some unknown creature deeper into its lair. There *is* a creature, dark and potent. But what?

Sometimes Velasquez, and sometimes Goya gives us a suggestion of these large, dark, unlighted eyes. And they go with fine, fleecy black hair—almost as fine as fur. I have not seen them north of Cagliari.

The q-b spies some of the blue-and-red stripe-and-line cotton stuff of which the peasants make their dress: a large roll in the doorway of a dark shop. In we go, and begin to feel it. It is just soft, thickish cotton stuff—twelve francs a metre. Like most peasant patterns, it is much more complicated and subtle than appears: the curious placing of the stripes, the subtle proportion, and a white thread left down one side only of each broad blue block. The stripes, moreover, run *across* the cloth, not lengthwise with it. But the width would be just long enough for a skirt—though the peasant skirts have almost all a band at the bottom with the stripes running round-ways.

The man—he is the esquimo type, simple, frank and amiable—says the stuff is made in France, and this the first roll since the war. It is the old, old pattern, quite correct—but the material not *quite* so good. The q-b takes enough for a dress.

He shows us also cashmeres, orange, scarlet, sky-blue, royal blue: good, pure-wool cashmeres that were being sent to India, and were captured from a German mercantile submarine. So he says. Fifty francs a metre—very, very wide. But they are too much trouble to carry in a knapsack, though their brilliance fascinates.

So we stroll and look at the shops, at the filigree gold jewelling of the peasants, at a good bookshop. But there is little to see and therefore the question is, shall we go on? Shall we go forward?

There are two ways of leaving Cagliari for the north: the State railway that runs up the west side of the island, and the narrow-gauge secondary railway that pierces the centre. But we are too late for the big trains. So we will go by the secondary railway, wherever it goes.

There is a train at 2:30, and we can get as far as Mandas, some fifty miles in the interior. When we tell the queer little waiter at the hotel, he says he comes from Mandas, and there are two inns. So after lunch—a strictly fish menu—we pay our bill. It comes to sixty odd francs—for three good meals each, with wine, and the night's lodging, this is cheap, as prices now are in Italy.

Pleased with the simple and friendly Scala di Ferre, I shoulder my sack and we walk off to the second station. The sun is shining hot this afternoon—burning hot, by the sea. The road and the buildings look dry and desiccated, the harbour rather weary and end of the world.

There is a great crowd of peasants at the little station. And almost every man has a pair of woven saddle-bags—a great flat strip of coarse-woven wool, with flat pockets at either end, stuffed with purchases. These are almost the only carrying bags. The men sling them over their shoulder, so that one great pocket hangs in front, one behind.

These saddle bags are most fascinating. They are coarsely woven in bands of raw black-rusty wool, with varying bands of raw white wool or hemp or cotton—the bands and stripes of varying widths going crosswise. And on the pale bands are woven sometimes flowers in most lovely colours, rose-red and blue and green, peasant patterns—and sometimes fantastic animals, beasts, in dark wool again. So that these striped zebra bags, some wonderful gay with flowery colours on their stripes, some weird with fantastic, griffin-like animals, are a whole landscape in themselves.

The train has only first and third class. It costs about thirty francs for the two of us, third class to Mandas, which is some sixty miles. In we crowd with the joyful saddlebags, into the wooden carriage with its many seats.

And, wonder of wonders, punctually to the second, off we go, out of Cagliari. En route again.

Suggestions for Study

COMPARE this selection with a passage from Ruskin's *Stones of Venice* and with one from Norman Douglas' *Old Calabria.* The exercise will give you an idea of what has happened to English prose since it began to escape from the Victorians. It is the comparative freedom of modern prose that allows Lawrence to concentrate on sensuous details and to project, through the energy of his sentences, his own protest against repression, which is expressed in the highly artful primitivism (sometimes it is almost barbarism) of his attitude and style.

Lawrence builds his descriptions out of many little pictures, all extremely accurate and simple, though there are many adjectives which express the author's attitude rather than the appearance of the scene. On the whole, in spite of the unconventionality of the style, these details are arranged with all the formality of landscape painting. Following one of these descriptions, there will often be a paragraph or so of comment, or a paragraph that records Lawrence's feelings.

The rhythm of the chapter is irregular, varying from the easy swiftness of the picture of the harbor to the nervous, ejaculatory description of and comment on the peasant and his costume. This latter effect results from the number of elliptical constructions and sentence fragments, and from the suppression of merely functional predications. The whole is rough and garrulous, but very powerful.

Go through the chapter and find evidence that will justify this analysis.

In the section that begins "One sees a few fascinating faces in Cagliari," (p. 543) Lawrence alludes to all the major ideas (or attitudes) that form his feeling for Cagliari. Analyze the section to prove this statement.

Piano in the Band

OTIS FERGUSON (1907–1943)

THEY BURIED Bessie Smith just the other day. She was a great handsome chunk of a woman and still so much in her prime you'd never dream her fifty years; but they picked her out of an automobile smash-up in Memphis and put her in the ground, and now there is nothing left of Bessie, who was the great girl they called the Empress of the Blues. And so I think it is a good idea to speak about the good musicians who are left, as quickly as we can, while they are still among us.

When you go to hear the great Benny Goodman band in New York (the word is great; and you'd better go), you will notice after a time that the band has someone it uses for playing the piano. This piano player will never steal the spotlight. He is slight, youngish, but with a shot of gray in his absolutely straight black hair, and with a sort of funny Irish face, usually absorbed. He is getting a permanent hook in his back from reading scores off a

PIANO IN THE BAND by Otis Ferguson is reprinted from *New Republic*, November 24, 1937, by permission of Dorothy Chamberlain.

flat piano top (he knows most of them by heart; just studies them to pass the time now), and his natural attitude is one of a kid doing algebra homework, dutiful and patient but cribbing the answers—he snickers to himself, for example, when he finds a little hole Benny hasn't plugged up and drives a minor third into it. He is a Chicago musician, from the old-time big-time; his name is Jess Stacy.

If you move up closer you will hear him come in for a little digging now and then, Gene Krupa giving him that extra *bum bum* on the foot pedal, "Hey, Jess," and Benny raising his eyebrows in the signal for what-the-hell-goes-on-here, or coming over to buzz a couple of high clarinet tones right in Jess's ear, and Harry looking down from the bass like the full moon. Jess proves to be just the butt for that sort of thing, because his face begins to get red and flustered, he ducks his head a little lower, which makes his eyes bug a little as he tries to keep everybody in sight and the score too, and he twitches as though one of the girls had tickled him in a severely unmentionable place just as the curtain was going up (Aw, *fellers*, cut it out will you?), and you can see his hands begin to hop. But if you are that close, you can hear how that big band piano is getting played.

Jess Stacy is above everything else a band pianist, the hands powerful on the full heavy chords, the fingers trained down to steel in bringing out both ends of an octave at once through any din, wrists, hands and fingers quick and skimming in a working musician's economy of motion. In such a job, some play a style that is clearly expressed in the term "ump-ah," and some in the butterfly style—i. e., you don't do much until the orchestra pauses for breath, when you immediately play a little right-hand fiddle-dee-diddle of notes above the staff, spattering the place with Duchin, in brief.

Jess plays neither style or all of them, for he uses the piano as both an orchestra in miniature and a linking force among its separate parts, tying the chorded beat of the rhythm section into the melodic line, providing a sort of common base as between brass and reeds, filling out the chords of each. His own summing up of it has the true clarity of one who must find words for his meaning, not a meaning for his words: "What I try to do—" Jess says. "Look, I try to *melt* with the band." It is a simple word, but all the meanings are there in it: nuance, mood, touch, attack, phrasing, harmonic direction, what not. Because it is still in the unspoiled charm of its youth, this jazz music has never troubled to build a complicated breastwork of definitions. Jess and the rest have an *active* knowledge of how a tune may run, of how the value of a chord may be shifted—by its place in the general pattern (where it rises from and leads to), by its attack, duration, the color of its key and measure of its contrast, the sonority dependent on which of its notes are uppermost.

All these things are in his ears and head and fingertips, that is what he's up to as he sits on the bench there, with his head craned over and his hands hopping, his ear sharpened for all the voicing of instruments, building up under the soloists or falling away to quiet backgrounds, letting a good chord bang out against the beat. Unless you sit under the piano you might not notice him at all in his general place, because he does not shoot cuffs or shake his hair down, and never bounces up off the keyboard as though it were a balloon tire and caught him by surprise. But then the band comes down to the release and Benny holds up one finger and Jess nods, Yes, he'll take it;—someone floods the spot over, the faces on the floor turn, and 1, 2, 3, 4—1, 2 . . . *Jess!* And there is Jess out in the open all by himself. At which time he seems to draw into the piano, very small behind its bulk and in all that light, and his hands begin to fly both ways from the center —and you'd think he had been waiting all his life to catch a piano and this one was going to fade away in another minute. On a quiet night you will be close enough to watch his face, as red and foolish as ever and a little more, because the lines around his mouth twitch and his long nose gets a sort of wrinkle, and he takes on the silliest look as he sneaks up on some special close harmony and holds off everything else to make it ring like a gong, and then pretends to play off away from it, and then pounces back onto it, driving it in cross-rhythms three, four, five times over.

If you listen with some love of the stuff you will hear many things in the spare phrasing and calculated attack of this music. There are echoes from way back, and there is a special background in music—the attitude toward it and way of playing it developed by the boys around Chicago years ago, when jazz was coming up the Mississippi from New Orleans and shifting its center. Krupa is from that center, Benny and Harry Goodman are too; but Jess Stacy is a man who goes back farther, older than any of them though still in his creative youth. He goes back to James P. Johnson and Pine Top Smith, beyond the time Louis Armstrong left the riverboats to work in Chicago and New York. And you can hear not only the new beauty of each figure as he plays it, but the overtones of the tradition it is played in, what he gathered from the best men and now plays in memory of their genius.

Jess Stacy was born (1904) in Cape Girardeau, Missouri, a town 150 miles down the river from St. Louis. He started on piano when he was twelve. His family being respectable Irish and poor, he went to high school and scrabbled around at odd jobs between times—jerking sodas, playing small non-union dates, at one time working as a hand in a barrel factory. He got within a few credits of graduation and then went on working. Finally, at the age of twenty, he got his first really professional job, $35 a week and room and board, with the band on a riverboat.

The boats came into town with as much gala as possible, inviting passengers to go aboard for an evening of dancing on the river, to the strains of their absolutely superior dance orchestra (Jess got $5 extra a week for playing the calliope as the boat came in around the bend). Up and down the river and all its navigable tributaries, from town to town, for thousands of miles. He covered the whole network before he was through. All the time he was hearing musicians; long before, he had gone to hear Fate Marable's band when it played his home town, with Louis Armstrong riding his silver horn, with Babe and Johnny Dodds; and that was the time when "Whispering" came out. And after a while he noticed, when they played a certain town, a little old round-faced kid who came aboard nightly to listen, his eyes wide and cheeks still like an apple—a shorty kid who'd never more than heard of a bottle then, but had such music in his heart that in the brief years before the bottle got him he released some of the finest notes in the country—Jess saw Bix Beiderbecke and sat in with him later, and still in 1937 speaks his name with reverence and happy memory, for he will endure no other trumpet player before him. Bix sat in with Carlisle Evans in Moline, Illinois, and later played the Greystone Ballroom in Detroit with Jean Goldkette; and at that time his peer, Louis, was at the Sunset Café in Chicago.

Jess kept playing and listening, getting nowhere much himself but going as high as $95 a week in Chicago music. Then the down grade ("bye and bye hard times"), and all the miserable salary cuts, lack of notice. He actually got down as low as $21 at the Subway Café when John Hammond came across him there. He had lost all hope, with all his friends dead or forgetfully famous, playing his fine music as uncompromisingly then as he always had—but who was there to hear it, outside of the night's handful of stumblebums? He got back up to $55 by the time Hammond got onto Goodman, and Goodman got an opening, and gave Jess the call.

About any musician who has to pull it out of himself as he goes along, the same thing is true as of poets: there are stretches of stuff that any competent man could have done, and then the burst of something that till now was never done, never imagined, lovely with the dew on it. On the latest Hampton record of "After You've Gone," for example, Stacy's solo is good average piano for the first six bars—and then there is this thing the boys mean when they say "out of this world," running strong through four bars, gradually tapering off through the last ten. Analyzed, it is simply the old piano blues style (a sort of *oink*-ily, *oink*-ily, *oink*-

ily effect), but it comes in at just the spot in just the register to mix pleased recognition with delighted surprise, banking two separate phrases against each other to link them inextricably. With his Quartet, incidentally, Teddy Wilson does the same sort of thing in a double-faced record called "In a Mood," a blues. In this case it is a man carrying 48 bars that are beautiful throughout, but rising even above that in his sixth and seventh. Both of them, one Negro and one white, are playing the same instrument at the top of their field, working in the same organization. Otherwise they are two different men. Wilson is more creative and his own melodist; Stacy is more the man who swings the band, always listening.

Jess Stacy has had those comical ears of his spread for music so long that it is a pleasure and a means of correction to go over musicians with him. "He doesn't make it sing like Bix," I say; and "You know a thing about Bix? He didn't give a *damn*," Jess says; and we each know what the other is talking about.

And when Teddy is playing between sets or with the quartet, Jess has his ear turned sideways and his mind remote from the chatter around the table. He once copied off a Wilson solo broadcast from the playback, note for note ("to see if I could just find what makes that man so *good*"). I'm not talking about surface poses, arms over shoulders for the camera, etc.; I mean from long hard day to long hard day. "Anybody I *really* admire," Jess is liable to blurt out any time of the night and off the record, "it's that little old Wilson." It is rather funny to see them independently, both quiet at their work, the younger man (Jess was learning the trade when Teddy was three) getting all the limelight of the quartet work and gathering fame about him like heat lightning, the veteran playing longer hours for less attention, and none of this rushing to the head or bile of either. Presently the band is up and Teddy comes to sit behind Jess's piano, to watch his hands. "Only wish I could work up a hand like that," Teddy says, spreading his fingers out in a full octave chord on the table to illustrate reach and power, nodding in Jess's rhythm with a sort of admiring regret. It is funny to see them, but there is also something restful, unique and sweet about this open delight in another man's worth. It is common only to the best artists and even among these (take a look around, just take a look around you), it seems to open out most easily in those arts, no matter how ragamuffin on the surface, that are nearest to the best in life, the men living their work without any fuss.

From the deep background of the blues and from his own feeling, mind and hand, Jess made twelve bars of piano on a record that John Hammond supervised for English Parlophone, "The Blues of Israel." That one is a sport all through, but after a few playings the piano stands out as much as anything. It has so completely that old-time pensive mood in the treble, the slurred second and the close three-finger chord hanging a mood of nostalgia around such a simple progression as sol, fa, mi, re; it is given so thorough a support in the constant working bass, whose left hand mingles intimately with what the right is doing. The song hangs on a trill, doubles the time for a swinging phrase, and slows to an ending of sustained chords, beautifully voiced. The analysis is simple, but the effect runs over into those complexities of the musical spirit that cannot be rightly described—and so it may be wiser just to say what the boys would say, speaking out like an infield: "*Play* that piano there, you Jess. It sure is pretty."

He is a great fellow for the blues, but in his fourteen working years, up and down the country, in and out of pavilions and barrel houses, he has taken all the styles discovered into his own style: the complex running bass of Pine Top Smith's boogie-woogie, a sort of reverse boogie-woogie he remembers from Lucky Roberts, way back; the Earl Hines and James P. Johnson of the old days; some single-note trumpet phrases from Bix and Louis; forgotten derivations from some chance genius of the honkey-tonks—above all the free, steady drive of the drums-guitar-bass part of a band (no good rhythm man may follow the beat, but must lead it, have the swing in him to carry it and the iron to hold it against gathering tension and fatigue).

So he runs from "The Blues of Israel" to the terrific and back-breaking tempo that Gene Krupa and a bunch of madmen held on the Victor recording of "Swing Is Here." He runs from the sophistication of a solo on Benny Goodman's "Madhouse" to the jazzy Dixieland blare of the "Maple Leaf Rag" (Paul Mares and his Friars' Society Orchestra). About the best of all is the way he used to eat up the choruses on "Sing, Sing, Sing," getting higher with each one and beyond himself, truly wonderful piano. (Benny, like the swell musician he is, would stand beaming and silent through all of them, but when they recorded it somebody was wrong, because there is everything on the double-side twelve-inch release except that perishable triumph.) The first time I heard it was at the New York Paramount, and when I began cheering afterward backstage, all Jess would say was "Oh, you mean that old A-minor-chord thing; it's all right, that chord." And much later they were playing some sad backwater where the bloods were yelling for "Casa Loma Stomp" and failed to get the idea of a solo and bawled for brass. And Jess dug in and took about five in a row, so mad they couldn't get him out of it, and it was beautiful—they didn't want to take him out. All he said after that was, "I'll teach them what to holler for, the icky bastards." (*You know a thing about Bix? He didn't give a damn.*)

But those are the recordings, the outstanding flash parts; and Jess Stacy more than almost any musician of his rank has little to show there. The deep consistent music of his piano still comes out best only to those who play over it or sit there under its sounding board. About which words lead only to more words—so go to hear him in town, or when the band plays a one-night stand in some town near. And when he plays, you listen; and when he possibly comes over to your table afterward and talks, you listen; and when he says, Let's sneak out and get a blast out of that jug the man has over at the bar, you go along. You will for once be near the singing tradition of this country and its people, nearer than you know.

The Picador

ERNEST HEMINGWAY (1898–   )

You read of bulls in the old days accepting thirty, forty, fifty and even seventy pics from the picadors while to-day a bull that can take seven pics is an amazing animal, and it seems as though things were very different in those days and the bullfighters must have been such men as were the football players on the high-school team when we were still in grammar school. Things change very much and instead of great athletes only children play on the high-school teams now and if you sit with the older men at the café you know there are no good bullfighters now either; they are all children without honor, skill or virtue, much the same as those children who now play football, a feeble game it has become, on the high-school team and nothing like the great, mature, sophisticated athletes in canvas-elbowed jerseys, smelling vinegary from sweated shoulder pads, carrying leather headguards, their moleskins clotted with mud, that walked on leather-cleated shoes that printed in the earth along beside the sidewalk in the dusk, a long time ago.

There were always giants in those days and the bulls really did accept that many pics, the contemporary accounts prove, but the pics were different. In the oldest old days the pic had a very small steel triangular tip so wrapped and protected that only that small tip could go into the bull. The picadors received the bull with their horse straight toward him, drove the pic at him and as they held him off pivoted the horse to the left freeing him from the charge and letting the bull go by. A bull, even a modern bull, could accept a large number of those pics since the steel did not cut into him deeply and it was a move of address on the part of the picador rather than a deliberately sought shock and punishment.

The present pic is very destructive even though properly placed. It is especially destructive since the picador does not place it, shoot the stick it is called, until the bull has reached the horse. The bull must then make the effort of lifting the horse at the same time the man is leaning his weight on the shaft and driving the steel into the bull's neck muscle or his withers. If all of the picadors were as skillful as a few are there would be no need to let the bull reach the horse before shooting the stick. But the majority of the picadors, because it is a poorly paid occupation that leads only to concussion of the brain, are not even capable of sinking the pic into a bull properly. They rely on a lucky drive and the certain effort the bull must make in tossing horse and rider to tire the bull's neck muscles and do the work that a real picador could accomplish without losing either his horse or his seat in the saddle. The wearing of protective mattresses by the horses has made the picadors' work much more difficult and hazardous. Without the mattress the bull's horn can get into the horse and he can lift him, or, sometimes, satisfied with the damage he is doing with his horn, be held off by the man's pic; with the mattress he butts into the horse, there is nothing for his horn to go into and he crashes horse and rider over in a heap. The use of the protective mattress has led to another abuse in bullfighting. Horses that are no longer killed in the ring may be offered by the horse contractor again and again. They are so afraid of the bulls and become so panic stricken on smelling them that they are almost impossible to manage. The new government regulation provides that the picadors may refuse such horses and that they must be marked so that they cannot be used or offered by any horse contractor, but since the picador is so poorly paid, this regulation too will probably be destroyed by the propina, or tip, which makes up a regular part of the picador's income and which he accepts from the contractor for riding the animals he is given the right and duty, by the government regulations, to refuse.

The propina is responsible for almost every horror in bullfighting. The regulations provide for the size, sturdiness and fitness of the horses used in the bull ring and if proper horses are used and the picadors well trained there would be no need for any horses to be killed except accidentally and against the will of the riders as they are killed, for instance, in steeple-chasing. But the enforcing of these regulations for his own protection is left to the picador as the most interested party and the picador is so poorly paid for the danger he undergoes that, for a small addition to this pay, he is willing to accept horses that make his work even more difficult and dangerous. The horse contractor must furnish or have available thirty-six horses for each fight. He is paid a fixed sum no matter what happens to his horses. It is to his interest to furnish the cheapest animals he can get and see that as few of them are used as possible.

This is about how it works out; the picadors arrive the day before the fight or in the morning of the fight at the corrals of the bull ring to choose and test the horses they are to ride. There is a piece of iron set in the stone wall of the corral that marks the minimum height at the shoulder that a horse must have to be accepted. A picador has the big saddle put on a horse, mounts, tests whether the horse minds bit and spur, backs, wheels and riding toward the corral wall drives against it with the shaft of a pic to see if the horse is sound and solid on his feet. He then dismounts and says to the contractor, "I wouldn't risk my life on that lousy skate for a thousand dollars."

"What's the matter with that horse?" says the contractor. "You'll go a long way before you'll find a horse like that."

"Too long a way," says the picador.

"What's the matter with him? That's a handsome little horse."

"He's got no mouth," the picador says. "He won't back. Besides he's short."

"He's just the right size. Look at him. Just the right size."

"Just the right size for what?"

"Just the right size to ride."

"Not me," says the picador turning away.

"You won't find a better horse."

"I believe that," says the picador.

"What's your real objection?"

"He's got glanders."

"Nonsense. That isn't glanders. That's just dandruff."

"You ought to spray him with flit," says the picador. "That would kill him."

"What's your real objection?"

"I have a wife and three children. I wouldn't ride him for a thousand dollars."

"Be sensible," the contractor says. They talk in low tones. He gives the picador fifteen pesetas.

"All right," says the picador. "Mark up the little horse."

So, in the afternoon you see the picador ride out the little horse and if the little horse gets ripped and, instead of killing him, the red-jacketed bull ring servant runs with him toward the horse gate to get him back where he can be patched up so the contractor can send him in again, you may be sure the bull ring servant has received or been promised a propina for every horse he can bring alive out of the ring, instead of killing them mercifully and decently when they are wounded.

I have known some fine picadors, honest, honorable, brave and in a bad business, but you may have all the horse contractors I have ever met, although some of them were nice fellows. If you wish and will take them, you may have all the bull ring servants too. They are the only people I have found in bullfighting that are brutalized by it and they are the only ones who take an active part who undergo no danger. I have seen several of them, two especially that are father and son, that I would like to shoot. If we ever have a time when for a few days you may shoot any one you wish I believe that before starting out to bag various policemen, Italian statesmen, government functionaries, Massachusetts judges, and a couple of companions of my youth I would shove in a clip and make sure of that pair of bull ring servants. I do not want to identify them any more closely because if I ever should bag them this would be evidence of premeditation. But of all the filthy cruelty I have ever seen they have furnished the most. Where you see gratuitous cruelty most often is in police brutality; in the police of all countries I have ever been in, including, especially, my own. These two Pamplona and San Sebastian monosabios should be, by rights, policemen and policemen on the radical squad, but they do the best they can with their talents in the bull ring. They carry on their belts puntillas, broad-headed knives, with which they can give the gift of death to any horse that is badly wounded, but I have never seen them kill a horse that could possibly be gotten on his feet and made to move toward the corrals. It is not only a question of the money they could make by salvaging horses to be taxidermed while alive so they may be reintroduced into the ring, for I have seen them refuse to kill, until forced to by the public, a horse there was no hope of getting onto his feet or of bringing back into the ring purely from pleasure in exerting their power to refuse to perform a merciful act as long as possible. Most bull ring servants are poor devils that perform a miserable function for a mean wage and are entitled to pity if not sympathy. If they save a horse or two that they should kill they do it with fear that outruns any pleasure and earn their money as well as the men do who pick up cigar butts, say. But these two that I speak of are both fat, well-fed and arrogant. I once succeeded in landing a large, heavy one-peseta-fifty rented, leather cushion alongside the head of the younger one during a scene of riotous disapproval in a bull ring in the north of Spain and I am never at the ring without a bottle of Manzanilla which I hope yet I will be able to land, empty, on one or the other at any time rioting becomes so general that a single bottle stroke may pass unperceived by the authorities. After one comes, through contact with its administrators, no longer to cherish greatly the law as a remedy in abuses, then the bottle becomes a sovereign means of direct action. If you cannot throw it at least you can always drink out of it.

In bullfights now a good pic is not one in which the picador, pivoting, protects his horse completely. That is what it should be, but you might go a long time and never see one. All you can expect in a good pic now is that the picador will place his stick properly, that is drive the point into the morillo, or hump of muscle that rises from the back of the bull's neck to his shoulders, that he will try to hold the bull off and that he will not twist his pic or turn it to try and make a deep wound in the bull in order that he may lose blood and so weaken, to make the danger less for the matador.

A bad pic is one that is placed anywhere else but in the morillo, one which rips or opens a big wound, or one in which the picador lets the bull reach the horse, then when the horn is in, pushes, drives and twists on the pic which is in the bull and tries to give the impression he is protecting his horse when he is really only injuring the bull to no good purpose.

If picadors had to own their own horses and were well paid they would protect them and the horse part of bullfighting would become one of the most brilliant and skillful of all rather than a necessary evil. For my own part if horses are to be killed the worse the horses are the better. For the picadors' part an old horse with big feet is much more useful to them in the way they pic now than would be a thoroughbred in good condition. To be useful in the bull ring a horse must be either old or well-tired. It is as much to tire the horses as to provide transportation for the picadors that the animals are ridden from the ring into town to the picadors' boarding house and back. In the provinces the bull ring servants ride the horses in the morning to tire them. The rôle of the horse has become that of providing something the bull will charge so that his neck muscles will be tired and of supporting the man who receives the charge and places his pic in such a manner as to force the bull to tire those muscles. His duty is to tire the bull rather than weaken him by wounds. The wound made by the pic is an incident rather than an end. Whenever it becomes an end it is censurable.

Used for this purpose the worst horses possible, that is those past any other usefulness, but which are solid on their feet and moderately manageable, are the best. I have seen thoroughbreds killed in their prime in other places than the bull ring and it is always a sad and disturbing business. The bull ring is a death's business for horses and the worse horses they are the better.

As I say, having the picadors own their own horses would change the whole spectacle. But I would rather see a dozen old worthless horses killed on purpose than one good horse killed by accident.

What about the Old Lady? She's gone. We threw her out of the book, finally. A little late you say. Yes, perhaps a little late. What about the horses? They are what people always like to talk about in regard to the bullfight. Has there been enough about the horses? Plenty about the horses, you say. They like it all but the poor horses. Should we try to raise the general tone? What about higher things?

Mr. Aldous Huxley writing in an essay entitled "Foreheads Villainous Low" commences: "In [naming a book by this writer] Mr. H. ventures, once, to name an Old Master. There is a phrase, quite admirably expressive [here Mr. Huxley inserts a compliment], a single phrase, no more, about 'the bitter nail-holes' of Mantegna's Christs; then quickly, quickly, appalled by his own temerity, the author passes on (as Mrs. Gaskell might hastily have passed on, if she had somehow been betrayed into mentioning a water-closet), passes on, shamefacedly, to speak once more of Lower Things.

"There was a time, not so long ago, when the stupid and uneducated aspired to be thought intelligent and cultured. The current of aspiration has changed its direction. It is not at all uncommon now to find intelligent and cultured people doing their best to feign stupidity and to conceal the fact that they have received an education"—and more; more in Mr. Huxley's best educated vein which is a highly educated vein indeed.

What about that, you say? Mr. Huxley scores there, all right, all right. What have you to say to that? Let me answer truly. On reading that in Mr. Huxley's book I obtained a copy of the volume he refers to and looked through it and could not find the quotation he mentions. It may be there, but I did not have the patience nor the interest to find it, since the book was finished and nothing to be done. It sounds very much like the sort of thing one tries to remove in going over the manuscript. I believe it is more than a question of the simulation or avoidance of the appearance of culture. When writing a novel a writer should create living people; people not characters. A *character* is a caricature. If a writer can make people live there may be no great characters in his book, but it is possible that his book will remain as a whole; as an entity; as a novel. If the people the writer is making talk of old masters; of music; of modern painting; of letters; or of science then they should talk of those subjects in the novel. If they do not talk of those subjects and the writer makes them talk of them he is a faker, and if he talks about them himself to show how much he knows then he is showing off. No matter how good a phrase or a simile he may have if he puts it in where it is not absolutely necessary and irreplaceable he is spoiling his work for egotism. Prose is architecture, not interior decoration, and the Baroque is over. For a writer to put his own intellectual musings, which he might sell for a low price as essays, into the mouths of artificially constructed characters which are more remunerative when issued as people in a novel is good economics, perhaps, but does not make literature. People in a novel, not skillfully constructed *characters*, must be projected from the writer's assimilated experience, from his knowledge, from his head, from his heart and from all there is of him. If he ever has luck as well as seriousness and gets them out entire they will have more than one dimension and they will last a long time. A good writer should know as near everything as possible. Naturally he will not. A great enough writer seems to be born with knowledge. But he really is not; he has only been born with the ability to learn in a quicker ratio to the passage of time than other men and without conscious application, and with an intelligence to accept or reject what is already presented as knowledge. There are some things which cannot be learned quickly and time, which is all we have, must be paid heavily for their acquiring. They are the very simplest things and because it takes a man's life to know them the little new that each man gets from life is very costly and the only heritage he has to leave. Every novel which is truly written contributes to the total of knowledge which is there at the disposal of the next writer who comes, but the next writer must pay, always, a certain nominal percentage in experience to be able to understand and assimilate what is available as his birthright and what he must, in turn, take his departure from. If a writer of prose knows enough about what he is writing about he may omit things that he knows and the reader, if the writer is writing truly enough, will have a feeling of those things as strongly as though the writer had stated them. The dignity of movement of an ice-berg is due to only one-eighth of it being above water. A writer who omits things because he does not know them only makes hollow places in his writing. A writer who appreciates the seriousness of writing so little that he is anxious to make people see he is formally educated, cultured or well-bred is merely a popinjay. And this too remember; a serious writer is not to be confounded with a solemn writer. A serious writer may be a hawk or a buzzard or even a popinjay, but a solemn writer is always a bloody owl.

Suggestions for Study

THERE ARE more famous pieces in Hemingway's work than this chapter from *Death in the Afternoon;* the description of the retreat from Caporetto in *Farewell to Arms* or the description of the smell of death in *For Whom the Bell Tolls* are rather more obviously great prose than this passage, which only talks about a process that most of its readers have not seen and are not likely to be much interested in. But the chapter seemed worth including for two reasons. It shows that a careful writer, who is willing to keep his eye on the world in front of him, can make something artistic and exciting out of just plain reporting. And it contains an important statement on the business of writers; and even in a book about reading, there ought to be something about writers, from a writer, for these days it sometimes seems as if we had forgotten all about the writers and their ideas, their notions of what they're supposed to be doing.

The core of this chapter is the analysis of the work of the picador; and this is taken care of quickly enough, with a description of the pic, a discussion of its use, and a couple of paragraphs that distinguish between good pics and bad. But the body and life of the chapter, the characteristic tone and movement, are supplied by Hemingway's reflections on the giants in the old days, the "fine picadors, honest, honorable, brave and in a bad business," Massachusetts judges, police brutality, the propina that corrupts the picadors, and the usefulness of the law. Experience is a complicated thing is what the chapter suggests; and the writer must write "from his knowledge, from his head, from his heart and from all there is of him."

But Hemingway does not write as if he saw the complexity of experience, or as if he wanted his reader to take it in as complicated. He uses the simplest words: "Things change very much"; "There are some things which cannot be learned quickly and time, which is all we have, must be paid heavily for their acquiring." His adjectives often seem to be mere counter words, though this effect is overcome by their arrangement (the rhythm, which gives the tone and thus the emotion to the expression), as in the series "honest, honorable, brave and in a bad business." His sentences are often, perhaps mostly, deliberately unsophisticated in pattern, even when they are dealing with rather involved ideas:

"They are the simplest things and because it takes a man's life to know them the little new that each man gets from life is very costly and the only heritage he has to leave." Most of the time he talks about things he has seen, and he does not bother much to analyze the experience: The police in all lands are brutal, he is willing to say, for he has noticed this fact. But the fact is enough, and reasons or causes are for some other writer.

Yet the effect of the chapter is not just that of a factual report. Take the concluding movements of a number of his sentences. ". . . that walked on leather-cleated shoes in the dusk, a long time ago." ". . . without being ruined both physically and in bravery." ". . . instead of killing them mercifully and decently when they are wounded." ". . . the little new that each man gets from life is very costly and the only heritage he has to leave." Here one notices at once that none of these sentences comes to a full, defined end; the effect is rather of a voice suspended, as if there were more to say. And of course there is more to say; there is all of Hemingway's feeling about life; and it is clear that he is not talking about picadors or brutal policemen or cruel monosabios. Instead he is asking you to feel with him that curiously mixed feeling of his that has so often been commented on but never so well, perhaps, as in Steig's cartoon symbol—a brawny stevedore's arm, holding with utmost delicacy a single rose.

Jean le Nègre

E. E. CUMMINGS (1894–)

ON A CERTAIN day, the ringing of the bell and accompanying rush of men to the window facing the entrance gate was supplemented by an unparalleled volley of enthusiastic exclamations in all the languages of La Ferté Macé—provoking in me a certainty that the queen of fair women had arrived. This certainty thrillingly withered when I heard the cry: "*Il y a un noir!*" Fritz was at the best peep-hole, resisting successfully the onslaughts of a dozen fellow-prisoners, and of him I demanded in English, "Who's come?"—"Oh, a lot of girls," he yelled, "and there's a NIGGER too"—hereupon writhing with laughter.

I attempted to get a look, but in vain; for by this at least two dozen men were at the peep-hole, fighting and gesticulating and slapping each other's backs with joy. However, my curiosity was not long in being answered. I heard on the stairs the sound of mounting feet, and knew that a couple of *plantons* would before many minutes arrive at the door with their new prey. So did everyone else—and from the farthest beds uncouth figures sprang and rushed to the door, eager for the first glimpse of the *nouveau:* which was very significant, as the ordinary procedure on arrival of prisoners was for everybody to rush to his own bed and stand guard over it.

Even as the *plantons* fumbled with the locks I heard the inimitable, unmistakable divine laugh of a negro. The door opened at last. Entered a beautiful pillar of black strutting muscle topped with a tremendous display of the whitest teeth on earth. The muscle bowed politely in our direction, the grin remarked musically; "*Bo'jour, tou'l'monde*"; then came a cascade of laughter. Its effect on the spectators was instantaneous: they roared and danced with joy. "*Comment vous appelez-vous?*" was fired from the hubbub.—"*J'm'appelle Jean, moi,*" the muscle rapidly answered with sudden solemnity, proudly gazing to left and right as if expecting a challenge to this statement: but when none appeared, it relapsed as suddenly into laughter—as if hugely amused at itself and everyone else including a little and tough boy, whom I had not previously noted, although his entrance had coincided with the muscle's.

Thus into the *misère* of La Ferté Macé stepped lightly and proudly Jean Le Nègre.

Of all the fine people in La Ferté, Monsieur Jean ("*le noir*" as he was entitled by his enemies) swaggers in my memory as the finest.

Jean's first act was to complete the distribution (begun, he announced, among the *plantons* who had escorted him upstairs) of two pockets full of Cubebs. Right and left he gave them up to the last, remarking carelessly, "*J'ne veux, moi.*"

Après la soupe (which occurred a few minutes after *le noir's* entry) B. and I and the greater number of prisoners descended to the *cour* for our afternoon promenade. The cook spotted us immediately, and desired us to "catch water"; which we did, three cartfulls of it, earning our usual *café sucré*. On quitting the *cuisine* after this delicious repast (which as usual mitigated somewhat the effects of the swill that was our official nutriment) we entered the *cour*. And we noticed at once a well-made figure standing conspicuously by itself, and poring with extraordinary intentness over the pages of a London *Daily Mail* which it was holding upside-down. The reader was culling choice bits of news of a highly sensational nature, and exclaiming from time to time—"*Est-ce vrai! V'la, le roi d'Angleterre est malade. Quelque chose!—Comment? La reine aussi? Bon Dieu! Qu'est-ce que c'est?—Mon père est mort! Merde!—Eh, b'en! La guerre est fini. Bon.*"—It was Jean Le Nègre, playing a little game with himself to beguile the time.

When we had mounted *à la chambre*, two or three tried to talk with this extraordinary personage in French; at which he became very superior and announced: "*J'suis anglais, moi. Parlez anglais. Comprends pas français, moi.*" At this a crowd escorted him over to B. and me—anticipating great deeds in the English language. Jean looked at us critically and said, "*Vous parlez anglais? Moi parlez anglais.*"—"We are Americans, and speak English," I answered.—"*Moi anglais,*" Jean said. "*Mon père, capitaine de gendarmerie, Londres. Comprends pas français, moi. SPEE-Kingliss*" —he laughed all over himself.

At this display of English on Jean's part the English-speaking Hollanders began laughing. "The son of a bitch is crazy," one said.

And from that moment B. and I got on famously with Jean.

His mind was a child's. His use of language was sometimes exalted fibbing, sometimes the purely picturesque. He courted above all the sound of words, more or less disdaining their meaning. He told us immediately (in pidgin-French) that he was born without a mother because his mother died when he was born, that his father was (first) sixteen (then) sixty years old, that his father *gagnait cinq cent francs par jour* (later, *par année*), that he was born in London and not in England, that he was in the French army and had never been in any army.

He did not, however, contradict himself in one statement: "*Les français sont des cochons*"—to which we heartily agreed, and which won him the approval of the Hollanders.

The next day I had my hands full acting as interpreter for "*le noir qui comprend pas français.*" I was summoned from the *cour* to elucidate a great grief which Jean had been unable to explain to the *Gestionnaire*. I mounted with a *planton* to find Jean in hysterics; speechless; his eyes starting out of his head. As nearly as I could make out, Jean had had sixty francs when he arrived, which money he had given to a *planton* upon his arrival, the *planton* having told Jean that he would deposit the money with the *Gestionnaire* in Jean's name (Jean could not write). The *planton* in question, who looked particularly innocent, denied this charge upon my explaining Jean's version; while the *Gestionnaire* puffed and grumbled, disclaiming any connection with the alleged theft and protesting sonorously that he was hearing about Jean's sixty francs for the first time. The *Gestionnaire* shook his thick piggish finger at the book wherein all financial transactions were to be found—from the year one to the present year, month, day, hour and minute (or words to that effect). "*Mais c'est pas là,*" he kept repeating stupidly. The *Surveillant* was uh-ahing at a great rate and attempting to pacify Jean in French. I myself was somewhat fearful for Jean's sanity and highly indignant at the *planton.* The matter ended with the *planton's* being sent about his business; simultaneously with Jean's dismissal to the *cour*, whither I accompanied him. My best efforts to comfort Jean in this matter were quite futile. Like a child who has been unjustly punished he was inconsolable. Great tears welled in his eyes. He kept repeating "Sees-tee franc—*planton voleur,*" and—absolutely like a child who in anguish calls itself by the name which has been given itself by grown-ups—"steel Jean munee." To no avail I called the *planton* a *menteur*, a *voleur*, a *fils de chienne* and various other names. Jean felt the wrong itself too keenly to be interested in my denunciation of the mere agent through whom injustice had (as it happened) been consummated.

But—again like an inconsolable child who weeps his heart out when no human comfort avails and wakes the next day without an apparent trace of the recent grief—Jean Le Nègre, in the course of the next twenty-four hours, had completely recovered his normal buoyancy of spirit. The sees-tee franc were gone. A wrong had been done. But that was yesterday. To-day—

And he wandered up and down, joking, laughing, singing:

"*après la guerre fini.*" . . .

In the *cour* Jean was the mecca of all female eyes. Handkerchiefs were waved to him; phrases of the most amorous nature greeted his every appearance. To all these demonstrations he by no means turned a deaf ear; on the contrary, Jean was irrevocably vain. He boasted of having been enormously popular with the girls wherever he went and of having never disdained their admiration. In Paris one day—(and thus it happened that we discovered why *le gouvernement français* had arrested Jean)—

One afternoon, having *rien à faire*, and being flush (owing to his success as a thief, of which vocation he made a great deal, adding as many ciphers to the amounts as fancy dictated) Jean happened to cast his eyes in a store window where were displayed all possible appurtenances for the *militaire*. Vanity was rooted deeply in Jean's soul. The uniform of an English captain met his eyes. Without a moment's hesitation he entered the store, bought the entire uniform, including leather puttees and belt (of the latter purchase he was especially proud), and departed. The next store contained a display of medals of all descriptions. It struck Jean at once that a uniform would be incomplete without medals. He entered this store, bought one of every decoration—not forgetting the Colonial, nor yet the Belgian Cross (which on account of its size and colour particularly appealed to him)—and went to his room. There he adjusted the decorations on the chest of his blouse, donned the uniform, and sallied importantly forth to capture Paris.

Everywhere he met with success. He was frantically pursued by women of all stations from *les putains* to *les princesses*. The police salaamed to him. His arm was wearied with the returning of innumerable salutes. So far did his medals carry him that, although on one occasion a gendarme dared to arrest him for beating in the head of a fellow English officer (who being a mere lieutenant, should not have objected to Captain Jean's stealing the affections of his lady), the *sergent de gendarmerie* before whom Jean was arraigned on a charge of attempting to kill refused to even hear the evidence, and dismissed the case with profuse apologies to the heroic Captain. "'*Le gouvernement français, Monsieur*, extends to you through me its profound apology for the insult which your honour has received.' *Ils sont des cochons, les français*," said Jean, and laughed throughout his entire body.

Having had the most blue-blooded ladies of the capital cooing upon his heroic chest, having completely beaten up with the full support of the law whosoever of lesser rank attempted to cross his path or refused him the salute—having had "great fun" saluting generals on *les grands boulevards* and being in turn saluted ("*tous les généraux, tous*, salute me, Jean have more medal"), and this state of affairs having lasted for about three months—Jean began to be very bored ("me *très ennuyé*"). A fit of temper ("me *très fâché*") arising from this ennui led to a *rixe* with the police, in consequence of which (Jean, though outnumbered three to one, having almost killed one of his assailants) our hero was a second time arrested. This time the authorities went so far as to ask the heroic captain to what branch of the English army he was at present attached; to which Jean first replied, "*Parle pas français, moi*," and immediately after announced that he was a Lord of the Admiralty, that he had committed robberies in Paris to the tune of sees-meel-i-own franc, that he was a son of the Lord Mayor of London by the Queen, that he had lost a leg in Algeria, and that the French were *cochons*. All of which assertions being duly disproved, Jean was remanded to La Ferté for psychopathic observation and safe keeping on the technical charge of wearing an English officer's uniform.

Jean's particular girl at La Ferté was "LOO-Loo." With Lulu it was the same as with *les princesses* in Paris—"me no *travaille, ja MAIS. Les femmes travaillent*, geev Jean mun-ee, sees, sees-tee, see-*cent francs. Jamais travaille, moi*." Lulu smuggled Jean money; and not for some time did the woman who slept next Lulu miss it. Lulu also sent Jean a lace embroidered handkerchief, which Jean would squeeze and press to his lips with a beatific smile of perfect contentment. The affair with Lulu kept Mexique and Pete the Hollander busy writing letters; which Jean dictated, rolling his eyes and scratching his head for words.

At this time Jean was immensely happy. He was continually playing practical jokes on one of the Hollanders, or Mexique, or the Wanderer, or in fact anyone of whom he was particularly fond. At intervals between these demonstrations of irrepressibility (which kept everyone in a state of laughter) he would stride up and down the filth-sprinkled floor with his hands in the pockets of his stylish jacket, singing at the top of his lungs his own version of the famous song of songs:

après la guerre fini,
soldat anglais parti
mademoiselle que je laissai en France
avec des pickaninee. PLENTY!

and laughing till he shook and had to lean against a wall.

B. and Mexique made some dominoes. Jean had not the least idea of how to play, but when we three had gathered for a game he was always to be found leaning over our shoulders, completely absorbed, once in a while offering us sage advice, laughing utterly when some one made a cinque or a multiple thereof.

One afternoon, in the interval between *la soupe* and promenade, Jean was in especially high spirits. I was lying down on my collapsible bed when he came up to my end of the room and began showing off exactly like a child. This time it was the game of *l'armée française* which Jean was playing.—"*Jamais soldat, moi. Connais toute l'armée française.*" John the Bathman, stretched comfortably in his bunk near me, grunted. "*Tous,*" Jean repeated.—And he stood in front of us; stiff as a stick in imitation of a French lieutenant with an imaginary company in front of him. First he would be the lieutenant giving commands, then he would be the Army executing them. He began with the manual of arms.

"*Com-pag-nie . . .*" then, as he went through the manual holding his imaginary gun—"htt, htt, htt."—Then as the officer commending his troops: "*Bon. Très bon. Très bien fait*"—laughing with head thrown back and teeth aglitter at his own success. John Le Baigneur was so tremendously amused that he gave up sleeping to watch. *L'armée* drew a crowd of admirers from every side. For at least three-quarters of an hour this game went on. . . .

Another day Jean, being angry at the weather and having eaten a huge amount of *soupe*, began yelling at the top of his voice "*MERDE à la France*," and laughing heartily. No one paying especial attention to him, he continued (happy in this new game with himself) for about fifteen minutes. Then The Sheeney With The Trick Raincoat (that undersized specimen, clad in feminine-fitting raiment with flashy shoes), who was by trade a pimp, being about half Jean's height and a tenth of his physique, strolled up to Jean—who had by this time got as far as my bed—and, sticking his sallow face as near Jean's as the neck could reach, said in a solemn voice: "*Il ne faut pas dire ça.*" Jean, astounded, gazed at the intruder for a moment; then demanded, "*Qui dit ça? Moi? Jean? Jamais, ja-MAIS. MERDE à la France!*" nor would he yield a point, backed up as he was by the moral support of every one present except the Sheeney—who found discretion the better part of valour and retired with a few dark threats; leaving Jean master of the situation and yelling for the Sheeney's particular delectation: "*MAY-RRR-DE à la France!*" more loudly than ever.

A little after the epic battle with stovepipes between The Young Pole and Bill the Hollander, the wrecked *poêle* (which was patiently waiting to be repaired) furnished Jean with perhaps his most brilliant inspiration. The final section of pipe (which conducted the smoke through a hole in the wall to the outer air) remained in place all by itself, projecting about six feet into the room at a height of seven or eight feet from the floor. Jean noticed this; got a chair; mounted on it, and by applying alternately his ear and his mouth to the end of the pipe created for himself a telephone, with the aid of which he carried on a conversation with The Wanderer (at that moment visiting his family on the floor below) to this effect:

—Jean, grasping the pipe and speaking angrily into it, being evidently nettled at the poor connection—"Heh-loh, hello, hello, hello"—surveying the pipe in consternation—"*Merde. Ça marche pas*"—trying again with a deep frown—"heh-LOH!"—tremendously agitated—"HEH-LOH!"—a beatific smile supplanting the frown—"hello *Barbu. Est-ce que tu es là? Qui? Bon!*"—evincing tremendous pleasure at having succeeded in establishing the connection satisfactorily—"*Barbu? Est-ce que tu m'écoutes? Qui? Qu'est-ce que c'est Barbu? Comment? Moi? Qui, MOI? JEAN? jaMAIS! jamais, jaMAIS, Barbu. J'ai jamais dit que vous avez des puces. C'était pas moi, tu sais. JaMAIS, c'était un autre. Peut-être c'était Mexique*"—turning his head in Mexique's direction and roaring with laughter—"Hello, HEH-LOH. *Barbu? Tu sais, Barbu, j'ai jamais dit ça. Au contraire, Barbu. J'ai dit que vous avez des totos*"—another roar of laughter—"*Comment? C'est pas vrai? Bon. Alors. Qu'est-ce que vous avez, Barbu? Des poux—OHHHHHHHHH. Je comprends. C'est mieux*"—shaking with laughter, then suddenly tremendously serious—"Hellohellohellohello HEHLOH!"—addressing the stovepipe—"*C'est une mauvaise machine, ça*"—speaking into it with the greatest distinctness—"HEL-L-LOH. *Barbu? Liberté, Barbu. Oui. Comment? C'est ça. Liberté pour tou'l'monde. Quand? Après la soupe. Oui. Liberté pour tou'l'monde après la soupe!*"—to which jest astonishingly reacted a certain old man known as the West Indian Negro (a stocky, credulous creature with whom Jean would have nothing to do, and whose tales of Brooklyn were indeed outclassed by Jean's *histoires d'amour*) who leaped rheumatically from his *paillasse* at the word "*Liberté*" and rushed limpingly hither and thither inquiring Was it true?—to the enormous and excruciating amusement of The Enormous Room in general.[1]

There was another game—a pure child's game—which Jean played. It was the name game. He amused himself for hours together by lying on his *paillasse*, tilting his head back, rolling up his eyes, and crying in a high quavering voice—"JAW-neeeeeee." After a repetition or two of his own name in English, he would demand sharply "*Qui m'appelle?* Mexique? *Est-ce que tu m'appelle*, Mexique?" and if Mexique happened to be asleep, Jean

[1] The next paragraph of the original text is omitted here.

would rush over and cry in his ear shaking him thoroughly—"*Est-ce tu m'appelle, toi?*" Or it might be *Barbu*, or Pete the Hollander, or B. or myself, of whom he sternly asked the question—which was always followed by quantities of laughter on Jean's part. He was never perfectly happy unless exercising his inexhaustible imagination. . . .

Of all Jean's extraordinary selves, the moral one was at once the most rare and most unreasonable. In the matter of *les femmes* he could hardly have been accused by his bitterest enemy of being a Puritan. Yet the Puritan streak came out one day, in a discussion which lasted for several hours. Jean, as in the case of France, spoke in dogma. His contention was very simple: "*La femme qui fume n'est pas une femme.*" He defended it hotly against the attacks of all the nations represented; in vain did Belgian and Hollander, Russian and Pole, Spaniard and Alsatian, charge and counter-charge—Jean remained unshaken. A woman could do anything but smoke—if she smoked she ceased automatically to be a woman and became something unspeakable. As Jean was at this time sitting alternately on B.'s bed and mine, and as the alternations became increasingly frequent as the discussion waxed hotter, we were not sorry when the *planton's* shout, "*A la promenade les hommes!*" scattered the opposing warriors. Then up leaped Jean (who had almost come to blows innumerable times) and rushed laughing to the door, having already forgotten the whole thing.

Now we come to the story of Jean's undoing, and may the gods which made Jean Le Nègre give me grace to tell it as it was.

The trouble started with Lulu. One afternoon, shortly after the telephoning, Jean was sick at heart and couldn't be induced either to leave his couch or to utter a word. Every one guessed the reason—Lulu had left for another camp that morning. The *planton* told Jean to come down with the rest and get *soupe*. No answer. Was Jean sick? "*Oui*, me seek." And steadfastly he refused to eat, till the disgusted *planton* gave it up and locked Jean in alone. When we ascended after *la soupe* we found Jean as we had left him, stretched on his couch, big tears on his cheeks. I asked him if I could do anything for him; he shook his head. We offered him cigarettes—no, he did not wish to smoke. As B. and I went away we heard him moaning to himself, "Jawnee no see Loo-Loo no more." With the exception of ourselves, the inhabitants of La Ferté Macé took Jean's desolation as a great joke. Shouts of Lulu! rent the welkin on all sides. Jean stood it for an hour; then he leaped up, furious; and demanded (confronting the man from whose lips the cry had last issued)—"Feeneesh Loo-Loo?" The latter coolly referred him to the man next to him; he in turn to some one else; and round and round the room Jean stalked, seeking the offender, followed by louder and louder shouts of Lulu! and Jawnee! the authors of which (so soon as he challenged them) denied with innocent faces their guilt and recommended that Jean look closer next time. At last Jean took to his couch in utter misery and disgust.—The rest of *les hommes* descended as usual for the promenade—not so Jean. He ate nothing for supper. That evening not a sound issued from his bed.

Next morning he awoke with a broad grin, and to the salutations of Lulu! replied, laughing heartily at himself, "FEENEESH LooLoo." Upon which the tormentors (finding in him no longer a victim) desisted; and things resumed their normal course. If an occasional Lulu! upraised itself, Jean merely laughed, and repeated (with a wave of his arm) "FEENEESH." Finished Lulu seemed to be.

But *un jour* I had remained upstairs during the promenade, both because I wanted to write and because the weather was worse than usual. Ordinarily, no matter how deep the mud in the *cour*, Jean and I would trot back and forth, resting from time to time under the little shelter out of the drizzle, talking of all things under the sun. I remember on one occasion we were the only ones to brave the rain and slough—Jean in paper-thin soled slippers (which he had recently succeeded in drawing from the *Gestionnaire*) and I in my huge sabots—hurrying back and forth with the rain pouring on us, and he very proud. On this day, however, I refused the challenge of the *boue.*

The promenaders had been singularly noisy, I thought. Now they were mounting to the room making a truly tremendous racket. No sooner were the doors opened than in rushed half a dozen frenzied friends, who began telling me all at once about a terrific thing which my friend the *noir* had just done. It seems that The Sheeney With The Trick Raincoat had pulled at Jean's handkerchief (Lulu's gift in other days) which Jean wore always conspicuously in his outside breast pocket; that Jean had taken the Sheeney's head in his two hands, held it steady, abased his own head, and rammed the helpless Sheeney as a bull would do —the impact of Jean's head upon the Sheeney's nose causing that well-known feature to occupy a new position in the neighbourhood of the right ear. B. corroborated this description, adding the Sheeney's nose was broken and that everyone was down on Jean for fighting in an unsportsmanlike way. I found Jean still very angry, and moreover very hurt because every one was now shunning him. I told him that I personally was glad of what he'd done; but nothing would cheer him up. The Sheeney now entered, very terrible to see, having been patched up by Monsieur Richard with copious plasters. His nose was not broken, he said thickly, but only bent. He hinted darkly of trouble in store for *le noir;* and received the commiserations of everyone present except Mexique, The Zulu, B. and me. The Zulu, I remember, pointed to his own nose (which was not unimportant), then to Jean, then made a *moue* of excruciating anguish, and winked audibly.

Jean's spirit was broken. The wellnigh unanimous verdict against him had convinced his minutely sensitive soul that it had done wrong. He lay quietly, and would say nothing to anyone.

Some time after the soup, about eight o'clock, The Fighting Sheeney and The Trick Raincoat suddenly set upon Jean Le Nègre à propos nothing; and began pommelling him cruelly. The conscience-stricken pillar of beautiful muscle—who could have easily killed both his assailants at one blow—not only offered no reciprocatory violence but refused even to defend himself. Unresistingly, wincing with pain, his arms mechanically raised and his head bent, he was battered frightfully to the window by his bed, thence into the corner (upsetting the stool in the *pissoir*), thence along the wall to the door. As the punishment increased he cried out like a child: "*Laissez-moi tranquille!*"—again and again; and in his voice the insane element gained rapidly. Finally, shrieking in agony, he rushed to the nearest window; and while the Sheeneys together pommelled him yelled for help to the *planton* beneath.—

The unparalleled consternation and applause produced by this one-sided battle had long since alarmed the authorities. I was still trying to break through the five-deep ring of spectators—among whom was The Messenger Boy, who advised me to desist and got a piece of advice in return—when with a tremendous crash open burst the door, and in stepped four *plantons* with drawn revolvers, looking frightened to death, followed by the *Surveillant* who carried a sort of baton and was crying faintly: "*Qu'est-ce que c'est!*"

At the first sound of the door the two Sheeneys had fled, and were now playing the part of innocent spectators. Jean alone occupied the stage. His lips were parted. His eyes were enormous. He was panting as if his heart would break. He still kept his arms raised as if seeing everywhere before him fresh enemies. Blood spotted here and there the wonderful chocolate carpet of his skin, and his whole body glistened with sweat. His shirt was in ribbons over his beautiful muscles.

Seven or eight persons at once began explaining the fight to the *Surveillant*, who could make nothing out of their accounts and therefore called aside a trusted older man in order to get his version. The two retired from the room. The *plantons*, finding the expected wolf a lamb, flourished their revolvers about Jean and threatened him in the insignificant and vile language which *plantons* use to anyone whom they can bully. Jean kept repeating dully, "*Laissez-moi tranquille. Ils voulaient me tuer.*" His chest shook terribly with vast sobs.

Now the *Surveillant* returned and made a speech, to the effect that he had received independently of each other the stories of four men, that by all counts *le nègre* was absolutely to blame, that *le nègre* had caused an inexcusable trouble to the authorities and to his fellow-prisoners by this wholly unjustified conflict, and that as a punishment the *nègre* would now suffer the consequences of his guilt in the *cabinot*.—Jean had dropped his arms to his sides. His face was twisted with anguish. He made a child's gesture, a pitiful hopeless movement with his slender hands. Sobbing, he protested: "*C'est pas ma faute, monsieur le surveillant! Ils m'attaquaient! J'ai rien fait! Ils voulaient me tuer! Demandez à lui*"—he pointed to me desperately. Before I could utter a syllable the *Surveillant* raised his hand for silence: *le nègre* had done wrong. He should be placed in the *cabinot*.

—Like a flash, with a horrible tearing sob, Jean leaped from the surrounding *plantons* and rushed for the coat which lay on his bed screaming—"AHHHHH—*mon couteau!*"—"Look out or he'll get his knife and kill himself!" some one yelled; and the four *plantons* seized Jean by both arms just as he made a grab for his jacket. Thwarted in this hope and burning with the ignominy of his situation, Jean cast his enormous eyes up at the nearest pillar, crying hysterically: "*Tout le monde me fout au cabinot parce que je suis noir.*"—In a second, by a single movement of his arms, he sent the four *plantons* reeling to a distance of ten feet; leaped at the pillar: seized it in both hands like a Samson, and (gazing for another second with a smile of absolute beatitude at its length) dashed his head against it. Once, twice, thrice he smote himself, before the *plantons* seized him—and suddenly his whole strength wilted; he allowed himself to be overpowered by them and stood with bowed head, tears streaming from his eyes—while the smallest pointed a revolver at his heart.

This was a little more than the *Surveillant* had counted on. Now that Jean's might was no more, the bearer of the *croix de guerre* stepped forward and in a mild placating voice endeavoured to soothe the victim of his injustice. It was also slightly more than I could stand, and slamming aside the spectators I shoved myself under his honour's nose. "Do you know," I asked, "whom you are dealing with in this man? A child. There are a lot of Jeans where I come from. You heard what he said? He is black, is he not, and gets no justice from you. You heard that. I saw the whole affair. He was attacked, he put up no resistance whatever, he was beaten by two cowards. He is no more to blame than I am."—The *Surveillant* was waving his wand and cooing, "*Je comprends, je comprends, c'est malheureux.*"—"You're god damn right it's *malheureux*," I said, forgetting my French. "*Quand même*, he has resisted authority." The *Surveillant* gently continued: "Now, Jean, be quiet, you will be taken to the *cabinot.* You may as well go quietly and behave yourself like a good boy."

At this I am sure my eyes started out of my head. All I could think of to say was: "*Attends, un petit moment.*" To reach my own bed took but a second. In another second I was back, bearing my great and sacred pelisse. I marched up to Jean. "Jean," I remarked with a smile, "*tu vas au cabinot, mais tu vas revenir tout de suite. Je sais bien que tu as parfaitement raison. Mets cela*"—and I pushed him gently into my coat. "*Voici mes cigarettes, Jean; tu peux fumer comme tu veux*"—I pulled out all I had, one full *paquet jaune* of Marylands and half a dozen loose ones, and deposited them carefully in the right-hand pocket of the pelisse. Then I patted him on the shoulder and gave him the immortal salutation—"*Bonne chance, mon ami!*"

He straightened proudly. He stalked like a king through the doorway. The astounded *plantons* and the embarrassed *Surveillant* followed, the latter closing the doors behind him. I was left with a cloud of angry witnesses.

An hour later the doors opened, Jean entered quietly, and the doors shut. As I lay on my bed I could see him perfectly. He was almost naked. He laid my pelisse on his mattress, then walked calmly up to a neighbouring bed and skilfully and unerringly extracted a brush from under it. Back to his own bed he tiptoed, sat down on it, and began brushing my coat. He brushed it for a half-hour, speaking to no one, spoken to by no one. Finally he put the brush back, disposed the pelisse carefully on his arm, came to my bed, and as carefully laid it down. Then he took from the right-hand outside pocket a full *paquet jaune* and six loose cigarettes, showed them for my approval, and returned them to their place. "*Merci*," was his sole remark. B. got Jean to sit down beside him on his bed and we talked for a few minutes, avoiding the subject of the recent struggle. Then Jean went back to his own bed and lay down.

It was not till later that we learned the climax—not till *le petit belge avec le bras cassé*, *le petit balayeur*, came hurrying to our end of the room and sat down with us. He was bursting with excitement, his well arm jerked and his sick one stumped about and he seemed incapable of speech. At length words came.

"*Monsieur Jean*" (now that I think of it, I believe some one had told him that all male children in America are named Jean at their birth) "*j'ai vu QUELQUE CHOSE! le nègre, vous savez?—il est FORT! Monsieur Jean, c'est un* GÉANT, *croyez moi! C'est pas un homme, tu sais? Je l'ai vu, moi*"—and he indicated his eyes.

We pricked our ears.

The *balayeur*, stuffing a pipe nervously with his tiny thumb said: "You saw the fight up here? So did I. The whole of it. *Le noir avait raison.* Well, when they took him downstairs, I slipped out too—*Je suis le balayeur, savez-vous?* and the *balayeur* can go where other people can't."

—I gave him a match, and he thanked me. He struck it on his trousers with a quick pompous gesture, drew heavily on his squeaky pipe, and at last shot a minute puff of smoke into the air; then another, and another. Satisfied, he went on; his good hand grasping the pipe between its index and second fingers and resting on one little knee, his legs crossed, his small body hunched forward, wee unshaven face close to mine—went on in the confidential tone of one who relates an unbelievable miracle to a couple of intimate friends.

"Monsieur Jean, I followed. They got him to the *cabinot*. The door stood open. At this moment *les femmes descendaient*, it was their *corvée d'eau, vous savez*. He saw them, *le noir*. One of them cried from the stairs, Is a Frenchman stronger than you, Jean? The *plantons* were standing around him, the *Surveillant* was behind. He took the nearest *planton*, and tossed him down the corridor so that he struck against the door at the end of it. He picked up two more, one in each arm, and threw them away. They fell on top of the first. The last tried to take hold of Jean, and so Jean took him by the neck"—(the *balayeur* strangled himself for our benefit)—"and that *planton* knocked down the other three, who had got on their feet by this time. You should have seen the *Surveillant*. He had run away and was saying, 'Capture him, capture him.' The *plantons* rushed Jean; all four of them. He caught them as they came and threw them about. One knocked down the *Surveillant*. The *femmes* cried '*Vive, Jean*,' and clapped their hands. The *Surveillant* called to the *plantons* to take Jean, but they wouldn't go near Jean; they said he was a black devil. The women kidded them. They were so sore. And they could do nothing. Jean was laughing. His shirt was almost off him. He asked the *plantons* to come and take him, please. He asked the *Surveillant*, too. The women had set down their pails and were dancing up and down and yelling. The *Directeur* came down and sent them flying. The *Surveillant* and his *plantons* were as helpless as if they had been children. Monsieur Jean—*quelque chose*."

I gave him another match. "*Merci*, Monsieur Jean." He struck it, drew on his pipe, lowered it, and went on:

"They were helpless, and men. I am little. I have only one arm, *tu sais*. I walked up to Jean and said, 'Jean, you know me, I am your friend.' He said, 'Yes.' I said to the *plantons*, 'Give me that rope.' They gave me the rope that they would have bound him with. He put out his wrists for me. I tied his hands behind his back. He was like a lamb. The *plantons* rushed up and tied his feet together. Then they tied his hands and feet together. They took the lacings out of his shoes for fear he would use them to strangle himself. They stood him up in an angle between two walls in the *cabinot*. They left him there for an hour. He was supposed to have been in there all night; but The *Surveillant* knew that he would have died, for he was almost naked, and *vous savez*, Monsieur Jean, it was cold in there. And damp. A fully-clothed man would have been dead in the morning. And he was naked . . . Monsieur Jean—*un géant!*"

—This same *petit belge* had frequently protested to me that *Il est fou, le noir*. He is always playing when sensible men try to sleep. The last few hours (which had made of the *fou* a *géant*) made of the scoffer a worshipper. Nor did "*le bras cassé*" ever from that time forth desert his divinity. If as *balayeur* he could lay hands on a *morceau de pain* or *de viande*, he bore it as before to our beds; but Jean was always called over to partake of the forbidden pleasure.

As for Jean, one would hardly have recognized him. It was as if the child had fled into the deeps of his soul, never to reappear. Day after day went by, and Jean (instead of courting excitement as before) cloistered himself in solitude; or at most sought the company of B. and me and *Le Petit Belge* for a quiet chat or a cigarette. The morning after the three fights he did not appear in the *cour* for early promenade along with the rest of us (including The Sheeneys). In vain did *les femmes* strain their necks and eyes to find the *noir qui était plus fort que six français*. And B. and I noticed our bed-clothing airing upon the window-sills. When we mounted, Jean was patting and straightening our blankets, and looking for the first time in his life guilty of some enormous crime. Nothing however had disappeared. Jean said, "Me feeks, *lits tous les jours*." And every morning he aired and made our beds for us, and we mounted to find him smoothing affectionately some final ruffle, obliterating with enormous solemnity some microscopic crease. We gave him cigarettes when he asked for them (which was almost never) and offered them when we knew he had none or when we saw him borrowing from some one else whom his spirit held in less esteem. Of us he asked no favours. He liked us too well.

When B. went away, Jean was almost as desolate as I.

About a fortnight later, when the grey dirty snow-slush hid the black filthy world which we saw from our windows, and when people lived in their ill-smelling beds, it came to pass that my particular *amis*—The Zulu, Jean, Mexique—and I and all the remaining misérables of La Ferté descended at the decree of Cæsar Augustus to endure our bi-weekly *bain*. I remember gazing stupidly at Jean's chocolate-coloured nakedness as it strode to the tub, a rippling texture of muscular miracle. *Tout le monde* had *baigné* (including The Zulu, who tried to escape at the last minute and was nabbed by the *planton* whose business it was to count heads and see that none escaped the ordeal) and now *tout le monde* was shivering all together in the ante-room, begging to be allowed to go upstairs and get into bed—when *Le Baigneur*, Monsieur Richard's strenuous successor that is, set up a hue and cry that one *serviette* was lacking. The Fencer was sent for. He entered; heard the case; and made a speech. If the guilty party would immediately return the stolen towel, he, The Fencer, would guarantee that party pardon; if not, everyone present should be searched, and the man on whose person the *serviette* was found *va attraper quinze jours de cabinot*. This eloquence yielding no results, The Fencer exhorted the culprit to act like a man and render to Cæsar what is Cæsar's. Nothing happened. Everyone was told to get in single file and make ready to pass out the door. One after one we were searched; but so general was the curiosity that as fast as they were inspected the erstwhile bed-enthusiasts, myself included, gathered on the side-lines to watch their fellows instead of availing themselves of the opportunity to go upstairs. One after one we came opposite The Fencer, held up our arms, had our pockets run through and our clothing felt over from head to heel, and were exonerated. When Cæsar came to Jean, Cæsar's eyes lighted, and Cæsar's hitherto perfunctory proddings and pokings became inspired and methodical. Twice he went over Jean's entire body, while Jean, his arms raised in a bored gesture, his face completely expressionless, suffered loftily the examination of his person. A third time the desperate Fencer tried; his hands, starting at Jean's neck, reached the calf of his leg—and stopped. The hands rolled up Jean's right trouser leg to the knee. They rolled up the underwear on his leg—and there, placed perfectly flat to the skin, appeared the missing *serviette*. As The Fencer seized it, Jean laughed—the utter laughter of old days—and the onlookers cackled uproariously, while with a broad smile The Fencer proclaimed: "I thought I knew where I should find it." And he added, more pleased with himself than anyone had ever seen him—"*Maintenant, vous pouvez tous monter à la chambre.*" We mounted, happy to get back to bed; but none so happy as Jean le Nègre. It was not that the *cabinot* threat had failed to materialize—at any minute a *planton* might call Jean to his punishment: indeed this was what everyone expected. It was that the incident had absolutely removed that inhibition which (from the day when Jean *le noir* became Jean *le géant*) had held the child, which was Jean's soul and destiny, prisoner. From that instant till the day I left him he was the old Jean—joking, fibbing, laughing, and always playing—Jean L'Enfant.

And I think of Jean Le Nègre . . . you are something to dream over, Jean; summer and winter (birds and darkness) you go walking into my head; you are a sudden and chocolate-coloured thing, in your hands you have a habit of holding six or eight *plantons* (which you are about to throw away) and the flesh of your body is like the flesh of a very deep cigar. Which I am still and always quietly smoking: always and still I am inhaling its very fragrant and remarkable muscles. But I doubt if ever I am quite through with you, if ever I will toss you out of my heart into the sawdust of forgetfulness. Kid, Boy, I'd like to tell you: *la guerre est finie.*

O yes, Jean: I do not forget, I remember Plenty; the snow's coming, the snow will throw again a very big and gentle shadow into The Enormous Room and into the eyes of you and me walking always and wonderfully up and down. . . .

—Boy, Kid, Nigger with the strutting muscles—take me up into your mind once or twice before I die (you know why: just because the eyes of me and you will be full of dirt some day). Quickly take me up into the bright child of your mind, before we both go suddenly all loose and silly (you know how it will feel). Take me up (carefully; as if I were a toy) and play carefully with me, once or twice, before I and you go suddenly all limp and foolish. Once or twice before you go into great Jack roses and ivory—(once or twice Boy before we together go wonderfully down into the Big Dirt laughing, bumped with the last darkness).

The New Way of Writing

BONAMY DOBRÉE (1891-   )

CAN WE say that there is, definitely, "a new way of writing"? Is there such a thing as *modern* prose, with characteristics the older prose does not possess? [1] It may seem at first sight that the question cannot reasonably be put, for if we are agreed that style is the personal voice—which pierces through even the "im-

THE NEW WAY OF WRITING, from *Modern Prose Style* by Bonamy Dobrée, is reprinted by permission of the Clarendon Press, Oxford.

[1] I may suggest to begin with, that had I been writing thirty years ago, I would probably have felt constrained to write "with characteristics *which* the older . . ."

personal" manner—and that the voice is the man; and if we assume, as we plausibly can, that man does not alter except over very long periods, can we talk of a modern as opposed to an old-fashioned style?

One can make two answers to this. The first is, that though time may not change man physically, nor perhaps mentally, leaving his vocal chords and what he wants to do with them still the same, two things do change: the social being, and with him the method of speech he must use to be effective with other social beings. Man as a social animal alters in tune with what we call, since a better term is lacking, "the spirit of the age," which we gauge by the different approaches men make to the external universe, and, more important perhaps, to their own emotions. Man may be fundamentally unchanged, but in the social process of his time, different facets are polished, unfamiliar aspects emerge. To take a simple example: How would a fourteenth-century man react if he were asked to think of "the wonders of the deep" compared with the way a twentieth-century man would react? Today we should at once let our minds turn to what we might roughly call "scientific marvels," that is to various detailed manifestations of fish life, or of corals. The fourteenth-century man would shudder deliciously at a vision of leviathans, appallingly, even incredibly shaped, of mermaids, of ghostly inhabitants. Not only, then, will men of various ages wish to *ex*press different things, but they will wish to *im*press men differently. What would be the good, for instance, of a member of the House of Lords rising up and saying:

> My Lords, this ruinous and ignominious situation, where we cannot act with success nor suffer with honour, calls upon us to remonstrate in the strongest and loudest language of truth, to rescue the ears of majesty from the delusions which surround it.

We can imagine a peer having similar feelings about, perhaps, the situation in India, but such language, used by Chatham in 1777, would have no result whatever now, though in its way it is splendid, and in its own age was no doubt very effective indeed. Our second answer arises out of the first: since the needs of the voice have changed, the instrument has been altered: we no longer use the same tool as our ancestors did to move other people. And there is still another consideration. If we use a different tool it is that our emotions have changed, or at any rate, if our emotions do not change, our attitude towards them differs with the age in which we live. These things, however, interact upon each other. We know, as once we did not know, that our emotions vary with the language we use in describing them: the spirit of an age may not only be reflected in its prose, it may be, indeed it is, to some extent conditioned by it. This, however, is an issue which would take us too far outside the bounds of our subject; nor am I qualified to pursue it.

Let us now take two passages, dealing with much the same range of ideas, written by men who were each in their day stylists. We have already done something of the sort in the Introduction, but we can use another example to reinforce the argument of the first. This time one writer is Sir Thomas Browne, the other William James, and I am taking Browne at his most straightforward.

Let thy studies be free as thy thoughts and contemplations: but fly not only upon the wings of imagination; join sense unto reason, and experiment unto speculation, and so give life unto embryon truths, and verities yet in their chaos. There is nothing more acceptable unto the ingenious world, than this noble eluctation of truth; wherein, against the tenacity of prejudice and prescription, this century now prevaileth.

That is from *Christian Morals:* now let us take this from *The Will to Believe:*

On the whole, then, we must conclude that no philosophy of ethics is possible in the old-fashioned absolute sense of the term. Everywhere the ethical philosopher must wait on facts. The thinkers who create the ideals come he knows not whence, their sensibilities are evolved he knows not how; and the question as to which of two conflicting ideals will give the best universe then and there, can be answered by him only through the aid of the experience of other men.

I take it that anybody, even neglecting Browne's obsolete forms, would at once recognize the first passage as belonging to the seventeenth century, and the second to our own time. Can we put our finger on where exactly the difference lies?

It is pretty obvious that the difference lies in the rhythm, but that is too easy a thing to say: and as a matter of fact, if we analyse these two passages into "prose rhythms" in the way that Saintsbury did in his fascinating book, they are not, prosodically speaking at least, so different after all. Are not such cadences as

embryon/truths, and/verities/yet in their/chaos,

and

old-fashioned/absolute/sense of the/term,

of much the same order? Both are, in a sense, dactylic. What is different is the way the metres are used. In modern writing there is far less insistence on the rhythms; the unit into which the rhythms are woven, that is to say the phrase, is far more flexible, on the whole longer. The antithetical balance has gone. But what is more significant is that the written language to-day is much nearer the spoken language, with implications we shall follow up in a moment. But first I must dispose of two possible objections. The first and lesser one is that for the seventeenth century example we have a very conscious stylist. That is true, but Jeremy Taylor or Milton will give much the same result. Why do we remember, except for its insistence on rhythm, Milton's "rousing herself like a strong man after sleep, and shaking her invincible locks"? But how do I know, it will be asked in the second place, that the older people did not speak as they wrote? The suggestion is often made, most notably by Mr. Gordon Bottomley, that in the seventeenth century, especially in Shakespeare's time, the rhythms of everyday speech were more accentuated, approached even those of blank verse, or of obviously cadenced speech. Let us look at something from a contemporary of Sir Thomas Browne's:

> Up, and by water, stopping at Michell's, and there saw Betty, but could have no discourse with her, but there drank. To White Hall, and there walked to St. James's, where I find the Court mighty full, it being the Duke of York's birthday; and he mighty fine, and all the musick, one after another, to my great content.

Pepys, you see at once, was not writing literary English: he was setting down his doings as he might have chatted about them to his wife—if, of course, he had been a brave enough man to do so.

It is fairly certain, I think, that the written language of the seventeenth century was farther from the spoken language than the written language of to-day is from our conversation, a division which probably began with Caxton. John Donne, one can be sure, never spoke at home in the way that he thundered from the pulpit. The proof is to be found in the correspondence of the time, much of which has been collected by Professor Wyld in his *History of Modern Colloquial English*, largely for this purpose; and what comes out is that the language of the Elizabethans was not essentially unlike our own. Here, for one example, is Sir Philip Sidney writing to Edward Molyneux:

> Few words are best. My letters to my father have come to the eyes of some. Neither can I condemn any but you for it. If it be so you have played the very knave with me; and so I will make you know if I have good proof of it. But that for so much as is past. For that is to come, I assure you before God, that if ever I know you do so much as read any letter I write to my father, without his commandment, or my consent, I will thrust my dagger into you. And trust to it, for I speak it in earnest. In the mean time, farewell.

The sentiments of this prose (we trust) are not ours, and the forms are not quite so, but the ring of it is. If we were to say that sort of thing, we should say it in that kind of way. Sidney's prose here, we see, is altogether different from what he wrote for the press, his "Sidneyan showers of sweet discourse." Here is another example; and making allowance for stage speech, does it sound very quaint or old-fashioned, or very heavily rhythmed?

> Thou art so fat-witted, with drinking of old sack, and unbuttoning thee after supper, and sleeping upon benches after noon, that thou hast forgotten to demand that truly which thou wouldst truly know. What a devil hast thou to do with the time of the day. . . .

Prince Hal probably spoke fairly current English; and the journalists of the time, Nashe, Greene, Dekker, wrote much in the way Prince Hal spoke, for they were not labouring after fine style, but trying to write as men talked. What appears to have happened is that in the seventeenth century a profound division developed between the spoken and the written language, a division bridged by the journalists and the comic writers. What seems to have occurred afterwards was, to cut a long story short, that the journalists, forgetting Dryden, deserted to the written side: one has only to think of Addison, and then of Dr. Johnson, who, far from trying to write as he naturally spoke, did his best to model his conversation on his writing. Everybody remembers how he let slip the remark about *The Rehearsal* not having wit enough to keep it sweet, and then, recoiling in horror from so natural an expression, hurriedly amended the phrase to "has not vitality enough to preserve it from corruption." The stylists of the eighteenth century seem to have taken their writing farther and farther away from their speech—Gibbon, Burke, Smollett. This process went on through the nineteenth century; we have only to think of Carlyle or Pater, though it is true that some people all the while kept up the spoken tradition, Defoe, Sterne, and even Lamb, for though Lamb's style is artificial as regards words, his rhythms are those of his talk, or at any rate of his possible talk. What I think is going on at the present day is a return to speech rhythms: the conscious stylists are, so to speak, ridding themselves of "style": not "style," but *a* style is what they are aiming at, a style that will faithfully reflect their mind as it utters itself naturally. What is curious is that now it is the leading authors who write naturally, style, so-called, being left to the journalists. I take the opening sentence of the first leading article of *The Times* of the day on which I happened to be taking notes for this chapter (19 August 1933): "As soon as it was announced, on the morrow of Parliament's rising. . . ." One need not go on. Who would dream of *saying* "on the morrow of Parliament's rising"? It is jargon. What we would probably say is, "the day after Parliament rose." Not that this *pompier* "style" is confined to the august heights of journalism: it runs all through, and not long ago *The Daily Worker* printed with regard to certain prisons: "No sound comes from out those walls." Does the man who wrote those words habitually say "from out"? Why does this happen? Why do people write forms which are dead, which they would never utter? In both the examples quoted one is tempted to diagnose insincerity of thought, or at least mental laziness.

Does it not seem, then, that the modern prosewriter, in returning to the rhythms of everyday speech, is trying to be more honest with himself than if he used, as is too wreckingly easy, the forms and terms already published as the expression of other people's minds? "Style . . . is not an ornament; it is not an exercise, not a caper, nor complication of any sort. It is the sense of one's self, the knowledge of what one wants to say, and the saying of it in the most fitting words." [2] And that is why it is extremely hard to achieve *a* style, for all these three things are very difficult to attain. Take only the last task, the saying of what one wants to say in the most fitting words. It seems almost impossible, for every time we speak we have virtually to re-create the instrument if we want to be faithful to our idea or feeling. Everywhere the words and phrasing of past generations interpose themselves between us and the reality. "It is . . . a true and

[2] Introduction to *The London Book of English Prose*, by Herbert Read and Bonamy Dobrée, Eyre and Spottiswoode, 1931.

lamentable fact that, in ultimate analysis, one cannot speak about anything without altering it to some extent." [3] It is the realization of this, a realization possibly new in our day, which impels authors to try to write as they speak in ordinary life on ordinary physical matters, for it is only in this way that one can achieve fidelity to one's self: otherwise the language and style of the literary tradition assert themselves. But the modern writer must not think of style: the man who thinks first of style is lost: the primary thing to do—this is an old observation—is to think clearly. As M. Jean Cocteau says, writing for modern authors: "Style cannot be a starting point: it happens. What is style? For a great many people it is a complicated way of saying very simple things. From our point of view it is a very simple way of saying complicated things." [4] How does a modern writer tackle this problem? Here, I think, is a good example:

> I had great ambitions. I have none now—and have not even the fear of failing. What matters to me and to many of the survivors of my generation is only that which is common to us all, our fear for our children. If it were not for that, I should know how to act in what remains of my life—that would be to withdraw as far as possible from the little world of writing and talking about books which is a microcosm of the whole, its values no finer than those accepted by the rest of the world, and only valid on the assumption that to a writer success means precisely what it means to a stockbroker or a multiple grocer. That is, material wealth, and the respect paid to it. This seems to me a denial of all the writer, the "clerk," should stand for, but I can do nothing to alter it, and therefore I ought to run away for my life.
>
> After all that turbulence of desire and ambitions it seems strange I should believe now that very little in me is real except the absolute need, intellectual and spiritual, for withdrawal, for resolving to satisfy in my life only the simple wants. It is as strange as that I am only just learning to write and don't care to.
>
> There are days when I retract all this, and think how queer I shall grow if I live alone, and think too that what is needed is some effort to

[3] *The Theory of Speech and Language,* by A. H. Gardiner, Oxford, 1932.
[4] *A Call to Order,* Allen and Unwin, trs. 1933.

create cells inside the body social, groups of angry, last-minute saints. That would be no good. I should weary in a week of the company of persons who thought and felt no differently from myself. [5]

That, as prose, is simple, easy, fluent, and flexible; what is important, however, is that it is written, apparently, in the *tones* of every day, though here and there we can detect traces of literary forms—"only that which" instead of "only what": "how to act" instead of "what to do": it is extraordinarily difficult to rid one's self of terms of that kind. But to show how new the tone is, here is a passage from another autobiography written, one always thought, in a natural, confidential manner:

There were perhaps twenty boys in the school at most, and often fewer. I made the excursion between home and school four times a day; if I walked fast, the transit might take five minutes, and, as there were several objects of interest on the way, it might be spread over an hour. In fine weather the going to and from school was very delightful, and small as the scope was, it could be varied almost indefinitely.[6]

There are, we see immediately, one or two obvious "literary" turns in that passage: "I made the excursion between home and school," instead of "I went to and from school": "If I walked fast, the transit might take five minutes," instead of "I could get there or back (or do the journey) in five minutes": "objects of interest," with others of the same sort. And the general run, which is the important thing, though simple and easy, and we might perhaps admit fluent, is not flexible. Each sentence contains an idea and completes it. The mind comes to a full stop at the end of each phrase. But our minds in life do not work in that way; they are always ready to frame the next sentence, carried on by the impetus of the last. Gosse, in common with the older writers, was concerned, not to follow the movements of his mind, but to present something concrete.

To say, then, that the hall-mark of good modern prose style

[5] From *No Time Like the Present*, by Storm Jameson, Cassell, 1933.
[6] From *Father and Son*, by Edmund Gosse, Heinemann, 1907.

is an essential fidelity does not imply that writers of previous generations were charlatans and liars, only that they owed fidelity to other things. And it is here that the spirit of our age imposes itself upon our style. All the previous ages whose writers have been quoted or referred to here had something they could take for granted, and it never occurred to the older writers that they could not take themselves for granted. We can be sure of nothing; our civilization is threatened, even the simplest things we live by: we are on the verge of amazing changes. In our present confusion our only hope is to be scrupulously honest with ourselves, so honest as to doubt our own minds and the conclusions they arrive at. Most of us have ceased to believe, except provisionally, in truths, and we feel that what is important is not so much truth as the way our minds move towards truths. Therefore, to quote M. Cocteau again, "Form must be the form of the mind. Not a way of saying things, but of thinking them." Perhaps that is why we nowadays instinctively mistrust any one who pontificates: and, as a matter of experience, if we examine the writings of the pontificators, people skilled in "a way of saying things," we invariably find that their style is bad, that falsity has crept in somewhere. The writer is not being faithful to the movement of his mind; he is taking things for granted, and he fills us of to-day with uneasiness.

We have, then, to judge of the integrity of a modern writer by this sense of himself that we feel he has. If we are to respond, he must (we suppose) be aware of himself as something a little uncertain in this shifting universe: he also is part of the material which he has to treat with respect: he must listen to himself, so to speak, to hear what he has to say. He must not prejudge, or force an issue: we must be able to imagine that he is talking to himself. In no other way can he achieve *a* style, which is the sound of his voice, which is the man himself.

It is not so simple as it sounds for a man to watch his own mind; it is as difficult as writing in the way you ordinarily talk: literary habits continually get in the way. Nor must a man write as he might lazily talk, and it is more important than ever for him to reject the dead metaphor which can never be more than an approximation, to choose the exact, the expressive word, to rid his style of fat, to make it athletic. What he must really do, as the first essential, is to keep his awareness athletic, especially his awareness of himself. And he must not watch his mind idly; he must watch it as he might a delicate piece of machinery doing its work, and he must watch it, not flickering about in every direction, as an active mind does, but only in the direction he wants it to go. Otherwise the result may be disastrous. Even the following extremely clever attempt seems to me an object-lesson:

The problem from this time on became more definite.

It was all so nearly alike it must be different and it is different, it is natural that if everything is used and there is a continuous present and a beginning again and again if it is all so alike it must be simply different and everything simply different was the natural way of creating it then.

In this natural way of creating it then that it was simply different everything being alike it was simply different, this kept on leading one to lists. Lists naturally for a while and by lists I mean a series. More and more in going back over what was done at this time I find that I naturally kept simply different as an intention. Whether there was or whether there was not a continuous present did not then any longer trouble me there was or there was, and using everything no longer troubled me if everything is alike using everything could no longer trouble me and beginning again and again could no longer trouble me because if lists were inevitable if series were inevitable and the whole of it was inevitable beginning again and again could not trouble me so then with nothing to trouble me I very completely began naturally since everything is alike making it as simply different naturally as simply different as possible. I began doing natural phenomena what I call natural phenomena and natural phenomena naturally everything being alike natural phenomena are making things be naturally simply different. This found its culmination later, in the beginning it began in a center confused with lists with series with geography with returning portraits and with particularly often four and three and often with five and four. It is easy to see that in the beginning such a conception as everything being naturally different would be very inarticulate and very slowly it began to emerge and take the form of anything, and then naturally if anything that is simply different is simply different what follows will follow.[7]

One cannot say whether Miss Stein's mind really moves like that: possibly it does, and possibly most of our minds move more like that than we are aware of, or at any rate are prepared to admit. What is clear is that the mere following of the mind, its echoes and repetitions, does not really give its shape; and this makes us realize that to write naturally as the mind would wish to utter, is just as much an art—or an artifice—as to write in what we call an artificial style, say that of a Pater or Meredith. What has happened is that the modern writer is faced with new material, and what he has to do is to discover the new form that this material requires.

But because this new form can only be an adaptation of the old, it takes consummate art to prevent literature interposing itself between us and life. The problem, no doubt, has always existed, but if it has been realized the solution has rarely, if ever, been hit on. Yet there is Sterne, and what Mrs. Woolf has to say about him is illuminating:

. . . With the first words—They order, said I, this matter better in France—we are in the world of *Tristram Shandy*. It is a world in which anything may happen. We hardly know what jest, what jibe, what flash of poetry is not going to glance suddenly through the gap which this astonishingly agile pen has cut in the thick-set hedge of English prose. Is Sterne himself responsible? Does he know what he is going to say next for all his resolve to be on his best behaviour this time? The jerky disconnected sentences are as rapid and it would seem as little under control as the phrases that fall from the lips of a brilliant talker. The very punctuation is that of speech, not writing, and brings the sounds and associations of the speaking voice in with it. The order of the ideas, their suddenness and irrelevancy, is more true to life than

[7] From *Composition as Explanation*, by Gertrude Stein, Hogarth Press, 1926.

to literature. . . . Under the influence of this extraordinary style the book becomes semi-transparent. The usual ceremonies and conventions which keep reader and writer at arm's length disappear. We are as close to life as we can be.[8]

That passage is not quoted as being characteristic of Mrs. Woolf: to hear her real voice one must go to the novels: it is quoted as an aid to my argument. And it serves it in two ways, because of what it says, and because of the way it says it, for if the prose is not markedly Mrs. Woolf's, it is obviously modern: the voice that is speaking is a voice of to-day: I shall not be misunderstood, I hope, if I say that any one might have written it. Now let us compare this with the way Bagehot wrote about Sterne in the *National Review* in 1864:

But here the great excellence of Sterne ends as well as begins. In *Tristram Shandy* especially there are several defects which, while we are reading it, tease and disgust us so much that we are scarcely willing even to admire as we ought to admire the refined pictures of human emotion. The first of these, and perhaps the worst, is the fantastic disorder of the form. It is an imperative law of the writing art, that a book should go straight on. A great writer should be able to tell a great meaning as coherently as a small writer tells a small meaning. . . .

and so it goes on. That is typical nineteenth-century prose: we get something very like it in Matthew Arnold, or Huxley, and in its way it is excellent. But the rhythms and inflexions are quite different from those of to-day: it consists, not of thoughts closely followed, not of ideas suggested, but of utterances, of pronouncements. Again, as with Gosse, we have the end-stopped phrase: there is a door banged at the end of each, and we feel as though we were on parade receiving orders.

What seems to us to be lacking in the older prose is the sense of the uninterrupted flow of the mind: Bagehot, for example, appears to cut off this continuum, shall we call it, into arbitrary lengths, as we slice chunks off a cucumber. This is to force on our minds a logic that is not of their own making; and though it may

[8] *The Common Reader*, ii, Hogarth Press, 1932.

be true that, as T. E. Hulme said, "All styles are only means of subduing the reader," we must not feel that our minds are being forced, and therefore distorted. Perhaps it was George Moore's principal achievement to give this sense of flow: there is hardly an instant's pause in his mental processes. His style is very distinctive; all the time one hears a voice, a personal utterance, though pursued to the lengths to which he took it, or allowed it to carry him, it becomes in the end monotonous. The mind runs on too much; it has no form but that of a stream: no solid shape emerges. But the sort of flow we are talking about can, and sometimes does, take form. Here is an extract from Henry James, whose whole being was directed to following the movement of his mind, and who gave form to this movement, not indeed in a language natural to us, but one which seems to have been natural to him, a way which he could not have escaped from even if he had wanted to:

> Momentary side-winds—things of no real authority—break in every now and then to put their inferior little questions to me; but I come back, I come back, as I say, I all throbbingly and yearningly and passionately, oh mon bon come back to this way that is clearly the only one in which I can do anything now, and that will open out to me more and more, and that has overwhelming reasons pleading all beautifully in its breast. What really happens is that the closer I get to the problem of the application of it in any particular case, the more I get *into* that application, so that the more doubts and torments fall away from me, the more I know where I am, the more everything spreads and shines and draws me on and I'm justified in my logic and my passion. . . . Causons, causons, mon bon—oh celestial, soothing, sanctifying process, with all the high sane forces of the sacred time fighting, through it, on my side! Let me fumble it gently and patiently out—with fever and fidget laid to rest—as in all the old enchanted months! It only looms, it only shines and shimmers, *too* beautiful and too interesting, it only hangs there too rich and too full and with too much to give and to pay; it only presents itself too admirably and too vividly, too straight and square and vivid, as a little organic and effective Action.[9]

[9] *Letters*, Macmillan.

We may think that artificial, but we do not feel, complicated as it is, that this is a literary language. It is the language of Henry James's speech; it reflects his mind accurately, a mind with a very definite form. James, if you like, had a tortuous way of thinking, but he had broken down the barriers between his mind and the expression of it.

What we look for, however, is a style which shall be as free and individual as in that passage, but which smacks less of idiosyncrasy, for something we might all use, though, no doubt, not so well as our model, for something which does not give us, as some recent prose does, the uneasy effect of submitting us to a laboratory experiment. Perhaps this is what we want:

> The trouble with her ship was that it would *not* sail. It rode waterlogged in the rotting port of home. All very well to have wild, reckless moods of irony and independence, if you have to pay for them by withering dustily on the shelf.
>
> Alvina fell again into humility and fear: she began to show symptoms of her mother's heart trouble. For day followed day, month followed month, season after season went by, and she grubbed away like a housemaid in Manchester House, she hurried round doing the shopping, she sang in the choir on Sundays, she attended the various chapel events, she went out to visit friends, and laughed and talked and played games. But all the time, what was there actually in her life? Not much. She was withering towards old-maiddom. Already in her twenty-eighth year, she spent her days grubbing in the house, whilst her father became an elderly, frail man still too lively in mind and spirit. Miss Pinnegar began to grow grey and elderly too, money became scarcer and scarcer, there was a black day ahead when her father would die and the home be broken up, and she would have to tackle life as a worker.
>
> There lay the only alternative: in work. She might slave her days away teaching the piano, as Miss Frost had done: she might find a subordinate post as nurse: she might sit in the cash-desk of some shop. Some work of some sort would be found for her. And she would sink into the routine of her job, as did so many women, and grow old and die, chattering and fluttering. She would have what is called her in-

dependence. But, seriously faced with that treasure, and without the option of refusing it, strange how hideous she found it.

Work!—a job! More even than she rebelled against the Withams did she rebel against a job. . . .[10]

It is clear, I imagine, that that could not have been written in the last century; it speaks with the authentic voice of this. It has the ring of what we hear around us every day: it has no air of "style," yet it is extremely expressive. Certain liberties are taken, such as leaving out "It is . . ." before "all very well . . ." in the first paragraph. Here and there we feel just a touch of literary formulas, and we wish they were not there: "as did so many women" instead of "as so many women did," but these things are very rare in Lawrence. We feel that he is nearly always completely free of "literature" and can be himself. We follow his mind working—and he speaks as it works. Or, at least, that is the impression we get. It is not true, of course: but at least he is using his material (part of which is his mind) with complete freedom, and finding a form which will make it tell.

Suppose that, before we go on to discuss experiments, we try to prophesy what direction our prose will take. We might perhaps say that it will be in that of greater flexibility and a more curious following of our mental processes, with, sometimes, violence offered to our old notions of syntax wherever we find them distorting or cumbrous. One would like to think that all of us will come to the stage of refusing to write what we would not, indeed could not, say, though that, of course, is not to limit our writing to what we actually do say. This is not to claim for a moment that by writing as we speak we shall achieve a style; before we do that we must go through at least three fundamental disciplines. First there is that of fidelity to thought, the extremely difficult task of complete honesty; we must not, as is so easy, allow language to condition our thought: then there is the labour of finding the exact words and the exact inflexion of phrase to carry the whole sense, the emotional colour, of the words; and

[10] From *The Lost Girl,* by D. H. Lawrence, Secker, 1920.

thirdly, it is over and above these things that we have to model our prose to give it what seems to be the run and structure of our usual speaking. That is where the artifice comes in, and that is where we can achieve the art.

Ladies' and Gentlemen's Guide to Modern English Usage

JAMES THURBER (1894–)

WHICH

THE RELATIVE pronoun "which" can cause more trouble than any other word, if recklessly used. Foolhardy persons sometimes get lost in which-clauses and are never heard of again. My distinguished contemporary, Fowler, cites several tragic cases, of which the following is one: "It was rumoured that Beaconsfield intended opening the Conference with a speech in French, his pronunciation of which language leaving everything to be desired . . ." That's as much as Mr. Fowler quotes because, at his age, he was afraid to go any farther. The young man who originally got into that sentence was never found. His fate, however, was not as terrible as that of another adventurer who became involved in a remarkable whichmire. Fowler has followed his devious course as far as he safely could on foot: "Surely what applies to games should also apply to racing, the leaders of which being the very people from whom an example might well be looked for . . ." Not even Henry James could have successfully emerged from a sentence with "which," "whom," and "being" in it. The safest way to avoid such things is to follow in the path of the American author, Ernest Hemingway. In his youth he was trapped in a which-clause one time and barely escaped with his mind. He was going along on solid ground until he got into this: "It was the one thing of which, being very much afraid—for whom has not been warned to fear such things—he . . ." Being a young and powerfully built man, Hemingway was able to fight his way back to where he had started, and begin again. This time he skirted the treacherous morass in this way: "He was afraid of one thing. This was the one thing. He had been warned to fear such things. Everybody has been warned to fear such things." Today Hemingway is alive and well, and many happy writers are following along the trail he blazed.

What most people don't realize is that one "which" leads to another. Trying to cross a paragraph by leaping from "which" to "which" is like Eliza crossing the ice. The danger is in missing a "which" and falling in. A case in point is this: "He went up to a pew which was in the gallery, which brought him under a colored window which he loved and always quieted his spirit." The writer, worn out, missed the last "which"—the one that should come just before "always" in that sentence. But supposing he had got it in! We would have: "He went up to a pew which was in the gallery, which brought him under a colored window which he loved and which always quieted his spirit." Your inveterate whicher in this way gives the effect of tweeting like a bird or walking with a crutch, and is not welcome in the best company.

It is well to remember that one "which" leads to two and that two "whiches" multiply like rabbits. You should never start out with the idea that you can get by with one "which." Suddenly they are all around you. Take a sentence like this: "It imposes a problem which we either solve, or perish." On a hot night, or after a hard day's work, a man often lets himself get by with a monstrosity like that, but suppose he dictates that sentence bright and early in the morning. It comes to him typed out by his stenographer and he instantly senses that something is the matter with it. He tries to reconstruct the sentence, still clinging to the "which," and gets something like this: "It imposes a problem which we either solve, or which, failing to solve, we must perish on account of." He goes to the water-cooler, gets a drink, sharpens his pencil, and grimly tries again. "It imposes a problem which we either solve or which we don't solve and . . ." He begins once more: "It imposes a problem which we either solve, or which we do not solve, and from which . . ." The more times he does it the more "whiches" he gets. The way out is simple: "We must either solve this problem, or perish." Never monkey with "which." Nothing except getting tangled up in a typewriter ribbon is worse.

THE SPLIT INFINITIVE

Word has somehow got around that a split infinitive is always wrong. This is of a piece with the sentimental and outworn notion that it is always wrong to strike a lady. Everybody will recall at least one woman of his acquaintance whom, at one time, or another, he has had to punch or slap. I have in mind a charming lady who is overcome by the unaccountable desire, at formal dinners with red and white wines, to climb up on the table and lie down. Her dinner companions used at first to pinch her, under cover of the conversation, but she pinched right back or, what is even less defensible, tickled. They finally learned that they could make her hold her seat only by fetching her a smart downward blow on the head. She would then sit quietly through the rest of the dinner, smiling dreamily and nodding at people, and looking altogether charming.

A man who does not know his own strength could, of course, all too easily overshoot the mark and, instead of producing the delightful languor to which I have alluded, knock his companion completely under the table, an awkward situation which should be avoided at all costs because it would leave two men seated next each other. I know of one man who, to avert this *faux pas*, used to punch his dinner companion in the side (she would begin to cry during the red-wine courses), a blow which can be executed, as a rule, with less fuss, but which has the disadvantage of almost always causing the person who is struck to shout. The hostess, in order to put her guest at her ease, must shout too, which is almost certain to arouse one of those nervous, high-strung men, so common at formal dinners, to such a pitch that he will begin throwing things. There is nothing more deplorable than the spectacle of a formal dinner party ending in a brawl. And yet it is surprising how even the most cultured and charming people can go utterly to pieces when something is unexpectedly thrown at table. They instantly have an overwhelming desire to "join in." Everybody has, at one time or another, experienced the urge to throw a plate of jelly or a half grapefruit, an urge comparable to the inclination that suddenly assails one to leap from high places. Usually this tendency passes as quickly as it comes, but it is astounding how rapidly it can be converted into action once the spell of dignity and well-bred reserve is broken by the sight of, say, a green-glass salad plate flying through the air. It is all but impossible to sit quietly by while someone is throwing salad plates. One is stirred to participation not only by the swift progress of the objects and their crash as they hit something, but also by the cries of "Whammy!" and "Whoop!", with which most men accompany the act of hurling plates. In the end someone is bound to be caught over the eye by a badly aimed plate and rendered unconscious.

My contemporary, Mr. Fowler, in a painstaking analysis of the split infinitive, divides the English-speaking world into five classes as regards this construction: those who don't know and don't care, those who don't know and do care, those who know and approve, those who know and condemn, and those who know and discriminate. (The fact that there was no transition at all between the preceding paragraph and this one does not mean that I did not try, in several different ways, to get back to the split infinitive logically. As in a bridge hand, the absence of a reëntry is not always the fault of the man who is playing the hand, but of the way the cards lie in the dummy. To say more would only make it more difficult than it now is, if possible, to get back to Mr. Fowler.) Mr. Fowler's point is, of course, that there are good split infinitives and bad ones. For instance, he contends that it is better to say "Our object is to further cement trade relations," thus splitting "to cement," than to say "Our object is further to cement trade relations," because the use of "further" before "to cement" might lead the reader to think it had the weight of "moreover" rather than of "increasingly." My own way out of all this confusion would be simply to say "Our object is to let trade relations ride," that is, give them up, let them go. Some people would regard the abandonment of trade relations, merely for the purpose of avoiding grammatical confusion, as a weak-kneed and unpatriotic action. That, it seems to me, is a matter for each person to decide for himself. A man who, like myself, has no knowledge at all of trade relations, cannot be expected to take the same interest in cementing them as, say, the statesman or the politician. This is no reflection on trade relations.

Who Is Loyal to America?

HENRY STEELE COMMAGER (1902–)

On May 6 a Russian-born girl, Mrs. Shura Lewis, gave a talk to the students of the Western High School of Washington, D.C. She talked about Russia—its school system, its public health pro-

Who Is Loyal to America? is reprinted from *Harper's Magazine*, September 1947, by permission of Henry Steele Commager.

gram, the position of women, of the aged, of the workers, the farmers, and the professional classes—and compared, superficially and uncritically, some American and Russian social institutions. The most careful examination of the speech—happily reprinted for us in the *Congressional Record*—does not disclose a single disparagement of anything American unless it is a quasi-humorous reference to the cost of having a baby and of dental treatment in this country. Mrs. Lewis said nothing that had not been said a thousand times, in speeches, in newspapers, magazines, and books. She said nothing that any normal person could find objectionable.

Her speech, however, created a sensation. A few students walked out on it. Others improvised placards proclaiming their devotion to Americanism. Indignant mothers telephoned their protests. Newspapers took a strong stand against the outrage. Congress, rarely concerned for the political or economic welfare of the citizens of the capital city, reacted sharply when its intellectual welfare was at stake. Congressmen Rankin and Dirksen thundered and lightened; the District of Columbia Committee went into a huddle; there were demands for housecleaning in the whole school system, which was obviously shot through and through with Communism.

All this might be ignored, for we have learned not to expect either intelligence or understanding of Americanism from this element in our Congress. More ominous was the reaction of the educators entrusted with the high responsibility of guiding and guarding the intellectual welfare of our boys and girls. Did they stand up for intellectual freedom? Did they insist that high-school children had the right and the duty to learn about other countries? Did they protest that students were to be trusted to use intelligence and common sense? Did they affirm that the Americanism of their students was staunch enough to resist propaganda? Did they perform even the elementary task, expected of educators above all, of analyzing the much-criticized speech?

Not at all. The District Superintendent of Schools, Dr. Hobart

Corning, hastened to agree with the animadversions of Representatives Rankin and Dirksen. The whole thing was, he confessed, "a very unfortunate occurrence," and had "shocked the whole school system." What Mrs. Lewis said, he added gratuitously, was "repugnant to all who are working with youth in the Washington schools," and "the entire affair contrary to the philosophy of education under which we operate." Mr. Danowsky, the hapless principal of the Western High School, was "the most shocked and regretful of all." The District of Columbia Committee would be happy to know that though he was innocent in the matter, he had been properly reprimanded!

It is the reaction of the educators that makes this episode more than a tempest in a teapot. We expect hysteria from Mr. Rankin and some newspapers; we are shocked when we see educators, timid before criticism and confused about first principles, betray their trust. And we wonder what can be that "philosophy of education" which believes that young people can be trained to the duties of citizenship by wrapping their minds in cotton-wool.

Merely by talking about Russia Mrs. Lewis was thought to be attacking Americanism. It is indicative of the seriousness of the situation that during this same week the House found it necessary to take time out from the discussion of the labor bill, the tax bill, the International Trade Organization, and the world famine, to meet assaults upon Americanism from a new quarter. This time it was the artists who were undermining the American system, and members of the House spent some hours passing around reproductions of the paintings which the State Department had sent abroad as part of its program for advertising American culture. We need not pause over the exquisite humor which congressmen displayed in their comments on modern art: weary statesmen must have their fun. But we may profitably remark the major criticism which was directed against this unfortunate collection of paintings. What was wrong with these paintings, it shortly appeared, was that they were un-American.

"No American drew those crazy pictures," said Mr. Rankin. Perhaps he was right. The copious files of the Committee on Un-American Activities were levied upon to prove that of the forty-five artists represented "no less than twenty were definitely New Deal in various shades of Communism." The damning facts are specified for each of the pernicious twenty; we can content ourselves with the first of them, Ben-Zion. What is the evidence here? "Ben-Zion was one of the signers of a letter sent to President Roosevelt by the United American Artists which urged help to the USSR and Britain after Hitler attacked Russia." He was, in short, a fellow-traveler of Churchill and Roosevelt.

The same day that Mr. Dirksen was denouncing the Washington school authorities for allowing students to hear about Russia ("In Russia equal right is granted to each nationality. There is no discrimination. Nobody says, you are a Negro, you are a Jew") Representative Williams of Mississippi rose to denounce the *Survey-Graphic* magazine and to add further to our understanding of Americanism. The *Survey-Graphic*, he said, "contained 129 pages of outrageously vile and nauseating anti-Southern, anti-Christian, un-American, and pro-Communist tripe, ostensibly directed toward the elimination of the custom of racial segregation in the South." It was written by "meddling un-American purveyors of hate and indecency."

All in all, a busy week for the House. Yet those who make a practice of reading their *Record* will agree that it was a typical week. For increasingly Congress is concerned with the eradication of disloyalty and the defense of Americanism, and scarcely a day passes that some congressman does not treat us to exhortations and admonitions, impassioned appeals and eloquent declamations, similar to those inspired by Mrs. Lewis, Mr. Ben-Zion, and the editors of the *Survey-Graphic*. And scarcely a day passes that the outlines of the new loyalty and the new Americanism are not etched more sharply in public policy.

And this is what is significant—the emergence of new patterns of Americanism and of loyalty, patterns radically different from those which have long been traditional. It is not only the Congress that is busy designing the new patterns. They are outlined in President Truman's recent disloyalty order; in similar orders formulated by the New York City Council and by state and local authorities throughout the country; in the programs of the D.A.R., the American Legion, and similar patriotic organizations; in the editorials of the Hearst and the McCormick-Patterson papers; and in an elaborate series of advertisements sponsored by large corporations and business organizations. In the making is a revival of the red hysteria of the early 1920's, one of the shabbiest chapters in the history of American democracy; and more than a revival, for the new crusade is designed not merely to frustrate Communism but to formulate a positive definition of Americanism, and a positive concept of loyalty.

What is the new loyalty? It is, above all, conformity. It is the uncritical and unquestioning acceptance of America as it is—the political institutions, the social relationships, the economic practices. It rejects inquiry into the race question or socialized medicine, or public housing, or into the wisdom or validity of our foreign policy. It regards as particularly heinous any challenge to what is called "the system of private enterprise," identifying that system with Americanism. It abandons evolution, repudiates the once popular concept of progress, and regards America as a finished product, perfect and complete.

It is, it must be added, easily satisfied. For it wants not intellectual conviction nor spiritual conquest, but mere outward conformity. In matters of loyalty it takes the word for the deed, the gesture for the principle. It is content with the flag salute, and does not pause to consider the warning of our Supreme Court that "a person gets from a symbol the meaning he puts into it, and what is one man's comfort and inspiration is another's jest and scorn." It is satisfied with membership in respectable organizations and, as it assumes that every member of a liberal organization is a Communist, concludes that every member of a conservative one is a true American. It has not yet learned that not everyone who saith Lord, Lord, shall enter into the kingdom of Heaven. It is designed neither to discover real disloyalty nor to foster true loyalty.

II

What is wrong with this new concept of loyalty? What, fundamentally, is wrong with the pusillanimous retreat of the Washington educators, the barbarous antics of Washington legislators, the hysterical outbursts of the D.A.R., the gross and vulgar appeals of business corporations? It is not merely that these things are offensive. It is rather that they are wrong—morally, socially, and politically.

The concept of loyalty as conformity is a false one. It is narrow and restrictive, denies freedom of thought and of conscience, and is irremediably stained by private and selfish considerations. "Enlightened loyalty," wrote Josiah Royce, who made loyalty the very core of his philosophy,

> means harm to no man's loyalty. It is at war only with disloyalty, and its warfare, unless necessity constrains, is only a spiritual warfare. It does not foster class hatreds; it knows of nothing reasonable about race prejudices; and it regards all races of men as one in their need of loyalty. It ignores mutual misunderstandings. It loves its own wherever upon earth its own, namely loyalty itself, is to be found.

Justice, charity, wisdom, spirituality, he added, were all definable in terms of loyalty, and we may properly ask which of these qualities our contemporary champions of loyalty display.

Above all, loyalty must be to something larger than oneself, untainted by private purposes or selfish ends. But what are we to say of the attempts by the NAM and by individual corporations to identify loyalty with the system of private enterprise? Is it not as if officeholders should attempt to identify loyalty with their own party, their own political careers? Do not those corporations which pay for full-page advertisements associating Americanism with the competitive system expect, ultimately, to profit from that association? Do not those organizations that deplore, in the name of patriotism, the extension of government operation of hydro-electric power expect to profit from their campaign?

Certainly it is a gross perversion not only of the concept of loyalty but of the concept of Americanism to identify it with a particular economic system. This precise question, interestingly enough, came before the Supreme Court in the Schneiderman case not so long ago—and it was Wendell Willkie who was counsel for Schneiderman. Said the Court:

> Throughout our history many sincere people whose attachment to the general Constitutional scheme cannot be doubted have, for various and even divergent reasons, urged differing degrees of governmental ownership and control of natural resources, basic means of production, and banks and the media of exchange, either with or without compensation. And something once regarded as a species of private property was abolished without compensating the owners when the institution of slavery was forbidden. Can it be said that the author of the Emancipation Proclamation and the supporters of the Thirteenth Amendment were not attached to the Constitution?

There is, it should be added, a further danger in the willful identification of Americanism with a particular body of economic practices. Many learned economists predict for the near future an economic crash similar to that of 1929. If Americanism is equated with competitive capitalism, what happens to it if competitive capitalism comes a cropper? If loyalty and private enterprise are inextricably associated, what is to preserve loyalty if private enterprise fails? Those who associate Americanism with a particular program of economic practices have a grave responsibility, for if their program should fail, they expose Americanism itself to disrepute.

The effort to equate loyalty with conformity is misguided because it assumes that there is a fixed content to loyalty and that this can be determined and defined. But loyalty is a principle, and eludes definition except in its own terms. It is devotion to the best interests of the commonwealth, and may require hostility to the particular policies which the government pursues, the particular practices which the economy undertakes, the particular institutions which society maintains. "If there is any fixed star in our Constitutional constellation," said the Supreme Court in the Barnette case, "it is that no official, high or petty, can prescribe what shall be orthodox in politics, nationalism, religion, or other matters of opinion, or force citizens to confess by word or act their faith therein. If there are any circumstances which permit an exception they do not now occur to us."

True loyalty may require, in fact, what appears to the naïve to be disloyalty. It may require hostility to certain provisions of the Constitution itself, and historians have not concluded that those who subscribed to the "Higher Law" were lacking in patriotism. We should not forget that our tradition is one of protest and revolt, and it is stultifying to celebrate the rebels of the past—Jefferson and Paine, Emerson and Thoreau—while we silence the rebels of the present. "We are a rebellious nation," said Theodore Parker, known in his day as the Great American Preacher, and went on:

> Our whole history is treason; our blood was attainted before we were born; our creeds are infidelity to the mother church; our constitution, treason to our fatherland. What of that? Though all the governors in the world bid us commit treason against man, and set the example, let us never submit.

Those who would impose upon us a new concept of loyalty not only assume that this is possible, but have the presumption to believe that they are competent to write the definition. We are reminded of Whitman's defiance of the "never-ending audacity of elected persons." Who are those who would set the standards of loyalty? They are Rankins and Bilbos, officials of the D.A.R.

and the Legion and the NAM, Hearsts and McCormicks. May we not say of Rankin's harangues on loyalty what Emerson said of Webster at the time of the Seventh of March speech: "The word honor in the mouth of Mr. Webster is like the word love in the mouth of a whore."

What do men know of loyalty who make a mockery of the Declaration of Independence and the Bill of Rights, whose energies are dedicated to stirring up race and class hatreds, who would straitjacket the American spirit? What indeed do they know of America—the America of Sam Adams and Tom Paine, of Jackson's defiance of the Court and Lincoln's celebration of labor, of Thoreau's essay on Civil Disobedience and Emerson's championship of John Brown, of the America of the Fourierists and the Come-Outers, of cranks and fanatics, of socialists and anarchists? Who among American heroes could meet their tests, who would be cleared by their committees? Not Washington, who was a rebel. Not Jefferson, who wrote that all men are created equal and whose motto was "rebellion to tyrants is obedience to God." Not Garrison, who publicly burned the Constitution; or Wendell Phillips, who spoke for the underprivileged everywhere and counted himself a philosophical anarchist; not Seward of the Higher Law or Sumner of racial equality. Not Lincoln, who admonished us to have malice toward none, charity for all; or Wilson, who warned that our flag was "a flag of liberty of opinion as well as of political liberty"; or Justice Holmes, who said that our Constitution is an experiment and that while that experiment is being made "we should be eternally vigilant against attempts to check the expression of opinions that we loathe and believe to be fraught with death."

III

There are further and more practical objections against the imposition of fixed concepts of loyalty or tests of disloyalty. The effort is itself a confession of fear, a declaration of insolvency. Those who are sure of themselves do not need reassurance, and those who have confidence in the strength and the virtue of America do not need to fear either criticism or competition. The effort is bound to miscarry. It will not apprehend those who are really disloyal, it will not even frighten them; it will affect only those who can be labeled "radical." It is sobering to recall that though the Japanese relocation program, carried through at such incalculable cost in misery and tragedy, was justified to us on the ground that the Japanese were potentially disloyal, the record does not disclose a single case of Japanese disloyalty or sabotage during the whole war. The warning sounded by the Supreme Court in the Barnette flag-salute case is a timely one:

> Ultimate futility of such attempts to compel obedience is the lesson of every such effort from the Roman drive to stamp out Christianity as a disturber of pagan unity, the Inquisition as a means to religious and dynastic unity, the Siberian exiles as a means to Russian unity, down to the fast-failing efforts of our present totalitarian enemies. Those who begin coercive elimination of dissent soon find themselves exterminating dissenters. Compulsory unification of opinion achieves only the unanimity of the graveyard.

Nor are we left to idle conjecture in this matter; we have had experience enough. Let us limit ourselves to a single example, one that is wonderfully relevant. Back in 1943 the House Un-American Activities Committee, deeply disturbed by alleged disloyalty among government employees, wrote a definition of subversive activities and proceeded to apply it. The definition was admirable, and no one could challenge its logic or its symmetry:

> Subversive activity derives from conduct intentionally destructive of or inimical to the Government of the United States—that which seeks to undermine its institutions, or to distort its functions, or to impede its projects, or to lessen its efforts, the ultimate end being to overturn it all.

Surely anyone guilty of activities so defined deserved not only dismissal but punishment. But how was the test applied? It was applied to two distinguished scholars, Robert Morss Lovett and

Goodwin Watson, and to one able young historian, William E. Dodd, Jr., son of our former Ambassador to Germany. Of almost three million persons employed by the government, these were the three whose subversive activities were deemed the most pernicious, and the House cut them off the payroll. The sequel is familiar. The Senate concurred only to save a wartime appropriation; the President signed the bill under protest for the same reason. The Supreme Court declared the whole business a "bill of attainder" and therefore unconstitutional. Who was it, in the end, who engaged in "subversive activities"—Lovett, Dodd, and Watson, or the Congress which flagrantly violated Article One of the Constitution?

Finally, disloyalty tests are not only futile in application, they are pernicious in their consequences. They distract attention from activities that are really disloyal, and silence criticism inspired by true loyalty. That there are disloyal elements in America will not be denied, but there is no reason to suppose that any of the tests now formulated will ever be applied to them. It is relevant to remember that when Rankin was asked why his Committee did not investigate the Ku Klux Klan he replied that the Klan was not un-American, it was American!

Who are those who are really disloyal? Those who inflame racial hatreds, who sow religious and class dissensions. Those who subvert the Constitution by violating the freedom of the ballot box. Those who make a mockery of majority rule by the use of the filibuster. Those who impair democracy by denying equal educational facilities. Those who frustrate justice by lynch law or by making a farce of jury trials. Those who deny freedom of speech and of the press and of assembly. Those who press for special favors against the interest of the commonwealth. Those who regard public office as a source of private gain. Those who would exalt the military over the civil. Those who for selfish and private purposes stir up national antagonisms and expose the world to the ruin of war.

Will the House Committee on Un-American Activities interfere with the activities of these? Will Mr. Truman's disloyalty proclamation reach these? Will the current campaigns for Americanism convert these? If past experience is any guide, they will not. What they will do, if they are successful, is to silence criticism, stamp out dissent—or drive it underground. But if our democracy is to flourish it must have criticism, if our government is to function it must have dissent. Only totalitarian governments insist upon conformity and they—as we know—do so at their peril. Without criticism abuses will go unrebuked; without dissent our dynamic system will become static. The American people have a stake in the maintenance of the most thorough-going inquisition into American institutions. They have a stake in nonconformity, for they know that the American genius is nonconformist. They have a stake in experimentation of the most radical character, for they know that only those who prove all things can hold fast that which is good.

IV

It is easier to say what loyalty is not than to say what it is. It is not conformity. It is not passive acquiescence in the status quo. It is not preference for everything American over everything foreign. It is not an ostrich-like ignorance of other countries and other institutions. It is not the indulgence in ceremony—a flag salute, an oath of allegiance, a fervid verbal declaration. It is not a particular creed, a particular version of history, a particular body of economic practices, a particular philosophy.

It is a tradition, an ideal, and a principle. It is a willingness to subordinate every private advantage for the larger good. It is an appreciation of the rich and diverse contributions that can come from the most varied sources. It is allegiance to the traditions that have guided our greatest statesmen and inspired our most eloquent poets—the traditions of freedom, equality, democracy, tolerance, the tradition of the higher law, of experimentation, co-operation, and pluralism. It is a realization that America was born of revolt, flourished on dissent, became great through experimentation.

Independence was an act of revolution; republicanism was something new under the sun; the federal system was a vast experimental laboratory. Physically Americans were pioneers; in the realm of social and economic institutions, too, their tradition has been one of pioneering. From the beginning, intellectual and spiritual diversity have been as characteristic of America as racial and linguistic. The most distinctively American philosophies have been transcendentalism—which is the philosophy of the Higher Law—and pragmatism—which is the philosophy of experimentation and pluralism. These two principles are the very core of Americanism: the principle of the Higher Law, or of obedience to the dictates of conscience rather than of statutes, and the principle of pragmatism, or the rejection of a single good and of the notion of a finished universe. From the beginning Americans have known that there were new worlds to conquer, new truths to be discovered. Every effort to confine Americanism to a single pattern, to constrain it to a single formula, is disloyalty to everything that is valid in Americanism.

Suggestions for Study

For beginning writers the most interesting aspect of the essay is the firmness with which it is blocked out. Commager begins with a section devoted to examples of the new red hysteria and comment on their significance: the first five paragraphs concern Mrs. Lewis, the content of her speech, the reaction of Washington educators; the next four paragraphs discuss other examples of the hunt and comment on its general significance. In the last paragraph of this section, Commager defines the new loyalty. The first six paragraphs of the second section criticize the new loyalty as wrong "morally, socially, and politically." The last three paragraphs attempt by allusion to suggest the qualities of true loyalty. In the third section Commager offers "further and more practical objections" to the loyalty tests: they are futile (paragraphs one and two); they are pernicious because they do not reach the right people (paragraphs three, four, and five). In the last section Commager attempts a definition of true loyalty by referring to American history and to the American character.

Although generally energetic and forceful, the style in this essay sometimes betrays its academic origin. Commager is not always careful to avoid the jargon of his profession, as for example when he speaks of "a quasi-humorous reference," or of Americanism being "equated" with competitive capitalism. He lets an archaic word ("hapless") slip in where, if any adjective at all is necessary, one from the middle level of the vocabulary would be better; or he will use a conspicuously heavy word like "animadversions," which may be only partly justified by its humorous (or quasi-humorous) effect. Sometimes he takes the easy way out by using a cliché: "created a sensation" or "tempest in a tea-pot." (A writer like Otis Ferguson would have strengthened the first and freshened the second expression.) He uses a good many rather heavy and abstract constructions: "we have learned not to expect either intelligence or understanding of Americanism from this element in our Congress"; "It is indicative of the seriousness of the situation"; "There are further and more practical objections against the imposition."

When Commager gets going, this academic fuzziness is pretty well forgotten. And what we finally remember is his contemptuous tone as he parades the names of the defenders of Americanism, or the hard-hitting questions and answers with which he celebrates the great American tradition of revolt. Both passages are more incantation than argument, and they are good illustrations of the powerful effect that well-chosen allusions may have.

Pointe du Hoe: The German Night Attack

CHARLES H. TAYLOR (1899–   )

[THE SELECTION is from "Pointe du Hoe," one of the combat actions treated in *Small Unit Actions* (Historical Division, War Department, 1946). Colonel Taylor has generously supplied the following introduction:

On 6 June, 1944, two divisions of V Corps of the U.S. First Army assaulted a three-mile stretch of sand in Normandy henceforth famous as "Omaha Beach." Losses were heavy, progress was slow, and at nightfall the units of V Corps were barely beyond the beach, miles short of their day's objectives.

As a part of the assault, three companies (D, E, and F) of the 2d Ranger Battalion had a special and isolated mission on D Day. At 0700, about 200 strong, they landed under the cliffs at Pointe du Hoe, four miles west of the Omaha sector. Against German fire from above, the Rangers scaled the ninety-foot cliffs to capture a fortified area supposed to contain six medium guns (155's) that could endanger the Allied transport area. But the guns had been moved. During the next hour small groups of Rangers worked half a mile inland to the main coastal highway; here they set up a roadblock and watched for the arrival of main assault forces coming from Omaha. Their patrols found the six German guns, abandoned in a farm lane.

Back at Pointe du Hoe, Lieutenant-Colonel James E. Rudder, Commander of the Ranger group, had no communications with higher headquarters and knew nothing of what had happened at Omaha Beach. Nearly a third of his men were casualties. German counterattacks twice threatened to recapture Pointe du Hoe, and his communications with the roadblock were limited to passage

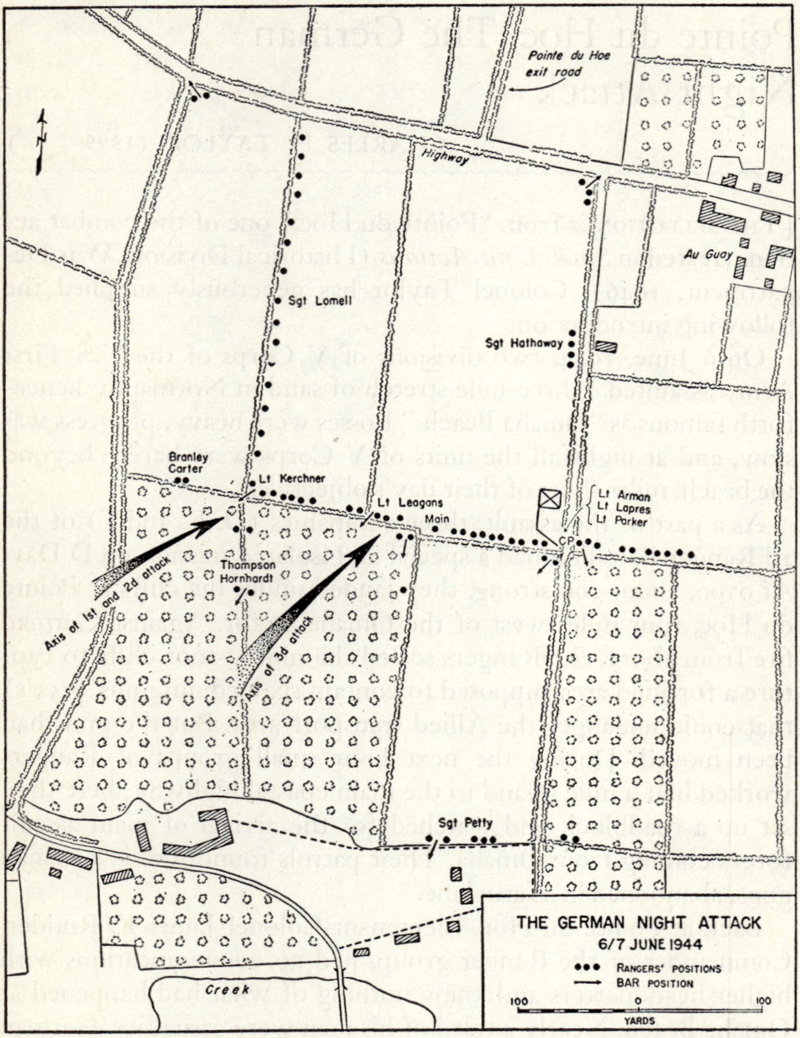
Pointe du Hoe exit road
Highway
Au Guay
Sgt Lomell
Sgt Hathaway
Branley
Carter
Lt Kerchner
Lt Leagans
Lt Arman
Lt Lapres
Lt Parker
Main
CP
Thompson
Hornhardt
Axis of 1st and 2d attack
Axis of 3d attack
Sgt Petty
Creek
THE GERMAN NIGHT ATTACK
6/7 JUNE 1944
RANGERS' POSITIONS
BAR POSITION
100 0 100
YARDS

of an occasional runner. However, in the early evening a platoon of 5th Rangers reached the roadblock after fighting across country from Omaha. They believed that the 29th Division was close behind. On the strength of that, Colonel Rudder decided to leave his advance party near the highway. During the long twilight, the 85 men, representing elements of four companies and commanded by lieutenants, organized for night defense.]

THE GERMAN NIGHT ATTACK: FIRST PHASE

Twilight in early June, on reckoning by British War Time, lasted until 2300. As night approached, and still no word came from Omaha Beach, Colonel Rudder faced a difficult command decision with regard to disposition of his limited force. Of his original 200 men over a third were casualties, though many of the lightly wounded (including Colonel Rudder) were staying in action. Ammunition was low, especially in grenades and mortar shells. The Germans were still holding the antiaircraft position close to the Point on the west, and had shown themselves in some force on the eastern flank as well. Communications between the Point and the highway group had always been precarious, and the latter force, numbering more than half of the Rangers, would be particularly exposed to counterattack that might cut it off from the shore. Either of the two Ranger positions was in danger; Colonel Trevor, the Commando officer, remarked casually in the CP [1] that "never have I been so convinced of anything as that I will be either a prisoner of war or a casualty by morning."

Colonel Rudder decided to leave the highway force in place. He was still expecting the arrival of the 5th Rangers and 116th Infantry units along the Vierville road, carrying out the D-Day program, and this expectation had been strengthened when Colonel Rudder heard that Parker's platoon had actually arrived, reporting (erroneously) that the rest of the 5th Rangers were probably just behind them. It was important, Colonel Rudder thought, to maintain the block on the Grandcamp highway

[1] Editors' note: CP = Command Post; BAR = Browning Automatic Rifle.

and so deny that vital road to the enemy. Even though German resistance had stiffened during the day, their counterattacks against the weaker force on the Point had been ineffective, and they had made no efforts against the highway position. As a final consideration, Colonel Rudder and his staff had very strong fears (proved by the next day's experience to be unfounded) of the danger from German artillery if his force were concentrated in a restricted area at the Point. Lieutenant Lapres, who had reached the Point with a patrol just before dark, went back inland with orders to hold the position.

Out beyond the highway, the Rangers made a few alterations in their positions to get ready for night defense. The main indications of enemy strength were to the south and west, and the greater number of the 85 men at hand (including Lieutenant Parker's platoon of 5th Rangers) were disposed to guard against attacks from those quarters.

The day positions of Company D were obviously too extended for safety, and its 20 men were drawn in to form the right flank of the main Ranger position, on a hedgerow that ran south from the highway to Company E's fox holes. Lieutenant Kerchner and a BAR man were at the angle formed by intersecting hedgerows where E and D joined; Sergeant Lomell was near the center of D's line. Two men were put out west of Kerchner's post, about half way to the lane bordering the next field. Another outpost of two Rangers, one with a BAR, was in the angle where that lane met the blacktop. The rest of Kerchner's men were strung out at wide intervals along the 300 yards of hedgerow, in a ditch running along the embankment.

Company E's 30 men held their day positions on the hedgeline running east toward the main CP. Some half dozen of the 5th Ranger men were distributed along their front. A few yards south of the angle where E and D connected, two riflemen were posted in the orchard that sloped away gently toward the creek; two more Rangers, one a BAR man, were 75 yards further out. The post of Lieutenant Leagans (2d Platoon) was in a German-prepared dugout near the middle of E's hedgerow, with a BAR man and a rifleman in the corner of the orchard on the other side of the hedgerow, and another rifleman 50 yards south on the boundary between the orchard and a wheatfield. A third BAR man was 20 yards west of Leagans' station. Between Leagans and the angle where Company D's line began, about 10 riflemen occupied fox holes north of the hedge, one group fairly close to the angle and the rest bunched near Leagans, an arrangement thought better for purposes of communication. From east of Leagans' post over to the main CP on the lane, the 1st Platoon of Company E and some 5th Rangers continued the hedgerow line, with main strength near the CP, where the Rangers were placed two to a fox hole for greater safety in night fighting. Sergeant Robey with a BAR was in the corner of the wheatfield just south of the CP, with a good field of fire to the southwest. In addition to their own four BAR's, Company E platoons had found and set up three German machine guns (two model '34's and one '42), for which ammunition was available.

East from the CP, the line that Company F had held in daylight was shortened to 100 yards. Near the lane that ran back from CP to highway, three Rangers with a BAR were placed in a trench that gave them a field of fire through a gateway into the orchard southeast of the CP. Beyond them were two men of Company F and some 5th Battalion Rangers. Sergeant Petty and seven men, including some 5th Rangers, still held an outpost along the stone wall at the foot of the wheatfield. Their advantages of observation from this position would be sharply reduced at night, and Petty was under orders to withdraw if an attack developed in his vicinity.

The main Ranger position thus formed a right angle, facing southwest, with equal sides about 300 yards long on two fields that ran back to the highway. The 30 or 40 German prisoners were put in fox holes in these fields, not far from the CP, and two Rangers were regarded as sufficient guard. Little concern was felt for the open flank to the east, protected by three men with a

BAR near the highway, and by a half dozen of Parker's 5th Rangers along the lane between the CP and the road.

Certain features of the night arrangements are worth noting, in view of later developments. The 5th Ranger platoon of 23 men had been scattered in small batches at various points and did not operate as a tactical unit under Lieutenant Parker. He and his assistant, 1st Lt. Stanley D. Zelepsky, were at the main CP with Arman and Lapres. Command functions in the Ranger force, made up of elements of four companies, were not centralized. During the day, the D, E, and F parties had cooperated on a more or less informal basis, with coordination secured by consultation of the four officers, Lieutenants Kerchner (D), Leagans and Lapres (E), and Arman (F). When plans had to be made in the morning as to positions for the day, Lieutenant Arman was the senior officer at hand and seems to have made the decisions. After that he did not consider himself in command in any formal sense. The decision to shorten up and tighten the defenses for the night was taken when Lieutenant Kerchner came over to Arman's post and reported seeing Germans in some strength to the southwest. Arman, Lapres, and Kerchner talked it over and agreed as to readjustment of positions.

As they settled in for night defense, the main worry of the Rangers was their ammunition supply, now running short, especially for the BAR's. Very few U.S. grenades were left; although a plentiful supply of German "potato-mashers" were found in prepared positions around the CP, the Rangers had a poor opinion of their effectiveness. A few Rangers had lost their rifles and were using German weapons, for which ammunition was in good supply. Companies D and E had three Tommy guns each, and E had three German machine guns. The Rangers had had nothing to eat since leaving ship except the individual D-bars, but in the excitement and activity of the day few men had felt the need for food.

Even before Lieutenant Kerchner's report, the officers had felt particularly apprehensive about the area southwest of their angle position. At the bottom of the little valley to the south, a country road ran more or less parallel to the Ranger lines, west from a bridge close by Sergeant Petty's outpost and then northwest toward the highway. From their higher ground, the Rangers could watch this road during daylight, but at night it was too far away for good observation. Houses, hedgerows, and orchards along it would give cover for assembly of troops. It was in this area, a few hundred yards southwest of the angle in the Rangers' right position, that Lieutenant Kerchner had observed German activity at dusk.

Despite a moon nearly full and only partly obscured by clouds, the Rangers found visibility poor in front of their angle, particularly into the orchards on the south. Here the ground sloped off 30 feet in 300 yards, and the fields of fire had been good for a daylight action.

About 2330 the Rangers posted in front of the D-E corner were startled by a general outburst of whistles and shouts, close by on the orchard slope. Enemy fire opened immediately and in considerable volume. Sgt. Michael J. Branley and Pfc. Robert D. Carty, in position west of the corner, saw tracer fire from a machine gun to their right and only 25 yards from Company D's side of the angle. South of the corner, in Company E's outpost, the men spotted another machine gun to the west, about 50 yards from Company E's defensive line. Neither outpost had seen or heard the enemy approach through the orchard. At the angle, and along E's front, the Rangers returned the enemy fire at once, the BAR's firing in full bursts. Carty and Branley started back toward the corner to get better firing positions; Carty was killed by a grenade, and his companion, hit in the shoulder by a bullet, managed to crawl to the hedgerow.

In the Company E outpost, Corporals Thompson and Hornhardt were almost walked over by a group of Germans who came suddenly around a hump in the north-south hedgerow dividing the orchard. Thompson saw their silhouettes against the sky, so the Rangers got in their fire first at point-blank range and knocked down three of the enemy. The others went flat and threw grenades, one of them exploding in Thompson's face and cutting him badly. He gave his BAR to Hornhardt and they started back for the corner.

Only a few minutes after the firing began, an immense sheet of flame shot up over to the west, near the position of the abandoned German guns. (The Rangers' guess was that, somehow, more powder charges had been set off in the ammunition dump.) The orchard slopes were fully lit up, and many Germans could be seen outlined against the glare. The flare died almost at once, and the firing ended at the same time. It is possible that the powder explosion had disconcerted the Germans and ended their effort, but more probably the attack was only a preliminary probe by combat patrols, trying to locate Ranger positions by drawing their fire.

This brief action brought about a few changes in the Ranger positions, affecting the outposts and the west side of the angle (Company D). Certain things that happened began to show some of the difficulties of night fighting. Thompson and Hornhardt got back to the corner and found nobody at that position; when they called for Sergeant Rupinski there was no answer. (He was 20 yards away, to the east, but did not hear them; there were two Company D men close by with a BAR, but Thompson missed seeing them too.) The outpost pair decided everybody must have pulled back across the field, so they started north along Company D's hedgerow and finally encountered Rangers in position near the highway end of the hedgerow. (They had passed others on the way without spotting them in their holes under the hedgerow.)

Lieutenant Kerchner and Sgt. Harry J. Fate were now at this end of the Company D line. When the firing began, with greatest concentration near Kerchner's post at the angle, he had the impression that the attack was going to roll right over them. So he and Fate went north along the hedgerow; as they started, Kerchner told Fate his plan. He would collect the D platoon near the highway, circle west and then south, and hit the German attack in the flank. Kerchner called to his men to follow as he ran along the hedgerow, but in the general uproar of the fire they failed to hear him. On reaching the highway he found only two men had joined up; the fire fight was already dying out, and the plan for a counterattack was given up. Lieutenant Kerchner decided to stay near the highway.

The net result of these shifts was to weaken the angle position toward which the German attack had come. Both outposts to south of it had come in, the two 5th Ranger men appearing at the main CP and telling Lieutenant Arman that they had been ordered to withdraw. (There is no way of tracing whether, why, or by whom such an order was given.) Two Rangers who had been near the angle were casualties; six others, including a BAR man and the only officer at that sector (Kerchner), had gone to other parts of the line. No information on these changes in strength at the angle seems to have reached Lieutenant Arman's CP. Neither Lieutenant Kerchner on D's thinly held front nor (apparently) Lieutenant Leagans in Company E made any move to strengthen the corner position. So far as can be determined no one visited the corner to see what the situation was.

On the east wing of the Rangers' position there had been no firing. Neither the first platoon of E (Lieutenant Lapres) nor the Company F men had been involved so far. Down near the creek, in Sergeant Petty's exposed outpost, the men were alarmed by the fire but couldn't locate it; they thought it was back near the highway, and some even believed it was the 116th pushing along the blacktop to relieve the Rangers at the Point. Petty, a little after the skirmish ended and quiet had settled down again, heard "clinking" sounds over toward the farm buildings west of his post. He put it down to noise made by farm animals. But after another short spell of quiet, a machine gun opened up from that flank, some of the shots ricocheting off a farm roller which Petty had placed against the stone wall for cover to his right. Petty's men stayed quiet, and after two short bursts the enemy fire stopped. Petty decided, in accordance with earlier instructions, that he should pull back up the slope to the CP. His group made the trip without drawing enemy fire. Petty with his BAR and Dix with a machine gun reinforced the CP position, while the rest of his men were put on the Company F line farther east.

At the CP, where Lieutenant Arman was stationed and to which other officers came occasionally, everything was quiet. After the fire fight ended, one or two Rangers from E's line reported in, and Lieutenant Lapres went over to the west to see what had happened. Two noncoms went along the E front to see if there were any casualties and if weapons were working properly. They passed word to expect more attacks. Lieutenant Arman was not informed in any detail of Company E's situation, and knew nothing about D. As far as Company F was concerned, he thought for a time of moving it south toward the creek, to bring flanking fire on any further German attack toward the angle, but decided against this idea because of the danger of firing on friendly positions. The group of German prisoners near the CP was moved farther out, into the middle of the field, and ordered to dig in for their own protection.

NIGHT ATTACK: SECOND PHASE

About 0100 the Germans came in with a stronger effort, hitting again from the south and southwest against the right of Company E's line. Once again, the Germans had got through the fields and orchard to within 50 yards of the Rangers without being spotted. The attack opened with whistles, followed by what seemed to be shouting of names up and down the front—a sort of "roll call." (Some Rangers believed the Germans were locating their men in relation to each other for beginning the assault, but the general view was that the enemy was trying to scare the defense.) The shouting was followed immediately by heavy firing, including machine guns and machine pistols. Much of the fire was tracer, somewhat high and inaccurate, designed for moral effect, but ball ammunition was spraying the hedgerow eastward from the angle. Wild mortar fire was put into the field behind the hedgerow, and some Rangers reported the enemy threw in a few mortar shells by hand. The Germans also used grenades.

Beyond this general characterization of the attack, the survivors' recollections of this action are confused and hard to fit into any clear pattern. Lieutenant Arman, at the CP to the east of the main fighting, had the impression of two distinct stages in the attack: first, a period of intense but wild fire; then, after a short pause, another burst of whistles and shouts followed by an assault. The main weight of the attack certainly came near the angle in the Rangers' lines, but—and this is a measure of the lack of communications during this night action—nobody knew then, or was sure later, what happened at the corner position. Of the survivors interviewed, Tech. 5 John S. Burnett was about 25 yards east of the angle and Branley (wounded) had crawled about 30 yards north of it, along Company D's hedgerow. Branley reports hearing Tech. 5 Henry S. Stecki's BAR open up from the corner (other Rangers, farther away, confirm this) and fire almost continuously for about two minutes. Then grenades exploded near the corner; after a short lull, the BAR fired again, there were some more grenades, and then Germans could be heard talking near the position.

Burnett at first made the same report, pointing to the conclusion that the Germans had occupied the corner. Later, he changed his story and insisted that the Ranger's BAR (Stecki) was still in action after the second German attack. Lieutenant Zelepsky (5th Ranger officer at Arman's CP) remembers being told that the enemy had broken into the Ranger lines, and recalls the impression of men at the CP that the angle was lost and the Germans were in the field. Lieutenant Arman has the same recollection, and thinks the BAR fire at the corner was not heard after the opening of the second attack. The weight of the evidence, pending information from Rangers who were later taken prisoner, suggests that the enemy had captured the angle, held only by a BAR man and one rifleman.

It is much more clear that, whatever happened at the angle, nobody at any distance north or east of that position knew, after the attack, just what the situation was. North of the corner, Company D's men (who had so far not taken part in the fire fight) lay quiet and did not investigate. Twenty-five yards eastward, Burnett and Sergeant Rupinski made no move to find out what had taken place. Over at the main CP, Lieutenant Lapres and Lieutenant Arman had agreed that Company D's hedgerow was overrun; they were discussing plans for withdrawal if the Germans made another attack. They had no communication with Company D, and did not try to send it word of their plan. The officers of the 5th Ranger platoon (Parker and Zelepsky) were supposedly told of the plan, but they do not recall hearing about it before it was carried out.

Near the middle of Company E's line, a Ranger remembers that word was passed down the line to avoid wild firing. Ammunition was running low.

NIGHT ATTACK: FINALE

The third German attack came at some time near 0300. In general character, this one developed like the second: the same whistles and roll calling to start with, then heavy and inaccurate fire, involving several machine guns and burp guns which sprayed the hedgerow and the fields beyond. Mortar fire, somewhat increased in volume, was falling in the area where the prisoners were grouped.

This time the enemy pressure extended farther east, reaching into the wheatfield south of the CP. From different accounts, machine guns were spotted in the orchard below the 2d Platoon of E and also directly south of the CP. An officer at the CP had the impression that machine-gun fire also came from the field inside the Rangers' positions, near the angle. This observation fits the theory that the Germans had captured the angle earlier, but the report might be based on high fire from a gun west of the angle, in the orchard where one was spotted in the first attack. The only certainty is that there was a great deal of fire, much of it indirect, and that it had the result of confusing the defense; some Rangers even believed that the enemy were in the rear of their position, near the blacktop.

Lieutenant Arman reports that (as in the second attack) the preliminary burst of shooting was followed by a brief pause, preceding the real assault. Whatever the sequence, the western half of Company E's line was overrun in a short time after the attack began. Only a few incidents of the action can be recovered from survivors who were in or near that area. There is enough evidence to suggest that, even if the angle had been taken earlier, the main penetration now came near the middle of E's hedgerow and rolled up the Ranger positions west from there to the angle.

One fox hole east of Lieutenant Leagans' post at the junction of the two platoons, Pfc. Harold D. Main (who had been wounded by a grenade) heard the Germans coming up close in the wheat just beyond the hedgerow. After a pause following the heavy opening fire, they rushed the hedgerow to Main's right, and Crook's BAR went silent. Minutes later, Main could hear Germans talking on his side of the hedge and knew what had happened. He crawled under the thick tangle of vines and briars into the middle of the hedgerow. Hidden there, he heard S/Sgt. Curtis A. Simmons surrender, only 15 feet away, but the Germans came no farther east.

Burnett, still in his fox hole 25 yards east of the corner, confirms the impression that the decisive action was not on his right, toward the angle, but left, toward Lieutenant Leagans' post. Near Burnett the Germans had worked through the orchard close to the Rangers, and their automatic fire ripped through the hedgerow, keeping the defenders down. The Rangers had plenty of German grenades and used them freely in a close-range exchange. To Burnett, the fight seemed to go on an hour (it can only have been minutes). He became aware that Sergeant Boggetto's BAR, to the left, had stopped firing; then a burst of German fire began to sweep along the Ranger side of the hedge, coming from the east and enfilading the 2d Platoon's fox holes. Burnett and the man next to him were wounded. The enemy had evidently broken into the field to their left. Burnett could also spot them to his right in the angle. He heard Sergeant Rupinski arguing with a few Rangers, trying to decide whether they could fight it out. The talk ended by Rupinski shouting "Kamerad." The Germans moved in and rounded up the survivors, many of them wounded, including Burnett. Lieutenant Leagans was dead. About 20 Rangers were taken off the field, nearly all from Leagans' platoon of E, and moved to a German CP a mile to the south. Here, Burnett [2] saw a force, estimated at a company, coming by the CP from the south, and judged the post was a battalion CP because of the presence nearby of an aid station.

From the varied and sometimes irreconcilable stories of the Rangers who were near Lieutenant Arman's CP, one gets a fair reflection of the confusion that existed under the difficulties of this last phase in a night battle. Arman reports that after the opening fire he, Lapres, and the 5th Ranger officers went ahead with the plan to withdraw, already agreed on. Arman had no idea whether Leagans of Company D knew the plan. According to Lieutenant Zelepsky (5th Rangers), there was little or no prearranged plan: men began to come in from E's line to the west, reporting the Germans had broken the position, and the report was confirmed by enemy fire that seemed to come from the field inside the angle. This led to a hasty decision to withdraw. Sgt. Lawrence Lare remembers a man running across the field from the west to report that Company D was wiped out. Smith and Tech. 5 Charles H. Dunlap, who had been near Main's fox hole, came in to the CP (because their guns had jammed) to report that there were no Rangers left between their former position and

[2] Burnett escaped a few days later by killing a guard, was helped by the French Underground, and succeeded in getting back to the Allied lines after they reached Rouen in August.

the CP. Some of the 5th Ranger men who had been in the Company E line later said that the 2d Rangers "pulled out and left them there."

According to plan or not, a withdrawal took place from the CP area. Just before it started, that wing of the Ranger line saw some action for the first time that night. Following the first burst of German fire, which indicated the enemy were now south of the CP in the wheatfield, some more Rangers were put into the northeast corner of that field to strengthen the group already there. The reinforcements included Sergeant Petty with his BAR, S/Sgt. Frederick A. Dix with a German machine gun, and some Company F riflemen. A German party came eastward crossing the upper end of the wheatfield; they were starting through the hedgerow embankment into the lane when Dix saw them only a few feet away from his post in the lane. He turned around to use the captured machine gun. It jammed on the first round, and a rifle bullet from some Ranger firing down the lane behind Dix hit a glancing blow on his helmet, stunning him. Recovering, and starting to crawl along the hedgerow ditch back to the CP, Dix heard Petty yell "Down!" just before opening with his BAR on Germans coming up the lane. Sergeant Robey's BAR joined in, and this fire broke up the only attack that came close to the CP. One German was caught crawling along the hedgerow into the CP area, and was killed by a grenade that landed directly under his chest. Plenty of fire was coming across the wheatfield from the west, but no assault was tried from that quarter.

As the volume of enemy fire built up again from south and west, indicating a new rush was at hand, hasty and informal measures were taken to pass the word around for withdrawal back to the highway and the Point. Some Rangers failed to get the notice and were temporarily left behind. Petty and Robey were told to bring up the rear and cover the withdrawal with their BAR's. Noncommissioned officers tried hurriedly to round up their men. Once started, movement was fast. S/Sgt. Richard N. Hathaway of the 5th Rangers had been posted halfway back to the highway, along the lane. His first notice of what was happening came when men ran by toward the north. Hathaway stuck his head through the hedgerow and shouted "Hey! What's up? Where you going?" The nearest man stopped running, put his rifle in Hathaway's face, and demanded the password. Hathaway was so rattled that he could just remember the word in time. Told "the Germans are right behind us—get out quick to the Point!" he collected part of his group (he couldn't find some, but they came in later), and went north. There could be no question of bringing back the prisoners.

As the parties arrived at the blacktop, there was no sign of any pursuit, and an effort was made to reorganize those Rangers at hand and to see that none were left. A hasty check-up showed that the Company F men were nearly all there, but only a scattering of E and none from D. Lieutenant Arman figured that the Germans might have infiltrated between the highway and the Point, so sent one party over to the east and then into the Point across fields. Lieutenant Arman and a second party, including some of Company E, went back by the exit road. The 5th Ranger men made their way through the completely unfamiliar terrain in scattered parties (and were afterward resentful of their having been cast adrift, though what happened was probably inevitable under the circumstances of night withdrawal). All told, about 50 men got back to the Point, shortly after 0400, and were put at once into an improvised defensive line from gun position No. 5 to gun position No. 3. Very little could be done to organize the position before daylight.

Colonel Rudder was told that the rest of the force had been destroyed. "Neutralized" would have been a more exact word. All Company E Rangers from Main's fox hole to the angle had been killed or captured, and a few men of D near the corner had been included in the disaster. But from about 30 yards north of the angle and on to the highway, the rest of D's contingent (some dozen men) were still in their original positions, scattered along 250 yards of hedgerow. They had no notice of a withdrawal. When they realized it was under way, they had no chance to move, with Germans in the fields to their rear and flanks. Daylight was near, and the 12 men stayed in the deep drainage ditch, overhung with the heavy vegetation of the hedgerow. They had delivered no fire during the attacks and could only hope the Germans had not spotted their positions.

On the east-west hedgerow, between the breakthrough area and the CP, three more Rangers had been left behind in the confusion of withdrawal. Main was one. Another was Tech. 5 Earl Theobold, who had been in the field guarding prisoners. During the final attack he came over to the hedgerow near Main "to help out." He could find no Rangers, and soon heard German voices near the CP, so he hid in the ditch. Pfc. Loring L. Wadsworth, in the same sector and about 75 yards from Main, had missed the word of withdrawal. When he finally called to his nearest neighbor, who had been only a few yards off, Wadsworth got no answer, and stayed put under a tangle of briars.

Both Theobold and Wadsworth were caught during the next two days. Wadsworth was spotted early in the morning. Theobold lay quiet for most of the day, then thought he was seen by a passing German and bolted out toward the highway, without drawing fire. He hid again in a ditch near the highway, for the night. On the morning of D + 2 firing came close to his hideout along the road. It was the 116th Infantry, attacking to relieve the Point, but Theobold could not know that. Leaving the highway and cutting south, he was captured by a machine-gun post near the creek. Main spent D + 1 watching German patrols go by, and a machine gun being set up in the field near his hedgerow. That night he crawled out, threw a grenade in the general direction of the machine gun, and "lit out for the point" without drawing enemy fire.

The Company D men lay hidden all the next day under their hedgerow. No enemy search of the area was made, and they saw only a few Germans during the period. Their main cause of worry was fire from naval guns, supporting the beleaguered Point; from time to time, friendly shells came close enough to "bounce the men around" in their holes, but there were no losses. Late in the day their hopes were raised and then dashed. Four Sherman tanks rolled down the highway toward Grandcamp within sight of the Rangers. But no infantry followed, and in a short while the tanks came back and went off eastward. Germans reappeared in the field at dusk and set up machine-gun positions; the isolated Ranger group settled in for another night. They were freed next morning by the 116th Infantry.

On D + 1 Colonel Rudder's force at Pointe du Hoe consisted of about 90 men able to bear arms. Restricted to a few acres, including only a part of the fortified area, they expected to be the target for heavy concentrations of artillery, and for assault by enemy ground forces. With the support of strong naval fire the Rangers held out during the day, and that afternoon their situation was improved by the landing of a craft with food, ammunition, and a platoon of reinforcements. By night they were in touch with patrols of a relief force that had reached St.-Pierre-du-Mont, only 1,000 yards away. The relief of the Point came next morning, on D + 2.[3]

That All Problems Are Merely Verbal

BARROWS DUNHAM (1905–)

THE NINETEEN-THIRTIES began in hunger and ended in blood. The lines of men before soup kitchens gave way to lines of pickets around factories and stores, and these in turn gave way to lines of troops moving into battle. The nineteen-thirties, a

[3] For an outline account of the relief of Pointe du Hoe, see *Omaha Beachhead*. in the *American Forces in Action* series.

decade conveniently marked in time, were part of a vaster epoch of social change, which had existed before them and continues to exist after them. Nevertheless, they had a nature of their own, and they generated doctrines appropriate to it. Among these was the belief that all problems are merely verbal. This doctrine is not, I think, very widely diffused throughout the population, most of which, indeed, could not possibly survive by any such notion. It is, however, common enough among the intelligentsia —a social class in which membership is voluntary and is apparently attained by simple declaration of arrival. If any readers feel themselves outside this class, they may dispense with further reading, and thus remain in profitable ignorance of at least one social superstition. But if they know themselves to be members, then I am bound to think that the discussion will be useful.

When Hitler entered Austria in 1938, he drove into exile, among other talented intellectuals, certain members of a philosophical school known as the *Wienerkreis*. This school, the Vienna Circle, developed in the mid-nineteen-twenties, basing itself on the work of Ernst Mach in the nineteenth century and on the philosophical criticism of Hume in the eighteenth. The school was primarily interested in logic and scientific method. It believed that most, if not all, of the major philosophical problems had arisen from an inaccurate use of language, and it therefore set itself the task of removing from philosophy all ambiguities of syntax and definition. Such was the origin of Logical Positivism.

The lives of the founders have not been easy. Moritz Schlick was murdered by a student, before *Anschluss*. The war itself pursued Wittgenstein to England and Carnap to America. Moreover, the Positivist movement, which had preceded them westward, had taken a form they perhaps did not intend. Its newer devotees had begun to treat social problems as if these, too, were purely verbal, as if the struggle against fascism involved no more than a definition of terms. While "the round earth's imagined corners" flamed with horror and sacrifice, there grew soberly under new hands what Carnap had called "*der logische Aufbau der Welt.*"

Why, at such a time and for so long a time, should one interest oneself in rearing "the logical structure of the world"? I am not suggesting that the task is unimportant; rather, the task, even if imperfectly achieved, would throw much light on all other problems. But when men assert, as these do, that such is philosophy's only task, that philosophy itself is only "the critique of language," [1] then we may well inquire why so faint and diffident a theory has prospered in so violent an age.

The answer would be something like this. Suppose you are living in the midst of a disaster which involves the whole community. If you think that society can recoup its losses, you will find yourself committed to several philosophical assumptions, such as that the universe is not static and hence that social change is possible, or that society can be an object of knowledge and, by that knowledge, be controlled. But if you hold that the disaster is beyond repair, your philosophical views are modified accordingly. You may decide to endure things patiently, and thus embrace stoicism; you may decide upon a cautious pursuit of pleasure, and thus embrace epicureanism; you may decide that all accepted values are in fact contemptible, and thus embrace cynicism; you may persuade yourself that knowledge is quite impossible, that we cannot even be sure we are unhappy, and thus embrace scepticism. All four of these views flourished in Greece after the Macedonian conquest. They form an ideological pattern for all times of general catastrophe.

If, however, a society finds the means of recovery, these philosophies begin to disappear, partly because they have no longer any use and partly because the daily experience of people will seem to contradict them. The solution of social problems convinces men that they do have knowledge; hence scepticism fades. Solution means a greater abundance and a better distribution of

[1] Ludwig Wittgenstein: *Tractatus Logico-Philosophicus,* Harcourt, Brace & Co., New York, 1922, p. 63.

goods; hence there are more pleasures available, fewer shocks have to be endured, and the accepted values tend to be confirmed. Epochs of expansion are alive with confidence and large in ideas. The gains of each new day confound the sceptics; success charms cynics out of their cynicism; pleasure seekers slough off their ill-borne caution; and stoics exchange patience under adversity for eagerness under hope. There is a brilliance lighting all prospects; and it would never occur to anyone to think that philosophy, hovering over a renascent world, is but the breath of speech about speech.

Yet if recovery delays and will not come round the expected corner, if, on the contrary, a slow, morose deterioration sets in, the dynamic of philosophy moves in another direction. On the one hand, we have a social crisis which endangers us all; on the other, we have perplexity and frustration in our search for remedies. Perhaps this is due to our not having searched far enough; nevertheless our failure is plain. We begin to think we were looking for the wrong kind of solution. We are confused: perhaps our confusion issued from misty syntax and unclear definition. We are unhappy: perhaps if we knew how the word "unhappiness" is to be defined, we should discover that we are happy after all. There is no money in our bank account: perhaps if we really understood the syntax of "there is" and the negativity of "no" we should find ourselves rich. All perplexity is frustrated speech. All problems are merely verbal.

The beauty of this solution is its ease. Anybody of reasonable intelligence can do it or understand it when it is done by someone else. There may have to be trips to the library in search of the larger dictionaries, the treatises on grammar, and the considerable bulk of Korzybski's *Science and Sanity*, which Mr. Stuart Chase says he read "completely through three times, and portions of it up to a dozen times." [2] The whole enterprise is a little

[2] Chase, *The Tyranny of Words*, Harcourt, Brace & Co., New York, 1938, p. 94. Mr. Chase goes on to add, with charming wistfulness, "Large sections are still blank in my mind. A book on the clarification of meaning should not be so difficult to understand."

like increasing your circle of friends by counting the names in a telephone directory.

When so gentle a solution is placed beside so terrible a problem, the contrast is spectacular. Social catastrophes are extremely violent, whereas nothing can be calmer than semantics. Men, it seems, must be made to kill one another over mistaken syntax and cloudy definition. Every devout semanticist regards himself as an island of sense in an ocean of absurdity. He frames his sentences correctly and establishes the meaning of each word. If violence engulfs him, well, he cannot help that. His abstention from the conflict is not only permitted, it is enjoined, by his philosophy. He is commanded to escape.

It is doubtless a long way from the sophistications of Wittgenstein to their applications by Mr. Chase, but the passage is direct. What Wittgenstein exhibits as critique of language Mr. Chase exhibits as social program. From the disciple and amateur we learn the new meaning of the master and sage. It will be found in Mr. Chase's discussion of the Spanish Civil War, that clear and terrible fire whose light made plain where everybody stood. Mr. Louis Fischer had written in the *Nation* of March 27, 1937, as follows:

> At this moment a brazen invasion of Spain is going on. The fascist powers, in undisguised violation of their own signatures, of every canon of international law, of every principle of decency and humanity, are trying to crush the Spanish people and their democratically elected, legally constituted government. Apparently that does not matter to us. We sit idly and contentedly, denying Spanish democracy the means to defend itself. Neutrality followed to its logical conclusion has made America effectively pro-fascist.

Mr. Chase quotes this passage, and on it makes the following observation:

> Thus we find an emotive content similar to that of 1916, similar slogans, a similar call to cherish democracy. Mr. Fischer, I take it, is

prepared, if necessary, to go to war to defend Russia. I am not. I am one of the greatest idle and contented sitters-by you ever saw.[3]

Remember the historical context: German and Italian troops were in Spain, trying out the new weapons, testing the new tactics, and, above all, winning an advantageous position for the future world war. The fall of Madrid was followed in a little more than a year by the fall of Paris. Another year, and the invasion of Russia began; six more months, and there were planes over Pearl Harbor. The world hung, for a dreadful moment, within the grasp of Axis fascism. Spain had been the first line of defense, and Mr. Fischer's plea was for a defense of that line. Yet Mr. Chase could see nothing but "an emotive content similar to that of 1916." Accordingly, he professes himself "one of the greatest idle and contented sitters-by you ever saw." Such is the proper, the inevitable, conclusion of a belief that all problems are verbal. Such is the social program (if sitting-by can be called a program) which that belief is intended to justify. Upon that belief and the sitters-by whom it has engendered lies part of the responsibility for the death and the agony of recent years.

Thus the semantic philosophy, like Milton's Belial,

> . . . with words clothed in reason's garb,
> Counselled ignoble ease and peaceful sloth,
> Not peace . . .

The effect upon the history of our times has been exactly that of witch doctoring upon disease. A medicine man is bound to believe that his failure is due to an error in the incantation. He has therefore to improve his language, sharpening and rearranging the words. Yet all this does nothing to stay the progress of bacteria. On the contrary, it assists that progress, because it makes impossible the intervention of genuine medical treatment. German and Italian fascism could not be destroyed by the mere

[3] *Ibid.*, p. 340.

assertion that "fascism" is a vague or meaningless term. On the contrary, the more meaningless the term was said to be, the more the movement itself thrived, since people cannot be organized against an enemy they are told is nonexistent. The future state of man will be as absurd as desperate, if the fascist remnants throughout the world are permitted to multiply again, on the excuse that there are no persons corresponding to the term.

Unfortunately, just this result is becoming observable. Whenever a man or a movement exhibits all or most of the usual fascist ideas and is named accordingly, some semanticist is sure to arise and pronounce the naming meaningless. The left wing has its labels, he will say, no less than the right; and both sets of labels lack content. Such "impartiality" is mere show. In reality it protects the fascists by enabling them to escape public identification, and it injures the anti-fascists by an accusation of word-mongering. It is now scarcely possible to gather men together on behalf of human welfare, without someone's blocking the whole program by a complaint of "semantic confusion." If we were to apply to the semantic philosophy one of its own favorite tests, the operational, we should find that its real meaning, abundantly demonstrated in practice, is defense of things as they are.

The theory is, indeed, a source of general paralysis, not creeping but swift. It invades all areas of thought and action, and everywhere it immobilizes. If the effect of its criticism were to enlighten men rather than to leave them in doubt and indecision, there could be no objection. But, as things are, the semanticist attack on logic has subverted all the techniques of acquiring knowledge, and the attack on ethics has deprived men of the rational ground for making choices. How, then, can a man act, if he must remain wholly unsure what circumstances he acts in and what values are to mold his decision? To avoid the paralysis, we shall have to repel the attacks. This is the main business of our discussion.

THE ATTACK UPON LOGIC

The villain in the semanticist drama is no less a person than the Father of Logic himself, Aristotle. It is, I suppose, one of the penalties of greatness to be abused by later and lesser intellects. With Aristotle, however, the inevitable penalty has been compounded, because he had the ill luck to undergo a sort of secular canonization during the Middle Ages. All the faults of scholastic philosophy have therefore been attributed to him, and the man who did rather more observing of facts than most of his contemporaries has come to be regarded as the great exemplar of men who do no such observing at all. In the seventeenth century Lord Bacon led an anti-Aristotelian movement on behalf of empirical science, although the basic principles of scientific method were laid down by Aristotle himself. In the twentieth century Count Korzybski proposes a complete regeneration of science under the universal heading, "Non-Aristotelian Systems." [4] We shall find, upon analysis, that the Count's complaints touch Aristotle just about as closely as the Viscount's.

In Korzybski's view, the root of error is the law of identity, which he understands to mean "Whatever is, is." Now, says he (and Mr. Chase after him), everything in the world is a process, and therefore whatever is is in the act of becoming something else. But if it is becoming something else, then it cannot be what it is—certainly not always, nor even at any given moment. Mr. Chase's examples are calculatedly familiar:

> A rocket is always the same rocket. True for words, but not for that non-verbal event in space-time which blazes in glory and falls a charred stick as we watch it; not for a mushroom full-blown today and underground yesterday; not for a rose, withered now and lovely a week ago; not for an ice-cream cone five minutes in the sun.[5]

[4] Korzybski's symbol for these systems is $\bar{A}$, pronounced "A-bar." The bar indicates the negation of everything indicated by the symbol beneath it. Thus $\bar{A}$= Non-Aristotelian. The device has been borrowed from the Boolean Algebra.

[5] Chase, *op. cit.*, p. 228.

"Change and decay in all around I see"! In the world of space and time this is certainly true. What I wonder is: Who are the thinkers who have ever denied it? The nearest ones would be those rather early Greeks, Parmenides and Zeno, who held that the evidence of our senses gives opinion rather than knowledge, or the more recent Hegelians who distinguish between appearance and reality.[6] Parmenides can perhaps be convicted of arguing from logic to fact, since he says that "thought and being are one." But before we ascribe such a view to the "infantile," or Aristotelian, period, as Korzybski does,[7] we had better reflect that Parmenides had a contemporary and an opponent named Heraclitus, whose account of the nature of change is far more accurate and profound than anything provided by the semanticists. And we may remark, also, that both our critics seem to be arguing without benefit of dates. Parmenides and Heraclitus belong to the late sixth century B.C.; Aristotle (and with him formal logic as such) belongs to the fourth century B.C. Between them lies the whole flowering of Greek philosophy, and early in that flowering stands a man, Protagoras, who is the true historical ancestor of the semantic philosophy itself. Zeal for a new philosophy flames hotter the more ignorant we are of the old.

Whatever errors there may have been in man's early philosophizing, the law of identity does not now have the meaning Korzybski gives it, and did not have that meaning even in Aristotle. As applied to terms and statements, the law asserts that, throughout any given stretch of reasoning, each term and each statement must retain one and the same meaning. Clearly, it must; the alternative is chaos. Suppose that Korzybski's "Ā" means one thing in the first chapter, something different in the second, something yet different in the third, and so on. What conclusions could Korzybski draw about the virtues of "Ā"? None, for he

[6] It is interesting to observe that Mr. Chase believes Zeno's paradoxes to be a "sardonic thrust at the absurdities of formal logic" (*op. cit.*, p. 73). The historical tradition is that Zeno was supporting Parmenides's concept of a static universe.

[7] Alfred Korzybski: *Science and Sanity*, The Science Press, Lancaster, Pa., 1933, p. 194.

would be talking about one thing in the premises and another thing in the conclusion.

Does this logical requirement correspond to the nature of the world around us? It does, and indeed it must, for otherwise there could be no correspondence between the world and our statements about it. What reference could "Ā" have, if the philosophies it denotes suddenly ceased to be non-Aristotelian, or (more paradoxically yet) at one and the same time possessed and did not possess the character of being non-Aristotelian? Rockets, mushrooms, roses, and ice-cream cones are undoubtedly processes, but each of them is a particular process with its own special nature and history. Each of them is exactly what it is, and is not other than it is. This is the whole meaning of the law of identity. I think we may defy semanticists to alter it.

The attack upon the law of contradiction fares no better. Now, contradictory statements exist always and only as pairs, and they are any two statements which cannot both be true and cannot both be false. Thus, for example, "There are no rosebushes in my garden" and "There is at least one rosebush in my garden." These statements cannot both be true; yet one of them must be, since if it is false that there are no rosebushes in my garden, there must be at least one rosebush there, and if it is false that there is at least one rosebush in my garden, then there cannot be any there.

An attack upon the law of contradiction might take the form of denying that such pairs of statements exist. But, on such a view, what would become of Korzybski's and Chase's arguments? They are both attacking a certain theory which they call Aristotelian. This theory, they say, is false. Now, suppose someone asserts that this theory is true. Korzybski and Chase have got to deny this statement; but, if the law of contradiction does not hold, their mightiest efforts will be in vain. They may heap argument upon argument on behalf of the statement "This theory is false"; but, unless the statement "This theory is false" *actually contradicts* the statement "This theory is true," Chase and Korzybski might as well save their ink. Unless contradiction is possible, denial is impossible; and it will not even be possible to deny that denial is possible.

Well, perhaps Chase and Korzybski don't mean this. They are fond of distinguishing between what is possible for words and what is possible for things. They might say that, though verbal contradictories exist, real ones do not; in other words, that there are no situations in the world of space and time which exclude other situations. I find this view hard to comprehend. Every situation in the world of space and time excludes, simply by existing, all the situations which might have been but are not. You are, let us say, a full-time student at X University in the year 1945–1946. This state of affairs excludes both your being a full-time student elsewhere in 1945–1946 and your not being a full-time student at all. The statement "You are a full-time student at X University in the year 1945–1946" expresses the actual objective fact. The statement "You are not a full-time student at X University in the year 1945–1946" expresses the eliminated possibilities. The contradiction between the statements is an accurate reflection of the incompatibility of the facts.

With this in mind, we may pass to a discussion of the law of excluded middle, which arouses in semanticists a special horror. This law has to do with the second aspect of contradictory statements, namely that they cannot both be false, i. e. one of them must be true. In all such circumstances you have just two alternatives; you cannot have both, you must have one, and you cannot have any third. It is one or the other, thus:

Either

Aristotle is guilty of all the errors charged to him,

Or

Aristotle is not guilty of all the errors charged to him.

Either

You are a full-time student at X University in 1945–1946,

Or

You are not a full-time student at X University in 1945–1946.

Chase and Korzybski call this structure "two-valued." Korzybski is willing to admit it as a "limiting case." This admission evidently occurs in a part of the book which Chase read only three times, for Chase is unwilling to admit the structure at all. As against the "two-valued" and the yet more primitive "one-valued," our semanticists urge the "many-valued" structure as infinitely superior. Such a structure alone is capable, they think, of recording the marvelous variety of possible events. The world is so full of a number of things that Chase and Korzybski are happy as kings. Here is a set of examples from Mr. Chase:

One-valued: Contemporary events make communism inevitable in America.

Two-valued: Events make either communism or fascism inevitable in America. (This is the vicious "either-or" pair.)

Many-valued: The American Government may evolve into one of a variety of political forms, some of them more dictatorial, some less so than the present government.[8]

Let us take a look at the second (or "vicious") example. I will grant that the alternatives there set forth are more than a little hair-raising. That quality, however, is purely esthetic, and we are concerned with the logic of the structure alone. "Events make either communism or fascism inevitable in America." Now, it happens that "communism" and "fascism" are opposites, but not contradictories; they exclude each other, but they do not exhaust between them all the political possibilities. It is therefore erroneous to assert that you must have one or the other. But, plainly, the error lies not in the either-or relation, but in the choice of terms which are thus related. Indeed, it is the very integrity of the either-or structure which reveals the error in the choice of terms. Mr. Chase's example, so far from proving that structure "vicious," proves only that he cannot tell the difference between contraries and contradictories. And as if to strengthen this latter revelation, the third example, which purports to illustrate the many-valued structure, actually illustrates the two-valued: "some

[8] Chase, *op. cit.*, pp. 234–235.

of them more dictatorial, some less so," the third possibility ("equally dictatorial") being by implication eliminated.

It is clear, therefore, that Mr. Chase is totally unaware of the logic which actually exists in his illustrations. The connections which he has in mind and which he mistakes for logical ones are really connections of quite another sort. They are connections in his feeling, not in his thinking. He sets up two alternatives, fascism and communism. He knows he doesn't want either, and he imagines that his readers don't want either. The emotional recoil from two specific alternatives he transforms into a recoil from all pairs of alternatives, contradictories included. It is a remarkable example of how nothing is immune to the influence of ideology. Because Mr. Chase opposes both fascism and communism, we are to abandon the basic principles of rational thought. "Because thou art virtuous, shall there be no more cakes and ale?"

The social reasons for attacking logic are perfectly obvious. Indecisive people, or people who want to appear liberal while avoiding the results of liberalism, have an extreme distaste for the either-or construction, because in practical life it presents them with problems they cannot evade. Abstaining from one alternative has the effect of enforcing the other, and this condition is intolerable to men who wish to abstain from both. In their agony they dream of other possibilities; and, when these prove nebulous, they begin to reflect, very philosophically, that nothing is really this or that. "Either-or" is a hoax of the logicians, a conspiracy by dogmatists.

But these desertions of logic on behalf of political needs must end in disaster. If we abandon the either-or construction, we shall lose the means of rigorous discrimination among choices. The world becomes a plate of noodles, which, turn it how you will, is still noodles. If we abandon the principle of contradiction, all statements will be reduced to a level of equal validity, and it will be impossible to distinguish any of them as true from others which are false. Such a nightmare world, in which all rational criteria have been thrown away, is full of lurid gleams and strident voices. You cannot think, for there is no method of thinking. There is nothing to do but feel. Thus the way is prepared for a swift passage into fascist ideology. One understands more clearly why semanticists sat by during the Spanish Civil War.

THE ATTACK UPON ETHICS

A large part of our lives is spent in debating whether such-and-such an act is good to do, whether this other act should be abstained from, whether so-and-so's policies are justifiable. Questions like these are moral questions; they can always be recognized by the presence of words like "good," "bad," "right," "wrong," "ought," "should." When you use such words, you are not merely stating a fact; you are evaluating something, passing judgment on it. For example, to say that "One atomic bomb is capable of destroying fifty thousand people" is to state a fact. To say "It is a bad thing to destroy fifty thousand people" is to evaluate the fact, to judge it according to certain standards.

Human experience seems to show that everyone finds the moral life somewhat burdensome, except perhaps those people who contrive by one means or another to set themselves up as censors, from which eminence they are able to prescribe law rather than obey it. Ethics is by no means a purely negative discipline, yet it does seem inordinately fond of prohibitions. One harried mortal, whom morality had strained beyond endurance, was heard to cry, "Everything I like is either illegal or unhealthful or immoral!" Every honest man, I think, will hear in his own heart an echo of that complaint.

Well, if human beings have been lecturable by moralists, they have also been inventive of compromises with morality. In adjusting the standard to the wish all men are pretty skillful; and if intelligence tests were based upon that sort of wit, the number of genius-intellects would be found enormously increased. Not until the twentieth century, however, had it occurred to anyone to criticize ethical theory on the ground that value-judgments are syntactically confused.

For this ingenious effect we must turn away from Chase and Korzybski to a certain British adaptation of Logical Positivism, made in the mid-'thirties. Now, the early Positivists had suggested that all statements might be divided into two great classes: the meaningful and the meaningless. Meaningful statements are (1) those which are tautological—i. e. their predicates are definitions of their subjects—and (2) those which can be tested by possible sense experience. Thus, "A triangle is a three-sided rectilinear plane figure" is a meaningful statement, because its predicate defines its subject; and "Smith is wearing a brown suit" is meaningful, because it can be tested by a glance at Smith.

When applied, for example, to ethics or theology, this principle has remarkable effects. "God is a Triune Spiritual Being" would be a meaningful statement, for that is the definition of God, at least according to the Athanasian Creed. But "God exists" is a meaningless statement, since no such being can be the object of any possible sense experience. Theologians, who were long hardened to objections that their statements were false, were left breathless before this new charge that they had, for the most part, been saying nothing at all.

Even more startling is the effect of this notion upon ethics. We said, a moment ago, that the statement "One atomic bomb is capable of destroying fifty thousand people" is a statement of fact. It is verifiable by sense experience (though I hope never to verify it), and Logical Positivists would say that it is meaningful. But our other statement, "It is a bad thing to destroy fifty thousand people," is a statement not of fact but of evaluation. I can observe the killing, but I cannot observe the badness. I am talking, not about the event, but about my attitude towards it. The word "bad" adds nothing to the factual content of the statement; it merely evinces my feeling about the fact. It is as if I had said in a tone of horror, "One atomic bomb is capable of destroying fifty thousand people!"

Now, suppose we have another man who thinks such destruction excellent. This, too, would be an evincing statement, as if he had said in tones of satisfaction, "One atomic bomb is capable of destroying fifty thousand people!" Most of us will quite naturally suppose that the two men have contradictory ethical opinions which they can rationally discuss—although, if I were the first man, I should prefer to take the second to the nearest psychiatrist. But, according to the new theory, no question of truth or falsity exists between the horrified gasp of the one and the delighted sigh of the other: there is no disputing about grunts. Mr. A. J. Ayer, the "*enfant terrible* of Oxford," puts the case thus:

Another man may disagree with me about the wrongness of stealing, in the sense that he may not have the same feeling about stealing that I have. . . . But he cannot, strictly speaking, contradict me. . . . There is plainly no sense in asking which of us is in the right. For neither of us is asserting a genuine proposition.[9]

So now we know where we are: Jones says that stealing is morally wrong, Brown says that stealing is morally admirable, and both Jones and Brown are uttering sounds of very limited significance.

Well! But suppose that instead of "stealing" (an illustration which smells damply of the academic cloister) we take something less obvious and trite. Let it be the sort of happening which verbalists have done so little to prevent. Ella Winter tells of a ten-year-old Russian boy, who came to a hospital for treatment. Under anesthesia he suddenly began to relive the experiences of three years before, when the Nazis captured his village and hanged his uncle. The things he had never described poured from him:

"Don't cry," he sobbed, "don't cry, Grandmother. Go away. I don't want Uncle Vasya like that. Look what the Germans have done! Split open his whole head. . . . God sees everything. . . .

[9] Alfred J. Ayer, *Language, Truth and Logic*, Oxford University Press, New York, 1936, p. 159. Mr. Ayer received his appellation in the *New Statesman and Nation* for March 27, 1937.

"When they took him down and buried him, look how he is all stiff, you can't even put him in the coffin. I will lie down with him in the coffin. Oh look, what a good Uncle Vasya.

"I will never forget Uncle Vasya [crying bitterly] . . . I will kill the Germans. Hurry up, Russians, kill the Germans! I want Uncle Vasya to be alive. Let God return him from the grave. Granny, don't cry or the Germans will kill you. . . .

"Grandmother, your heart can break with sorrow." [10]

I will pass over what the Nazis did to Uncle Vasya, whose only crime was rescuing a wounded Russian soldier. I will pass over what the Nazis did to other children, whose tongues they cut out, whose ears they cut off, whose bodies they used for target practice. I will even pass over that horrible pile of infants' shoes at the Maidanek death camp. I will turn to those philosophers who maintain that moral judgments express no more than personal feeling, and ask them to consider Vitya's wild cry: "Grandmother, your heart can break with sorrow." Then, having caught the attention of these somewhat timid moralists, I will say, "Gentlemen, I consider it demonstrably true that it is evil, vilely evil, to use children thus. Have I asserted a genuine proposition?" And the moralists in question will answer, "No, you have not." Then I shall have to say, "Gentlemen, I have a son of about Vitya's age, and my son has friends of about that age, and some of my friends have children of about that age. I do not think that the welfare of children can be a matter of personal taste."

It is at once absurd and fitting that at just that moment of history when the most exquisite torments have been inflicted and the greatest agonies endured there should exist a philosophy which holds moral judgments to be capable of no proof. One might think that philosophers of such mind would recoil from the consequences of their theory and re-examine the postulates which had generated such folly. For the consequences are that one cannot *rationally* choose (i. e. choose on the basis of argu-

[10] Ella Winter, *I Saw The Russian People*, Little, Brown & Co., Boston, 1945, p. 208.

ment) between death camps and liberation; one can only "evince" approval or disapproval. One cannot demonstrate that fascist practices are evil; one can only express dislike of them. No philosophy would better please the fascists themselves, since moral questions could then be safely left in the hands of the police.

The absurdity of all this arises from a peculiar philosophical bias. Ayer's view is that factual statements and tautological statements are the *only* meaningful ones, and consequently that, if ethical statements are to mean anything, they must merely express a psychological fact. But no proof is ever given for this "only"; it remains, from first to last, a simple assumption. It is an assumption which results from taking science and mathematics seriously, while indulging an emancipated scepticism toward ethics. The sense of what is triumphs over the sense of what ought to be.

Thus men like Ayer will seem to take ethics rather frivolously. I do not mean that they are morally frivolous; when they leave your house, you don't have to count your spoons. They are philosophically frivolous, however, because they simply pay no attention to what an ethical statement actually asserts. When I said, "It was an evil thing for Nazis to torture children," I was certainly doing more than asserting that the Nazis did torture children. Ayer would say that the "more" which I did was to grunt my personal disapproval. Well, I will allow the grunt, but I must insist that my original assertion contained still more than the fact plus the grunting. It contained the further assertion that everybody ought to disapprove the torture of children by the Nazis (or, for that matter, by anybody else). For the whole point of ethical statements is their claim to be binding upon *all* men. This claim upon all cannot possibly be exhausted by the grunts of any *one*. Therefore, ethical statements contain more than Ayer is willing to admit, and this additional content is in fact their proper meaning. They are therefore meaningful in a sense which makes them susceptible of argument and hence of verification.

It may be worth while to add that if Ayer's Positivism is true, then the statements which express its main tenets are themselves meaningless. These statements are not definitions. If, then, they are to be meaningful, they must (according to the theory itself) be verifiable by some sense experience. But how can you verify by sense experience the statement that all meaningful, nontautological statements must be verifiable by sense experience? You cannot. As a matter of fact, sense experience *alone* will not tell you whether you have exhausted the meaning of any statement whatever, for, in order to tell a thing like that, you would have to compare the given sense experience with the given statement, the meaning of which you would have to know already.

We have, therefore, a theory which is reduced to meaninglessness by its own tests. On behalf of this theory, we are asked to abandon all moral judgments, to surrender, that is to say, every rational means by which good may be chosen and evil shunned. I think we shall require more than a frightened and self-defeated theory to lure us in any such direction. We may leave it to the verbalists to analyze gasps and breathings. For our part, let us continue to seek a better future for mankind.

THE ATTACK UPON SOCIAL CONCEPTS

Having thus indulged an excursion upon strange seas of thought, we may return to more familiar subjects. The damage done by the attack on logic and ethics is hidden, but the damage done by the attack on social concepts is obvious and great. Semanticists are full of admiration for science; they invoke it with a solemnity which was once reserved for religion alone. Nevertheless, it will not be difficult to show that, if the views of semanticists are correct, there can be no science of anything. And especially, there can be no science of society.

Any science is a system of *general* statements about the world. The statement which expresses the principle of gravitation, for example, does not confine itself to the two balls which Galileo is said to have dropped from the tower of Pisa. It asserts, rather, that, assuming a vacuum, all objects fall at the same rate. A science, therefore, deals with classes and kinds, not with individuals alone.

In the second place, a science deals with systems, with organizations, of things. In order to explain the behavior of any individual member of a system, it has to describe the nature of the system and the individual's relation to it. If we were to consider the heart in isolation from the lungs and the circulatory system, not very much could be known about so solitary an organ.

Now, if a science is to be really a science, its statements must correspond accurately to that portion of the world which it describes. But if classes and systems do not really exist in the world, most of the statements of any science will have nothing to correspond to. The science will then be locked within its own statements and will be pure fancy and artifice. No scientist, so far as he is a *scientist*, can fail to assume as a basic fact that classes and systems are as real as the individuals composing them.

This proposition, however, the semanticists deny. Their view is that individuals are real, but that classes and systems are abstractions. This *is* their view, despite the fact that they have carved in the granite dogma certain passages of escape. Korzybski, for example, says that on nonverbal levels "we deal exclusively with absolute individuals, in the sense that they are not identical." [11] Now, an absolute individual would be one which had no connections whatever with anything else; and we are said to deal with this "exclusively." But all this intransigeance of language melts away when "absolute" is defined as meaning merely that the given individual thing is not identical with others. Of course it isn't, and no one would suppose that it was. This obvious, indeed platitudinous, fact serves as an escape corridor when the fortress is stormed. For the essential question here is not whether individuals differ from one another, but whether, by the possession of common qualities, they form real classes.

The semanticists also give faint recognition to the presence of systems in the world by their concept of space as a "plenum." "When we have a plenum or fullness," says Korzybski, "it must

[11] Korzybski, *op. cit.*, p. 405. It happens that Aristotle also held the individual to be basically real. If Aristotelianism is "infantile," what are we to say to the semantic philosophy?

be a plenum of 'something,' 'somewhere,' at 'some time.' "[12] But there is very little system in this plenum, which speedily resolves itself into a sequence of individuals related like the knots in a string:

> All our experiences and all we know indicate definitely that ordinary materials ("objects") are extremely rare and very complex special cases of the beknottedness of the plenum; that the organic world and "life" represent extremely rare and still more complex special cases of the material world; and, finally, so-called "intelligent life" represents increasingly complex and still rarer cases of "life." [13]

In this passage the beknottedness of the plenum seems somewhat overmatched by the besottedness of the language, but it is nevertheless quite plain that Korzybski ignores the fact of things interacting with one another. Without this notion the term "system" is meaningless. Everything has been explained away into what Mr. Chase more poetically calls "a mad dance of atoms." The lunacy, however, is not in the atoms. They are not so mad as to avoid combining with one another to produce systems great and small, and thus to produce the world.

The effect of this relentless atomizing of the universe is to unsettle confidence in our knowledge of it. The old, deadly schism between "appearance" and "reality" is introduced once more; and the ordinary reader, as modest as he is unwary, begins to distrust even the most obvious teachings of experience. His enemies vanish beneath a transcendental disguise, only to reappear in the end miraculously, like Birnam Wood before Dunsinane. Let us observe how Mr. Chase accomplishes the process of dissolution, from philosophy to politics:

> There are no dogs-in-general in the world of experience, but only $Rover_1$, $Rover_2$, $Rover_3$, some gentle, some neutral, some vicious.[14]

[12] *Ibid.*, p. 229.
[13] *Ibid.*, p. 480.
[14] Chase, *op. cit.*, p. 51. The subnumerals are a semantic affectation which purports to emphasize the individuality of individuals.

There is no entity "mankind." Call as briskly as you may, "Hey, Mankind, come here!" and not an Adam will answer.[15]

No profit system exists as an entity in the real world. Instead one has to study the behavior of Adam$_1$, Adam$_2$, Morgan$_1$ and Morgan$_2$.[16]

Semantically there is no "party" as an entity. The referents of the term are individual voters more or less controlled by local bosses.[17]

Well, what does fascism mean? Obviously the term by itself means nothing. In one context it has some meaning as a tag for Mussolini, his political party, and his activities in Italy. In another context it might be used as a tag for Hitler, his party, and his political activities in Germany. The two contexts are clearly not identical, and if they are to be used one ought to speak of the Italian and German varieties as fascism$_1$ and fascism$_2$.[18]

To which let us add some remarks by Mr. Bernard DeVoto, who wrote admiringly of Mr. Chase, regretting only that Mr. Chase did not go further:

He [Chase] says that "more than one-third of the people in America are underfed, inadequately housed, and shoddily clothed." He has never counted them, no one has ever counted them, and his statement is not meaningful but emotionally useful. The only word in it that can be operationally examined is "underfed," and an inquiry by nutritionists (granting they could agree on tests) would possibly reveal a certain percentage of "blab." "Inadequately housed" is open at both ends —inadequately by what scale, in relation to what facts, in relation to what specifications and persons? "Shoddily clothed" is meaningless though it appears to refer to garments.[19]

There is no such thing as "truth." There is no such thing as "social justice."[20]

So now we see it all: there are no dogs-in-general, no mankind, no profit system, no parties, no fascism, no underfed people, no

[15] *Ibid.*, p. 102.
[16] *Ibid.*, p. 277.
[17] *Ibid.*, p. 347.
[18] *Ibid.*, p. 188. But if "there is no 'party' as an entity," how can Mussolini and Hitler each have had one?
[19] In *Harper's Magazine*, 176: pp. 222–223 (January, 1938).
[20] *Ibid.*, p. 224.

inadequate housing, no shoddy clothes, no truth, and no social justice. Such being the case, there can be no economic problem, no political problem, no fascist problem, no food problem, no housing problem, no "garment" problem, no scientific problem, and no social problem. By the simple exhalation of breath, Messrs. Chase and DeVoto have conjured out of existence every major problem which has vexed mankind throughout the entire history of the human race.

Of the five terms which Chase proscribes as meaningless, one ("dogs-in-general") is a class name, and the others are names of systems. Since classes differ very markedly from systems,[21] we may divide our commentary accordingly.

(1) It is remarkable that Mr. Chase, while denying the existence of dogs-in-general, nevertheless contrives to call his three dogs "Rover." The sub-numerals indicate that they are different dogs, but "Rover" indicates that all of them are dogs. How does Mr. Chase know that all of them are dogs? Because they all possess the essential canine characteristics. Mr. Chase appears to think that, though individual dogs exist, the class of dogs is merely an abstraction in his mind. But how can this be? $Rover_1$ will go right on resembling $Rover_2$ and $Rover_3$, whether Mr. Chase has a mind or not. The dogs are in the class and the class is in the dogs.

Let us put the case another way. Suppose you have upon your pantry shelf a jar of pickles, and suppose that on that jar there is a label which says PICKLES. According to Mr. Chase and the other semanticists, the pickles are real enough: there is $Pickle_1$, $Pickle_2$, $Pickle_3$, and so forth. But pickles-in-general is an abstraction, a sort of mental sign referring to the individual pickles exactly as the label PICKLES does on the jar. Well, I submit that no housewife has any such notion. She is not concerned with the pickleness that is in Mr. Chase's mind; she is concerned with the

[21] Individuals belong to classes by virtue of common characteristics. Individuals belong to systems by virtue of constant interaction with one another. "Party" is both a class name and the name of a system.

pickleness that is in the pickles. If it is not there, she has been wantonly deceived by her grocer, who was, perhaps, a semanticist.

(2) Now for the terms which signify systems. Mr. Chase says that there is no entity called "mankind," that if you were to summon mankind to you, no one would answer. Well, naturally. You might also cry out, "Hey, United States Army, come here!" Not a soldier would answer. Can we then infer that there is no entity called "The United States Army"? Obviously such reasoning is nonsense. What Mr. Chase has done is to assume that a system will behave like one of its members. An individual man would doubtless answer if you called, "Come here!" Mr. Chase expects the same behavior of "mankind," that is, of men taken collectively. Not finding that behavior, he infers the nonexistence of the system. His assumption was, of course, false: what is true of a part is not necessarily true of the whole. Logicians call this error the Fallacy of Composition, and it was first identified by Aristotle. Who, then, is more "infantile," the philosopher who discovered the fallacy or the writer who continues to commit it?

"No profit system exists as an entity in the real world." Mr. Chase urges us to study the behavior of various Adams and Morgans. Very well, let us study it. If $Adam_1$ goes to work in a factory, he enters a system of relationships so intimate that the product which comes off the assembly line cannot be supposed the work of any one man; it issues from the *collective* labor of hundreds of men. If we assume $Morgan_1$ to be an industrialist rather than a banker, then we know that he markets the products which $Adam_1$ has helped to make. $Morgan_1$ must sell the products for an amount greater than the costs of production, among which are $Adam_1$'s wages. The difference between the income on sales and the costs of production represents $Morgan_1$'s profits, and without these he cannot continue in business. Thus $Adam_1$ and $Morgan_1$ are members of a system which will operate only so long as profits are made. No profit system exists, then? Well, perhaps it is only a system by which people make profits.

The assertions about "party" and "fascism" are equally ludicrous. There are, to be sure, individual Democrats, but there certainly is also an entity known as the Democratic Party—an organization with an apparatus of functionaries, an organization capable of putting on campaigns. There are, to be sure, individual fascists; but there is also fascism—a definite, describable social and political system. Without this, indeed, it would be impossible to identify fascist_1 or fascist_2, for the individual fascists are fascists precisely because they strive to bring into existence, or to maintain in existence, that very system itself. If the term "fascism" means nothing by itself (in the same sense in which any other term has meaning by itself), then we can never recognize any regime as fascist, nor can we combat any movement to establish such a regime. The effect of Mr. Chase's argument is to blind us to our enemies.

As for the remaining "meaningless" terms, I confess I would enjoy imposing on semanticists their own operational test. If, like Mr. DeVoto, they find no meaning in "underfed," "inadequately housed," and "shoddily clothed," then I think it would be pleasant to watch their behavior on an unemployment allotment of, say, five dollars a week. And when, after months of this, they come to us with obvious symptoms of malnutrition, with bodies enfeebled by exposure to the elements, and on their backs the rags of ancient clothing, we may justly remind them that it was they who "proved" that no one can be ill-fed or ill-clothed or ill-housed, because all these are meaningless terms. And such is their passion for this preposterous dogma that I rather wonder whether they would not go away convinced and satisfied. At any rate, so long as the operational test is imposed only on other people, the semanticists will see no reason to change their minds.

In general, the social views of semanticists are what you would expect of men who are unable to perceive either the effects of poverty or the conspiracies of fascism. Korzybski's ethics is clearly that of an aristocrat, who hates above all things "commercialism," that is to say, the influence which capitalism has had upon art, science, and invention.[22] Chase is a smiling, and DeVoto a rather grim, conservative. Both of them find in semantics a means of combating the great anti-fascist movement of the past fifteen years. In this they are altogether correct, for the semantic philosophy has no other social reason to exist.

An attentive reader will also discern in the writings of some semanticists a faint murmur of racism. Ogden and Richards, whose *Meaning of Meaning* first made semanticism fashionable, tell a story which they call a "darky anecdote." [23] They also quote with obvious approval the sneering remarks of a certain Ingraham:

> We do not often have occasion to speak, as of an indivisible whole, of the group of phenomena involved or connected in the transit of a negro over a rail-fence with a melon under his arm while the moon is just passing behind a cloud.[24]

Korzybski tells us that the Aristotelian system was a semantic response "of the white race of more than two thousand years ago." [25] Evidently he believes that systems of thought are determined by the racial origins of thinkers. That appears to be the meaning, also, of the following passage:

> . . . When we explore the objective level . . . we must try to define every "meaning" as a conscious feeling of actual, or assumed, or wished, *relations* which pertain to first order objective entities, psychological included, and which can be evaluated by personal, varied, and racial—again unspeakable first order—psychophysiological effects.[26]

We must exempt Mr. Chase from any such charge, for he shows himself not lacking in a certain militancy against racism. But we have, at any rate, two semanticists who are contemptuous of

[22] See the remarkable Table of Standards, Korzybski: *op. cit.*, pp. 555–557.

[23] C. K. Ogden and I. A. Richards, *The Meaning of Meaning,* Harcourt, Brace & Co., New York, 1923, p. 347 *n.*

[24] *Ibid.*, p. 131.

[25] Korzybski, *op. cit.*, p. 555.

[26] *Ibid.*, p. 23. Except for the three dots to indicate omissions, the punctuation and italics are Korzybski's. I say "appears to be the meaning," because it strikes me as improbable that this passage can be clear in anybody's mind, including the author's.

Negroes, and one who regards race as a determinant of thought.

Lastly, we can learn something of these men by the authors they praise. Korzybski is lavish of compliments to Spengler,[27] whose work the Nazis drew upon, and who himself joined the Nazi Party. Chase repudiates Spengler, but falls instead into a citation of Alexis Carrel, the collaborationist, and of *Man, the Unknown*, which was in its day an important contribution to fascist ideology in America.[28] I do not for one moment suppose that these facts suffice to make fascists out of Korzybski and Chase; but they do show that our two authors either do not recognize fascism when they see it, or find some of its ideas congenial. In any case, the facts corroborate empirically what we deduced by theoretical analysis—that there is a decided kinship between the semantic philosophy and the whole world of fascist and reactionary ideas.

If the nineteen-thirties began in hunger and ended in blood, we must strive to prevent the nineteen-forties, which began in blood, from ending in hunger. But we shall never succeed in this task unless we recognize that the real world sets us real problems, and that the real problems are susceptible of real solutions. We have to repair a ravaged world, to feed and clothe and house its people, to liberate the yet oppressed, to deal justly with millions who have never known the touch of honest hands. It is inconceivable that even the smallest of these mercies can be visited, if we permit ourselves to think that the words which express them are meaningless and vain. Nor shall we succeed by imagining the contrary folly, that problems can be solved by a simple adjustment of language.

There is a problem of language, to be sure; but that is not our main concern. There is a need for speech of clarity and precision, but neither is that our final goal. What we shall find is that our speech will grow clearer in proportion as we solve the objective,

[27] *Ibid.*, p. 47.

[28] Chase, *op. cit.* Carrel is cited as an authority on page 194. The repudiation of Spengler is on page 222.

nonverbal problems; and that, so far as we fail to solve them, our speech will remain halting and obscure. It is precisely for this reason that semanticists cannot make themselves intelligible; and the semantic philosophy, a tower of confusion, warns us forever that men who forsake the care of humankind will lose all understanding from their hearts and all vision from their eyes.

The Mental Attitude of the Educated Classes

FRANZ BOAS (1858–1942)

When we attempt to form our opinions in an intelligent manner, we are inclined to accept the judgment of those who by their education and occupation are compelled to deal with the questions at issue. We assume that their views must be rational, and based on intelligent understanding of the problems. The foundation of this belief is the tacit assumption not only that they have special knowledge but also that they are free to form perfectly rational opinions. However, it is easy to see there is no type of society in existence in which such freedom exists.

I believe I can make my point clearest by giving an example taken from the life of a people whose cultural conditions are very simple. I will choose for this purpose the Eskimo. In their social life they are exceedingly individualistic. The social group has so little cohesion that we have hardly the right to speak of tribes. A number of families come together and live in the same village, but there is nothing to prevent any one of them from living and settling at another place with other families. In fact during a period of a lifetime the families constituting an Eskimo village community are constantly shifting about; and while they generally return after many years to the place where their relatives live, the family may have belonged to a great many different communities. There is no authority vested in any individual, no chieftaincy, and no method by which orders, if they were given, could be carried out. In short, so far as law is concerned, we have a condition of almost absolute anarchy. We might therefore say that every single person is entirely free, within the limits of his own mental ability, to determine his own mode of life and his own mode of thinking. Nevertheless it is easily seen that there are innumerable restrictions that determine his behavior. The Eskimo boy learns how to handle the knife, how to use bow and arrow, how to hunt, how to build a house; the girl learns how to sew and mend clothing and how to cook; and during all their life they use their tools in the way they learned in childhood. New inventions are rare, and the whole industrial life of the people follows traditional channels. What is true of industrial activities is no less true of their thoughts. Certain religious ideas have been transmitted to them, notions as to what is right and wrong, certain amusements, and enjoyment of certain types of art. Any deviation from these is not likely to occur. At the same time it never enters into their minds that any other way of thinking and acting would be possible, and they consider themselves as perfectly free in regard to all their actions. Based on our wider experience, we know that the industrial problems of the Eskimo may be solved in a great many other ways and that their religious traditions and social customs might be quite different from what they are. From the outside, objective point of view we see clearly the restrictions that bind the individual who considers himself free.

It is hardly necessary to give many instances of these occurrences. It seems desirable however to illustrate the great strength of these ideas that restrict the freedom of thought of the individual, leading to the most serious mental struggles when traditional social ethics come into conflict with instinctive reactions. Thus among a tribe of Siberia we find a belief that every person will live in the future life in the same condition in which he finds himself at the time of death. As a consequence an old man who begins to be decrepit wishes to die, in order to avoid life as a cripple in the endless future, and it becomes the duty of his son to kill him. The son believes in the righteousness of this command but at the same time feels the filial love for his father, and many are the instances in which the son has to decide between the two conflicting duties—the one imposed by the instinctive filial love, the other imposed by the traditional custom of the tribe.

Another interesting observation may be deduced from those somewhat more complex societies in which there is a distinction between different social classes. We find such a condition, for instance, in North America, among the Indians of British Columbia, in which a sharp distinction is made between people of noble birth and common people. In this case the traditional behavior of the two classes shows considerable differences. The social tradition that regulates the life of the nobility is somewhat analogous to the social tradition of our society. A great deal of stress is laid upon the strict observance of convention and upon display, and nobody can maintain his position in high society without an adequate amount of ostentation and without strict regard for conventional conduct. These requirements are so fundamental that an overbearing conceit and a contempt for the common people become social requirements of an important chief. The contrast between the social proprieties for the nobility and those for the common people is very striking. Of the common people are expected humbleness, mercy and all those qualities that we consider amiable and humane.

Similar observations may be made in all those cases in which, by a complex tradition, a social class is set off from the mass of the people. The chiefs of the Polynesian Islands, the kings in Africa, the medicine men of all countries present examples in which a social group's line of conduct and of thought is strongly modified by their segregation from the mass of the people. On the whole, in societies of this type, the mass of the people consider as their ideal those actions which we should characterize as humane; not by any means that all their actions conform to humane conduct, but their valuation of men shows that the fundamental altruistic principles which we recognize are recognized by them too. Not so with the privileged classes. In place of the general humane interest the class interest predominates; and while it would be wrong to say that their conduct is selfish, it is always so shaped that the interest of the class to which they belong prevails over the interest of society as a whole. If it is necessary to secure rank and to enhance the standing of the family by killing a number of enemies, there is no hesitation felt in taking life. If the interests of the class require oppression of the rest of the people, then they are oppressed. If the interest of the class requires that its members should not perform menial occupations but should devote themselves to art or learning, then all the members of the class will vie with one another in the attainment of these achievements. It is for this reason that every segregated class is much more strongly influenced by special traditional ideas than is the mass of the people; not that the multitude is free to think rationally and that its behavior is not determined by tradition, but that the tradition is not so specific, not so strictly determined in its range, as in the case of the segregated classes. For this reason it is often found that the restriction of freedom of thought by convention is greater in what we might call the educated classes than in the mass of the people.

I believe this observation is of great importance when we try to understand conditions in our own society. Its bearing upon the problem of the psychological significance of nationalism will at once be apparent; for the nation is also a segregated class, albeit segregated according to other principles; and the characteristic feature of nationalism is that its social ethical standards are considered as more fundamental than those that are general and human, or rather that the members of each nation like to assume that their ideals are or should be the true ideals of mankind. At the same time it illustrates clearly that we should make a fundamental mistake if we should confound class selfishness and individual selfishness; for we find the most splendid examples of unselfish devotion to the interests of the nation, heroism that has been rightly praised for thousands of years as the highest virtue, and it is difficult to realize that nevertheless the whole history of mankind points in the direction of a *human* ideal as opposed to a *national* ideal. And indeed may we not continue to admire the self-sacrifice of a great mind, even if we transcend to ideals that were not his, and that perhaps, owing to the time and place in which he lived, could not be his?

Our observation has also another important application. The industrial and economic development of modern times has brought about a differentiation within our population that has never been equaled in any primitive society. The occupations of the various parts of a modern European or American population differ enormously; so much so, that in many cases it is almost impossible for people speaking the same language to understand one another when they talk about their daily work. The ideas with which the scientist, the artist, the tradesman, the business man, the laborer operate are so distinctive that they have only a few fundamental elements in common. Here it may again be observed that those occupations which are intellectually or emotionally most highly specialized require the longest training, and training always means an infusion of historically transmitted ideas. It is therefore not surprising that the thought of what we call the educated classes is controlled essentially by those ideals which have been transmitted to us by past generations. These ideals are always highly specialized, and include the ethical tendencies, the aesthetic inclinations, the intellectuality, and the expression of volition, of past times. Their control may find expression in a dominant tone which determines our whole mode of thought and which, for the very reason that it has come to be ingrained into our whole mentality, never rises into our consciousness.

In those cases in which our reaction is more conscious, it is either positive or negative. Our thoughts may be based on a high valuation of the past, or they may be a revolt against it. When we bear this in mind we may understand the characteristics of the behavior of the intellectuals. It is a mistake to assume that their mentality is, on the average, appreciably higher than that of the rest of the people. Perhaps a greater number of independent minds find their way into this group than into some other group of individuals who are moderately well-to-do; but their average mentality is surely in no way superior to that of the workingmen, who by the conditions of their youth have been compelled to subsist on the produce of their manual labor. In both groups mediocrity prevails; unusually strong and unusually weak individuals are exceptions. For this reason the strength of character and intellect that is required for vigorous thought on matters in which intense sentiments are involved is not commonly found—either among the intellectuals or in any other part of the population. This condition, combined with the thoroughness with which the intellectuals have imbibed the traditions of the past, makes the majority of them in all nations conventional. It has the effect that their thoughts are based on tradition, and that the range of their vision is liable to be limited. Even the apparent exception of the Russian intellectuals, who have been brought up under the influence of West European ideas, does not contradict our general conclusion.

There are of course strong minds among the intellectuals who rise above the conventionalism of their class, and attain that freedom that is the reward of a courageous search for truth, along whatever path it may lead.

In contrast to the intellectuals, the masses in our modern city populations are less subject to the influence of traditional teaching. They are torn away from school before it can make an indelible impression upon their minds and they may never have known the strength of the conservative influence of a home in which parents and children live a common life. The more heterogeneous the society in which they live, and the more the constituent groups are free from historic influences, or the more they represent different historic traditions, the less strongly will they be attached to the past.

It would be an exaggeration if we should extend this view over all aspects of human life. I am speaking here only of those fundamental concepts of right and wrong that develop in the segregated classes and in the masses. In a society in which beliefs are transmitted with great intensity the impossibility of treating calmly the views and actions of the heretic is shared by both groups. When, through the progress of scientific thought, the foundations of dogmatic belief are shaken among the intellectuals and not among the masses, we find the conditions reversed and greater freedom of traditional forms of thought among the intellectuals—at least in so far as the current dogma is involved. It would also be an exaggeration to claim that the masses can sense the right way of attaining the realization of their ideals, for these must be found by painful experience and by the application of knowledge. However, neither of these restrictions touches our main contention, namely, that the desires of the masses are in a wider sense more human than those of the classes.

It is therefore not surprising that the masses of the people—whose attachment to the past is comparatively slight and who work—respond more quickly and more energetically to the urgent demands of the hour than the educated classes, and that the ethical ideals of the best among them are human ideals, not those of a segregated class. For this reason I should always be more inclined to accept, in regard to fundamental human problems, the judgment of the masses rather than the judgment of the intellectuals, which is much more certain to be warped by unconscious control of traditional ideas. I do not mean to say that the judgment of the masses would be acceptable in regard to every problem of human life, because there are many which, by their technical nature, are beyond their understanding. Nor do I believe that the details of the right solution of a problem can always be found by the masses; but I feel strongly that the problem itself, as felt by them, and the ideal that they want to see realized, is a safer guide for our conduct than the ideal of the intellectual group that stands under the ban of an historical tradition that dulls their feeling for the needs of the day.

One word more, in regard to what might be a fatal misunderstanding of my meaning. If I decry unthinking obedience to the ideals of our forefathers, I am far from believing that it will ever be possible, or that it will even be desirable, to cast away the past and to begin anew on a purely intellectual basis. Those who think that this can be accomplished do not, I believe, understand human nature aright. Our very wishes for changes are based on criticism of the past, and would take another direction if the conditions under which we live were of a different nature. We are building up our new ideals by utilizing the work of our ancestors, even where we condemn it, and so it will be in the future. Whatever our generation may achieve will attain in course of time that venerable aspect that will lay in chains the minds of the great mass of our successors and it will require new efforts to free a future generation of the shackles that we are forging. When we once recognize this process, we must see that it is our task not only to free ourselves of traditional prejudice, but also to search in the heritage of the past for what is useful and right, and to endeavor to free the mind of future generations so that they may not cling to our mistakes, but may be ready to correct them.

The Hickman Story

JOHN BARTLOW MARTIN (1915–)

THE OLDEST son of the Hickman family, Willis, twenty years old, went to the barber shop after work and got home about 8:15, and then they all were home who were coming home that night, the seven children and the parents. Another son was working. The father, James Hickman, a cleancut Negro of thirty-nine, serious of mien and small but tightly-knit of body, was getting ready to go to his night job. He "had bad feet" and he sent Willis to the floor below to get a bucket of water to bathe them. (The Hickmans had no running water in their attic room atop the tenement.) About nine o'clock, Hickman left for the steelmill. He was the head of this family.

Willis, and Charles, who was nineteen, and their mother helped the younger children with their lessons. The three in school—Leslie, fourteen, Elzena, nine, and Sylvester, seven—were really studying and Velvena was playing at studying, though she was only four. After a half hour Mrs. Hickman, a thin quiet woman, went to bed. Soon the four younger children crawled in with her. Willis and Charles got into the other bed, first turning off the kerosene heater, cookstove, and lamp. They all fell asleep. It was then about 10:00 P. M. on January 16, 1947.

An hour and a half later Mrs. Hickman was wakened by fire. "I heard the paper popping" in the ceiling. She ran to the door to the only stairway and "the fire and smoke hit me, fire came right to me, in the face," and she slammed the door and went to get the children up. Charles leaped through the fiery doorway naked and escaped down the stairs. Mrs. Hickman was about to collapse. Willis wakened; "fire was over my head, in the door, I threw the cover back, and burned my hand." He rolled out of bed, crawled beneath the smoke to the front window, kicked it out, started out, hesitated, looked back.

Dimly through the smoke and flame he saw his mother huddled in the corner near her four smallest children. The flames were upon them. He pulled her to the window. It was three floors straight down the bare face of the old brick tenement to the street. He straddled the sill and hung her outside and told her to kick out the window glass on the third floor below. She was too short, so Willis climbed out and, hanging by one hand, lowered her down. She scrambled to the second-floor window. He grabbed the third-floor window frame but it gave way and he fell to the ground, breaking his collar bone and leaving her dangling. A man below yelled to her to let go, and she did, and he caught her. Later a fire chief said, "I cannot understand how she escaped . . . it was a miracle," and the coroner said, "The Lord was with her." But her four children were dead.

The night was cold, snow lay on the ground, but a great crowd gathered, this was a slum fire. Other tenants of the building streamed out, maybe forty of them. Neighbors took Mrs. Hickman and Willis to the hospital. The fire chief recalled, "It was a holocaust, it was one mass of fire rolling across that roof." But the firemen put it out in five minutes. Soon the street in the slum was deserted again.

Hours later, about 7:30 in the morning, gray daylight, a man alone came walking up the street, James Hickman, the father. He had been told at work that he "had trouble in my home." Out in front of the tenement a man was tinkering with an automobile, he had the hood up, and another man was pouring water over the steps of the building. Hickman started upstairs; ". . . a policeman hailed me and asked where I was going. I said I was going upstairs where I live. 'You can't go up there,' he said. 'Man, you tell me I can't go up there, what's the trouble? I am James Hickman, I live there.' " The policeman asked cautiously what floor he lived on. "I said the fourth and he said, 'Ah, you can't go up there, we had a big fire.' I asked him where were my children, he said he didn't know." Another tenant had appeared. "He said, 'Mr. Hickman, I hate to tell you this, four of your children is burnt to death.' And I weakened down to the ground." They carried him into the basement. Presently, Hickman recalls, "my mind referred back." He remembered that his landlord, David Coleman, had threatened to burn down the building if the tenants didn't clear out. A neighbor recalls, "Mr. Hickman was walking back and forth. He said nothing. There were tears in his eyes. Mr. Hickman looked pretty bad, like he was losing his mind. After about one half-hour, some officers helped Mr. Hickman away."

Our story is about James Hickman, a Negro. It is about his landlord, David Coleman, likewise a Negro, and their combat. It is also about slums and housing and race discrimination, the plight of the Negroes in the northern ghettos, the segregation that keeps them there and generates explosions, explosions like this fire and what came after it.

James Hickman, a man of rich brown color, was born February 19, 1907, "in the country" near Louisville, Mississippi. His mother and father were sharecroppers raising cotton and corn. They lived in a four-room shack. He was the youngest of four children; one was killed, the others left. At ten he went to work in the fields. At twelve he experienced a religious conversion. Forever after he was deeply religious. His mother and father separated when he was fourteen and he quit school. At sixteen he married a neighbor girl, Annie Davis. They lived with his mother and took care of her; she had tuberculosis. (She died in 1926 and for half a year Hickman grieved.) Their first child was born August 2, 1924. They named her Arlene, and Hickman made a vow to God: "I was the head of this family and had to make a support for them, I was a guardian to see for them as long as the days I should live on the land." He was then seventeen.

They moved to Fern Spring, "sharecropping cotton and corn, and vegetables for ourselves," his wife remembers. "We started farming at sun-up and stopped at sun-down. We were in the hilly part of Mississippi. I chopped cotton myself. . . ." They moved often, making a crop and giving birth to a child, then moving on, trying to better their lot. Some owners were fair, some were not. "We never could own the land." They moved to the Delta, land of milk and honey. They farmed the Delta seventeen years. One year, 1942, they made $935, their greatest earnings in the South. Before the war they often made only $100, one year $28, some years nothing at all. When they had a bad year "the boss-men . . . claimed that the cotton prices had failed." "When we got paid, Smith and Wiggins took their money first for food, clothes, fertilizer." Hickman says, "The landlord furnished everything. But you pays for it. And he don't work."

After the children were eight or nine, they rarely attended school more than four or five months a year, sometimes only one; for if the parents didn't send them to the fields, Hickman recalls, "the landlord'd be a-grumblin'. He'd say, get 'em busy, your grass is growin', this, that, or else he'd put a bunch in the fields and it'd come out of your pay in the fall. Work is all they look for you to do. They don't look for no school. The plow and hoe and such'll keep knowledge out of a person's head." Mrs. Hickman says, "We was very anxious to get up North where they had the opportunity to go to school and all these privileges," meaning by "privileges" freedom for a black person.

Nine children were born and the Hickmans reared them all, an achievement for Negroes in the South. One, Corene, was born blind and never talked, the only one afflicted. Hickman said, "We couldn't help her but I loved her just like I loved the rest of them." Hickman was stern with his children but he loved them with a surpassing love. Upon the birth of each he had repeated his vow to God to protect them and set them free. He wanted to take them North. He felt they were destined for great things. The ones born first disappointed him. "The oldest one was taken in the Army. The next one was kicked out of school. The daughter married.

I said all right. These youngest children—I had told them all one night—'It seems like I can see a future for you.' I see in those four children that they possibly would be great men and great women some day. . . . I had a vision and the spirit said they would be great. . . ."

The Navy ordered Hickman to report for induction April 12, 1944, but the day before, men of his age were exempted "until further notice." He didn't know what to do, but the North had been tugging at him for a long time, so he went up there, worked ten months in a shipyard, went back South, then in the spring of 1945 went alone to Chicago, intending to find a job and a home and to bring his family North to stay.

How did Chicago look to this countryman? He'd visited Southern cities but Chicago was different. Bigger, of course, but more than that. "Here, it was quite different when I'd see peoples riding in the cars together, buses—in the banks and post office colored would be working," he said recently in his slow, deep, deliberate voice. His oldest daughter, who had married, was living in Chicago and Hickman stayed with her. "A gentman picking up labor carried us over to a place to work"; Hickman thought it was the factory where his son-in-law worked but it was the stockyards, and he left. He got a job at Wisconsin Steel, far out at the Indiana line. He worked "on the crib," guiding the hot steel as it came off the hotbed. He was paid about $1.25 an hour, an awful lot to him. Better still, "I could see what I was gittin'. On the farm I'd be charged for a lot of things, I couldn't see what it was for. In the factory work it come to my hand."

But soon the pleasures of earning good money and riding white men's buses palled. "I would see so many old raggedy buildings, I'd say my goodness, I see so many nice buildings and then others just propped, folks livin' in just to have some place to live." He was hunting a place for his family. Finding one proved difficult. Hickman was bucking what may be the nation's worst housing problem.

Chicago's Black Belt is a narrow strip of land seven miles long and a mile and a half wide on the South Side, in spots almost—but not quite—touching the gilded lakefront. This is America's second biggest Negro city. Here, and in several scattered communities, dwell almost 400,000 Negroes, a tenth of Chicago's population. When a housing project of 1,658 units was opened in 1941, more than 19,000 people applied to live in it. Since then about 100,000 more Negroes, drawn by the war boom and Northern freedom, have come to live in Chicago. Why do they all crowd into this one area? Poverty? Yes, to a certain extent; but well-to-do Negroes live here too. The law? No, our laws imply the opposite, freedom. Ethnological attraction, then, which draws any immigrant group together? Again, yes, to a certain extent. Ah, but here we can see the truth: the European immigrants, as their earnings and adaptation increased, scattered throughout the city, disappearing into the general population. "Disappearing"—how can a black man disappear? He is not wanted. He is condemned to inhabit the areas that nobody else wants. Around the Negroes we have welded an iron ring of restrictive covenants and less formalized segregation enforced by violence. Thus trapped they turn upon one another. In this artificially restricted market, people of means bid high for hovels; rentals skyrocket; landlords gouge. Some of the landlords are white, some are black, all profit by the race-hate that makes their hovels desired. The Black Belt landlords squeeze tighter and tighter, and sometimes an eruption occurs, as in the Hickman case.

James Hickman got off the night shift at the steelmill at 7:00 A.M. "I would leave the job and just ride, hunting for a place for my folks," till dark, rest a few hours, then go back to work. "Ride and ride, walk and walk. I'd knock on a door and ask. Workin' and lookin'." Ignorant of Chicago, he often got into strange neighborhoods. "Sometimes I'd get to where they wasn't nothin' but white folks, I'd be the only colored man walkin' down the street. I'd see houses and I didn't know who was living there till I'd knock on the door and they'd say white folks only. They'd tell me which hundred block was for colored. I'd catch the car and go back and get off there." Did he experience any unpleasantness? "My race talked more rougher than the other race. I was born in a country where there's nothin' but white folks and I knowed how to talk and carry myself and they treated me mighty fine."

He found plenty of empty flats. "But they didn't want nobody with children." Even a public housing project refused him because he had so many children. Real estate offices took his money and produced nothing. Their usual fee was between $1 and $5 "to enlist," plus a month's rent if they found you a place. One landlord wanted to rent a four-room flat for $45 a month and sell the furniture for $1,200. Another asked "a thousand dollars down and $55 for twenty-five years, I didn't have that kind of money." But he had saved $260 since coming to Chicago and he was willing to pay up to $100 a month rent.

After six months, a barber offered to rent him a room in his own home. Hickman paid him a month's rent, $30, and sent train fare to his wife. She arrived with all the children on January 10, 1946, and Hickman met them at the station and took them out to their daughter's flat. Next day their furniture arrived from Mississippi, all their belongings, "meat and lard and everything but bread."

But the barber said the room wasn't ready yet. They put their furniture in their daughter's basement. Time passed. The Hickmans began looking for another place. A "real estate lady" found them one and they gave her $25 and paid the landlady $25 but the landlady returned their money; they couldn't have the apartment. They resumed their search, streetcars, pavements, want ads, realtors, all spring long. In June the barber called: they could have the room. They hired a truck for $18 and took their belongings to the barber's home. The barber's wife met them. She said they couldn't move in; "she was the boss." They went away. They put the furniture in a warehouse. And started all over again, looking.

Hickman's daughter's landlord said there were too many of them, they'd have to get out. "We scattered," he recalls. On August 19, their daughter heard about a five-room basement flat where children were acceptable. Immediately Mr. and Mrs. Hickman caught a streetcar to the real estate office, paid $5 a room "for listing"—$23 cash and $2 owed—received the landlord's address, 2720 Prairie, and hurried there by taxi. It proved to be a stone relic of Gold Coast splendor, drawing rooms and even butler's pantries now rented out as "apartments." Far at the back, in a recess dark even at noonday, lived the man the Hickmans had come to see, David Coleman. He only rented a room here, this was not his building. He took them outdoors to talk things over. They sat down in his half-brother's two-tone Buick taxicab parked in the glass-strewn street in front of the mansion's big iron gates.

Coleman was a very black man, twenty-five years old, about five-feet-ten, solidly built. He asked $200 rent in advance. Hickman said he couldn't pay so much. Coleman asked if he could pay $150. "Then he stopped, he looked at me, he said you look like I see you somewhere Hickman." They had lived only about three miles apart in the Delta. Coleman said. "Well now. Maybe we can get together. You can give me $100, can't you?" Hickman said he could but he wanted to see the apartment first. The three of them caught a streetcar.

II

Now David Coleman had been born January 12, 1922, at a flagstop on the railroad in the Mississippi Delta. He was the last of eleven children; all but three of them died in infancy. "They just died," his mother says. "I don't know what of." He went to the fields full-time at twelve; later got a job driving a truck; married and had a child; and in 1943, lured by tales of freedom and high wartime wages, drove with his family to Chicago. They got along fine. The mother says, "We had a good job and a place to live. Nobody can do better." They came earlier than the Hickmans, before the housing screws were tightened quite so much, and they had fewer children. Coleman's wife died in bearing his second child. He married again; learned arc welding and once earned $2.10 an hour; liked to think of himself as a business man and tried to dress like one.

In July 1946, he met a woman with a building to sell. He borrowed money and leased the building and later he bought it "on contract" for $8,000, paying $300 down, the rest monthly. He had a lot of trouble over this deal, as we shall see; indeed, it led to his death.

The building is on the West Side in an area once called Little Italy but now almost solidly Negro except for a few Mexicans. The best buildings are the churches and the factories. The buildings where people live are high brick tenements, patched-up wooden tenements, sheds. In between are vast wastelands, desolate open areas where buildings have collapsed or been torn down, the excavations partly filled with rubble. Broad Roosevelt Road, busy with traffic, cuts the section cleanly. A half block south is Washburne Street, our scene. It is a quiet street. A man is sitting idly on the iron railing in front of a house, tossing a pair of dice into the air and catching them, and a woman is sweeping the sidewalk with a broom, and now and then a child skates past, and that is all. The doorways of many houses are open, open onto a black void, the doors may be open or they may have vanished, and the houses look abandoned; but a woman is leaning on the railing, a hint of humanity packed inside. At the streetcorners are a Jewish delicatessen, a drugstore selling "Dream Books," the Temptation Cleaners, the iron structure of the El. In midblock, one of many in a row, is No. 1733, David Coleman's building. It is old, perhaps forty or fifty years old. It is high and narrow—it stands three stories high above an English basement but, built on a twenty-five-foot lot, it is only thirty-one brick-lengths wide. Two perpendicular rows of windows run up its face; in each is a panel of stained glass. To reach the upstairs flats you have to walk down a narrow gangway and enter a doorway halfway back along the side.

It was to this building on August 20, 1946, that David Coleman, as landlord, took Mr. and Mrs. Hickman. He showed them the basement apartment, offered at $50 a month. Hickman recalls, ". . . the water was half a leg deep in the basement . . . no windows, no lights, no nothing in there." A man who has since visited it says, "It was a woodshed really. The only impression it made on me was, this is how rats live." Hickman said it wouldn't do. Coleman said that in nine days a flat on the second floor would be available at $50 a month, and in the meanwhile they could have a room in the attic for $6 a week. Hickman testified later: "We walked up the stairs, it was so dark . . . we almost had to feel our way. . . . I am walking around looking at it, I don't like this. She said, I don't neither but surely we can stay here because we ain't got no place." They went outdoors and Hickman paid Coleman $30 "to hold us." He went to the South Side, withdrew $70 from his postal savings, and took it to Coleman. He got his furniture out of storage and that night he and his wife hired a taxi and took their six youngest children there—the two older boys moved in later—and they all slept there that night.

And so now, after more than a year, they had a home. It was an attic room about fourteen by twenty-one feet but the roof sloped so that you could stand up only in a fourteen-foot-square space. The three smallest children slept with Mr. and Mrs. Hickman and the rest slept in the other bed. There was no electricity; they used a kerosene lamp. There was no gas; they used a stove and heater burning kerosene. There was one window. There was no water; they had to go down to the third floor to use the toilet or to get water for washing or cooking. But it was shelter, and a place they could all be together with their things. And it was, they thought, only temporary.

The nine days passed, however, and ten more, and Hickman asked Coleman about the second-floor flat. "He said, Hickman, wait until the 18th and if those folks don't move out, I'll give you back your $100." Hickman agreed. But "on September 18th, he dodged me." Hickman began to suspect a runaround. Other tenants told him they'd had trouble with Coleman. On September 22 Hickman caught up with Coleman. He asked for his $100 so he could use it to find another place to live. Coleman replied, "I won't pay you until I get ready." Hickman recalls, "I said I'd go to the law and make him give it back. He said he had a man on the East Side ready to burn the place up if . . . I had him arrested. . . . He said go ahead and have me arrested, I would be sorry. And," Hickman now says, "I really was sorry." But that day he said nothing, he went back upstairs. "I looked at my family, looked at my small children. . . . I . . . told my wife what David Coleman told me downstairs, I said I wanted peace, I have lived in peace for forty years, I asked her if there was laws in Chicago to take care of men like that, she said yes." On September 24 they got a warrant for Coleman's arrest. But the police never served it.

Coleman had leased the building July 27 from the owner, Mrs. Mary Porter Adams, a county social worker. About October 7 he took possession under his purchase contract. He had paid a rather high price and to meet the monthly payments he decided to cut the building up into more lucrative "kitchenette" apartments. He sent a contractor to the building, but the tenants obstructed him. Coleman arrived. An argument ensued. If he wanted to cut up the flats, they said, he would have to have the court evict them first. One recalled later, "He said: 'I am the owner, I don't have to go to Court to do that, I will get everybody out of here when I want to if it takes fire.' "

Another family man, Albert Jones, had rented the dismal basement for $300, six months at $50 a month. Coleman had promised to repair it but he didn't. The main water line into the building was broken and so the water ran onto the floor of Jones's "apartment"; to alleviate this condition the other tenants turned off the main valve outside the building, and by prearrangement one of them would go outdoors and turn on the valve for a few minutes each day while the others flushed all the toilets and drew water into slop jars and buckets.

The Hickmans took their blind backward child, Corene, to a State hospital at Lincoln, Illinois. That left nine Hickmans in the room. "I worried about it day and night. I did not want to bring them up in such living conditions." Hickman later testified that he never had lived so poorly in Mississippi as he had to live in Chicago.

Coleman refused to make repairs. Perhaps he hoped that hardship would drive the tenants out. Many bitter wrangles ensued. The tenants appealed to the OPA, the police, the fire department, the board of health, the water inspector. The only results: a policeman "come and looked and said it was awful," and the waterman shut off the water (probably because the bill wasn't paid). Nor was all this anything new; one tenant said, "We had been calling [the authorities] for the last few years," and violation of fire or building regulations—including insufficient fire exits—had been charged against various owners of this building but only one fine—of $25—had been levied. In December 1946, after a routine department inspection, Mrs. Adams was ordered to make certain repairs and to remove papers, lumber, rags, and combustible rubbish, and a little later the city building department ordered her and Coleman to exterminate rats, reduce illegal overcrowding, repair the plumbing, and "place premises in habitable condition or vacate same." But nothing was done and there is no evidence that the building department took any steps toward enforcement—until after the fire.

As we have seen, Coleman had bought the building on a shoestring. In November he leased it to Anthony Lee Barnett, Jr., who paid him $425. But then Barnett discovered that Jones already had a lease on the basement and Hickman had a $100 claim, so Barnett went to the State's Attorney and was advised to get a warrant for Coleman's arrest. Coleman fell behind in his monthly payments to Mrs. Adams. She visited the building about January 1, 1947, and was surprised to learn of Barnett's lease. The thing was a terrible muddle. That Sunday there was a fire in the flue. It did little damage but it aroused the tenants. They telephoned Mrs. Adams. She too wanted to get them out. One of them testified that she said, "Well, you are not paying enough rent there. . . . I am not going to fix anything. . . . It is not my fault because you got children. . . . Just find yourself another place." Another tenant told Mrs. Adams he was going to have the plumbing fixed "and pay it out of the rents." She sent him an eviction notice. She told the Hickmans there were too many of them in one room. Hickman said he didn't know what to do; and she suggested he find another home.

That same week the fire chief, on a routine inspection, found nineteen people living in the attic: another family had moved into the rear room. The chief ordered this other family out, and they went.

On three nights that week the Hickmans heard "somebody tipping up the stairs to the door and tipping down." Hickman asked his wife, "I wonder what they are up to. Do you reckon that somebody would burn us up here?" Coleman had lived for a time in a small room at the head of the stairs and had left an old bed-frame and mattress and a trunk; now he came up and moved his trunk away. But he left the old bed-frame and the mattress, the mattress rolled up in the corner. A week later the fire started where the mattress was.

III

Hickman was at work when the fire occurred. The police telephoned the steelmill and the foreman called for Hickman and a white man named Hicks went home by mistake. Not till almost 4:00 A. M. did they reach the right person. They told him he was wanted at the DesPlaines Street police station. The streetcar motorman told him where to get off but it was the wrong place and he walked around, lost. A man told him to go back to State Street and take a car up to Roosevelt Road and transfer. He still couldn't find the station so he went home.

The police investigation was lackadaisical (a deputy coroner remarked: "If this fire happened over on Sheridan Road some place, we would have half the police force in here"). Coleman denied having threatened to burn the building. There was no direct evidence that he had had it set afire. But nobody could figure out an innocent origin and evidence indicated a strong possibility of arson. In the little room at the head of the stairs, investigators found a five-gallon can that nobody in the building recognized and it was half full of kerosene; one witness had seen a strange man running down the stairs the night of the fire; Coleman had removed his trunk a week earlier; firemen thought the fire moved suspiciously fast. But the coroner's jury, while "vigorously" condemning the condition of the building, confessed itself unable to determine whether the fire was accident or arson and recommended that the State's Attorney investigate further. The State's Attorney's investigation was feeble. The Coroner dropped the case. Nothing at all resulted. In April Coleman was fined $350 and costs and Mrs. Adams was fined $250 and costs for violations of the city building code—charges that could have been instituted months earlier, before the fire, but were not.

Hickman was convinced that Coleman had fired the building. And he felt justice had not been done. He was bitter. "Paper was made to burn, coal and rags. Not people. People wasn't made to burn." His son Willis remembers, "Before the fire he was outgoing. Not after the fire. He wouldn't eat. He had nothing to say. He would sit with his eyes closed, but was not asleep." One night in April, Willis heard him in the bedroom, "talkin' to Elzena," the child of nine who had burned to death, and to Velvena, the dead child of four. He talked "at first faintly and then excitedly." Then he jumped out of bed and cried, "The Lord have mercy," and ran from the room.

People of sympathy had got the Hickmans into a housing

project, and Hickman had gone back to work, but his wife remembers, "He used to carry on practically every day. He would come home from work, sit down, and start talking about the children. 'My children got no cause to be dead. Other children are playing. My children have a right to play too. They didn't do any harm.' The more we talked about it, the more I would get worried. He would say: 'I know what Coleman told me. After he said it would happen, it did happen.' " Coleman's threat "went through my mind like a clock, over and over again." He bought a thirty-two caliber automatic pistol, telling his wife it was "for home use"; he always had kept a gun around the house. A strike at the steelmill July 10 made him idle. He brooded more. "When I looked around, the oldest ones was gone and the youngest ones were too. It used to be if we wanted a drink of water the baby would get it. Now there was no one there. No one to say: 'Daddy, have you any candy?' There would be no happiness again until I would get in camp with God." He and his wife were officers of the Liberty Baptist Church. On July 15, Hickman said, "I got no mind to go to church," but they went. His wife recalls, "We had a Morning Star Club meeting." They got home about midnight. Hickman went to bed, got up, went into the boys' room, looked at them sleeping, looked at the pictures of the dead children. He got out his gun and polished it. He "turned the radio on—it didn't play so good. I started a verse to a hymn. I walked back and sat down on the studio couch. When I got to summing up my life, I saw my life was unhappy. I was in grief and sorrow." Next morning, his wife recalls, "he got up quiet."

Hickman remembers that day: "I drunk a half a cup of tea and part of a sandwich, I was filled up. I wasn't mad, I wasn't glad, I walked in the . . . living room, I reached under the bed in the cash box, I took the key off my side and unlocked it, reached in for this automatic, picked it up and laid it down. You just got to go through with it. I laid it down again. I walked back and sat down beside my wife, I ain't spoke nothing to her. I walked back to the cash box, I picked up this gun, I knocked the safety off of it and wanted to see if it would hang. I put it back down, I can't go through with this. The voice kept speaking, you know your promise." This "promise" was the vow he had made to God to protect his children. "The third time I picked up this gun, I put eight in the magazine, knocked the safety off and threw one in the barrel." Still he paced the house and yard in torment; once he got a block away. But he came back: "The word was so sharp it was cutting like a two edge sword. . . . The third time I didn't return no more."

He caught a bus, transferred to a streetcar, and got off at 26th and Indiana. Coleman lived a few blocks away. "I stood there on the street. I didn't want to go through with what it was telling me. . . . [But] this was a vow that I made to this family in 1923 . . . and the answer is I wouldn't back up. So I walked on down to Prairie." It was a little before 1:00 P.M. Out in front of the big dilapidated mansion at 2720 Prairie, David Coleman was sitting behind the wheel of his half-brother's big Buick taxicab, reading a newspaper, reading aloud an account of a raid to Percy Brown, who was leaning through the window.

Hickman came up the sidewalk. "He had some rent tickets in his lap. . . . I walked up to him and spoke to him and friendly talked. I wanted peace with all mankind. 'How do you do, how are you feeling this morning, Coleman?' 'What do you want with me?' 'I come to ask you something about this arrest warrant, of the $100 and causing this disturbance,' " that is, the fire. Coleman replied "Yes, but I ain't going to pay you." Hickman recalls, "My mind got scattered. I took out my automatic and blazed him twice. He said: 'I'll pay you.' I said: 'It's too late now. God is my secret judge.' I said: 'You started that fire.' He said: 'Yes, I did.' I shot him twice more. . . . I thought he was dead." He wasn't but he died three days later.

Hickman walked down the street and away, the automatic still in his hand. He missed a streetcar, walked on, farther than he needed. "I had put a heavy load down and a big weight fell off of me and I felt light." He took a streetcar home and asked his son Charles, "Where is your mother? He said, down to Arlene's. I said, 'Tell her to come here, I got something to tell her,' so she came. . . . She said . . . 'They will find you.' 'I know.' " He waited till 4:15 P.M. before the Homicide Squad arrived. They arrested him and took his gun. He confessed immediately. A coroner's jury bound him to the Grand Jury, which indicted him for first degree murder. He was jailed without bond. He had no money for a lawyer. It looked like at least fourteen years in the penitentiary and he could have been electrocuted.

IV

But suddenly to his rescue came some citizens—an organizer for the Socialist Workers party, Mike Bartell, and two labor union men, Willoughby Abner, a Negro and first vice president of the central CIO Council in Chicago, and Charles Chiakulas, president of a United Auto Workers (CIO) local. (Hickman was not then a CIO member.) Bartell had visited Hickman the day after the fire and at his behest a civil-rights lawyer, M. J. Myer, had represented Hickman at the inquest (subsequently, when Mrs. Adams had filed suits to evict the other tenants who kept on living in the burned building without paying rent, Myer and Leon M. Despres represented them, presenting the interesting defense that the building was unfit for human habitation and therefore no rent was due). Now Abner, Chiakulas, and Bartell formed a Hickman Defense Committee.

Myer, Despres, and William H. Temple agreed to defend Hickman. Abner recalls, "We had two objectives—to raise money for the defense and to educate the public to the horrible conditions these people lived in and the tragedies that can result." Others active were the Reverend James Luther Adams, a Unitarian minister and a board member of the Independent Voters of Illinois; Gerald Bullock, chairman of the Committee on Racial Equality; Franklin Fried, a unionist active in the AVC; and Sidney Lens, head of an AF of L local. Many such groups degenerate into luncheons and resolutions. Hickman's defenders worked hard, effectively, fast, and according to plan. One traveled all over the East on $100, setting up local committees. They held rallies (Tallullah Bankhead, the actress, appeared) and put donation jars in Black Belt stores. Each member obtained mailing lists, publicity, and money from organizations he had access to.

Hickman's trial began on November 10, 1947, before a white judge and a white jury, with four white lawyers out of five on both sides. The prosecution proved that Hickman killed Coleman, defense claimed he did so while temporarily insane. Hickman himself occupied the witness chair for a day and a half, a small black man behind an oak panel, speaking freely in flowing narrative, sometimes in language almost biblical.

He said: "My feelings was that I was mistreated without a cause. I felt that my children was without a guardian, that they suffered death, that they ought to be free on land and living."

He said: "This was God fixed this. I had raised these children up and God knowed that vow I made to him . . . that these children was a generation to be raised up. God wasn't pleased what happened to them."

His lawyer asked him about blind Corene who had been taken to an institution: "Mr. Hickman, while you were up in the attic before the fire, did one of the children leave the family and go live elsewhere?" and he said, "Leave the family? Yes, sir," and the lawyer said, "Will you describe her—when was she born, what happened to her?" and Hickman began, "She was born in June and she was beautiful."

His lawyer asked him to describe "your feelings" between the fire and the shooting, and he replied: "I had two sons and two daughters who would some day be great men and women, some day they would have married, some day they would have been fathers or mothers of children; these children would have children and then these children would have children and another generation of Hickmans could raise up and enjoy peace."

The jury was out for nineteen hours and then reported hopeless disagreement. All six men and one woman reportedly voted for acquittal, the other five women for conviction. The jury was discharged. Hickman was sent back to jail to await a new trial.

But by this time the Hickman Defense Committee's work had taken hold. Letters were rolling in on the State's Attorney from all over the United States. The Defense Committee finally reached an agreement with Assistant State's Attorney Samuel L. Freedman, and on December 16 Judge Rudolph F. Desort dismissed the murder charge, found Hickman guilty of manslaughter, and placed him on probation for two years. A few hours later he went home to his family for Christmas.

Before disbanding, the Defense Committee held its only luncheon meeting. Abner, a quiet softspoken man, recalls, "Mr. and Mrs. Hickman thanked us from the bottom of their hearts, said they were grateful." Abner said recently, "I don't know—at the start, you knew the thing was there, you couldn't just sit back and do nothing about it, it got inside you. We really felt good when it was over. It shows everything isn't in vain, it isn't all injustice, people will rally, it shows what can be done."

Not quite everybody had rallied. Some organizations declined to do so. The Communists and the organizations they control or influence would not participate. The American Civil Liberties Union felt that no civil-rights issue was involved and the National Association for the Advancement of Colored People that no race issue was involved. Attorney Myer said recently, "Sure Hickman and Coleman were both Negroes—but there wouldn't have been any fire or shooting either if it hadn't been for restrictive covenants and the Negro slums."

And in truth Coleman as well as Hickman seems the victim of a system. The system of segregation that creates such tremendous housing pressures also creates opportunity for men weak by nature to exploit their fellows. Coleman happened to be black but it was white man's race prejudice that enabled him to exploit Hickman. And he was only the last of many men who had oppressed Hickman because of Hickman's color. The white planters of Mississippi had driven him to Chicago. Here Coleman took over. And he was able to take over because of the prejudice of Northern whites. The North has failed the Negro no less than the South, there is no place in this country for a black man to go. In Chicago after the 1917–18 war the tremendous population pressure burst the bounds of the Black Belt despite bombings, arsons, and a major race riot. The same thing is happening today. And the greater the pressure of the blacks, the greater white resistance—more hurried meetings of "improvement" associations to draw new restrictive covenants, more rocks and bombs and "Molotov cocktails" thrown at newly-purchased Negro homes, more suspect fires that already within the past three years have killed a score of Negroes, more "street-car incidents" and "bathing beach incidents," more political speeches promising "racial purity." Even the government's efforts in the Negroes' behalf, public housing, have been resisted stoutly. It is profitable to rent firetraps. The vested—and highly respectable—real estate interests of this city draw the iron ring ever tighter. (Who cares if they are corroding away the heart of the city? They also are pandering to our own prejudices.) Chicago's postwar housing record is one of complete failure; indeed, despite innumerable editorials and civic luncheons, bond issues and tubthumping, in 1946 the city actually lost more dwelling units through fire and simple decay than it erected. The housing problem is bad everywhere in America, in no major city is it worse than in Chicago, and Negroes are at the bottom of the heap because we put them there and we keep them there. Now after a "people's war" Negroes are becoming restive; on at least one occasion since V-J Day only Negro restraint has prevented a major race riot; and the Mayor's Commission on Human Relations, which has done much to ease the dangerous tensions, has warned: "Unless more homes are provided, no one, regardless of good will or police power, can check the social conflicts which are inherent in this situation . . . we have all of the ingredients for social destruction."

The Defense Committee helped to get Hickman a new job. He and his wife and the remaining children, the three boys eighteen, twenty, and twenty-two, are living in a housing project near the airport, close to another project where in 1946 one of Chicago's most dangerous race flare-ups occurred. They intend to stay in Chicago. Mrs. Hickman says, "I like Chicago. I used to like it very much when I had my children."

A year after the fire the old building at 1733 Washburne was deserted. After the shooting the tenants had quit resisting eviction and moved away, and almost at once another fire gutted the building. The windows have been boarded up, the attic is open to the weather, charred black timbers and jagged bricks and boards askew against the sky. In the alley dirty newspapers blow gently by a wrecked car, a woman is burning trash in a salamander, and in the center lies a dead rat. On a little mound of rubble behind 1733, an old Negro squats amid piles of junk, hat brim up, shoes broken, denim jacket patched; he is tending a little fire to burn the wood from barrel hoops, burning tin cans and buckets clean with fire. He moved here in 1919 from the South Side, the only Negro in his block, and for a time white kids broke his windows, "though I guess their folks put them up to it." It isn't as nice here as on the South Side. Why do people move over here? "Looking for some place to go." There's talk that the owner of 1733 is going to fix the building up and sell it. Will people live in it? "Sure," and he laughs. "If they fix it up, they'll soon be lined up here, putting in their application. People got no place to go."

Suggestions for Study

NOTICE THE plan of "The Hickman Story." The essay deals with a complex social problem, which in a different magazine, directed toward a different audience, would have to be analyzed in great detail. But the readers of general magazines do not expect such articles; and so Martin is able to plan his article as almost purely emotive, with its main intention to arouse indignation, and perhaps ultimately to provoke action. Notice that Martin includes only a couple of paragraphs of analysis. He makes his case through the narrative of an event which exactly illustrates the complexity of the problem of the position of Negroes in this country, and which at the same time dramatizes the human significance of the problem.

This narrative is composed of short scenes and snatches of dialogue, the latter apparently drawn from the record at Hickman's trial, or perhaps from interviews. (In one way the article is like a newspaper report, but a newspaper report of a very superior kind.) Notice that these vignettes are not chronologically organized. Martin begins at the central event in his story, and then moves backward and forward in time, with his material organized for the emotional impact gained from the juxtaposition of scene and dialogue. The quick succession of scenes is occasionally interrupted by paragraphs of summary narration, which often seem to have been written to be spoken, like the narration accompanying a documentary film.

Perhaps the form of "The Hickman Story" can best be compared to that of a documentary film, for it is clear that this prose does not move because of its rhythm, its color, or the richness of its diction. Indeed, many of its sentences must strike the reader as rather flat, though of course consciously so. (On this point compare the essay by Mencken, in which the emotive effect is achieved by the sound and the brilliant diction of the prose.) In "The Hickman Story" the appeal is to the eye of the reader, who, as the title implies, is supposed to see the story of James Hickman; to feel it, and by feeling to comprehend it.

Horsefeathers Swathed in Mink

A. J. LIEBLING (1904–)

REPORTERS and headline writers have a way of cooking up descriptive titles for women involved in celebrated newspaper cases. To name a few that I can think of as I write, there was the Pig Woman, witness in the Hall-Mills murder inquest; the Woman in Red, who betrayed Dillinger to the law; the Bobbed-Hair Bandit, a lady stickup man of the twenties; the Broadway Butterfly, who was strangled to death in 1924; and the Black Dahlia, a young woman unpleasantly done in about a year ago in Los Angeles. Sometimes these inventions become generic labels for types of crime, as when, last summer, New York headline writers began calling the taking off of Mrs. Sheila Mannering a Butterfly Murder—an allusion to the similar taking off of Dorothy King, the Broadway Butterfly—and one of the tabloids recently referred to a local cadaver as a Black Dahlia Murder Victim because the killer had written on it with lipstick, in the manner of the dispatcher of the Black Dahlia out West.

New York newspapers added another title to their list a short while back when they invented the name the Lady in Mink for a woman who was reported to have received relief payments from the New York City Welfare Department though she was possessed of a mink coat. (It may be expected that "the Lady in Mink" will soon be contracted to just "Mink" and, as such, will become a part of headline language, like "Butterfly" or "Dahlia" or "Ripper" or "Raffles." In that event, the headline "Cops Collar Mink Suspect" will inform the hep newspaper reader that the police have arrested a man for asking alms while wearing clothes that once came from Brooks Brothers.) The Welfare Department is prevented by law from divulging the names of relief clients, and as a result the reporters felt justified in using the Lady in Mink sobriquet in practically every paragraph of every story they wrote about the case. On October 30th, the *Times* called her, on first acquaintance, merely the *woman* in mink, but on November 1st it yielded to the vogue and recognized her as a lady. The apparent triviality of the story did not prevent the *Times* from giving it, on the day it broke, the best spot in the paper—the right-hand column of the front page—under this three-column head:

WOMAN IN MINK WITH $60,000
LIVED ON RELIEF IN A HOTEL,
INQUIRY BY STATE DISCLOSES

(The Report of the President's Committee on Civil Rights, which was issued on the same day, got the second-best place—a three-column head on the left side of the page.) The drop under the *Times* "Mink" headline read:

42 CASES ANALYZED
INVESTIGATOR SAYS CITY AGENCY HELD
"CLIENT IS ALWAYS RIGHT"

ONE "FRONT FOR BOOKIES"
DEAL APPARENTLY INVOLVED HER LIVING ON
AID WHILE HUSBAND PAID $14,000
IN BAD CHECKS

The story that followed was written by a man named William R. Conklin. I discovered, on reading it, that the all-important "with $60,000" in the headline had been based only on the opening paragraph—a single sentence—of Conklin's report. This sentence read, "The story of a mink-coated, mink-hatted 'relief client' [the necessity for the quotation marks is obscure, since relief client is an accepted term in social-welfare work] who lived at city expense in a hotel at $7.50 a day despite assets of $60,000 was spread on the record of the State Board of Social Welfare yesterday as it opened an attack on administration of a $142,000,000 relief program by the New York City Welfare Department." Nothing in the rest of the piece supported the statement that the relief client had "assets of $60,000." The body of the story stated, beginning near the bottom of the first column, that in 1940 the woman had been awarded a divorce settlement of $40,000 in California, of which $3,400 had never been paid, and "in addition" had sold $20,000 worth of stocks in 1942. It was not made clear whether she had bought the stocks with part of the divorce settlement, nor did the story show that she had all, or any, of the $56,600, or $36,600, whichever it was, in June, 1946, when she applied for relief in New York. As a matter of fact, Benjamin Fielding, the newly appointed Welfare Commissioner, announced a couple of days later that he considered the woman, as she had reported herself to be, too poor to support her child. A fairer headline for the *Times'* story might have read:

WOMAN WHO ONCE HAD
$X NOW ON RELIEF

Conklin, of course, must have known that his story didn't bear out his lead, but some reporters do this sort of thing impulsively, like poker players who occasionally try to steal a pot. It is up to the editors to spot such discrepancies, especially in the case of stories to which they decide to give a big play.

The mink coat in the case—as most newspaper readers know by now, for Fielding showed a nice flair for publicity in his handling of this detail—was appraised by a fur expert of I. J. Fox & Co. The expert, a Mr. Herman Peroff, said that the coat was from six to eight years old, had a torn lining, and was worth about three hundred dollars at the present market. Fielding allowed news photographers to make shots of him and Mr. Peroff handling the coat—shots in which, after all the fuss, the coat looked so mangy that they proved irresistible to the picture editors of the two-cent tabloids, hostile though they were to the "pampering" of the poor. The *Times* very sportingly took cognizance of the appraisal in the last line but one of the last bank of the headline over its October 31st story—"One Coat Valued at $300," it said—and, on the next morning, gave the following handsome, though slightly equivocal, one-column display to Commissioner Fielding's announcement that the owner of the coat had no funds:

GRAND JURY TO SCAN
RELIEF; CITY BACKS
THE "LADY IN MINK"

I am aware that to half retract, in half of a one-column head, what you have fully stated in all of a three-column head is decidedly better than standard newspaper practice.

To return briefly to the Conklin story and the headings over it, the line "42 Cases Analyzed" did little to help the reader understand that this number represented only about one-thirteenth of one per cent of the Department's burden. (The forty-two cases involved a total of two hundred and seven persons, for whom social workers contended that only hotel lodgings could be found, out of the average of 263,000 persons on the Department's rolls in 1947.) As to the "Front for Bookies" line, the incident it referred to was completely refuted within a couple of days. And the lead sentence, beginning, "The story of a . . . 'relief client' who lived at city expense in a hotel at $7.50 a day," seems to me inexcusably ambiguous. It implies (1) that the woman was living alone in the hotel and (2) that she was paying $7.50 a day just for her room, whereas the fact is that she had her five-year-old daughter with her and the daily $7.50 was to provide for all expenses, including food and clothing, for the two of them. To be sure, you could learn about the existence of the daughter if you read far enough down in Conklin's story, even though he did make her four months old instead of five years—an error that I am willing to ascribe to inadvertence. If you read all the way off the first page and deep into the runover of the story, you found out that the woman and her daughter had long before been moved out of the hotel room they had been occupying and had since then been receiving only $162.20 a month from the Department.

The editors of the *Times,* if called upon to explain the play they gave this story, would doubtless say that they had been actuated not by the details of an isolated case but by the principle of the thing. It would be interesting in this instance to know the nature of the principle upon which the *Times* proceeded. I am afraid that a hint as to the answer may be contained in a further passage from Conklin's story, in which he wrote, "Explaining that state law forbids identifying relief clients by name and address, Mr. Shapiro [the state investigator] summarized twelve cases accepted as eligible for relief by the city's Welfare Department. They included a married woman indicted for grand larceny; a mother who entertained men in her hotel room while her children played in the lobby at all hours; alcoholics; a divorcee with an out-of-wedlock child; an unmarried mother with two children; a male bigamist [if he was a practicing one, why wasn't he in jail, or if he once served time for bigamy, was he returned by the law to both his spouses?]; and a man separated from his wife and three children who was living with another woman on city relief."

None of these descriptions has any legal relevance to an applicant's eligibility for relief. No law specifies that a woman must be blameless to qualify for a food grant at the prevailing rates of $16.45 a month if unemployed and living in a family group and $21.65 if pregnant—to cite a couple of examples of the "liberal" allowances referred to in a report put out by Commissioner Fielding himself last week as attracting relief cases to the city. All the woman in question has to be is without means. The principle involved in the treatment given the Mink story—if, indeed, it was a case of principle and not of sheer ineptness—seems to be that the poor are poor because of their sins and whatever they get is too good for them. In effect, the *Times*' story served to discredit, by implication, all applicants for relief and to provide an argument against increasing expenditures. (The Welfare Department's current allowances for food are based on prices prevalent in June, 1946.)

This is a lot of space to devote to one newspaper story, but I think that Conklin's piece and the headline over it justify detailed consideration. I was saddened by the whole thing because the *Times* is in many respects a sound newspaper, within the translucent mass of which one may occasionally discern the outlines of commendable purposes, fixed like strawberries in a great mold of jello, and of good men struggling feebly, like minnows within a giant jellyfish. The *Herald Tribune*, although officially Republican, covered this investigation by the State Board of Social Welfare (Republican) of the City Welfare Department (Democratic) with considerably more reserve. The *Sun* (Republican) was also more restrained than I had, perhaps unjustly, expected, even if it did at one point take a strong anti-gypsy position. "Gypsies, alcoholics, unmarried mothers, persons in difficulty with the law, neglectful parents and employables who would not work were maintained in hotels," the *Sun's* October 29th story began, as if Romany blood were per se a reason for reproach.

The *World-Telegram*, claiming credit on October 27th, the first day of the investigation, for having inspired all the commotion over the Welfare Department by its "revelations" last spring ("World-Telegram's Charges Confirmed by City's Report"), referred editorially to the since-resigned Commissioner Edward E. Rhatigan's "nervy request for an $82,000,000 boost in the $142,000,000 Welfare Department budget," which was, I imagine, getting rather near the *Telegram's* chief preoccupation with the matter. In view of a recent twenty-five-per-cent boost in the number of persons on relief, and an additional twenty-five-per-cent boost since March, 1945, in the cost of living for all of them, such a request would seem to me to be less than "nervy." It is true, however, that an increase in the Welfare Department's budget would bring nearer the day when the State Constitution will have to be amended to permit an increase in the city's real-estate taxes, and that obviously one of the most effective ways of keeping relief costs from rising is to shout that the people on relief don't deserve to be there and to imply that officials of the Welfare Department are Communists who are packing the relief rolls to run down free enterprise. "But," the *World-Telegram* editorial said, "we hope Mr. Fielding, who calls himself 'a plain blunt guy,' also sees the necessity of releasing key positions and policies in the Welfare Department from the grip of the Communist-dominated CIO Public Workers of America." Next day, the *Telegram* was announcing on its front page that a Republican city councilman had "assailed the appointment of Commissioner Fielding, who, he said, was a member of the Communist-dominated American Labor Party." On October 29th, the paper returned to the picayune cruelties of its original "revelations" by running this headline:

PROBE OF STATE
CONFIRMS W-T
WASTE EXPOSE
SHOWS WELFARE DEPT. PAMPERED
CHISELERS IN LUXURY HOTELS

and, under it, a story beginning, "Former convicts, alcoholics, neglectful parents, and women who entertained men in their rooms . . ." (All of these, of course, are types that are to be found in higher economic strata as well.) The reporter, Walter MacDonald, had evidently not heard about the gypsies. On November 1st, by which time even the *Journal-American* reached the conclusion, inconspicuously, that "the case of the celebrated 'Lady in Mink' apparently had fizzled today into just welfare routine," a *Telegram* headline read:

STATE AID ACCUSES FIELDING
OF SNIPING AT RELIEF PROBE
CITY'S DEFENSE OF RITZY DOLE
IS UNDER FIRE

This, by the way, was on the day that Mr. Fielding collapsed and was taken to a hospital as a result of overwork, causing veiled merriment among old-time Welfare Department employees, who told one another, "Now he knows what it's like to work here." The Department is chronically understaffed.

A day or so ago, I saw a *World-Telegram* advertisement in another newspaper. It was headed, "Sure, New York Has a Heart!," and read, in part, "There are three W-T staff writers in particular who are on most intimate terms with New York's tough-but-soft heart. Their roving job is to peer between the skyscrapers and under the chromium to find the hidden stories—the ones that have a special color all their own. Watch for their sketches of New York's real heartbeats." Maybe this trio, rather than Mr. MacDonald, ought to have been turned loose on the Welfare Department.

Out of sheer perverseness, I suppose, I have leaned backward in an effort not to give *PM* unduly frequent good marks in these random pieces about the press. Perhaps it is because the paper reminds me too often of the repulsive lines forced upon a young American actor, Penrod Schofield, in one of the books I like best to remember:

"I hight Sir Lancelot du Lake, the child,
Gentul-hearted, meek, and mild."

If *PM* were a girl, her face would be shiny, and she would be conscientiously and resolutely promiscuous and tell all her boy friends about their complexes. But on a story like this curious investigation *PM* does a beautiful job. "Buried obscurely in the testimony, which dealt exclusively with the now-famous 42 'hotel cases,'" John K. Weiss, of the *PM* staff, wrote after a day of "revelations," "were such details as these: many of the hotel cases involved mentally disturbed or depressed persons; press hysteria about the hotel cases forced many persons into sub-standard housing; one case concerned an immature mother who was moved from a hotel directly into a mental hospital. Not once during the day was the fact mentioned that the State had approved the hotel procedure." And Mr. Weiss's colleague on *PM*, Albert Deutsch, wrote, "Well, what does one do with such people, subject them to euthanasia? . . . Incompetence in public agency workers and inefficiency in public administration cannot be condoned. Periodic inquiries and exposures of maladministration can only be welcomed by the citizenry. But such inquiries must be conducted on the basis of fair play and sound judgment; it is a nasty business to make a political football out of public relief, and to run a headline-hunting campaign under the guise of a fact-finding inquiry." I can't fault him on that.

In Memoriam: W. J. B.

H. L. MENCKEN (1880–)

HAS IT BEEN duly marked by historians that the late William Jennings Bryan's last secular act on this globe of sin was to catch flies? A curious detail, and not without its sardonic overtones. He was the most sedulous fly-catcher in American history, and in many ways the most successful. His quarry, of course, was not

Musca domestica but *Homo neandertalensis.* For forty years he tracked it with coo and bellow, up and down the rustic backways of the Republic. Wherever the flambeaux of Chautauqua smoked and guttered, and the bilge of Idealism ran in the veins, and Baptist pastors dammed the brooks with the sanctified, and men gathered who were weary and heavy laden, and their wives who were full of Peruna and as fecund as the shad (*Alosa sapidissima*)—there the indefatigable Jennings set up his traps and spread his bait. He knew every country town in the South and West, and he could crowd the most remote of them to suffocation by simply winding his horn. The city proletariat, transiently flustered by him in 1896, quickly penetrated his buncombe and would have no more of him; the cockney gallery jeered him at every Democratic national convention for twenty-five years. But out where the grass grows high, and the horned cattle dream away the lazy afternoons, and men still fear the powers and principalities of the air—out there between the corn-rows he held his old puissance to the end. There was no need of beaters to drive in his game. The news that he was coming was enough. For miles the flivver dust would choke the roads. And when he rose at the end of the day to discharge his Message there would be such breathless attention, such a rapt and enchanted ecstasy, such a sweet rustle of amens as the world had not known since Johann fell to Herod's ax.

There was something peculiarly fitting in the fact that his last days were spent in a one-horse Tennessee village, and that death found him there. The man felt at home in such simple and Christian scenes. He liked people who sweated freely, and were not debauched by the refinements of the toilet. Making his progress up and down the Main street of little Dayton, surrounded by gaping primates from the upland valleys of the Cumberland Range, his coat laid aside, his bare arms and hairy chest shining damply, his bald head sprinkled with dust—so accoutred and on display he was obviously happy. He liked getting up early in the morning, to the tune of cocks crowing on the dunghill.

He liked the heavy, greasy victuals of the farmhouse kitchen. He liked country lawyers, country pastors, all country people. He liked the country sounds and country smells. I believe that this liking was sincere—perhaps the only sincere thing in the man. His nose showed no uneasiness when a hillman in faded overalls and hickory shirt accosted him on the street, and besought him for light upon some mystery of Holy Writ. The simian gabble of the cross-roads was not gabble to him, but wisdom of an occult and superior sort. In the presence of city folks he was palpably uneasy. Their clothes, I suspect, annoyed him, and he was suspicious of their too delicate manners. He knew all the while that they were laughing at him—if not at his baroque theology, then at least at his alpaca pantaloons. But the yokels never laughed at him. To them he was not the huntsman but the prophet, and toward the end, as he gradually forsook mundane politics for more ghostly concerns, they began to elevate him in their hierarchy. When he died he was the peer of Abraham. His old enemy, Wilson, aspiring to the same white and shining robe, came down with a thump. But Bryan made the grade. His place in Tennessee hagiography is secure. If the village barber saved any of his hair, then it is curing gall-stones down there to-day.

But what label will he bear in more urbane regions? One, I fear, of a far less flattering kind. Bryan lived too long, and descended too deeply into the mud, to be taken seriously hereafter by fully literate men, even of the kind who write school-books. There was a scattering of sweet words in his funeral notices, but it was no more than a response to conventional sentimentality. The best verdict the most romantic editorial writer could dredge up, save in the humorless South, was to the general effect that his imbecilities were excused by his earnestness—that under his clowning, as under that of the juggler of Notre Dame, there was the zeal of a steadfast soul. But this was apology, not praise; precisely the same thing might be said of Mary Baker G. Eddy, the late Czar Nicholas, or Czolgosz. The truth is that even Bryan's sincerity will probably yield to what is called, in other fields, definitive criticism. Was he sincere when he opposed imperialism in the Philippines, or when he fed it with deserving Democrats in Santo Domingo? Was he sincere when he tried to shove the Prohibitionists under the table, or when he seized their banner and began to lead them with loud whoops? Was he sincere when he bellowed against war, or when he dreamed of himself as a tin-soldier in uniform, with a grave reserved among the generals? Was he sincere when he denounced the late John W. Davis, or when he swallowed Davis? Was he sincere when he fawned over Champ Clark, or when he betrayed Clark? Was he sincere when he pleaded for tolerance in New York, or when he bawled for the faggot and the stake in Tennessee?

This talk of sincerity, I confess, fatigues me. If the fellow was sincere, then so was P. T. Barnum. The word is disgraced and degraded by such uses. He was, in fact, a charlatan, a mountebank, a zany without shame or dignity. His career brought him into contact with the first men of his time; he preferred the company of rustic ignoramuses. It was hard to believe, watching him at Dayton, that he had traveled, that he had been received in civilized societies, that he had been a high officer of state. He seemed only a poor clod like those around him, deluded by a childish theology, full of an almost pathological hatred of all learning, all human dignity, all beauty, all fine and noble things. He was a peasant come home to the barnyard. Imagine a gentleman, and you have imagined everything that he was not. What animated him from end to end of his grotesque career was simply ambition—the ambition of a common man to get his hand upon the collar of his superiors, or, failing that, to get his thumb into their eyes. He was born with a roaring voice, and it had the trick of inflaming half-wits. His whole career was devoted to raising those half-wits against their betters, that he himself might shine. His last battle will be grossly misunderstood if it is thought of as a mere exercise in fanaticism—that is, if Bryan the Fundamentalist Pope is mistaken for one of the bucolic Fundamentalists. There was much more in it than that, as everyone knows who saw him on the field. What moved him, at bottom, was simply hatred of the city men who had laughed at him so long, and brought him at last to so tatterdemalion an estate. He lusted for revenge upon them. He yearned to lead the anthropoid rabble against them, to punish them for their execution upon him by attacking the very vitals of their civilization. He went far beyond the bounds of any merely religious frenzy, however inordinate. When he began denouncing the notion that man is a mammal even some of the hinds at Dayton were agape. And when, brought upon Darrow's cruel hook, he writhed and tossed in a very fury of malignancy, bawling against the baldest elements of sense and decency like a man frantic—when he came to that tragic climax of his striving there were snickers among the hinds as well as hosannas.

Upon that hook, in truth, Bryan committed suicide, as a legend as well as in the body. He staggered from the rustic court ready to die, and he staggered from it ready to be forgotten, save as a character in a third-rate farce, witless and in poor taste. It was plain to everyone who knew him, when he came to Dayton, that his great days were behind him—that, for all the fury of his hatred, he was now definitely an old man, and headed at last for silence. There was a vague, unpleasant manginess about his appearance; he somehow seemed dirty, though a close glance showed him as carefully shaven as an actor, and clad in immaculate linen. All the hair was gone from the dome of his head, and it had begun to fall out, too, behind his ears, in the obscene manner of the late Samuel Gompers. The resonance had departed from his voice; what was once a bugle blast had become reedy and quavering. Who knows that, like Demosthenes, he had a lisp? In the old days, under the magic of his eloquence, no one noticed it. But when he spoke at Dayton it was always audible.

When I first encountered him, on the sidewalk in front of the office of the rustic lawyers who were his associates in the Scopes case, the trial was yet to begin, and so he was still expansive and amiable. I had printed in the *Nation*, a week or so before, an article arguing that the Tennessee anti-evolution law, whatever its wisdom, was at least constitutional—that the rustics of the State had a clear right to have their progeny taught whatever they chose, and kept secure from whatever knowledge violated their superstitions. The old boy professed to be delighted with the argument, and gave the gaping bystanders to understand that I was a publicist of parts. Not to be outdone, I admired the preposterous country shirt that he wore—sleeveless and with the neck cut very low. We parted in the manner of two ambassadors. But that was the last touch of amiability that I was destined to see in Bryan. The next day the battle joined and his face became hard. By the end of the week he was simply a walking fever. Hour by hour he grew more bitter. What the Christian Scientists call malicious animal magnetism seemed to radiate from him like heat from a stove. From my place in the courtroom, standing upon a table, I looked directly down upon him, sweating horribly and pumping his palm-leaf fan. His eyes fascinated me; I watched them all day long. They were blazing points of hatred. They glittered like occult and sinister gems. Now and then they wandered to me, and I got my share, for my reports of the trial had come back to Dayton, and he had read them. It was like coming under fire.

Thus he fought his last fight, thirsting savagely for blood. All sense departed from him. He bit right and left, like a dog with rabies. He descended to demagogy so dreadful that his very associates at the trial table blushed. His one yearning was to keep his yokels heated up—to lead his forlorn mob of imbeciles against the foe. That foe, alas, refused to be alarmed. It insisted upon seeing the whole battle as a comedy. Even Darrow, who knew better, occasionally yielded to the prevailing spirit. One day he lured poor Bryan into the folly I have mentioned: his astounding argument against the notion that man is a mammal. I am glad I heard it, for otherwise I'd never believe in it. There stood the man who had been thrice a candidate for the Presidency of the Republic—there he stood in the glare of the world, uttering stuff that a boy of eight would laugh at! The artful Darrow led him on: he repeated it, ranted for it, bellowed it in his cracked voice.

So he was prepared for the final slaughter. He came into life a hero, a Galahad, in bright and shining armor. He was passing out a poor mountebank.

The chances are that history will put the peak of democracy in America in his time; it has been on the downward curve among us since the campaign of 1896. He will be remembered, perhaps, as its supreme impostor, the *reductio ad absurdum* of its pretension. Bryan came very near being President. In 1896, it is possible, he was actually elected. He lived long enough to make patriots thank the inscrutable gods for Harding, even for Coolidge. Dullness has got into the White House, and the smell of cabbage boiling, but there is at least nothing to compare to the intolerable buffoonery that went on in Tennessee. The President of the United States may be an ass, but he at least doesn't believe that the earth is square, and that witches should be put to death, and that Jonah swallowed the whale. The Golden Text is not painted weekly on the White House wall, and there is no need to keep ambassadors waiting while Pastor Simpson, of Smithville, prays for rain in the Blue Room. We have escaped something—by a narrow margin, but still we have escaped.

That is, so far. The Fundamentalists, once apparently sweeping all before them, now face minorities prepared for battle even in the South—here and there with some assurance of success. But it is too early, it seems to me, to send the firemen home; the fire is still burning on many a far-flung hill, and it may begin to roar again at any moment. The evil that men do lives after them. Bryan, in his malice, started something that it will not be easy to stop. In ten thousand country towns his old heelers, the evangelical pastors, are propagating his gospel, and everywhere the yokels are ready for it. When he disappeared from the big cities, the big cities made the capital error of assuming that he was done for. If they heard of him at all, it was only as a crimp for real-estate speculators—the heroic foe of the unearned increment hauling it in with both hands. He seemed preposterous, and hence harmless. But all the while he was busy among his old lieges, preparing for a *jacquerie* that should floor all his enemies at one blow.

He did his job competently. He had vast skill at such enterprises. Heave an egg out of a Pullman window, and you will hit a Fundamentalist almost everywhere in the United States to-day. They swarm in the country towns, inflamed by their *shamans*, and with a saint, now, to venerate. They are thick in the mean streets behind the gas-works. They are everywhere where learning is too heavy a burden for mortal minds to carry, even the vague, pathetic learning on tap in little red schoolhouses. They march with the Klan, with the Christian Endeavor Society, with the Junior Order of United American Mechanics, with the Epworth League, with all the rococo bands that poor and unhappy folk organize to bring some light of purpose into their lives. They have had a thrill, and they are ready for more.

Such is Bryan's legacy to his country. He couldn't be President, but he could at least help magnificently in the solemn business of shutting off the Presidency from every intelligent and self-respecting man. The storm, perhaps, won't last long, as time goes in history. It may help, indeed, to break up the democratic delusion, now already showing weakness, and so hasten its own end. But while it lasts it will blow off some roofs.

The Pastons and Chaucer

VIRGINIA WOOLF (1892–1941)

THE TOWER of Caister Castle still rises ninety feet into the air, and the arch still stands from which Sir John Fastolf's barges sailed out to fetch stone for the building of the great castle. But now jackdaws nest on the tower, and of the castle, which once covered six acres of ground, only ruined walls remain, pierced by loop-holes and surmounted by battlements, though there are neither archers within nor cannon without. As for the "seven religious men" and the "seven poor folk" who should, at this very moment, be praying for the souls of Sir John and his parents, there is no sign of them nor sound of their prayers. The place is a ruin. Antiquaries speculate and differ.

Not so very far off lie more ruins—the ruins of Bromholm Priory, where John Paston was buried, naturally enough, since his house was only a mile or so away, lying on low ground by the sea, twenty miles north of Norwich. The coast is dangerous, and the land, even in our time, inaccessible. Nevertheless the little bit of wood at Bromholm, the fragment of the true Cross, brought pilgrims incessantly to the Priory, and sent them away with eyes opened and limbs straightened. But some of them with their newly-opened eyes saw a sight which shocked them—the grave of John Paston in Bromholm Priory without a tombstone. The news spread over the country-side. The Pastons had fallen; they that had been so powerful could no longer afford a stone to put above John Paston's head. Margaret, his widow, could not pay her debts; the eldest son, Sir John, wasted his property upon women and tournaments, while the younger, John also, though a man of greater parts, thought more of his hawks than of his harvests.

The pilgrims of course were liars, as people whose eyes have just been opened by a piece of the true Cross have every right to be; but their news, none the less, was welcome. The Pastons had risen in the world. People said even that they had been bondmen not so very long ago. At any rate, men still living could remember John's grandfather Clement tilling his own land, a hard-working peasant; and William, Clement's son, becoming a judge and buying land; and John, William's son, marrying well and buying more land and quite lately inheriting the vast new castle at Caister, and all Sir John's lands in Norfolk and Suffolk. People said that he had forged the old knight's will. What wonder, then, that he lacked a tombstone? But, if we consider the character of Sir John Paston, John's eldest son, and his upbringing and his surroundings, and the relations between himself and his father as the family letters reveal them, we shall see how difficult it was, and how likely to be neglected—this business of making his father's tombstone.

For let us imagine, in the most desolate part of England known to us at the present moment, a raw, new-built house, without telephone, bathroom, or drains, arm-chairs or newspapers, and one shelf perhaps of books, unwieldy to hold, expensive to come by. The windows look out upon a few cultivated fields and a dozen hovels, and beyond them there is the sea on one side, on the other a vast fen. A single road crosses the fen, but there is a hole in it, which, one of the farm hands reports, is big enough to swallow a carriage. And, the man adds, Tom Topcroft, the mad bricklayer, has broken loose again and ranges the country half-naked, threatening to kill any one who approaches him. That is what they talk about at dinner in the desolate house, while the chimney smokes horribly, and the draught lifts the carpets on the floor. Orders are given to lock all gates at sunset, and, when the long dismal evening has worn itself away, simply and solemnly, girt about with dangers as they are, these isolated men and women fall upon their knees in prayer.

In the fifteenth century, however, the wild landscape was broken suddenly and very strangely by vast piles of brand-new masonry. There rose out of the sandhills and heaths of the Norfolk coast a huge bulk of stone, like a modern hotel in a watering-place; but there was no parade, no lodging houses, and no pier at Yarmouth then, and this gigantic building on the outskirts of the town was built to house one solitary old gentleman without any children—Sir John Fastolf, who had fought at Agincourt and acquired great wealth. He had fought at Agincourt and got but little reward. No one took his advice. Men spoke ill of him behind his back. He was well aware of it; his temper was none the sweeter for it. He was a hot-tempered old man, powerful, embittered by a sense of grievance. But whether on the battlefield or at court he thought perpetually of Caister, and how, when his duties allowed, he would settle down on his father's land and live in a great house of his own building.

The gigantic structure of Caister Castle was in progress not so many miles away when the little Pastons were children. John Paston, the father, had charge of some part of the business, and the children listened, as soon as they could listen at all, to talk of stone and building, of barges gone to London and not yet returned, of the twenty-six private chambers, of the hall and chapel; of foundations, measurements, and rascally work-people. Later, in 1454, when the work was finished and Sir John had come to spend his last years at Caister, they may have seen for themselves the mass of treasure that was stored there; the tables laden with gold and silver plate; the wardrobes stuffed with gowns of velvet and satin and cloth of gold, with hoods and tippets and beaver hats and leather jackets and velvet doublets; and how the very pillow-cases on the beds were of green and purple silk. There were tapestries everywhere. The beds were laid and the bedrooms hung with tapestries representing sieges, hunting and hawking, men fishing, archers shooting, ladies playing on their harps, dallying with ducks, or a giant "bearing the leg of a bear in his hand." Such were the fruits of a well-spent life. To buy land, to build great houses, to stuff these houses full of gold and silver plate (though the privy might well be in the bedroom), was the proper aim of mankind. Mr. and Mrs. Paston spent the greater part of their energies in the same exhausting occupation. For since the passion to acquire was universal, one could never rest secure in one's possessions for long. The outlying parts of one's property were in perpetual jeopardy. The Duke of Norfolk might covet this manor, the Duke of Suffolk that. Some trumped-up excuse, as for instance that the Pastons were bondmen, gave them the right to seize the house and batter down the lodges in the owner's absence. And how could the owner of Paston and Mauteby and Drayton and Gresham be in five or six places at once, especially now that Caister Castle was his, and he must be in London trying to get his rights recognised by the King? The King was mad too, they said; did not know his own child, they said; or the King was in flight; or there was civil war in the land. Norfolk was always the most distressed of counties and its country gentlemen the most quarrelsome of mankind. Indeed, had Mrs. Paston chosen, she could have told her children how when she was a young woman a thousand men with bows and arrows and pans of burning fire had marched upon Gresham and broken the gates and mined the walls of the room where she sat alone. But much worse things than that had happened to women. She neither bewailed her lot nor thought herself a heroine. The long, long letters which she wrote so laboriously in her clear cramped hand to her husband, who was (as usual) away, make no mention of herself. The sheep had wasted the hay. Heyden's and Tuddenham's men were out. A dyke had been broken and a bullock stolen. They needed treacle badly, and really she must have stuff for a dress.

But Mrs. Paston did not talk about herself.

Thus the little Pastons would see their mother writing or dictating page after page, hour after hour, long, long letters, but to interrupt a parent who writes so laboriously of such important matters would have been a sin. The prattle of children, the lore of the nursery or schoolroom, did not find its way into these elaborate communications. For the most part her letters are the letters of an honest bailiff to his master, explaining, asking advice, giving news, rendering accounts. There was robbery and manslaughter; it was difficult to get in the rents; Richard Calle had gathered but little money; and what with one thing and another Margaret had not had time to make out, as she should have done, the inventory of the goods which her husband desired. Well might old Agnes, surveying her son's affairs rather grimly from a distance, counsel him to contrive it so that "ye may have less to do in the world; your father said, In little business lieth much rest. This world is but a thoroughfare, and full of woe; and when we depart therefrom, right nought bear with us but our good deeds and ill."

The thought of death would thus come upon them in a clap. Old Fastolf, cumbered with wealth and property, had his vision at the end of Hell fire, and shrieked aloud to his executors to distribute alms, and see that prayers were said "in perpetuum," so that his soul might escape the agonies of purgatory. William Paston, the judge, was urgent too that the monks of Norwich should be retained to pray for his soul "for ever." The soul was no wisp of air, but a solid body capable of eternal suffering, and the fire that destroyed it was as fierce as any that burnt on mortal grates. For ever there would be monks and the town of Norwich, and for ever the Chapel of Our Lady in the town of Norwich. There was something matter-of-fact, positive, and enduring in their conception both of life and of death.

With the plan of existence so vigorously marked out, children of course were well beaten, and boys and girls taught to know their places. They must acquire land; but they must obey their parents. A mother would clout her daughter's head three times a week and break the skin if she did not conform to the laws of behaviour. Agnes Paston, a lady of birth and breeding, beat her daughter Elizabeth. Margaret Paston, a softer-hearted woman, turned her daughter out of the house for loving the honest bailiff Richard Calle. Brothers would not suffer their sisters to marry beneath them, and "sell candle and mustard in Framlingham." The fathers quarrelled with the sons, and the mothers, fonder of their boys than of their girls, yet bound by all law and custom to obey their husbands, were torn asunder in their efforts to keep the peace. With all her pains, Margaret failed to prevent rash acts on the part of her eldest son John, or the bitter words with which his father denounced him. He was a "drone among bees," the father burst out, "which labour for gathering honey in the fields, and the drone doth naught but taketh his part of it." He treated his parents with insolence, and yet was fit for no charge of responsibility abroad.

But the quarrel was ended, very shortly, by the death (22nd May 1466) of John Paston, the father, in London. The body was brought down to Bromholm to be buried. Twelve poor men trudged all the way bearing torches beside it. Alms were distributed; masses and dirges were said. Bells were rung. Great quantities of fowls, sheep, pigs, eggs, bread, and cream were devoured, ale and wine drunk, and candles burnt. Two panes were taken from the church windows to let out the reek of the torches. Black cloth was distributed, and a light set burning on the grave. But John Paston, the heir, delayed to make his father's tombstone.

He was a young man, something over twenty-four years of age. The discipline and the drudgery of a country life bored him. When he ran away from home, it was, apparently, to attempt to enter the King's household. Whatever doubts, indeed, might be cast by their enemies on the blood of the Pastons, Sir John was unmistakably a gentleman. He had inherited his lands; the honey was his that the bees had gathered with so much labour. He had the instincts of enjoyment rather than of acquisition, and with his mother's parsimony was strangely mixed something of his father's ambition. Yet his own indolent and luxurious temperament took the edge from both. He was attractive to women, liked society and tournaments, and court life and making bets, and sometimes, even, reading books. And so life, now that John Paston was buried, started afresh upon rather a different foundation. There could be little outward change indeed. Margaret still ruled the house. She still ordered the lives of the younger children as she had ordered the lives of the elder. The boys still needed to be beaten into book-learning by their tutors, the girls still loved the wrong men and must be married to the right. Rents had to be collected; the interminable lawsuit for the Fastolf property dragged on. Battles were fought; the roses of York and Lancaster alternately faded and flourished. Norfolk was full of poor people seeking redress for their grievances, and Margaret worked for her son as she had worked for her husband, with this significant change only, that now, instead of confiding in her husband, she took the advice of her priest.

But inwardly there was a change. It seems at last as if the hard outer shell had served its purpose and something sensitive, appreciative, and pleasure-loving had formed within. At any rate Sir John, writing to his brother John at home, strayed sometimes from the business on hand to crack a joke, to send a piece of gossip, or to instruct him, knowingly and even subtly, upon the conduct of a love affair. Be "as lowly to the mother as ye list, but to the maid not too lowly, nor that ye be too glad to speed, nor too sorry to fail. And I shall always be your herald both here, if she come hither, and at home, when I come home, which I hope hastily within XI. days at the furthest." And then a hawk was to be bought, a hat, or new silk laces sent down to John in Norfolk, prosecuting his suit, flying his hawks, and attending with considerable energy and not too nice a sense of honesty to the affairs of the Paston estates.

The lights had long since burnt out on John Paston's grave. But still Sir John delayed; no tomb replaced them. He had his excuses; what with the business of the lawsuit, and his duties at Court, and the disturbance of the civil wars, his time was occupied and his money spent. But perhaps something strange had happened to Sir John himself, and not only to Sir John dallying in London, but to his sister Margery falling in love with the bailiff, and to Walter making Latin verses at Eton, and to John flying his hawks at Paston. Life was a little more various in its pleasures. They were not quite so sure as the elder generation had been of the rights of man and of the dues of God, of the horrors of death, and of the importance of tombstones. Poor Margaret Paston scented the change and sought uneasily, with the pen which had marched so stiffly through so many pages, to lay bare the root of her troubles. It was not that the lawsuit saddened her; she was ready to defend Caister with her own hands if need be, "though I cannot well guide nor rule soldiers," but there was something wrong with the family since the death of her husband and master. Perhaps her son had failed in his service to God; he had been too proud or too lavish in his expenditure; or perhaps he had shown too little mercy to the poor. Whatever the fault might be, she only knew that Sir John spent twice as much money as his father for less result; that they could scarcely pay their debts without selling land, wood, or household stuff ("It is a death to me to think of it"); while every day people spoke ill of them in the country because they left John Paston to lie without a tombstone. The money that might have bought it, or more land, and more goblets and more tapestry, was spent by Sir John on clocks and trinkets, and upon paying a clerk to copy out Treatises upon Knighthood and other such stuff. There they stood at Paston—eleven volumes, with the poems of Lydgate and Chaucer among them, diffusing a strange air into the gaunt, comfortless house, inviting men to indolence and vanity, distracting their thoughts from business, and leading them not only to neglect their own profit but to think lightly of the sacred dues of the dead.

For sometimes, instead of riding off on his horse to inspect his crops or bargain with his tenants, Sir John would sit, in broad daylight, reading. There, on the hard chair in the comfortless room with the wind lifting the carpet and the smoke stinging his eyes, he would sit reading Chaucer, wasting his time, dreaming—or what strange intoxication was it that he drew from books? Life was rough, cheerless, and disappointing. A whole year of days would pass fruitlessly in dreary business, like dashes of rain on the window pane. There was no reason in it as there had been for his father; no imperative need to establish a family and acquire an important position for children who were not born, or if born, had no right to bear their father's name. But Lydgate's poems or Chaucer's, like a mirror in which figures move brightly, silently, and compactly, showed him the very skies, fields, and people whom he knew, but rounded and complete. Instead of waiting listlessly for news from London or piecing out from his mother's gossip some country tragedy of love and jealousy, here, in a few pages, the whole story was laid before him. And then as he rode or sat at table he would remember some description or saying which bore upon the present moment and fixed it, or some string of words would charm him, and putting aside the pressure of the moment, he would hasten home to sit in his chair and learn the end of the story.

To learn the end of the story—Chaucer can still make us wish to do that. He has pre-eminently that story-teller's gift, which is almost the rarest gift among writers at the present day. Nothing happens to us as it did to our ancestors; events are seldom important; if we recount them, we do not really believe in them; we have perhaps things of greater interest to say, and for these reasons natural story-tellers like Mr. Garnett, whom we must distinguish from self-conscious story-tellers like Mr. Masefield, have become rare. For the story-teller, besides his indescribable zest for facts, must tell his story craftily, without undue stress or excitement, or we shall swallow it whole and jumble the parts together; he must let us stop, give us time to think and look about us, yet always be persuading us to move on. Chaucer was helped to this to some extent by the time of his birth; and in addition he had another advantage over the moderns which will never come the way of English poets again. England was an unspoilt country. His eyes rested on a virgin land, all unbroken grass and wood except for the small towns and an occasional castle in the building. No villa roofs peered through Kentish tree-tops; no factory chimney smoked on the hillside. The state of the country, considering how poets go to Nature, how they use her for their images and their contrasts even when they do not describe her directly, is a matter of some importance. Her cultivation or her savagery influences the poet far more profoundly than the prose writer. To the modern poet, with Birmingham, Manchester, and London the size they are, the country is the sanctuary of moral excellence in contrast with the town which is the sink of vice. It is a retreat, the haunt of modesty and virtue, where men go to hide and moralise. There is something morbid, as if shrinking from human contact, in the nature worship of Wordsworth, still more in the microscopic devotion which Tennyson lavished upon the petals of roses and the buds of lime trees. But these were great poets. In their hands, the country was no mere jeweller's shop, or museum of curious objects to be described, even more curiously, in words. Poets of smaller gift, since the view is so much spoilt, and the garden or the meadow must replace the barren heath and the precipitous mountain-side, are now confined to little landscapes, to birds' nests, to acorns with every wrinkle drawn to the life. The wider landscape is lost.

But to Chaucer the country was too large and too wild to be altogether agreeable. He turned instinctively, as if he had painful experience of their nature, from tempests and rocks to the bright May day and the jocund landscape, from the harsh and mysterious to the gay and definite. Without possessing a tithe of the virtuosity in word-painting which is the modern inheritance, he could give, in a few words, or even, when we come to look, without a single word of direct description, the sense of the open air.

And se the fresshe floures how they sprynge

—that is enough.

Nature, uncompromising, untamed, was no looking-glass for happy faces, or confessor of unhappy souls. She was herself; sometimes, therefore, disagreeable enough and plain, but always in Chaucer's pages with the hardness and the freshness of an actual presence. Soon, however, we notice something of greater importance than the gay and picturesque appearance of the mediæval world—the solidity which plumps it out, the conviction which animates the characters. There is immense variety in the *Canterbury Tales,* and yet, persisting underneath, one consistent type. Chaucer has his world; he has his young men; he has his young women. If one met them straying in Shakespeare's world one would know them to be Chaucer's, not Shakespeare's. He wants to describe a girl, and this is what she looks like:

Ful semely hir wimpel pinched was,
Hir nose tretys; hir eyen greye as glas;
Hir mouth ful smal, and ther-to soft and reed;
But sikerly she hadde a fair foreheed;
It was almost a spanne brood, I trowe;
For, hardily, she was nat undergrowe.

Then he goes on to develop her; she was a girl, a virgin, cold in her virginity:

I am, thou woost, yet of thy companye,
A mayde, and love hunting and venerye,
And for to walken in the wodes wilde,
And noght to been a wyf and be with childe.

Next he bethinks him how

Discreet she was in answering alway;
And though she had been as wise as Pallas
No countrefeted termes hadde she
To seme wys; but after hir degree
She spak, and alle hir wordes more and lesse
Souninge in vertu and in gentillesse.

Each of these quotations, in fact, comes from a different Tale, but they are parts, one feels, of the same personage, whom he had in mind, perhaps unconsciously, when he thought of a young girl, and for this reason, as she goes in and out of the *Canterbury Tales* bearing different names, she has a stability which is only to be found where the poet has made up his mind about young women, of course, but also about the world they live in, its end, its nature, and his own craft and technique, so that his mind is free to apply its force fully to its object. It does not occur to him that his Griselda might be improved or altered. There is no blur about her, no hesitation; she proves nothing; she is content to be herself. Upon her, therefore, the mind can rest with that unconscious ease which allows it, from hints and suggestions, to endow her with many more qualities than are actually referred to. Such is the power of conviction, a rare gift, a gift shared in our day by Joseph Conrad in his earlier novels, and a gift of supreme importance, for upon it the whole weight of the building depends. Once believe in Chaucer's young men and women and we have no need of preaching or protest. We know what he finds good, what evil; the less said the better. Let him get on with his story, paint knights and squires, good women and bad, cooks, shipmen, priests, and we will supply the landscape, give his society its belief, its standing towards life and death, and make of the journey to Canterbury a spiritual pilgrimage.

This simple faithfulness to his own conceptions was easier then than now in one respect at least, for Chaucer could write frankly where we must either say nothing or say it slyly. He could sound every note in the language instead of finding a great many of the best gone dumb from disuse, and thus, when struck by daring fingers, giving off a loud discordant jangle out of keeping with the rest. Much of Chaucer—a few lines perhaps in each of the Tales—is improper and gives us as we read it the strange sensation of being naked to the air after being muffled in old clothing. And, as a certain kind of humour depends upon being able to speak without self-consciousness of the parts and functions of the body, so with the advent of decency literature lost the use of one of its limbs. It lost its power to create the Wife of Bath, Juliet's nurse, and their recognisable though already colourless relation, Moll Flanders. Sterne, from fear of coarseness, is forced into indecency. He must be witty, not humorous. He must hint instead of speaking outright. Nor can we believe, with Mr. Joyce's *Ulysses* before us, that laughter of the old kind will ever be heard again.

> But, lord Christ! When that it remembreth me
> Up-on my yowthe, and on my Iolitee,
> It tikleth me aboute myn herte rote.
> Unto this day it doth myn herte bote
> That I have had my world as in my tyme.

The sound of that old woman's voice is still.

But there is another and more important reason for the surprising brightness, the still effective merriment of the *Canterbury Tales.* Chaucer was a poet; but he never flinched from the life that was being lived at the moment before his eyes. A farmyard, with its straw, its dung, its cocks and its hens is not (we have come to think) a poetic subject; poets seem either to rule out the farmyard entirely or to require that it shall be a farmyard in Thessaly and its pigs of mythological origin. But Chaucer says outright:

> Three large sowes hadde she, and namo,
> Three kyn, and eek a sheep that highte Malle;

or again,

> A yard she hadde, enclosed al aboute
> With stikkes, and a drye ditch with-oute.

He is unabashed and unafraid. He will always get close up to his object—an old man's chin—

> With thikke bristles of his berde unsofte,
> Lyk to the skin of houndfish, sharp as brere;

or an old man's neck—

> The slakke skin about his nekke shaketh
> Whyl that he sang;

and he will tell you what his characters wore, how they looked, what they ate and drank, as if poetry could handle the common facts of this very moment of Tuesday, the sixteenth day of April, 1387, without dirtying her hands. If he withdraws to the time of the Greeks or the Romans, it is only that his story leads him there. He has no desire to wrap himself round in antiquity, to take refuge in age, or to shirk the associations of common grocer's English.

Therefore when we say that we know the end of the journey, it is hard to quote the particular lines from which we take our knowledge. He fixed his eyes upon the road before him, not upon the world to come. He was little given to abstract contemplation. He deprecated, with peculiar archness, any competition with the scholars and divines:

> The answere of this I lete to divynis,
> But wel I woot, that in this world grey pyne is.

> What is this world? What asketh men to have?
> Now with his love, now in the colde grave
> Allone, withouten any companye,

he asks, or ponders

> O cruel goddes, that governe
> This world with binding of your worde eterne,
> And wryten in the table of athamaunt
> Your parlement, and your eterne graunt,
> What is mankinde more un-to yow holde
> Than is the sheepe, that rouketh in the folde?

Questions press upon him; he asks questions, but he is too true a poet to answer them; he leaves them unsolved, uncramped by the solution of the moment, thus fresh for the generations that come after him. In his life, too, it would be impossible to write him down a man of this party or of that, a democrat or an aristocrat. He was a staunch churchman, but he laughed at priests. He was an able public servant and a courtier, but his views upon sexual morality were extremely lax. He sympathised with poverty, but did nothing to improve the lot of the poor. It is safe to say that not a single law has been framed or one stone set upon another because of anything that Chaucer said or wrote; and yet, as we read him, we are of course absorbing morality at every pore. For among writers there are two kinds: there are the priests who take you by the hand and lead you straight up to the mystery; there are the laymen who imbed their doctrines in flesh and blood and make a complete model of the world without excluding the bad or laying stress upon the good. Wordsworth, Coleridge, and Shelley are among the priests; they give us text after text to be hung upon the wall, saying after saying to be laid upon the heart like an amulet against disaster—

Farewell, farewell, the heart that lives alone

He prayeth best that loveth best
All things both great and small

—such lines of exhortation and command spring to memory instantly. But Chaucer lets us go our ways doing the ordinary things with the ordinary people. His morality lies in the way men and women behave to each other. We see them eating, drinking, laughing, and making love, and come to feel without a word being said what their standards are and so are steeped through and through with their morality. There can be no more forcible preaching than this where all actions and passions are represented, and instead of being solemnly exhorted we are left to stray and stare and make out a meaning for ourselves. It is the morality of ordinary intercourse, the morality of the novel, which parents and librarians rightly judge to be far more persuasive than the morality of poetry.

And so, when we shut Chaucer, we feel that without a word being said the criticism is complete; what we are saying, thinking, reading, doing has been commented upon. Nor are we left merely with the sense, powerful though that is, of having been in good company and got used to the ways of good society. For as we have jogged through the real, the unadorned country-side, with first one good fellow cracking his joke or singing his song and then another, we know that though this world resembles, it is not in fact our daily world. It is the world of poetry. Everything happens here more quickly and more intensely, and with better order than in life or in prose; there is a formal elevated dullness which is part of the incantation of poetry; there are lines speaking half a second in advance what we were about to say, as if we read our thoughts before words cumbered them; and lines which we go back to read again with that heightened quality, that enchantment which keeps them glittering in the mind long afterwards. And the whole is held in its place, and its variety and divagations ordered by the power which is among the most impressive of all—the shaping power, the architect's power. It is the peculiarity of Chaucer, however, that though we feel at once this quickening, this enchantment, we cannot prove it by quotation. From most poets quotation is easy and obvious; some metaphor suddenly flowers; some passage breaks off from the rest. But Chaucer is very equal, very even-paced, very unmetaphorical. If we take six or seven lines in the hope that the quality will be contained in them it has escaped.

> My lord, ye woot that in my fadres place,
> Ye dede me strepe out of my povre wede,
> And richely me cladden, o your grace.
> To yow broghte I noght elles, out of drede,
> But feyth and nakedness and maydenhede.

In its place that seemed not only memorable and moving but fit to set beside striking beauties. Cut out and taken separately it appears ordinary and quiet. Chaucer, it seems, has some art by which the most ordinary words and the simplest feelings when laid side by side make each other shine; when separated lose their lustre. Thus the pleasure he gives us is different from the pleasure that other poets give us, because it is more closely connected with what we have ourselves felt or observed. Eating, drinking and fine weather, the May, cocks and hens, millers, old peasant women, flowers—there is a special stimulus in seeing all these common things so arranged that they affect us as poetry affects us, and are yet bright, sober, precise as we see them out of doors. There is a pungency in this unfigurative language; a stately and memorable beauty in the undraped sentences which follow each other like women so slightly veiled that you see the lines of their bodies as they go—

> And she set down hir water pot anon
> Biside the threshold in an oxe's stall.

And then, as the procession takes its way, tranquilly, beautifully, out from behind peeps the face of Chaucer, grinning, malicious, in league with all foxes, donkeys, and hens, to mock the pomp and ceremonies of life—witty, intellectual, French, at the same time based upon a broad bottom of English humour.

So Sir John read his Chaucer in the comfortless room with the wind blowing and the smoke stinging, and left his father's tombstone unmade. But no book, no tomb, had power to hold him long. He was one of those ambiguous characters who haunt the boundary line where one age merges in another and are not able to inhabit either. At one moment he was all for buying books cheap; next he was off to France and told his mother, "My mind is now not most upon books." In his own house, where his mother Margaret was perpetually making out inventories or confiding in Gloys the priest, he had no peace or comfort. There was always reason on her side; she was a brave woman, for whose sake one must put up with the priest's insolence and choke down one's rage when the grumbling broke into open abuse, and "Thou proud priest" and "Thou proud Squire" were bandied angrily about the room. All this, with the discomforts of life and the weakness of his own character, drove him to loiter in pleasanter places, to put off coming, to put off writing, to put off, year after year, the making of his father's tombstone.

Yet John Paston had now lain for twelve years under the bare ground. The Prior of Bromholm sent word that the grave cloth was in tatters, and he had tried to patch it himself. Worse still, for a proud woman like Margaret Paston, the country people murmured at the Pastons' lack of piety, and other families she heard, of no greater standing than theirs, spent money in pious restoration in the very church where her husband lay unremembered. At last, turning from tournaments and Chaucer and Mistress Anne Hault, Sir John bethought him of a piece of cloth of gold which had been used to cover his father's hearse and might now be sold to defray the expenses of his tomb. Margaret had it in safe keeping; she had hoarded it and cared for it, and spent twenty marks on its repair. She grudged it; but there was no help for it. She sent it him, still distrusting his intentions or his power to put them into effect. "If you sell it to any other use," she wrote, "by my troth I shall never trust you while I live."

But this final act, like so many that Sir John had undertaken in the course of his life, was left undone. A dispute with the Duke of Suffolk in the year 1479 made it necessary for him to visit London in spite of the epidemic of sickness that was abroad; and there, in dirty lodgings, alone, busy to the end with quarrels, clamorous to the end for money, Sir John died and was buried at Whitefriars in London. He left a natural daughter; he left a considerable number of books; but his father's tomb was still unmade.

The four thick volumes of the Paston letters, however, swallow up this frustrated man as the sea absorbs a raindrop. For, like all collections of letters, they seem to hint that we need not care overmuch for the fortunes of individuals. The family will go on whether Sir John lives or dies. It is their method to heap up in mounds of insignificant and often dismal dust the innumerable trivialities of daily life, as it grinds itself out, year after year. And then suddenly they blaze up; the day shines out, complete, alive, before our eyes. It is early morning and strange men have been whispering among the women as they milk. It is evening, and there in the churchyard Warne's wife bursts out against old Agnes Paston: "All the devils of Hell draw her soul to Hell." Now it is the autumn in Norfolk and Cecily Dawne comes whining to Sir John for clothing. "Moreover, Sir, liketh it your mastership to understand that winter and cold weather draweth nigh and I have few clothes but of your gift." There is the ancient day, spread out before us, hour by hour.

But in all this there is no writing for writing's sake; no use of the pen to convey pleasure or amusement or any of the million shades of endearment and intimacy which have filled so many English letters since. Only occasionally, under stress of anger for the most part, does Margaret Paston quicken into some shrewd saw or solemn curse. "Men cut large thongs here out of other men's leather. . . . We beat the brushes and other men have the birds. . . . Haste reweth . . . which is to my heart a very spear." That is her eloquence and that her anguish. Her sons, it is true, bend their pens more easily to their will. They jest rather stiffly; they hint rather clumsily; they make a little scene like a rough puppet show of the old priest's anger and give a phrase or two directly as they were spoken in person. But when Chaucer lived he must have heard this very language, matter of fact, unmetaphorical, far better fitted for narrative than for analysis, capable of religious solemnity or of broad humour, but very stiff material to put on the lips of men and women accosting each other face to face. In short it is easy to see, from the Paston letters, why Chaucer wrote not *Lear* or *Romeo and Juliet*, but the *Canterbury Tales.*

Sir John was buried; and John the younger brother succeeded in his turn. The Paston letters go on; life at Paston continues much the same as before. Over it all broods a sense of discomfort and nakedness; of unwashed limbs thrust into splendid clothing; of tapestry blowing on the draughty walls; of the bedroom with its privy; of winds sweeping straight over land unmitigated by hedge or town; of Caister Castle covering with solid stone six acres of ground, and of the plain-faced Pastons indefatigably accumulating wealth, treading out the roads of Norfolk, and persisting with an obstinate courage which does them infinite credit in furnishing the bareness of England.

The Whig World

DAVID CECIL (1902–   )

THE GREAT Whig country houses of the eighteenth and early nineteenth centuries are among the most conspicuous monuments of English history. Ornate and massive, with their pedimented porticoes, their spreading balustraded wings, they dominate the landscape round them with a magnificent self-assurance. Nor are their interiors less imposing. Their colonnaded entrance halls, whence the Adam staircase sweeps up beneath a fluted dome; their cream and gilt libraries piled with sumptuous editions of the classics; their orangeries peopled with casts from the antique; their saloons hung with yellow silk, and with ceiling and doorways painted in delicate arabesque by Angelica Kauffmann, all combine to produce an extraordinary impression of culture and elegance and established power.

Yet, they are not palaces. There is something easy-going and unofficial about them. Between library and saloon one comes on little rooms, full of sporting prints and comfortable untidiness; the bedrooms upstairs are friendly with chintz and flowered wallpaper. Even the great rooms themselves, with their roomy writing tables, their armchairs, their tables piled with albums and commonplace books, seem designed less for state occasions than for private life: for leisure and lounging, for intimate talk, and desultory reading. And the portraits that glow down from the walls exhibit a similar character. The gentlemen lean back in their hunting coats, the ladies stroll in their parks with spaniels snapping at the ribbons that dangle from the garden hats, slung on their arms. In big and in detail these houses convey an effect of splendid naturalness. In this they are typical of the society which was their creator.

The Whig aristocracy was a unique product of English civilization. It was before all things a governing class. At a time when economic power was concentrated in the landed interest, the Whigs were among the biggest landowners: their party was in office for the greater part of the eighteenth century; during this period they possessed a large proportion of the seats in the House of Commons; they produced more ambassadors and officers of state than the rest of England put together. And they lived on a scale appropriate to their power. "A man," said one of their latest representatives, "can jog along on £40,000 a year." And jog very well they did. They possessed, most of them, a mansion in London and two or three in the country; they moved through the world attended by a vast retinue of servants, of secretaries and chaplains, of companions, librarians and general hangers-on; they never travelled but in their own carriages; they kept open house to a continuous stream of guests, whom they entertained in the baroque and lavish style approved by their contemporaries.

For the elaboration of their life was increased by the period they lived in. The eighteenth century, that accomplished age, did not believe in the artless and the austere. In its view the good man or, as they would have phrased it, "the man of sense and taste," was he whose every activity was regulated in the light of a trained judgment and the experience of the wise in his own and former ages. From his earliest years the Whig nobleman was subjected to a careful education. He was grounded in the classics first by a tutor, then at Eton, then at the University. After this he went abroad for two years' grand tour to learn French and good manners in the best society of the continent. His sisters learnt French and manners equally thoroughly at home; and their demeanour was further improved by a course of deportment. The Whigs' taste was in harmony with the ideal that guided their education. They learnt to admire the grand style in painting, the "correct" in letters, the Latin tradition in oratory. And in everything they paid strict attention to form. Since life to them was so secure and so pleasant, the Whig aristocrats tended to take its fundamental values very much for granted; they concentrated rather on how to live. And here again, their ideal was not an artless one. Their customs, their mode of speech, their taste in decoration, their stylish stiff clothes, are alike marked by a character at once polished and precise, disciplined and florid. If one of them writes a note it is rounded with a graceful phrase, their most extempore speeches are turned with a flourish of rotund rhetoric.

Yet—and here it is that it differs from those of similar societies on the continent—theirs was not an unreal life; no Watteau-like paradise of exquisite trifling and fastidious idleness. For one thing it had its roots in the earth. Founded as their position was on landed property, the Whig aristocracy was never urban. They passed at least half the year in their country seats; and there they occupied themselves in the ordinary avocations of country life. The ladies interested themselves in their children, and visited the poor; the gentlemen looked after their estates, rode to hounds, and administered from the local bench justice to poachers and pilferers. Their days went by, active out-of-door, unceremonious; they wore riding-boots as often as silk stockings. Moreover, they were always in touch with the central and serious current of contemporary life. The fact that they were a governing class meant that they had to govern. The Whig lord was as often as not a minister, his eldest son an M.P., his second attached to a foreign embassy. So that their houses were alive with the effort and hurry of politics. Red Foreign Office boxes strewed the library tables; at any time of day or night a courier might come galloping up with critical news, and the minister must post off to London to attend a Cabinet meeting. He had his work in the country too. He was a landlord and magistrate, often a lord lieutenant. While every few years would come a general election when his sons, if not himself, might have to sally forth to stand on the hustings and be pelted with eggs and dead cats by the free and independent electors of the neighbouring borough. Indeed his was not a protected existence. The eighteenth century was the age of clubs; and Whig society itself was a sort of club, exclusive, but in which those who managed to achieve membership lived on equal terms; a rowdy, rough-and-tumble club, full of conflict and plain speaking, where people were expected to stand up for themselves and take and give hard knocks. At Eton the little dukes and earls cuffed and bullied each other like street urchins. As mature persons in their country homes, or in the pillared rooms of Brooks's Club, their intercourse continued more politely, yet with equal familiarity. While their House of Commons life passed in a robust atmosphere of combat and crisis and defeat. The Whigs despised the royal family; and there was certainly none of the hush and punctilio of court existence about them. Within the narrow limits of their world they were equalitarians.

Their life, in fact, was essentially a normal life, compounded of the same elements as those of general humanity, astir with the same clamour and clash and aspiration and competition as filled the streets round their august dwellings. Only, it was normal life played out on a colossal stage and with magnificent scenery and costumes. Their houses were homes, but homes with sixty bedrooms, set in grounds five miles round; they fought to keep their jobs, but the jobs were embassies and prime ministerships; their sons went to the same universities as humbler students, but were distinguished from them there by a nobleman's gold-tasselled mortarboard. When the Duke of Devonshire took up botany, he sent out a special expedition to the East Indies to search for rare plants; Lord Egremont liked pictures, so he filled a gallery with Claudes and Correggios; young Lord Palmerston was offered the Chancellorship of the Exchequer a year or two after entering Parliament.

This curiously blended life produced a curiously blended type of character. With so many opportunities for action, its interests were predominantly active. Most of the men were engaged in politics. And the women—for they lived to please the men—were political too. They listened, they sympathized, they advised; through them two statesmen might make overtures to each other, or effect a reconciliation. But politics then were not the life sentence to hard labour that in our iron age they have become. Parliament only sat for a few months in the year; and even during the session, debates did not start till the late afternoon. The Whigs had the rest of their time to devote to other things. If they were sporting they raced and hunted; if interested in agriculture they farmed on an ambitious scale; if artistic they collected marbles and medals; if intellectual they read history and philosophy; if literary they composed compliments in verse and sonorous, platitudinous orations. But the chief of their spare time was given up to social life. They gave balls, they founded clubs, they played cards, they got up private theatricals: they cultivated friendship, and every variety, platonic and less platonic, of the art of love. Their ideal was the Renaissance ideal of the whole man, whose aspiration it is to make the most of every advantage, intellectual and sensual, that life has to offer.

In practice, of course, this ideal was not so broad as it sounds. The Whigs could not escape the limitations imposed by the splendour of their circumstances. Like all aristocrats they tended to be amateurs. When life is so free and so pleasant, a man is not likely to endure the drudgery necessary to make himself really expert in any one thing. Even in those affairs of state which took up most of the Whigs' time, they troubled little with the dry details of economic theory or administrative practice. Politics to them meant first of all personalities, and secondly general principles. And general principles to them were an occasion for expression rather than thought. They did not dream of questioning the fundamental canons of Whig orthodoxy. All believed in ordered liberty, low taxation and the enclosure of land; all disbelieved in despotism and democracy. Their only concern was to restate these indisputable truths in a fresh and effective fashion.

Again, their taste was a little philistine. Aristocratic taste nearly always is. Those whose ordinary course of life is splendid and satisfying, find it hard to recognize the deeper value of the exercises of the solitary imagination; art to them is not the fulfilment of the soul, but an ornamental appendage to existence. Moreover, the English nobility were too much occupied with practical affairs to achieve the fullest intellectual life. They admired what was elegant, sumptuous and easy to understand; portraits that were good likenesses and pleasing decorations; architecture which appropriately housed a stately life. In books, they appreciated acute, wittily phrased observation of human nature, or noble sentiments expressed in flowing periods; Cicero, Pope, Horace, Burke. The strange and the harsh they dismissed immediately. Among contemporary authors they appreciated Jane Austen, condemned Crabbe, for the most part, as sordid and low; and neglected Blake almost entirely. If they had read him, they would not have liked him. For—it is another of their limitations—they were not spiritual. Their education did not encourage them to be; and, anyway, they found this world too absorbing to concern themselves much with the next. The bolder spirits among them were atheists. The average person accepted Christianity, but in a straightforward spirit, innocent alike of mysticism and theological exactitude.

Further, their circumstances did not encourage the virtues of self-control. Good living gave them zest; wealth gave them opportunity; and they threw themselves into their pleasures with an animal recklessness at once terrifying and exhilarating to a modern reader. The most respectable people often drank themselves under the table without shocking anyone. "Colonel Napier came in to-night as drunk as an owl," remarks Lady Sarah Napier, of the staid middle-aged gentleman who was her husband. And their drinking was nothing to their gambling. Night after night they played loo and faro from early evening till the candles guttered pale in the light of the risen sun. Lord Stavordale lamented he had not been playing higher, on a night when he won £11,000 in a single hand at hazard. Georgiana, Duchess of Devonshire, cost her husband nearly £1,000,000 in card debts. Rich as they were, they often ruined themselves. The letters of the time are loud with lamentations about the duns coming in and the furniture going out. Nor was their sexual life of a kind to commend them to an austere morality. "I was afraid I was going to have the gout the other day," writes Lord Carlisle to a friend, "I believe I live too chaste: it is not a common fault with me." It was not a common fault with any of them. In fact an unmarried man was thought unpleasantly queer, if he did not keep under his protection some sprightly full-bosomed Kitty Clive or Mrs. Bellamy, whose embraces he repaid with a house in Montpelier Square, a box at the opera, and a smart cabriolet in which to drive her down to Brighthelmstone for a week's amorous relaxation. Nor did he confine himself to professional ladies of pleasure. Even unmarried girls like Lady Hester Stanhope were suspected of having lovers; among married women the practice was too common to stir comment. The historian grows quite giddy as he tries to disentangle the complications of heredity consequent on the free and easy habits of the English aristocracy. The Harley family, children of the Countess of Oxford, were known as the Harleian Miscellany on account of the variety of fathers alleged to be responsible for their existence. The Duke of Devonshire had three children by the Duchess and two by Lady Elizabeth Foster, the Duchess one by Lord Grey; and most of them were brought up together in Devonshire House, each set of children with a surname of its own. "Emily, does it never strike you," writes Miss Pamela Fitzgerald in 1816, "the vices are wonderfully prolific among Whigs? There are such countless illegitimates, such a tribe of children of the mist." It is noteworthy that the author of this lively comment was a carefully brought up young lady of the highest breeding. The free habits of these days encouraged free speech. "Comfortable girls," remarks a middle-aged lady of her growing nieces, "who like a dirty joke." And the men, as can be imagined, were a great deal freer than the women. For all their polish the Whigs were not refined people in the Victorian sense of the word.

It appears in other aspects of their lives. They could be extremely arrogant; treating their inferiors with a patrician insolence which seems to us the reverse of good breeding. Lady Catherine de Bourgh was not the caricature that an ignorant person might suppose. Fashionable young men of refined upbringing amused themselves by watching fights where the Game Chicken battered the Tutbury Pet into unconsciousness with bare and blood-stained fists. And the pamphlets, the squibs, the appalling political cartoons that lay open in the most elegant drawing-rooms show that the ladies of the day were not squeamish either.

Still, unseemly as some of its manifestations were, one must admit that there is something extremely attractive in this earthy exuberance. And, as a matter of fact, it was the inevitable corollary of their virtues. English society had the merits of its defects. Its wide scope, its strong root in the earth, gave it an astounding, an irresistible vitality. For all their dissipation there was nothing decadent about these eighteenth century aristocrats. Their excesses came from too much life, not too little. And it was the same vitality that gave them their predominance in public life. They took on the task of directing England's destinies with the same self-confident vigour, that they drank and diced. It was this vigour that made Pitt Prime Minister at twenty-four years old,[1] that enabled the Foxites to keep the flag of liberty flying against the united public opinion of a panic-stricken nation. Nor did they let their pleasures interfere with these more serious activities. After eighteen hours of uninterrupted gambling, Charles Fox would arrive at the House of Commons to electrify his fellow members by a brilliant discourse on American taxation. Rakes and ladies of fashion intersperse their narratives of intrigue with discussions on politics, on literature, even on morals. For they were not unmoral. Their lapses came from passion not from principle; and they are liable at any time to break out in contrite acknowledgments of guilt, and artless resolutions for future improvement.

[1] Pitt diverged from the Whigs in later life: but he was brought up among them; and is, so far, representative of the Whig tradition.

Indeed it was one of the paradoxes created by their mixed composition that, though they were worldly, they were not sophisticated. Their elaborate manners masked simple reactions. Like their mode of life their characters were essentially natural; spontaneous, unintrospective, brimming over with normal feelings, love of home and family, loyalty, conviviality, desire for fame, hero-worship, patriotism. And they showed their feelings too. Happy creatures! They lived before the days of the stiff upper lip and the inhibited public school Englishman. A manly tear stood in their eye at the story of a heroic deed: they declared their loves in a strain of flowery hyperbole. They were the more expressive from their very unselfconsciousness. It never struck them that they needed to be inarticulate to appear sincere. They were equally frank about their less elevated sentiments. Eighteenth century rationalism combined with rural common sense to make them robustly ready to face unedifying facts. And they declared their impressions with a brusque honesty, outstandingly characteristic of them. From Sir Robert Walpole who encouraged coarse conversation on the ground that it was the only form of talk which everyone enjoyed, down to the Duke of Wellington who described the army of his triumphs as composed of "the scum of the earth, enlisted for drink," the Augustan aristocracy, Whig and Tory alike, said what they thought with a superb disregard for public opinion. For if they were not original they were independent-minded. The conventions which bounded their lives were conventions of form only. Since they had been kings of their world from birth they were free from the tiresome inhibitions that are induced by a sense of inferiority. Within the locked garden of their society, individuality flowered riotous and rampant. Their typical figures show up beside the muted introverts of to-day as clear-cut and idiosyncratic as characters in Dickens. They took for granted that you spoke your mind and followed your impulses. If these were odd they were amused but not disapproving. They enjoyed eccentrics; George Selwyn who never missed an execution, Beau Brummel who took three hours to tie his cravat. The firm English soil in which they were rooted, the spacious freedom afforded by their place in the world, allowed personality to flourish in as many bold and fantastic shapes as it pleased.

But it was always a garden plant, a civilized growth. Whatever their eccentricities, the Whig nobles were never provincial and never uncouth. They had that effortless knowledge of the world that comes only to those, who from childhood have been accustomed to move in a complex society; that delightful unassertive confidence possible only to people who have never had cause to doubt their social position. And they carried to the finest degree of cultivation those social arts which engaged so much of their time. Here we come to their outstanding distinction. They were the most agreeable society England has ever known. The character of their agreeability was of a piece with the rest of them; mundane, straightforward, a trifle philistine, largely concerned with gossip, not given to subtle analyses or flights of fancy. But it had all their vitality and all their sense of style. It was incomparably racy and spontaneous and accomplished; based solidly on a wide culture and experience, yet free to express itself in bursts of high spirits, in impulses of appreciation, in delicate movements of sentiment, in graceful compliments. For it had its grace; a virile classical grace like that of the Chippendale furniture which adorned its rooms, lending a glittering finish to its shrewd humour, its sharp-eyed observation, its vigorous disquisitions on men and things. Educated without pedantry, informal but not slipshod, polished but not precious, brilliant without fatigue, it combined in an easy perfection the charms of civilization and nature. Indeed the whole social life of the period shines down the perspective of history like some masterpiece of natural art; a prize bloom, nurtured in shelter and sunshine and the richest soil, the result of generations of breeding and blending, that spreads itself to the open sky in strength and beauty.

It was at its most characteristic in the middle of the century, it was at its most dazzling towards its close. By 1780 a new spirit was rising in the world. Ossian had taught people to admire ruins and ravines, Rousseau to examine the processes of the heart; with unpowdered heads and the ladies in simple muslin dresses, they paced the woods meditating, in Cowperlike mood, on the tender influences of nature. Though they kept the style and good sense of their fathers, their sympathies were wider. At the same time their feelings grew more refined. The hardness, which had marred the previous age, dwindled. Gainsborough, not Hogarth, mirrored the taste of the time; sensibility became a fashionable word. For a fleeting moment Whig society had a foot in two worlds and made the best of both of them. The lucid outline of eighteenth-century civilization was softened by the glow of the romantic dawn.

Dawn—but for them it was sunset. The same spirit that tinged them with their culminating glory was also an omen of their dissolution. For the days of aristocratic supremacy were numbered. By the iron laws which condition the social structure of man's existence, it could only last as long as it maintained an economic predominance. With the coming of the Industrial Revolution this predominance began to pass from the landlords to other ranks of the community. Already by the close of the century, go-ahead manufacturers in the north were talking of Parliamentary reform; already, in the upper rooms of obscure London alleys, working men met together to clamour for liberty, equality, and fraternity. Within forty years of its zenith, the Whig world was completely swept away. Only a few survivors lingered on to illustrate to an uncomprehending generation the charm of the past. Of these the most distinguished was William Lamb, second Viscount Melbourne.[2]

[2] *Editors' note:* "The Whig World" is the opening chapter of Cecil's biography of Lord Melbourne; hence this sentence, which is not so much a conclusion of the chapter as a forecast of the subject of the book.

Suggestions for Study

MOST OF this piece seems to be plain statement; Cecil only occasionally allows himself an obviously decorative sentence: "Night after night they played loo and faro from early evening till the candles guttered pale in the light of the risen sun"; or "Indeed the whole social life of the period shines down the perspective of history like some masterpiece of natural art; a prize bloom, nurtured in shelter and sunshine and the richest soil, the result of generations of breeding and blending that spreads itself to the open sky in strength and beauty." In each of these sentences there is a conspicuous heightening of the rhythm: *pale* (not *palely*) and *risen* in the first sentence, and the repeated *and*'s in "shelter and sunshine and the richest soil" in the second sentence were probably chosen for their effect on the rhythm. There is an archaic formality about both *pale* and *risen;* and this, along with the elaborate sentence pattern and the alliteration and assonance (e. g., "shelter and sunshine," "breeding and blending"), deepens the tone of these sentences, in an admirable contrast with the generally rather astringent style.

On the whole Cecil seems to write like a historian, telling us facts, giving us conclusions. The sentences are short, with a tone of finality; and we are not much aware of subsidiary clauses that might take the emphasis off the fact that each sentence carries. The paragraph beginnings seem to be part of a complex argument: "Yet they are not"; "For the elaboration of their life"; "Yet—and here it is that it differs"; "Their life, in fact, was essentially"; "In practice, of course, this ideal was not so broad"; and so on. Many abstract conceptions suggest a historian's appraisal of a period; but note how nicely these are balanced by concrete allusions and examples. Many abstract or Latinate words suggest the scholar's aridity of style; but again, note how these are balanced by concrete or English words.

Yet Cecil does not achieve his effect by the logic of his argument, or by the control of his style. For he is not really trying to convince us of some new interpretation of Whig society, or to present us with new facts about it. Rather he is asking us to understand this "masterpiece of natural art," to understand this paradox of "splendid naturalness." And when he says, "Here we come to their outstanding distinction," we are aware at last that we have been led, or cajoled, to accept his statement that "they were the most agreeable society England has ever known." Cecil's facts are indeed facts, but facts of an especially amusing or dramatic kind, which exemplify the incongruities of human nature while at the same time they record the special qualities of the Augustan age.

Cecil's sentences are indeed short and somewhat dry, but there is a wonderful variation in their attack and in their pattern. After several sentences that seem merely informative, we are given one like this: "Since life to them was so secure and so pleasant, the Whig aristocrats tended to take its fundamental values very much for granted; they concentrated rather on how to live," in which the argument is at once summed up and expanded. Or a sentence like this: "And general principles to them were an occasion for expression rather than thought," in which the wit and the epigrammatic structure compress a good deal of acute criticism of eighteenth-century thinking. Neither the style nor the content of the essay is florid or sentimental; there is about it only the "easy perfection" of civilization.

The English Tradition

THOMAS SHARP (1901–)

I. NEVER THE REAL *Urbs?*

IN A SKETCH called *Nottingham and the Mining Countryside*, written probably about 1929, D. H. Lawrence described English towns as "a great scrabble of ugly pettiness over the face of the land." "The English," he asserted, "are town birds through and through. Yet they don't know how to build a city, how to think of one, or how to live in one. They are all suburban, pseudo-cottagy, and not one of them knows how to be truly urban. . . . The English may be mentally and spiritually developed. But as citizens of splendid cities they are more ignominious than rabbits."

Those are hard words. But looking at most of our towns to-day, at the vast drab areas of mean streets and the dull engulfing suburbs around them, it is difficult to deny that the description is only a little exaggerated. We are the most urban nation in the world. Something like 80 per cent. of us live in urban areas. In the last twenty years we have added over four million houses to our towns. And yet, considered either as architectural compositions or as utilities for the collective living of any reasonable kind of social life, our towns fall miserably short of what they should be.

Our towns have been repulsive and inefficient for a hundred years and more—for so long, in fact, that most of us have become almost inured to their badness. Even those of us who are still aware of the possibility of a town's being an orderly, perhaps a beautiful creation, have come to regard the building of fine towns as a faculty which has somehow been denied to Englishmen. That opinion has been expressed innumerable times. Lawrence, in his Nottingham sketch, expressed it again. "England has had towns for centuries," he said. "But they have never been real towns, only clusters of village streets. Never the real *urbs.*"

Yet that is quite untrue. The English once built towns which, according to the standards of their times, were excellent instruments for the living of a good social life; which were altogether admirable essays in large-scale architectural composition. Those towns were at least as fine as any in their contemporary world. Incredible as it may seem now, they even held promise of our becoming the best of town-builders instead of what we have become —pretty nearly the worst.

Right up till a hundred years ago there was a remarkably strong and virile town tradition in England. That tradition was very different from the continental tradition. It was none the worse for that. But it is a curious thing that to-day not only the ordinary citizen, not only writers like Lawrence, but our professional men whose job it is to study and build towns, our architects and town-planners, are mostly unaware that such a tradition ever existed, and are content to belaud foreign towns and sigh plaintively because we have never built in precisely the same way in England.

Towns have sometimes been described as the physical expression of a nation's civilisation. The physical form of a town does in many ways reflect fairly accurately the social condition of the people who live in it, their mode of life, their cultural achievement, their economic status, the kind of government they possess. The town reflects these characteristics because it arises out of them. And it is, of course, precisely because of this that the English town tradition developed on its own individual lines.

Our fall from grace has been very deep during the last century. We are not very sensible, however, because of that, to forget that we once did, in fact, live and build in grace. It is, indeed, all the more necessary for us to remember. The English contribution to the art of building towns was once an original and a valuable one. It is important that this should be realised, for if we are ever again to build good towns we shall need to restore our lost confidence, and perhaps to re-establish something of the old tradition.

2. THE ENGLISH TRADITION IN THE TOWN

Even as early as mediæval times those factors that have been mentioned as influencing the physical form of the town—i. e., methods of government, economic organisation and the like—began to give the English town certain individual characteristics. Though in most countries in the mediæval period, and even later, the necessity for defence led to varying degrees of congestion within city walls, here a settled form of government and the natural protection of geographical isolation made walls unnecessary at a comparatively early date. Because of this it was possible for our towns to develop on a more spacious scale. Then with this lack of the necessity for defence there was coupled that early "industrial revolution" concerned with the production of wool and its manufacture into cloth, upon which so much of England's prosperity depended from the 15th right down to the 19th century. And this, besides making possible the development of the great number of country towns which is so pleasant a feature of England, resulted also in that lack of a sharp distinction between small town and village which is probably the real cause of people like Lawrence describing our towns as "clusters of village streets": for the fact is not so much that those towns are like villages, as that, in general, our villages, in spite of their many rural features, their greens, their occasional cottage gardens, their old trees, have nevertheless a certain air of urbanity, though not of urbanness, about them.

The most individual characteristics of the English town tradition, however, were expressed during that great period of town planning, the architectural Renaissance. The towns that were built or extended in England during the two hundred years of Renaissance building may be much less spectacular than many built at the same time in other parts of Europe; but the truth is, in spite of what Lawrence and his like maintain, they were generally far more genuine as towns. The English town was built for no other purpose than to house free citizens as comfortably and pleasantly as was possible according to the standards of the time, and with as much outward order and seemliness as could be achieved without the exercise of a tyrannical compulsion. It was a genuine utility, though in many ways a very imperfect one, for facilitating the collective living of a democratic body of people. The most admired of the finely planned quarters of certain continental towns of this period, on the other hand, were less utilities for collective living than symbolic expressions, material glorifications, of the power of the absolute monarchs, the autocratic princelings, the military dictators who dominated and exploited those towns.

Many of the principal European cities, including Paris and Vienna, were not even that. Paris, for example, less than a hundred years ago was nothing more than a vast, squalid, insanitary huddle of narrow, crooked streets and tumble-down houses, with a few bold squares and one or two magnificent vistas that had been vaingloriously planted on to it by a succession of dictators over a period of three hundred years and more. As a utility for collective living, it was very far from being the fine place that it is to-day. It was, in fact, wretchedly inadequate for any such purpose; and Lawrence's phrase about rabbits might with very considerable truth have been used of the Parisians of that time.

By comparison with this, London, as late as seventy-five or a hundred years ago, was a supremely civilised city. From the 17th century onwards it had developed in a fine tradition of domestic graciousness; and in some hundreds of squares and a multitude of streets it could lay claim to being far away the best-built capital city in the world. The early squares and streets of the 17th and the greater part of the 18th centuries were not perhaps perfectly unified architectural compositions. They were developed piecemeal, often over a considerable period—sometimes over twenty or thirty years and more. As a result, though all their buildings were informed by the common urbane spirit of the age and were "so far uniform as to be all sashed and all pretty nearly of an equal height," they fell somewhat short of formal architectural perfection. They were nevertheless extremely pleasant places to live in. Their very lack of any show of architectural monumentality, their quiet, gracious air of domesticity, helped them in this. These were places where people lived their own lives as citizens, not adjuncts of a court on perpetual parade.

If such pleasantness is not entirely sufficient to constitute the "real *urbs*," if perhaps architectural formality also is necessary, then the London squares that were built from about 1770 onwards till well on into the 19th century had that quality also.

The houses in the earlier squares had mostly been put up one or two at a time for individual clients. Now speculating builders began building whole squares at a single undertaking, whole *series* of squares, even, and the connecting streets between them. These squares and streets were not generally the work of "great" architects. Only occasionally was some well-known name connected with them, as the Adam brothers were associated with the Adelphi or John Nash with Regent Street. Ordinarily their builders were so little known as to be practically anonymous. They were just *builders:* speculators like Thomas Cubitt, who developed a great deal of Bloomsbury and most of Belgravia: men who were not in the least conscious of creating works of art, certainly not building monuments to themselves or to anyone else, but just building quarters for citizens to live in; and because the citizens of the time did not expect a flamboyant expression of their own individuality in their houses, but were content to subscribe to the principles of order and good design, building them simply and soberly, making them (to use the modern cant phrase) "machines for living in" rather than conscious masterpieces of architectural design.

Though they probably did not aim at great urban architecture, these unpretentious builders nevertheless achieved it. For sheer urbanity these London streets and squares of this later period have never been bettered anywhere. They are gracious, calm, reticent, perfectly civilized, admirable in their architectural refinement. In their simple, orderly composition, where no one house attempts domination over its neighbours, they are the perfect expression of citizenship, of the art of living in co-operative association.

Even so, however finely urbane might be their architecture, these squares would still have fallen short of providing the admirable solution they do provide of the problem of living comfortably in a great city had there not been another feature to add to their pleasantness. In all the earlier squares it had been the practice to leave the central area paved in the fashion of most continental squares. It was only later—towards the end of the 18th century—that it became the practice to lay out those central areas as gardens with lawns and free-growing trees. And so, at the very time when formality was the keynote for building, there was sufficient realisation of the psychological needs of the town-dweller for further aids to comfortable living to be planned for and provided.

It is difficult to conceive how it can be said that a people which has done these things has never known "how to build a city, how to think of one, or how to live in one." Compared with other contemporary cities, London a hundred years ago must have been a splendid city both to look at and to live in. It had these fine urbane streets and squares. It had abundantly the kind of facilities for social intercourse (at Vauxhall, Ranelagh and similar places) which we now associate only with continental towns. It had admirable cultural institutions. It had excellent parks and promenades (the one royal contribution). It had the countryside within easy walking distance of even its central districts. It had not, of course, the fine vistas, the imposing avenues, the boulevards, the monumental groupings of present-day Paris or Vienna. But, then, neither had Paris nor Vienna themselves: those features they were to acquire later, after London and all other English towns had been swamped by a heartless commercialism. Compared to Paris, Vienna, or any other large city in the world, London a hundred years ago must have seemed almost an ideal place.

The English provincial town, too, had nothing to fear in a comparison with continental provincial cities. The planned towns here were certainly not as monumental as some of their German and French counterparts. They had no spectacular vistas, no radiating avenues. They consisted generally of just a few streets and squares, not arranged in any very logically connected sequences, and lacking in grand climaxes. They were very pleasant towns for citizens to live in, nevertheless; real towns, not mere monuments to autocracy, as were so many continental planned palace suburbs: and they had at least a fine urbanity, if not a monumental splendour, in their architectural character.

It would be tedious to list a mere catalogue of the English towns which contain fine work in the excellent native tradition. A host of inland and seaside resorts, including Bath, Cheltenham, Brighton and Weymouth, to give particular examples; numbers of commercial towns like Bristol, Newcastle-on-Tyne, Plymouth, Liverpool, to mention a few that come immediately to mind: some Irish towns, too, and especially Dublin, with its gracious squares and streets that have fallen from their one-time glory into a wretched slumdom: and one or two Scottish towns, with Edinburgh New Town standing out importantly because of the mere bulk and the perfect coherence of the work there—in all these places the quarters that were developed in the 18th or early 19th century have a fine formal architectural unity. And besides these formally organised developments, most of the buildings in nearly all the towns of this period, in ports, country towns, small manufacturing towns, were so informed with the general spirit of the age, they subscribed so closely to the common architectural tradition, that, though formal compositional perfection might be lacking, they achieved, these individual buildings, such a similarity of expression, such a unity of spirit, that the towns which they formed had still, in spite of their unplanned growth, a general sense of order and a fine air of urbanity as well.

To say all this is not for a moment to suggest that the English town of this period was the *perfect* utility for collective living. It obviously was not. In it the poorer kind of citizen had no very great share of the pleasantness. He lived in cramped and congested quarters hidden away behind the spacious middle-class streets and squares. While the English town was not in any sense the instrument of a personal absolutism, many of its chief benefits were enjoyed only by one powerful section of the community. It was essentially the creation of its times: it could not be anything else: it was bound to reflect the social standards of the age—and they were a long way from perfection. Nor were the continental towns by any means all of the kind that have been suggested. Many of them were as free from the dictation of Absolutism as the English towns themselves, and were as pleasant to live in. Generalisations are easy and dangerous, and no doubt the generalisation that the English town of the 18th and 19th centuries was the best kind of town in its contemporary world, and that English architecture of that time was the most truly urbane, may seem to be as rash as it is unusual. But it is far less rash, and infinitely less absurd, than the assertion which has been repeated *ad nauseam*, that the English have never been good townsmen or good town-builders. Leaving aside all odious and dangerous comparisons, we can still say that the English up till a hundred years ago did this—they built towns that were comfortable to live in and extremely pleasant to look at: they regarded the town not as a mere spectacle: not at all as an opportunity for architectural bravura, not as a monument, not as a glorification of anybody or anything, but as something far superior to all these, simply as a home, the dwelling-place of a community (in so far as that conception was realised), a place designed for living in.

The Renaissance tradition did not last so long in England as it did elsewhere. It was a fine, singing, high-flying bird that was knocked to smithereens by two wretched missiles: one the smothering dough-lump of the Romantic Revival; the other the iron-hard money-bag of the Industrial Revolution.

We cannot go into the story of it here. It has been written in numbers of books, and only too solidly and inescapably in innumerable buildings that most of us must see every day of our lives in all the vast 19th-century quarters of our towns. It is sufficient to say that not only the characteristic English tradition, but the English town in its entirety, has never recovered from that dual blow.

First there came the degradation of the town: utter black and hopeless degradation. In foul slums and in deserts of dreary byelaw-standardised streets, in the sun-obscuring murk of factory chimneys, the very conception of the town *as a town* disappeared from English minds. By the end of the 19th century, so vilely had the English towns been built in the period of their greatest extension, the whole conception of the town as a home, as a utility for collective living of a good life, as a place where beauty might be created, whence enlightenment might emanate, had vanished into the anything but thin contemporary air. The town was no longer any of these things. It was a mere multiplication of that object of Victorian hate and fear—the workhouse: a hateful prison-workhouse, sordid, brutal, mean. The town should be an object of love and loyalty. The Victorian town was an object of indifference at best, of hatred and loathing at worst.

It was small wonder, then, that the majority of its inhabitants waited longingly, almost hopelessly, for the opportunity to escape. And when that opportunity did eventually come, with the invention of the motor-car, its was inevitable that they should escape in headlong flight—to the suburbs.

In one sense this flight to the suburbs is not entirely disconnected from the old tradition. The marked characteristic of that tradition was, as we have seen, an emphasis on the domestic rather than the monumental aspect of building. The emphasis is still on the home rather than the monument: it is, indeed, on it with a vengeance. But the new way of building is a dreadful debasement of the old tradition. The old emphasis was on the domestic character of the town. But it was on the *town*, not merely on the individual house. The town was domestic not so much because it was a collection of domestic units, as because its character was expressed through the use of those units for collective effect: whatever beauty and dignity it had was integral with its domestic character, and was not thrust upon it by external influences for non-civic, personal-monumental purposes. Now, however, in the new suburbs domesticity is everywhere and the town is nowhere at all. In reaction against the 19th-century degradation both of the whole and the part, that debasement both of the town and the house, it is individual not collective domesticity that is expressed in the partial renewal of the submerged tradition. The new suburban "town" is no longer a collective home, it is a mere collection of thousands of little individual homes. The new emphasis on individual domesticity has destroyed collective domesticity. The home is, in fact, being destroyed by the houses.

Now indeed Lawrence's description is only too true: "A great scrabble of ugly pettiness over the face of the land." Littleness, suburbanity, petty individualism triumphant. Truly the English "don't know how to build a city, how to think of one, how to live in one." Undeniably "they are all suburban, pseudo-cottagy and not one of them knows how to be truly urban." There is no use denying it: it is all too obviously written far and wide over the face of the land.

Yet we should remember for our souls' sake, and for the future's, that it wasn't always so.

3. WHO MADE THE COUNTRY?

The 20th-century Englishman has forgotten that Englishmen once built fine towns because his immediate predecessors murdered those towns. It is not improbable, if things go on as they have done for the last twenty years, that the 21st-century Englishman will have similar cause to forget that his countrymen once developed a beautiful countryside also.

We have almost forgotten it already. Even while widespread destruction of that countryside goes on, we still, paradoxically enough, like a man who absent-mindedly kills what he loves, profess pride in and derive deep enjoyment from its beauty. But how that beauty ever came about is a question which never occurs to anyone any more. If we think about it at all, it is with the thought that it is only proper that God should be specially good to us, that it is natural for him to look after his own. The fact that it was not God, but the Englishmen of the 18th century, who made the landscape (those very Englishmen who built the fine forgotten towns) has passed so completely out of mind that the suggestion seems almost like blasphemy.

The conception of the landscape as a thing of man-made beauty has vanished as completely as the conception of the town's being a creation capable of any beauty at all. And this, at bottom, is why that beauty is so rapidly being despoiled. For when once man ceases to acknowledge, or even to realise, his function as creator, there is little likelihood of his achieving beauty (or order, or even mere efficiency) in the things he unconsciously and thoughtlessly creates. Beauty rarely happens of itself in man-created or man-directed things. It generally has to be sought after. And while it may be present in infinite measure in entirely natural (i. e., primeval) landscapes, the extent of its measure in a man-inhabited landscape depends ultimately upon man's realisation of his function as creator or adapter: upon that and, of course, upon the scope and extent of his activity there.

It is obvious, if the matter is considered at all, that every civilised landscape must be largely man-made. Civilised man everywhere *must* alter and adapt the natural landscape to suit his mode of life. His very existence, his civilisation depends on it. Man would never have emerged from barbarism had he not done so. When once he left off his nomadic wanderings he immediately took up the rôle of creator. The first forest-clearing, wherever it might have been; the first surface scratching to raise some desired crop; the first raising of some burial-mound—these were all essays, though unconscious ones, in the creation of landscape. As the character of men's towns reflects their social condition, their economic status, their form of government—in short, their civilisation—so does the character of their countryside. It reflects them because it arises out of them.

The principle of it is something like this. The appearance of any cultural landscape is determined in two ways: by what man has inherited in the chaos of the landscape's first created form, and by what he has done with that heritage. He has inherited a complex structure of rocks (a geological formation) already moulded into hills, valleys and plains whose configuration he can do little to alter. Over these are laid soils of different natures according to the natures of the rocks themselves. These soils place certain limits on what he can grow on his landscape. Similarly he has to take as he gets it that other natural phenomenon, the weather. But given these materials and limitations he is free to do as he likes with his landscape, and although he cannot literally mould and shape it, he is always, consciously or unconsciously, adapting it to suit his own needs.

The primary purpose of landscape-adaptation everywhere is to produce the means of human subsistence: the primary motive is essentially economic. But there is another kind of adaptation that may be carried on alongside this economic one, and sometimes even independently of it—the adaptation of the landscape for æsthetic purposes, for the creation of a countryside which, besides producing the means of life, will be in itself a comfortable and a satisfying place to live in.

The primary economic motive has been the only motive in most parts of the world. Generally men have cleared the forest, drained the swamp, cultivated the land; that is all. Sometimes a utilitarian motive that produced æsthetic effect almost accidentally has crept in, as when, for example, in southern countries roadsides have been planted with avenues of trees for shade. And very generally, of course, the immediate surroundings of human habitations have been embellished by groupings of trees, by the planting of gardens. These activities and activities like them have softened and to some extent humanised the bald economic pattern in many landscapes. They have almost always, however, been restricted in scope and limited in scale.

It is only rarely that humanisation with a strong conscious

æsthetic motive has been practised on any large scale and applied to a whole tract of landscape. When it has been so practised and so applied it has in most countries been done for monumental effect. The great set-pieces of landscape design as much as those of civic design have generally been associated with the personal glorification of some autocrat. Thus a Versailles has been created; a stupendous landscape spectacle made at a colossal expenditure of money and human lives to satisfy the vanity of a Louis XIV: a dramatic show-piece set in a neglected countryside in much the same way as the squares and vistas of Paris were set in the midst of a squalid slum-city.

But here, in the landscape as in the town, we have taken our own individual line in England. Partly as a result of our social and political traditions, and partly because of our early developed love of natural beauty, we have created not merely a few spectacular show-pieces, the personal monuments of Absolutism, but a whole landscape that is everywhere enriched for the benefit of all those who dwell in it. And we have done so with such effect that whatever may have been thought of our towns, however humble a place our achievement in that direction may wrongly have been given, the beauty that has here been created in landscape has been so universally acknowledged that the English countryside may be claimed to be one of the supreme achievements of civilisation.

4. THE ENGLISH TRADITION IN THE COUNTRYSIDE

Up till towards the end of the 17th century the English countryside had much in common with most western European landscapes. There was, no doubt, a heavier proportion of grassland to arable than was general, for the great English woollen trade required extensive pasturage for its sheep, and the temperate climate provided it in excellent quality. Even so there was probably then a greater extent of arable land than there is now. This ploughland was nearly all cultivated on that open-field system of strip cultivation which had continued for nearly a thousand years since the Saxons developed it here, and which is still the agricultural economy in many parts of Europe. The open-field system meant an almost complete absence of hedges. There was, too, by the 17th century a great shortage of sizable trees, for the forests had long been cleared as more and more land was brought into cultivation, and a great deal of the remaining scattered timber had been used for industrial purposes such as iron-smelting and glass-making, and for the building of ships. Great parts of the English landscape at this time must have been bare and patchy in appearance, with immense windy open fields and unfenced commons, dotted only occasionally by a few spindly trees or a thicket of brushwood. It must have been a drab and unfriendly landscape not unlike some of the depressing landscapes of northern France to-day.

It was because of this very bareness and patchiness that beauty was eventually brought forth in abundance. A precise date can almost be put, if not upon the change in the landscape itself, at least upon the change in the Englishman's attitude towards it. In 1664, alarmed by the danger that the scarcity of timber implied for the future of the navy, John Evelyn published his book *Sylva.* That "trumpet call to the nation on the condition of their woods and forests" appealed so successfully to the patriotic feelings of Evelyn's countrymen that *Sylva* ran through edition after edition, and created everywhere enthusiasm for the practice of the new and exciting art of arboriculture. The English as a nation of tree-lovers may be said to date from this time. And this is the important part of it. For Evelyn's appeal and the nation's response were not from limited patriotic reasons alone. If they had been, the English landscape would probably have been very different from what it is to-day. But the appeal was founded as much on æsthetic as on patriotic grounds. It was addressed to "Noble Persons to adorn their goodly Mansions and Demesnes with trees of venerable shade" for beauty's as well as for the Navy's sake; and it was in this spirit of creating beauty, at least as much as from political and economic necessity, that the English landowners seized the opportunity which came a little later to refashion the landscape of England.

The opportunity came in the first years of the 18th century. By that time it had become obvious that the old agricultural methods of the common-field system were now quite hopelessly inefficient for producing the nation's food. Farmers had their open-field holdings in various small, narrow strips of land scattered wildly over all parts of a parish, and this inevitably involved waste of time and energy. It also obstructed the development of a more mechanical form of husbandry which recent advancements had made possible. The long, narrow shape of each strip had necessitated centuries of ploughing in the same direction, with the inevitable result of the impoverishment of the soil. The fact that the open fields were held in common for half the year obstructed the change from a three-course to a four-course rotation that promised to revolutionise farming. These and numerous other factors made the growing class of men who were interested in the improvement of the land impatient to be rid of the old enfeebled agricultural economy. Old methods were out-of-date. New knowledge demanded new forms for its expression. The old must give way to the new. Thus the final abandonment of the thousand-year-old agricultural system and the wholesale enclosure and redistribution of the land had become inevitable.

It was a wonderful opportunity and it was wonderfully utilised. Such an immense work as the complete alteration of large parts of the landscape of England could never, of course, have arisen save in economic and political necessity. And that is the glory of it. The adaptation of the old agricultural system to new requirements need not have led to any very great æsthetic improvement, even though the most satisfactory method of enclosure had itself the beauty of a living fence or hedgerow. The more rational distribution of the land was a mere matter of the alteration of the shape and size of parcels. That alone need have made little difference to the appearance of England. But the desire to create a new beauty, the desire to make a landscape that was more than economically efficient, that was, in fact, a home as well as a work-place, was there so strongly and vividly, awaiting merely an opportunity of expression, that, the opportunity occurring, the use of it for æsthetic purposes was at least as important in the minds of 18th-century Englishmen as its economic and political possibilities.

The æsthetic motive had developed rapidly from its first important expression in Evelyn's *Sylva*. The early tree-planting which followed Evelyn's appeal had been carried out in that planting of avenues that was so characteristic of French grand manner. But the English aversion for the grand manner and a growing appreciation of a "natural" beauty defeated this. Actually the "natural" beauty that was more favoured was that of the highly idealised landscapes of painters like Claude, Salvator Rosa, Poussin and others. It was not "natural" in that it was strictly an imitation of Nature (though later landscapists maintained that they aimed at this). It was natural only in that the landscape was not forced into formal patterns but was free, was modelled for pictorial rather than dragooned for monumental effect. What was aimed at by the great band of enthusiastic 18th-century landscapists who arose to seize the offered opportunity was the creation in actuality of something like those ideal landscapes that Claude and Poussin and others had imagined on canvas.

All this was no easy task to be undertaken lightly. It cost a vast amount of money and trouble. And there is this to be particularly remembered. The men who undertook this work could not hope to see it come to anything like full pictorial perfection. Working in natural slow-growing materials they could never hope themselves to see the scenes that they planned. They planned, they worked, they expended their money and energy to provide delight and profit for future generations, knowing full well that they would be forgotten by the time their labours materialised. It was a very noble work: a work of which we, two hundred years later, might well think with admiration and awe.

Beauty, of course, has many qualities and is of many kinds. It can be of a kind which, immediately stimulating in its grandeur or nobility, is nevertheless oppressive to live with perpetually. It can be of a kind that is too impersonal, too detached from human relationship to maintain a long and enduring appeal. It can be of a kind that in the long run is disturbing rather than comforting to the human spirit. Or it may be of that more intimate order that throws grace and serenity over vastness, that brings the might and the mystery of the world within easier human comprehension, that is a comfort and a solace to the perplexed human spirit.

It is this latter kind of beauty that has been given to the English countryside. The landscape has been humanised with natural materials. It has been given friendliness and a calm quality of security. It has been brought into a satisfying human relationship. The terrifying scale of Nature has been reduced. Distance has been conquered. Vastness has been reduced to a succession of small units. The apparently infinite has been rounded to a pattern, has been given a recognisable rhythm.

All this has been achieved by the simplest of means—merely by clothing the economic pattern of the landscape, by defining its units with solid visible boundaries of living hedges, by embellishing those hedges with trees that have been allowed to grow to their full maturity. It is these elements, the hedges and the hedgerow trees, that constitute the beauty of England. The woodlands and copses, the parklands of the great houses—these features also make their valuable contribution to the scene. But essentially this lovely English landscape is compounded of the modest use of simple elements: it is itself essentially simple: there is nothing grand or spectacular about it: it is, as William Morris described it, "neither prison nor palace, but a decent home."

A decent home. That is the crux of the matter. The English activity, the English tradition, has never been directed towards the creation of the monuments that delighted and still delight the Baroque mind. Theatricality and display, the love of the show-piece and the spectacle, have had little part in the national make-up. By nature we have tended to avoid the counterplay of high light and shadow and have striven to maintain a steady gleam. The unthinking intoxication of an occasional burst of wild extravagance does not, to us, compensate for a general average of dull impoverishment. So in our towns and our countryside, as in other things, we have concentrated, in our great days at least, on the more domestic virtues. But the town and the countryside are after all more a home than a playhouse, and the domestic virtues are in place there.

Here, then, is what it all comes to. In spite of everything that has been said, and that nowadays deserves to be said, against the English town, that town up till a hundred years ago, considered as a pure town—that is, as a place for citizens to live in—was one of the most successful creations of its kind in its contemporary world. The countryside created at that same time was even more successful for its own particular purpose. Both these parts of the national synthesis were admirably designed and developed to provide a worthy physical setting for human lives: they constituted a home where order and beauty in good measure facilitated the achievement of human happiness.

5. PAST AND PRESENT

That briefly is the story of the English achievement in town and countryside. It has not been told here from any promptings of smug patriotic satisfaction. It is a story to make us ashamed rather than proud to-day. History is chiefly of value in so far as we can learn from it anything that will help us to shape the future better; and from this we can get two aids for our future activity. One is the knowledge that the old resigned confession that the English have never built good towns is a foolish lie. This at least should encourage as well as shame us. The other is the knowledge that where the 18th-century Englishman succeeded was in his seizing of the opportunities for improvement which changing conditions offered, and that where the Victorian failed, and where we fail to-day, is in our incapacity to seize similar and even greater opportunities that have been offered to us.

In the last hundred years we have had marvellous opportunities for building good towns, and we have missed them all. The speed with which our towns have been newly built and extended has been used time and again as an excuse for their badness. Yet if our sense of values had not been utterly corrupted we would have *used* that speed as a heaven-sent opportunity. It is difficult to get order and organisation and architectural cohesion into a town that grows slowly, where only a house or a cottage is added here and there at long intervals over a course of several hundred years. But when a town or a new large quarter of a town is built as a single undertaking in a few years, then there is the perfect opportunity of obtaining all those qualities that make a town good to live in. All down the 19th century we had the most splendid opportunities for building fine towns; infinitely greater opportunities than any that occurred in the 18th century. Brutalised and corrupted in our values, we missed them most tragically. In the last twenty years we have had even greater opportunities, since local authorities have had power at hand to plan and control, and have themselves built hundreds of thousands of houses. Seduced by a trivial romanticism, we have again bungled the opportunity, and instead of fine towns we have built our squandering, tawdry, empty suburbs. We of this generation hold an awful responsibility there. Future generations will despise us as we despise the Victorians, and they will have even greater reason. Yet it is not too late to retrieve ourselves to some extent. The opportunity is not yet entirely gone. There are still great areas of slums, and far greater areas of sad and dreary though sanitary streets that cry out for rebuilding. If we set ourselves vigorously to seize this opportunity, to snatch from it every possibility of doing our work in the finest instead of the easiest way, then we may once again build towns that will be worthy of us, that will have beauty and order and all the facilities for the living of that good social and physical life which it is the prime purpose of the town to provide.

And as the town must change and develop, so must the countryside. The anxious cry of "Preserve the countryside" that has gone up of recent years is understandable in view of the damage that has been wrought on that lovely heritage. Yet it represents an unattainable hope—and a dangerous one. The countryside is not merely scenery: it is a place of industry as much as is the town, a place of social and economic activity. It is a living organism. And it is impossible to preserve any living organism in the condition at which it has arrived at any particular moment of time. To preserve it is merely to kill it.

All life involves change, growth, development. We must recognise that change cannot be stopped. It can, however, be directed. That is what we have got to remember when we set our hopes on the future of the countryside. And in remembering this we should remember, too, for our inspiration, that the countryside we now enjoy largely arose out of changing conditions that were comparable both in scale and in character to those which are operating so disastrously to-day.

The great changes which in the 18th century altered the face of England and turned it from a bare and patchy universality into its recent individual loveliness were, as we have seen, the results of social, economic and mechanical advancements. The reorganisation of the system of land tenure, the development of agriculture through the production of new types of crops and new methods of producing them, were changes as great as those that face us to-day. But the Englishmen of the 18th century did not try to ignore them. They didn't cry "Preserve, preserve." They accepted them joyfully and eagerly for what they really were—as opportunities for improvement. They set about deliberately adorning for their æsthetic satisfaction the new pattern which the social and economic changes had brought into the landscape. They created a new England from the one that was outworn.

We to-day shall have to admit similar changes. We cannot stop them even if we wish to. So long as the landscape is a scene of economic activity (which it must always be) we are bound to admit the expression of new forms of knowledge, the operation of new social and economic requirements. Once again agriculture is in decline, and new methods of farming may change the old pattern. Once again there is a great necessity for new tree-planting. Once again the system of land tenure is in need of rationalisation. Once more there are new mechanical advancements that require to be expressed, that need to be absorbed into the landscape. And in addition to these there is the greatest change of all, the new demands of the townsman for a place where he had none before. All these are disrupting factors now. But that is because we make no effort to direct them, to correlate them, to weld them into a great scheme for improvement. We stand miserably by, those of us who are conscious of the destruction that is being wrought, a small and ineffectual minority. We bemoan the change, make feverish little efforts here and there to save a "beauty spot." And all the while we betray our own littleness, our timidity, our lack of spirit. If we had any imagination we would realise how favoured is this generation in the opportunity it is given. If we had the will and the energy we would use our opportunity for the making of an English countryside far finer even than that we have inherited, finer because it would not only have, as the old countryside had, all its constituents organised in a sympathetic relationship to each other to make a splendid whole, but would have among those constituents the facilities necessary to enable the great new inventions to confer their immense potential benefits upon the 20th-century inhabitants of a 20th-century England.

This, then, is what the past offers us for the future. A fine tradition of developing town and countryside as a home, lovingly decorated, proudly yet modestly designed. A fine tradition of seizing the opportunities of social and economic change for the creation of new beauties and new possibilities of happiness. The lesson of this past is the necessity of looking forward: and not the necessity only, but the profit as well.

How to Criticize a Poem

(In the Manner of Certain Contemporary Critics)

THEODORE SPENCER (1902–1949)

1

I PROPOSE to examine the following poem:

Thirty days hath September,
April, June and November:
All the rest have thirty-one,
Excepting February alone,
Which has only eight and a score
Till leap-year gives it one day more.

2

The previous critics who have studied this poem, Coleridge among them, have failed to explain what we may describe as its fundamental *dynamic*. This I now propose to do. The first thing to observe is the order in which the names (or verbal constructs) of the months are presented. According to the prose meaning—what I shall henceforth call the prose-*demand*—"September" should not precede, it should follow "April," as a glance at the calendar will show. Indeed "September" should follow not only "April," it should also follow "June" if the prose-demand is to be properly satisfied. The prose order of the first two lines should therefore read: "Thirty days hath April, June, September and November." That is the only sequence consonant with prose logic.

HOW TO CRITICIZE A POEM by Theodore Spencer is reprinted from *New Republic*, December 6, 1943, by permission of New Republic.

3

Why then, we ask ourselves, did the poet violate what educated readers know to be the facts? Was he ignorant of the calendar, believing that September preceded April in the progress of the seasons? It is difficult to imagine that such was the case. We must find another explanation. It is here that the principle of dynamic analysis comes to our aid.

4

Dynamic analysis proves that the most successful poetry achieves its effect by producing an *expectation* in the reader's mind before his sensibility is fully prepared to receive the full impact of the poem. The reader makes a *proto-response* which preconditions him to the total response toward which his fully equilibrized organs of apperception subconsciously tend. It is this proto-response which the poet has here so sensitively manipulated. The ordinary reader, trained only to prose-demands, expects the usual order of the months. But the poet's sensibility knows that poetic truth is more immediately effective than the truth of literal chronology. He does not *state* the inevitable sequence; he *prepares* us for it. In his profound analysis of the two varieties of mensual time, he puts the *gentlest* month first. (Notice how the harsh sound of "pt" in "September" is softened by the "e" sound on either side of it.) It is the month in which vegetation first begins to fade, but which does not as yet give us a sense of tragic fatality.

5

Hence the poet prepares us, dynamically, for what is to follow. By beginning his list of the months *in medias res*, he is enabled to return later to the beginning of the series of contrasts which is the subject of his poem. The analogy to the "Oedipus Rex" of Euripides and the "Iliad" of Dante at once becomes clear. Recent criticism has only too often failed to observe that these works also illustrate the dynamic method by beginning in the middle of things. It is a striking fact, hitherto (I believe) unnoticed, that a Latin poem called the "Aeneid" does much the same thing. We expect the author of that poem to begin with the departure of his hero from Troy, just as we expect the author of our poem to begin with "April." But in neither case is our expectation fulfilled. Cato, the author of the "Aeneid," creates dynamic suspense by beginning with Aeneas in Carthage; our anonymous poet treats his readers' sensibilities in a similar fashion by beginning with "September," and then *going back* to "April" and "June."

6

But the sensibility of the poet does not stop at this point. Having described what is true of *four* months, he disposes of *seven* more with masterly economy. In a series of pungent constructs his sensibility sums up their inexorable limitations: they *All* (the capitalization should be noted) "have thirty-one." The poet's sensibility communicates a feeling to the sensibility of the reader so that the sensibility of both, with reference to their previous but independent sensibilities, is fused into that momentary communion of sensibility which is the final sensibility that poetry can give both to the sensibility of the poet and the sensibility of the reader. The texture and structure of the poem have erupted into a major reaction. The ambiguity of equilibrium is achieved.

7

Against these two groups of spatial, temporal and numerical measurements—one consisting of four months, the other of seven—the tragic individual, the sole exception, "February," is dramatically placed. February is "alone," is cut off from communion with his fellows. The tragic note is struck the moment "February" is mentioned. For the initial sound of the word "excepting" is "X," and as that sound strikes the sensibility of the reader's ear a number of associations subconsciously accumulate. We think of the spot, the murderous and lonely spot, which "X" has so frequently marked; we remember the examinations of our childhood where the wrong answers were implacably signaled with "X"; we think of ex-kings and exile, of lonely crossroads and executions, of the inexorable anonymity of those who cannot sign their names. . . .

8

And yet the poet gives us one ray of hope, though it eventually proves to be illusory. The lonely "February" (notice how the "alone" in line four is echoed by the "only" in line five), the solitary and maladjusted individual who is obviously the hero and crucial figure of the poem, is not condemned to the routine which his fellows, in their different ways, must forever obey. Like Hamlet, he has a capacity for change. He is a symbol of individualism, and the rhythm of the lines which are devoted to him signalize a gayety, however desperate, which immediately wins our sympathy and reverberates profoundly in our sensibility.

9

But (and this is the illusion to which I have previously referred) in spite of all his variety, his capacity for change, "February" cannot quite accomplish (and in this his tragedy consists) the *quantitative* value of the society in which circumstances have put him. No matter how often he may alternate from twenty-eight to twenty-nine (the poet, with his exquisite sensibility, does not actually *mention* those humiliating numbers), he can never achieve the bourgeois, if anonymous, security of "thirty-one," nor equal the more modest and aristocratic assurance of "thirty." Decade after decade, century after century, millennium after millennium, he is eternally frustrated. The only symbol of change in a changeless society, he is continually beaten down. Once every four years he tries to rise, to achieve the high, if delusive, level of his dreams. But he fails. He is always one day short, and the three years before the recurrence of his next effort are a sad interval in which the remembrance of previous disappointment melts into the futility of hope, only to sink back once more into the frustration of despair. Like Tantalus he is forever stretched upon a wheel.

10

So far I have been concerned chiefly with the dynamic *analysis* of the poem. Further study should reveal the *synthesis* which can be made on the basis of the analysis which my thesis has tentatively attempted to bring to an emphasis. This, perhaps, the reader with a proper sensibility can achieve for himself.

Appendix: Metrics

ANALYSIS of the technical aspects of a poem will illuminate its craftsmanship, but it is simply one step, not an end, in critical reading. A reader may be able to scan a poem without gaining a glint of its meaning or without feeling its power as a work of art. Yet if the craft (the verse technique) is considered as organic in the total effect of the poem, that is, one of the elements which make the poem an artistic experience and not just an ordinary, though perhaps useful, communication of fact or idea, then the analysis of sound and meter becomes a vital part of the understanding of poetry.

Basic in the study of the craft of poetry is an awareness of the rhythms, for verse has, in contrast to prose, more highly organized or more systematic arrangement of rhythm. (For comment on prose rhythm see the Dobrée selection, page 585.) The importance of rhythm in every aspect of the universe from the motion of the planets to the buzzing of an insect is clear to anyone who has looked at the world about him. Both the accentual quality and the very sound of English poetry derive from rhythm.

Since verse is rhythmically arranged sound, rhythm establishes through stress the arrangement or pattern which the reader will expect and recognize as it recurs. In the following stanza,

> Queen and huntress, chaste and fair,
> Now the sun is laid to sleep,
> Seated in thy silver chair,
> State in wonted manner keep:
>   Hesperus entreats thy light,
>   Goddess excellently bright.

the first line begins with a vocative, an address to the goddess Diana. The opening word "Queen" is stressed and is followed by "and," which receives far less stress. The rhythmical pattern is simple and clearly heard. The same pattern follows for the rest of the lines.

stress stress stress stress
Queen and huntress, chaste and fair,

The pattern thus set up (trochaic: ´ ˘) may continue in the reader's mind beyond the reading of the line to the point where it becomes a desired pattern for another experience like the first line. The poem does not disappoint this wish, for the rest of the lines follow the pattern. There are other elements, such as rhyme, which develop expected patterns, but these are not under discussion here.

But all verse is not just the fulfillment of established or expected rhythmic patterns. Within a poem the rhythmic movement may vary or "counterpoint" the expected pattern. Some of the most interesting rhythmical effects are produced by this "counterpointing," or apparent violation of the expected pattern. In such cases the poet may play against the rhythm which is being heard in the reader's mind. A simple parallel in music is syncopation; many of the interesting characteristics of modern dance music—swing and bebop—are built on variation of the basic rhythmic patterns set up in the listener's consciousness.

In the following stanza from Part IV of *The Ancient Mariner*, describing the water snakes, the first two lines set up a simple rhythmic pattern (iambic: ˘ ´) in which a stressed syllable regularly follows an unstressed syllable. (The stressed syllables are marked with an accent: ´.)

Withín the shádow of the shíp
I wátch'd their rích attíre:
Blúe, glóssy gréen, and vélvet bláck,
They cóil'd and swám; and évery tráck
Was a flásh of gólden fíre.

The third line comes as a kind of shock. It begins with stress on "Blue" and follows with another stressed syllable, "glóssy." The expected pattern is violated, but the effect created is dramatic; it draws attention to striking color. The fourth line returns to the iambic pattern, but the fifth line provides another variant of interest in opening with two unstressed syllables, "Was a," followed by a strong stress on "flash." The effect of this variation is to give a sense of speed to the line, in perfect accord with the picture Coleridge is creating.

For purposes of study some general features of rhythm in English verse, seen in broadest terms as alternation of stress and less stress or lack of stress in syllables, can be marked by accepted graphic symbols: ˘ for an unaccented syllable; ′ for an accented syllable. But the application of these signs to verse, a practice called scansion, only generally and loosely indicates the real quality and effects; and most of the descriptive terms, derived from classical Greek and Latin principles of versification, are, in fact, misnomers. Too often readers are content to think they have understood the craftmanship of a line of verse if they have scanned it or can say glibly, "iambic pentameter."

It is of basic importance to remember that in English verse, with certain exceptions, words take their normal speech accents. Thus in scanning English verse, the first step would be to mark the accents which the words would usually receive when pronounced with their full values; that is, as separate words, not as words in a context: the mul-ti-tu-di-nous seas in-car-na-dine. (Note that the passage does not "scan" when so marked. But it can be scanned as soon as one notices that in actual speech, the *i* of the penult does not receive its full value, so that we say *túd-nous.*) These normal speech accents will by no means give the actual rhythm of the passage, but they do provide the structure on which the rhythm is built. After this step, the words should be reread as part of the context, in order to determine to what extent the sense (rhetorical emphasis) of the passage modifies the usual speech accents. Here, of course, individual differences in interpretation will have their effect on the scansion.

Although no two people read a line of a poem the same way, intelligent reading aloud is an essential step toward understanding the craft of poetry. The ear must be used as the responsive, critical, and appreciative instrument it really is. Intelligent reading will reveal the main stresses or accents in the lines as no optical analysis will. Only after careful reading should a student begin a graphic though approximate record of the rhythm of the poem. No attempt should be made to fit iambic or trochaic or other measures and accents until the main accents are indicated. The opening stanza of Gray's "Elegy Written in a Country Churchyard" will serve as an example.

> The cúrfew tólls the knéll of párting dáy,
> The lówing hérd wind slówly o'ér the léa,
> The plówman hómeward plóds his wéary wáy,
> And léaves the wórld to dárkness ánd to mé.

The regularity of the movement should be immediately apparent when the unstressed syllables are also marked:

> Thĕ cúrfĕw tólls thĕ knéll ŏf pártĭng dáy.

Lines 3 and 4 show the same regularity. In line 2, properly read, the word "wind" seems to require greater stress than the unaccented words like "the," perhaps almost the same stress as "slowly." Here the slight variation from the plain iambic (˘ ´) pattern is also a matter of time as well as accent. The graphic symbol to mark the value of "wind" exactly does not exist. The necessary approach to it might be a secondary accent (`) or a full accent. The effect of slowness is strongly established and then reinforced by the rhythmical quality and the placing of the central words in the line. The line could thus be scanned: "Thĕ lówĭng hérd wìnd slówlў o'ĕr thĕ léa." Time values expressed by musical notes might give a more graphic idea of the line.

The lowing herd wind slowly o'er the lea.

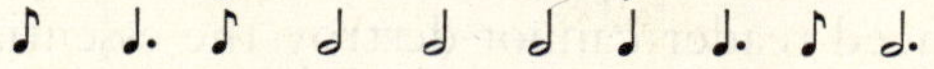

The whole stanza has a feeling of calmness and quiet, not only because of the details of atmosphere ("curfew tolls") or the pictorial details ("lowing herd," "plowman") but because of the regularity in iambic pentameter of the rhythm and because of various devices of sound (rhyme, *abab;* alliteration in "*pl*owman . . . *pl*ods"; "*w*eary *w*ay"; assonance in "l*ow*ing" and "sl*ow*ly," "slow*ly*" and "*lea*"; consonance in "*l*owing," "s*l*ow*l*y," "*l*ea").

The stanza contains almost no pauses within the line, the main caesuras (or pauses) coming regularly at the end of each line. In line 4, a light caesura after "darkness" gives a dramatic effect to the final verse. The suitability of the rhythm to the tone of the stanza is apparent. The rhythm in all its aspects is not *imposed* on the stanza. It is an integral part of the stanza.

Gray's stanza offers almost no metrical complexities; its atmosphere has been derived in part from the simplicity of its meter. The following song of Ben Jonson's from a masque called *Cynthia's Revels* (1601) is a good example of the use of a more complicated metrical and sound pattern to produce the dramatic effect of grief. The verses are Echo's song over the death of her love, Narcissus, who melted away into a spring and eventually, in Jonson's use of the legend, became a daffodil.

Slow, slow, fresh fount, keep time with my salt tears;
Yet slower yet, oh, faintly, gentle springs;
List to the heavy part the music bears,
Woe weeps out her division when she sings.
Droop herbs and flowers,
Fall grief in showers;
Our beauties are not ours.
Oh, I could still,
Like melting snow upon some craggy hill,
Drop, drop, drop, drop,
Since nature's pride is now a withered daffodil.

A reading of the poem will reveal how completely the poet has control over the mood and the movement of the poem. Even the least experienced reader cannot destroy the essentially deliberate slow tempo of the lines. The reason is that Jonson has made full use of devices of rhythm and sound.

In the first place Jonson has combined spondaic movement (´´) with a frequent use of strategically placed pauses or caesuras. The first six syllables of the ten in the opening line are almost equally stressed; three pauses occur: the first after the first syllable, the second after the second syllable and the third after the fourth syllable.

Slów, || slów, || | frèsh fóunt, || | kéep tíme | wĭth mý | sàlt téars; || |

The effect of the line is one of gravity and grief.

The second line intensifies the dramatic situation with a feeling of anxiety and pleading. The rhythm of the line differs from the first line, but the tempo is just as thoroughly controlled by the caesuras after "yet" and "faintly." Although the basic meter of the line is iambic, the secondary accent on "oh" and the ceasuras break up any completely iambic movement.

Yĕt slów | ĕr yét, || òh, fáint | lў, || gén | tlĕ spríngs; || |

The third line, essentially trochaic in movement, is a mild command to attention to the mournful quality of the fountain; and the fourth line by a combination of alliteration and consecutively stressed syllables produces an effect which exactly illustrates what is called for in line 3 and corresponds generally with the rhythmical characteristics of line 1.

Líst tŏ thĕ | héavў | párt thĕ | músic | béars, || |
Wóe wéeps | óut hĕr | dĭví | sĭon whĕn | shĕ síngs. || |

Repetition and assonance (Sl*ow*, sl*ow*, line 1; sl*ow*er, line 2; *Woe* in line 4;), and alliteration (*W*oe *w*eeps . . . *w*hen in line 4) are a few of the devices of sound which help to create here the emotional effect of grief.

The next three lines form a triplet in which the feminine rhymes (flowers, showers, ours; "ours" in line 7 is read as two syllables), the short lines, and the consequent quick return of the rhymes maintain the tone of the poem, but also seem to provide a contemplative quality by the formal tripartite division.

The last four lines contain a personal wish. Their outstanding sound device is, of course, the onomatopoetic words "Drop, drop, drop, drop" (line 10) with their even stresses and regular pauses. The last line, which gives the reason for the situation of grief, is the longest line of the poem, containing six feet, and has a conclusive effect because of its length and its iambic regularity.

Since nature's pride is now a withered daffodil.

Although this brief survey of the meter and sound of Jonson's poem may seem detailed to a critical reader at first, it does not attempt to cover all the technical aspects of the poem. Enough has been noticed, however, to show how carefully the small song is made and how effectively its technical qualities suit its delicacy, mood, and emotional effect.

The variety of effects which a line of verse or a stanza or a whole poem may have are in part attributable to the basic rhythmical and vocal qualities of the poem itself. These elements can be temporarily isolated for study but can be finally appreciated only in terms of the whole work; in a good poem, style, which involves craftmanship in meter and sound, cannot be separated from substance. Remember that the terms and symbols used to describe and scan verse are only approximate. A scientific record of anyone's reading of a line of verse could of course be made, but an oscillograph is not a necessary piece of equipment for the average reader.

For the sake of convenience the following list of terms and definitions is supplied. The arrangement is according to rhythm and meter and devices of sound.

RHYTHM AND METER

FOOT: The metrical unit of a poem; consists of one accented and one or more unaccented syllables. Common types of feet in English verse are:

IAMB (˘ ′ *compel*): An unaccented syllable followed by an accented syllable; the most common meter in English.

TROCHEE (′ ˘ *neatly*): One accented followed by one unaccented syllable.

ANAPEST (˘ ˘ ′ *interfere*): Two unaccented syllables followed by an accented syllable.

DACTYL (′ ˘ ˘ *happiness*): One accented syllable followed by two unaccented syllables.

SPONDEE (′ ′ *sunset*): The term really describes a foot in classical meter composed of two long syllables, but it is often used in English verse to describe a situation in which two accents or a secondary and a full accent are in succession.

And one | clear call | for me! |

VERSE: A line of poetry. A line of verse is composed of one or more feet.

One foot: monometer
Two feet: dimeter
Three feet: trimeter
Four feet: tetrameter
Five feet: pentameter
Six feet: hexameter or alexandrine
Seven feet: heptameter

CAESURA: The main pause in a line of verse, which is sometimes marked || to distinguish it from the mark used to designate a foot |. Other pauses are sometimes called secondary pauses.

> Tears, idle tears, || I know not what they mean,||
> Tears from the depth of some divine despair
> Rise in the heart, || and gather to the eyes, . . .

RUN-ON LINES: The carrying over of sense and grammatical structure from one verse to a succeeding one for completion; the process is often called enjambement. The opening lines of Shakespeare's 116th sonnet will illustrate:

> Let me not to the marriage of true minds
> Admit impediments. Love is not love
> Which alters when it alteration finds, . . .

END-STOPPED LINES: Lines of verse in which both the grammatical structure and the sense are complete at the end of the line. A couplet from Pope's *An Essay on Criticism* may serve:

> True ease in writing comes from art, not chance,
> As those move easiest who have learned to dance.

SOUND

The quality and relationships of sounds in poetry are often called *verse texture*. Among these relationships are alliteration, assonance, consonance, and rhyme.

ALLITERATION: Repetition of consonants, especially initial consonants, in a line. A stanza from Coleridge's *The Rime of the Ancient Mariner* gives examples:

> The *f*air breeze blew, the white *f*oam *f*lew,
> The *f*urrow *f*ollowed *f*ree;
> We were the *f*irst that ever burst
> Into that *s*ilent *s*ea.

ASSONANCE: The identity of vowel sounds in a line or stanza.

> To d*y*ing ears, when unto d*y*ing e*y*es, . . .

Consonance: The identity of consonant patterns in a line or stanza. Consonance is found more rarely than assonance in English verse. A line from Shelley's "To Night" illustrates consonance within a line:

Where *all* the *long* and *lon*e daylight

Onomatopoeia: The use of words which suggest their meaning through their pronunciation: *buzz, whirr, sizzle.*

And more to lull him in his slumber soft,
A *trickling* stream from high rock tumbling down
And *ever-drizzling* rain upon the loft,
Mixed with a *murmuring* wind, much like the sound
Of swarming bees, did cast him in a swoon:
No other noise, nor people's troublous cries,
As still are wont t'annoy the walled town,
Might there be heard: but careless Quiet lies,
Wrapped in eternal silence far from enemies.
(Spenser's *Faerie Queene*, Bk. I)

Rhyme: Actually the similarity or identity of sounds based on the vowels of accented syllables and the consonants and vowels following within a line or lines of verse. (Assonance, consonance, and alliteration may all be considered forms of rhyme.) The term *rhyme* is most often used to designate *end rhyme*, which occurs at the ends of the verses. *End rhyme* is often classified as *masculine rhyme*, in which the final syllable of the line is the rhymed syllable:

obey, decay

and *feminine*, in which the rhymed syllables are followed by identical unaccented syllables:

fighting, writing

This is sometimes called *double rhyme.* When the correspondence of sound occurs in three syllables it is called *triple rhyme:*

malicious, nutritious

RHYME SCHEME: The patterns of end rhymes in a stanza, usually designated by indicating each similar sound by the same letter of the alphabet. The pattern of the Spenserian stanza quoted under ONOMATOPOEIA is *ababbcbcc*.

STANZA FORMS

The most commonly used forms are defined briefly below:

COUPLET: A stanza of two lines. *Tetrameter couplet:* also called octosyllabic couplet; usually iambic tetrameter, *aa*. *Heroic couplet:* Usually iambic pentameter, *aa*.

TERCET: A stanza of three lines, a triplet, *aaa*.

TERZA RIMA: Iambic pentameter tercets in linked rhyme, *aba-bcb-cdc*, etc.

QUATRAIN: A stanza of four lines. Ballad measure; lines 1 and 3 have eight syllables each and lines 2 and 4 six syllables. Usually iambic; rhyme is *abcb*. The ordinary quatrain is iambic pentameter, *abab*, as in Gray's *Elegy*, but there are variants of the rhyme scheme, such as *abba*, *aaba*.

RHYME ROYAL: A stanza of seven lines, pentameter, *ababbcc*.

OTTAVA RIMA: A stanza of eight lines, pentameter, *abababcc*.

SPENSERIAN STANZA: A stanza of nine lines, pentameter, except for last line, which is an alexandrine, *ababbcbcc*.

SONNET: A stanza of fourteen lines, pentameter.

1. Italian sonnet, pentameter, *abbaabba cdecde*. The first eight lines, which usually present the theme of the sonnet, are called an *octave*. The last six lines, in which the conclusion of the theme is given, are called a *sestet*. The sestet often varies in rhyme scheme.
2. The Shakespearean (or English) sonnet, pentameter, *ababcdcdefefgg*. The division is by three quatrains and a concluding couplet. Often the proposition of

the poem is presented in the first three quatrains and concluded or commented on in the couplet, but the first two quatrains are sometimes used as the octave in the Italian sonnet.

Blank Verse: Not a stanza form. It is a line of unrhymed pentameter verse, usually iambic. It can of course form lines which may constitute a stanza pattern.

Free Verse: Verse which does not conform to any conventional or regular pattern.

Index of First Lines of Poems

Index of Authors and Titles